Fundamentals in Oncologic Ultrasound

O. Catalano • A. Nunziata • A. Siani

Fundamentals in Oncologic Ultrasound

Sonographic Imaging and Intervention in the Cancer Patient

Foreword by David Cosgrove

Springer

Orlando Catalano
1st Department of Radiology
National Cancer Institute
"Fondazione G. Pascale"
Naples, Italy

Alfredo Siani
1st Department of Radiology
National Cancer Institute
"Fondazione G. Pascale"
Naples, Italy

Antonio Nunziata
Department of Radiology
"S. Bellone" Center
DSB50, ASL NA1
Naples, Italy

Additional material to this book can be downloaded from http://extras.springer.com.

Completely revised and updated edition of the volume:
Ecografia in Oncologia
Testo-Atlante di ultrasonologia diagnostica e interventistica dei tumori
Orlando Catalano, Alfredo Siani

Translation: Alexander Cormack, Trieste, Italy

ISBN 978-88-470-5804-0 ISBN 978-88-470-1355-1 (eBook)
DOI 10.1007/978-88-470-1355-1
Springer Milan Berlin Heidelberg New York

Springer is a part of Springer Science+Business Media
springer.com

Softcover reprint of the hardcover 1st edition 2009

Cover image credit: NASA/JPL-Caltech/Harvard-Smithsonian Center for Astrophysics

Typesetting: Compostudio, Cernusco s/N (Milan), Italy
Printing and binding: Printer Trento S.r.l., Trento, Italy

Springer-Verlag Italia S.r.l., Via Decembrio 28, I-20137 Milan, Italy

Foreword

It is a remarkable observation that human creativity can be fostered by spectacular scenery, itself usually the result of tectonic activity which raises mountains of beauty but carries the sting of earthquakes and eruptions. Think of Silicon Valley in California or of the Tokyo-Kyoto corridor in Eastern Japan. Another is the glorious Amalfi coast around Naples, where the authors of this new textbook work in the shadow of Mount Vesuvius. Is it the beauty that inspires or the tension of knowing that one's life may be shattered at any moment if a volcanic or tectonic disaster strikes? Whatever the explanation, these authors' passion for their subject shines through and their work carries not only their enthusiasm but also a rare beauty in its construction/format, for it is a joy to hold and behold with its beautiful all-colour printing and abundant illustrations of excellent quality, mainly, of course, ultrasound images but also corresponding CT scans and numerous elegant diagrams.

But, is there a need for a textbook on ultrasound in oncology? Doesn't everyone accept that CT or PET/CT (and sometimes MR) have nailed the problem of oncologic imaging? Well, while CT is undoubtedly the core imaging technique for the detection, staging, treatment planning and follow-up of tumours, there remain many applications for modern ultrasound, as readers of this textbook will be persuaded. It has the advantages of availability and ready repeatability and, in some situations, the lack of ionizing radiation is an advantage, even in oncology. Furthermore, it provides functional information, especially about blood flow, that may be critical in some oncology problems (choriocarcinoma is an example). It is also the best imaging modality for guiding interventional procedures.

The content of *Fundamentals in Oncologic Ultrasound* goes far beyond a narrow interpretation of the title, in that a wide range of non-tumour conditions is included and illustrated – in fact, wherever a non-tumour mass should be considered as part of the differential diagnosis, it is covered in detail here. This means that it will be indispensable to all clinics using ultrasound in general imaging. A wide-ranging introductory section covers the basics of ultrasound interpretation, including grey scale and Doppler, as well as microbubble contrast agents. In addition, unusually, there is a detailed discussion of the pros and cons of ultrasound compared with other imaging techniques, and a discussion of the benefits and dangers of screening, a topic that is often short-changed. There is also an important discussion of the use of imaging in evaluating response to treatment. As well as sections on the abdomen and superficial structures such as the head and neck, and the breast, there are sections on the genito-urinary tract and one on the use of ultrasound to guide interventional procedures, including ablation techniques.

The authors are justifiably renowned for their careful, detailed and precise work in general ultrasound over many years. Their passion for the subject is evident in the detailed descriptions of the wide range of pathologies it includes, both adult and paediatric.

I congratulate Drs. Catalano, Nunziata and Siani on their labour of love and commend this excellent textbook to you.

London, February 2009

David Cosgrove
Imperial College, London UK

Preface

Unlike other volumes of oncologic imaging, ours is not encyclopedic. It does not aim to analyze organ by organ every tumor which may be found there, with a systematic description regarding the etiopathogenetic, epidemiologic, clinical, diagnostic and therapeutic features of the disease. It does not begin, therefore, with a predetermined diagnosis but rather from the clinical problems that may lead there, because this is the reality of daily clinical practice. The volume is therefore structured in seven broad chapters.

Chapter 1. An analysis is made of the general relations between diagnostic imaging modalities, with particular reference to ultrasound, and the principal fields of oncology. An initial presentation is made of the advantages and limitations of US, the knowledge of which is essential for any clinical application of the technique, and therefore also for the study of cancer. The focus then shifts to the different phases in which US and the oncologic disease interact: secondary prevention, intrinsic characteristics of the cancer (with particular reference to neoangiogenesis), cancer staging, the evaluation of response to different types of anticancer treatments, short- and long-term monitoring, and the identification of disease recurrence. Only with an adequate understanding of these features of malignant disease can diagnostic imaging make a truly effective contribution. Chapter 1 also takes into consideration the examination techniques of US, spectral Doppler, color Doppler, power Doppler and contrast-enhanced US (CEUS), with particular reference to the study of neoplastic diseases in their superficial and deep locations. The presentation especially focuses on the current possibility of optimizing the US instrumentation and exploration technique, with the aim of maximizing the detection and morphofunctional analysis of neoplastic lesions. The sections dealing with the examination technique alternate with a presentation of the principal imaging characteristics: although tumors arising in different organs may display different features, the discussion aims to underline the common imaging characteristics so they can be applied from time to time to the various anatomic regions and clinical problems.

Chapters 2–6. The clinical problems connected either directly or indirectly to neoplastic disease of the different body regions are many and varied and can be included in a single volume only in part. Instead of an encyclopedic approach, with systematic discussion of the epidemiologic, clinical, diagnostic and imaging characteristics of the different neoplasms in different body regions, we preferred to begin with the basic clinical problem, which is how the disease is presented to the diagnostic imaging specialist. This approach involves, first of all, an illustration of the general appearance and then the imaging characteristics, first and foremost US, but also CD, spectral Doppler and CEUS.

Chapter 7. The current range of extravascular interventional procedures is extremely broad and constantly on the increase. This chapter describes the main US-guided procedures used in the cancer patient: diagnostic sampling of superficial and deep lesions (both cytologic – FNAC, and histologic – core biopsy), vacuum-assisted biopsy in breast cancer, placement of presurgical markers, drainage of collections, cysts and liquefactive masses, percutaneous ablation (with special reference to percutaneous ethanol injection and radiofrequency thermal ablation, and especially with regard to focal hepatic lesions). It should, nonetheless, be borne in mind that the number of US-guided interventional procedures is much greater, ranging from biliary drainage to nephrostomy and nerve block for anesthesia or pain management to venous catheterization. US guidance, either alone or in combination with other modalities; this allows all of these procedures to be performed more effectively and with greater safety for the patient than with a "blind" approach". An increasingly widespread diffusion of the technique can therefore be reasonably expected.

In this text the term color Doppler and its abbreviation CD are used, except where specifically stated, in reference to the Doppler techniques in general and therefore including power Doppler. In all cases where the description refers specifically to power Doppler this term will be expressly stated.

The term contrast-enhanced US (CEUS) is always used to refer specifically to gray-scale study with injection of sonographic contrast medium. When the intention is to indicate CD with contrast medium this is always expressly stated and should not be considered associated with the idea of US contrast enhancement.

Throughout the volume the term "US-guided" is a general reference to all procedures performed with US guidance, regardless of the type of transducer used, whether dedicated to the intervention or not. The specific meaning attributed to the terms "freehand", "US-assisted" and "US-guided" is discussed at the beginning of Chapter 7.

Lastly, throughout the text, the term "biopsy" is used as a general indication of diagnostic sampling, both cytologic and microhistologic, where not otherwise specified. The difference between the former (aspirated with a fine needle, with the abbreviation FNAC) and true biopsy (indicated as "core biopsy") is also thoroughly illustrated in Chapter 7. We preferred not to use the well-known abbreviation FNAB at all to avoid confusion in terms.

We thought it useful to provide a compact disc with video material of US examinations performed with various techniques. The choice appears appropriate especially given the difficulty in encapsulating in static images characteristics that can only be fully appreciated in real time, especially with regard to CEUS studies and interventional procedures.

Orlando Catalano
Antonio Nunziata
Alfredo Siani

Contents

Contributors

Orlando Catalano 1st Department of Radiology, National Cancer Institute "Fondazione G. Pascale", Naples, Italy

Flavio Fazioli Department of Soft-tissue Tumor Surgery, National Cancer Institute "Fondazione G. Pascale", Naples, Italy

Gaetano Massimo Fierro "Medicina Futura" Laboratory, Acerra, Italy

Mauro Mattace Raso 1st Department of Radiology, National Cancer Institute "Fondazione G. Pascale", Naples, Italy

Antonio Nunziata Department of Radiology, "S. Bellone" Center, DSB50, ASL NA1, Naples, Italy

Fabio Sandomenico 1st Department of Radiology, National Cancer Institute "Fondazione G. Pascale", Naples, Italy

Sergio Venanzio Setola 1st Department of Radiology, National Cancer Institute "Fondazione G. Pascale", Naples, Italy

Alfredo Siani 1st Department of Radiology, National Cancer Institute "Fondazione G. Pascale", Naples, Italy

Paolo Vallone 1st Department of Radiology, National Cancer Institute "Fondazione G. Pascale", Naples, Italy

Abbreviations

3D	three-dimensional
μg	microgram
μm	micrometer
ABBI	advanced breast biopsy instrumentation
ACR	American College of Radiology
ACS	American Cancer Society
ACTH	adrenocorticotropic hormone
AFP	α-fetoprotein
AI	acceleration index
AIDS	acquired immunodeficiency syndrome
BCLC	Barcelona Clinic Liver Cancer
BI-RADS	breast imaging reporting and data system
CA	cancer antigen
CD	color Doppler
CEA	carcinoembryonic antigen
CEUS	contrast-enhanced ultrasound
cm	centimeter
CT	computed tomography
CUP	cancer of unknown primary (tumor)
CVC	central venous catheter
dB	decibel
DPI	Doppler perfusion index
DRE	digital rectal examination
EFOV	extended field of view
EUS	endoscopic ultrasound
FDG	fluorodeoxyglucose
FIGO	International Federation of Gynecology and Obstetrics
F/M	female/male
FNAB	fine-needle aspiration biopsy
FNAC	fine-needle aspiration cytology
FNH	focal nodular hyperplasia
FOV	field of view
G	gauge
GIST	gastrointestinal stromal tumor
HBV	hepatitis B virus
HCC	hepatocellular carcinoma
HCG	human chorionic gonadotropin
HCV	hepatitis C virus
HIAA	hydroxy-indoleacetic acid
IOUS	intraoperative ultrasound
IU	international unit

IV	intravenous
Kg	kilogram
kHz	kiloHertz
L	liter
LABC	locally advanced breast cancer
LDH	lactic dehydrogenase
M/F	male/female
MALToma	tumor from mucous-associated lymphoid tissue
MEN	multiple endocrine neoplasm
mg	milligram
MHz	megaHertz
MI	mechanical index
MIBI	methoxyisobutylisonitrile
mL	milliliter
mm	millimeter
mmHg	millimeters of mercury
mPa	milliPascal
MRCP	magnetic resonance cholangiopancreatography
MR	magnetic resonance
MSCT	multislice computed tomography
MVD	microvessel density
ng	nanogram
NHL	non-Hodgkin's lymphoma
PACS	pictures archiving and communication system
PAT	percutaneous ablation therapy
PC	personal computer
PD	power Doppler
PEI	percutaneous ethanol injection
PET	positron emission tomography
PET-CT	PET and CT fusion
PI	pulsatility index
PIN	prostatic intraepithelial neoplasm
PLAP	placental alkaline phosphatase
PRF	pulse repetition frequency
PSA	prostate specific antigen
PSAD	prostate specific antigen density
PT	prothrombin time
PTT	partial thromboplastin time
QUART	quadrantectomy, axillectomy, radiation therapy
RCC	renal cell carcinoma
RECIST	response evaluation criteria in solid tumors
RF	radiofrequency
RFTA	radiofrequency thermal ablation
RI	resistive index
RIS	radiologic information system
ROI	region of interest
ROLL	radio-guided occult lesion localization
s	second
SD	standard deviation
SF_6	sulfur hexafluoride
SPECT	single photon emission computed tomography
SUV	standardized uptake value
TACE	transcatheter arterial chemoembolization
Tc	technetium
Tis	tumor in situ
TNM	tumor – node – metastasis

TRUS	transrectal ultrasound
TSH	thyroid-stimulating hormone
TUR	transurethral resection
TVUS	transvaginal ultrasound
US	ultrasound
VB	vacuum-assisted biopsy
VEGF	vascular endothelial growth factor
V_{max}	maximal velocity
V_{m}	mean velocity
V_{min}	minimal velocity
vs.	versus
WHO	World Health Organization

General Considerations 1

1.1 Advantages of Ultrasound in Oncology

US has a number of characteristics which make it a very useful diagnostic technique both for general application and for oncology in particular. First of all, US is a simple technique. This **simplicity**, which is sometimes confused with ease of use, is related to the way the examination is performed. No preliminary analysis or special preparation is required and it can always be immediately carried out, making it much more accessible in any hospital setting than the "heavy" devices of CT and MR. The **immediacy** of the image is another advantage, whereby the clinical picture may be clarified at the very time the US transducer is placed on the skin in the anatomic area in question. In addition, the **rapidity** of the examination is an important characteristic, particularly in other areas, such as emergency medicine. In oncology, however, a careful and comprehensive study is recommended, which slowly and repeatedly explores all the anatomic areas involved in the examination in question. This is particularly important in the "positive" patient: a pathologic finding indicating malignancy in a particular organ should increase the level of attention of the US operator due to the elevated probability that there are other associated findings. Special attention should therefore be paid to confirmation of diagnostic suspicions once a specific pathologic finding has been identified.

The possibility of studying normal and pathologic masses in **real time** is a prerogative of US, which in this sense is unique among imaging modalities. Echoscopy is able to visualize anatomic structures and their pathologic alterations "in vivo", with the possibility of studying organ function, e.g. intestinal peristalsis, diaphragm motility, contraction of muscular-tendinous structures, cardiac kinesis, etc. Furthermore there are interventional applications, where real-time US guidance in general terms is preferable, wherever possible, to methods such as CT and MR that are usually characterized by discontinuous scan.

The **multiplanar capabilities** of the technique, i.e. the possibility of obtaining any scan plane by simply rotating the transducer, is a characteristic that is only partly shared with other tomographic imaging modalities. With the advent of multislice devices, CT has achieved true multiplanar capabilities, albeit in the form of electronic reconstructions, whereas MR has always been multiplanar in acquisition, but clearly with the need to obtain the images each time according to a specific scan plane.

The **high spatial resolution** achievable with high-frequency transducers is far superior to other imaging modalities. The possibility of identifying and characterizing the morphologic and vascular structure of small lesions to the skin, the subcutaneous layers, the thyroid, the lymph nodes or other superficial structures is undoubtedly much higher than can be obtained with CT or MR. For example, in the preoperative identification and evaluation of superficial satellite metastases from melanoma, US is able to identify a larger number of nodules than other imaging modalities. Whereas CT and MR rely mainly on the criteria of size, with regard to structures such as superficial lymph nodes, US provides a more detailed study, being able to identify metastatic lymph nodes as small as 3–4 mm, or metastatic foci <1 cm within lymph nodes with an otherwise normal appearance.

US is **transportable** and can therefore be performed at the patient's bedside or in the operating room, a feature which significantly facilitates the study of fatigued patients in an advanced tumor stage. This characteristic is also beneficial in the early postoperative period, as well as during US-guided diagnostic and therapeutic procedures performed at the operating table (not to mention IOUS proper).

US is also highly **repeatable**, and is thus particu-

O. Catalano, A. Nunziata, A. Siani, *Fundamentals in Oncologic Ultrasound.*

larly indicated for serial studies such as the monitoring over time of known findings or in follow-up examinations, as well as in screening. The repeatability is also a consequence of the low costs, simplicity and low level of **invasiveness** of the technique, the latter being associated with the use of nonionizing radiation and the technique generally being performed without intravenous contrast media.

The possibility of **doctor–patient interaction** is greater than with other modalities, with an "ongoing" patient history becoming more specific as the findings appear on the US monitor.

US is a very **diffuse** technique, with a widespread distribution both geographically and in the hospital setting, where numerous devices are present in various departments.

The **costs** are lower than those of other imaging modalities, making it the ideal technique for large-scale or serial applications.

Undoubtedly, from a number of points of view, US is underutilized in oncology, where there is a greater tendency towards more sophisticated modalities such as CT, MR, PET and image co-registration. However, many more or less simple clinical queries can be resolved with US or CEUS. For example, US can often be effectively used as a problem solver in cases of a discrepancy between findings of different imaging modalities or between clinical laboratory findings and radiologic or instrumental findings. An initial and accurate US study in patients with a nonoperable advanced-stage tumor can avoid the need for further more invasive and costly examinations. In general, when hypothesizing a diagnostic investigation to clarify a specific clinical problem, it is worth considering whether the problem can be solved with US or whether more complex modalities are required.

1.2 Limitations of Ultrasound in Oncology

The presence of a number of limitations should be borne in mind not only by physicians prescribing US examinations but by US operators themselves, who are naturally led to "overestimate" the capabilities of "their own" technique with which they clearly have the utmost confidence.

The limited **panoramic view** is definitely the major limitation of US. This limitation should be understood in a number of ways. First of all, air and dense anatomic structures such as bone hinder the evaluation of structures lying deep to them, such that the cranial-encephalic, pulmonary-mediastinal and skeletal structures are barely accessible if at all with US, at least in the adult. It is therefore not materially possible to perform a whole-body US scan in the way that is possible with CT or MR. In addition, the technique only "sees" the body region where the transducer is placed. Therefore, a structure such as a lower limb, which in theory can be panoramically explored in all its soft parts with US, is better defined with multislice CT or MR. For example, in a surgical patient with extensive compartmental excision due to a malignancy of the lower limb, a CT or MR study appears more rational, at least in most cases, with the possibility of detailed targeted evaluation with US rather than vice versa. In special cases US can be used to demonstrate malignant lesions in multiple anatomic regions, either individually and on a single image or in highly specialized anatomic sites, which normally would suggest limited or no application of the technique (Figs. 1.1–1.7, Video 1.1). Nonetheless, US is unable to achieve the possibilities of a CT or MR multidistrict study. Lastly, the **field of view** of US is limited and therefore for diagnostic and interventional purposes only partial visualization of the anatomic structures of the area in question is possible in comparison to CT and MR. Particularly voluminous superficial lesions can be difficult to include in the FOV and to measure on a single image, even when high-frequency transducers with a wide field (e.g. 5 cm) are used or when the visualized area is electronically widened with a trapezoidal FOV. As an alternative, spacer pads can be used or an abdominal transducer, although their lower resolution can render visualization of the margins of the mass difficult and therefore hinder its correct measurement from another perspective.

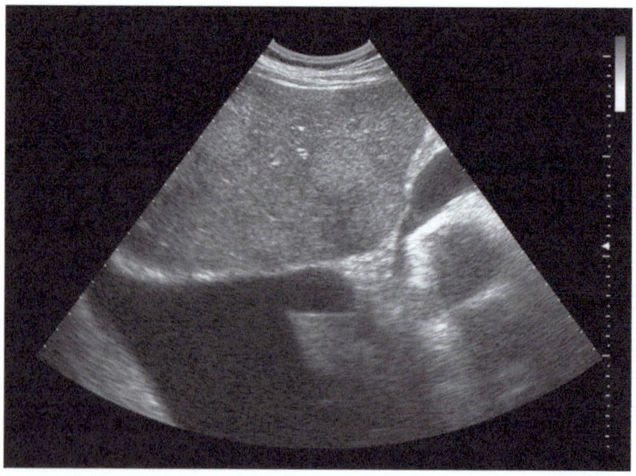

Fig. 1.1 Liver metastases from pulmonary carcinoma associated with pleural and pericardial effusion. Panoramic demonstration in a single US scan of the hepatic lesions, the pericardial fluid layer and the moderate pleural effusion with parenchymal atelectasis. In general, however, US is not a very panoramic technique

The **spatial resolution** is also lower than that of CT and MR with regard to deep structures, which require the use of low-frequency transducers.

US is very accurate in discriminating between solid and fluid-filled structures. In cases where CT is often nonspecific, e.g. demonstrating a near-liquid appearance (visibly or with the measurement of attenuation coefficients), US often is able to demonstrate a solid

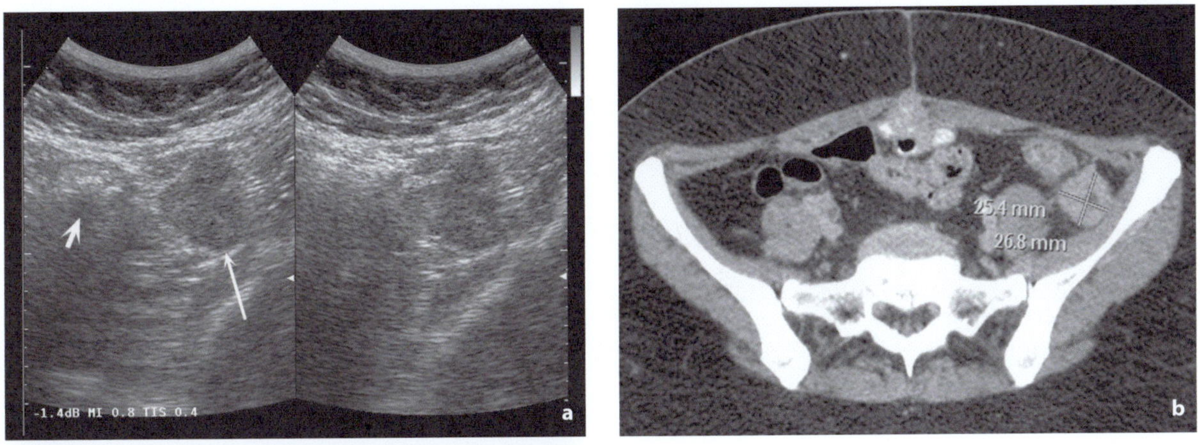

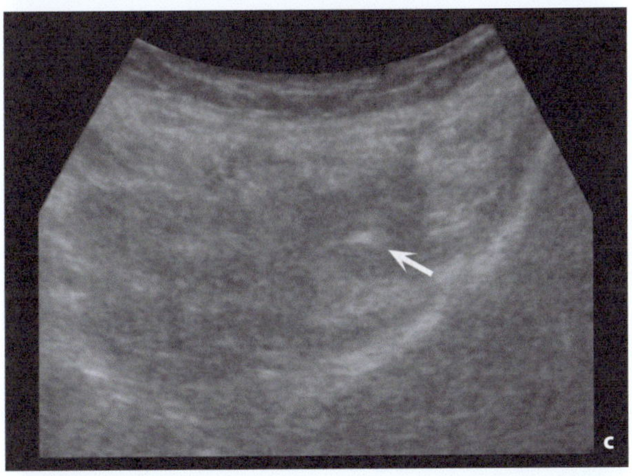

Fig. 1.2a-c Recurrence of cervical cancer. US study (**a**) shows a heterogeneous hypoechoic nodulation in the left iliac fossa (*long arrow*) adjacent to the descending colon (*short arrow*) confirmed by CT (**b**) as well as PET and US-guided biopsy. The finding of this single lesion in an unusual location was possible because of a thorough abdominal-pelvic US study, whereas the finding is immediately recognizable on CT. Confirmation with FNAC (**c**, *arrow*)

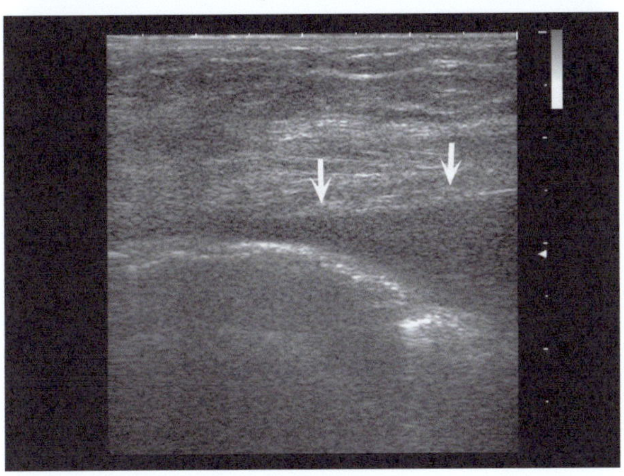

Fig. 1.3 Pleural effusion identified during US study of the thoracic wall. US study of the thoracic wall following radical mastectomy revealed an unexpected underlying pleural effusion (*arrows*)

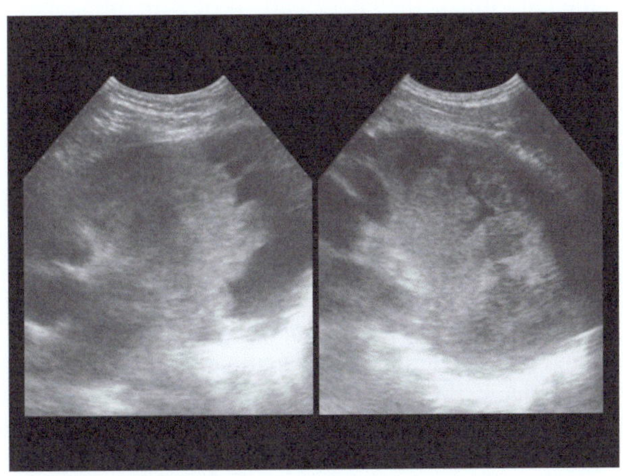

Fig. 1.4 Primary yolk sac tumor of the mediastinum. Heterogeneous echoic mass with hypo-anechoic areas at the level of the anterior mediastinum

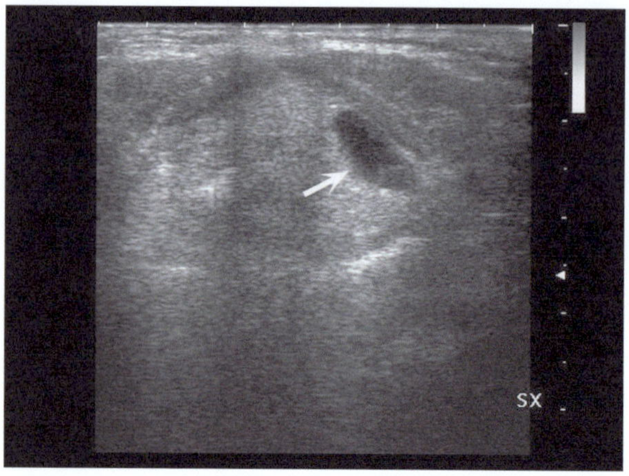

Fig. 1.5 Laryngeal metastasis from melanoma. The targeted US study of the neck in a patient with radiotracer uptake at PET shows a moderately hypoechoic heterogeneous nodulation immediately dorsal to the left thyroid cartilage (*arrow*). The lesion in this site would probably not have been identified without the guidance of the PET finding

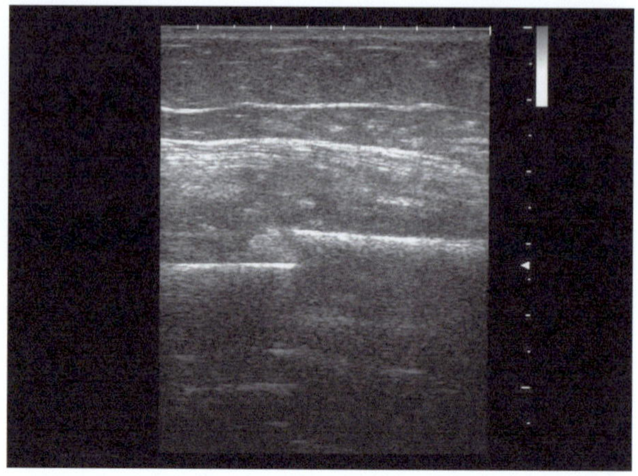

Fig. 1.6 Pathologic fracture of the humerus due to breast cancer metastasis. The examination, performed on indication of a tenderness of the arm, shows the unexpected interruption of the humeral cortex with heterogeneity of the adjacent soft tissue

formation. In addition, fine intralesional alterations can go unrecognized on CT images, especially due to the partial volume effect. Complex cystic formations, for example, can appear homogeneously liquid on CT images, but with fine septations or with internal corpuscular material on US. That being said, it should be underlined that US has low **contrast resolution** and therefore, indirectly, a lower ability to **characterize tissue** than that of CT and MR. Therefore distinguishing between different solid and fluid structures, recognizing necrotic phenomena and identifying fine vasculature are all features which are more difficult, if not impossible, with US.

The US image is not immediately interpretable for clinicians, unless they personally deal with ultrasonography. In general, those who are not involved with diagnostic imaging have greater **confidence** with radiographic images, CT or, to a lesser extent, MR than with US images.

Not unlike other imaging modalities, US requires **adequate information** regarding the clinical setting of the individual patient so that the examination can be correctly focused and the sensitivity maximized. Knowing that CT has identified a suspicious area in a specific hepatic segment, or that PET has demonstrated radiotracer uptake in a particular anatomic area, is completely different from acting without this knowledge. The availability of RIS and PACS, coupled with the possibility of analyzing prior reports, and the images regarding the different examinations performed, only partially overcomes the notorious lack of communication between requesting physicians and those performing diagnostic imaging.

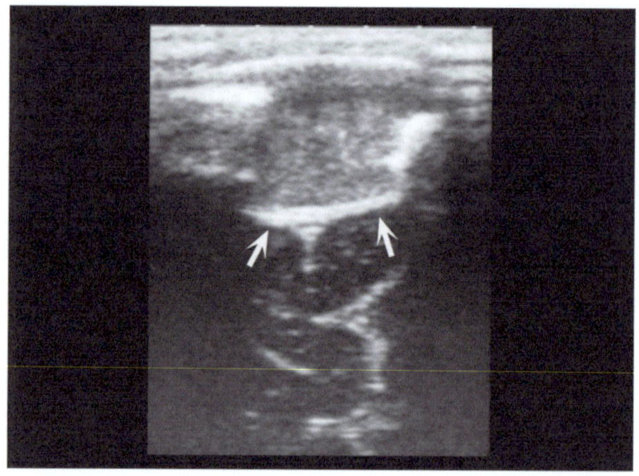

Fig. 1.7 Eosinophilic granuloma of the parietal bone, in a pediatric patient with referred palpable mass of the head. Interruption of the skull due to the presence of an echogenic mass bounded deeply by the meninges (*arrows*)

One of the main risks of diagnostic imaging in oncology, and not only in US, is being influenced by the clinical setting, e.g. considering a finding definitely or probably malignant simply because it is identified in a subject with a prior or current history of cancer. Complicating the problem is the nature of the malignant disease itself, which often exhibits unpredictable behavior, for example in terms of distribution (e.g. unusual site or “skip” of specific lymph node stations or specific parenchymas – as in the case of pulmonary metastases from gastrointestinal tumors in the absence of demonstrable liver metastases) or timing (e.g. metastasis many years after treatment of the primary tumor). A further complication is the existence of "second" malignancies which develop in patients already treated for malignant disease.

US is a less **objective** technique than other imaging modalities. The imaging findings included in the report, despite being plentiful and detailed with writing and pictures on the images indicating the anatomic area of the findings identified, certainly cannot express what the observation was in real time. When confronted with a small lesion identified with CT, the previous CT examination can be reviewed to understand whether the lesion was already present, whereas this is absolutely impossible with US. Even with the use of video recordings of the examinations performed, the US study remains a not completely objective examination, and this creates problems, especially for trials and off-site evaluations.

However, this should not suggest that US is a subjective technique or, as is commonly stated, **operator dependent**. The findings of any diagnostic examination are in fact dependent on the experience and dedication of the operator. Incorrect timing of the various phases of hepatic contrast in CT or a failure to perform a particular sequence in MR can be dependent on the operator just as much as a failure to identify a US finding. The difference, in terms of reliability, is that a technically suboptimal CT or MR examination can still be recognized after a retrospective evaluation of the images, something which in US can only occur to a much lesser extent. It cannot be demonstrated that US implies a degree of intraobserver or interobserver **reproducibility** of the measurements performed or of the diagnostic results achieved; reproducibility is lower than the other imaging modalities. The problem of variability of measurement in oncology is of undoubted importance in the setting both of clinical trials and diagnostic practice, and to all of the imaging modalities [1].

A more significant problem than the presumed operator dependence, and one which is often underestimated, is **patient dependence**. This is certainly greater in US than in other imaging modalities. Even with the current equipment, patients who are highly obese, with interference from gas (aerated lung, intestinal gas, pneumoperitoneum, subcutaneous emphysema, etc.), with overlying skeletal structures or with particular conformations of the ribcage are a significant limitation for the US study. However, in thin patients visualizing exceptional anatomic detail is possible, e.g. with the use of high-frequency transducers for exploration of the abdomen, the study of internal structures in subjects who are large in build is rather inexact, especially if the structures are deep. Irregularities and hardening of the skin surface associated with prior surgery, radiation therapy, edema (venous or lymphatic) and/or tumor infiltration can create difficulties for the positioning of the transducer – especially with wide transducers – and can therefore hinder optimal US exploration. The prescribing physician, when requesting the examination, and the US operator, when writing the report, should always ask themselves whether that particular patient and that particular problem are effectively accessible with US. Individuals with a considerable body mass should, in general, be investigated with other imaging modalities.

Doppler technique should also be mentioned. The first major problem in this field regards the quality of the equipment, which can significantly influence the sensitivity for low intralesional flows. A nodule may appear avascular with a low-level device and hypervascular with a high-quality device. In addition, the sensitivity depends on the setting of the equipment and the experience of the operator, which becomes an even more important parameter than it already is for grayscale US. With a PRF which is too high or with excessive compression of the transducer against the skin, flow can be totally cancelled even in a highly vascular lesion. An intrinsic limitation of Doppler techniques regards the impossibility of demonstrating slow flows in the parenchymal capillary network and intralesional neoangiogenic vessels, although these limitations can be largely overcome with CEUS.

1.3 Ultrasound and Cancer Screening

Cancer **screening** indicates an array of diagnostic procedures used in the study of more-or-less selected asymptomatic subjects for the early identification of a possible malignancy. This is prompted by the premise that early diagnosis and treatment can positively modify the natural history of the cancer in the individual patient. This is different from the concept of **surveillance**, which is used for asymptomatic individuals at high risk of developing a malignancy and therefore subject to a closer evaluation [2,3].

The aim of secondary prevention in oncology, in terms of both screening and surveillance, is therefore the systematic search of a malignancy in the preclinical phase, i.e. in asymptomatic individuals. The endpoint is the prevention/delay, within reasonable costs and through early treatment, of the advanced stage of the disease itself, thus reducing morbidity and mortality [4–6]. The concept of **natural history** is fundamental. When a subject develops a malignancy during his life, the tumor will first have a preclinical phase, which begins at the time of the biologic development of the disease itself. This is followed by a clinical phase, which begins with the onset of symptoms and ends with the death of the individual (either due to the disease or from other causes) [7]. The **detectable preclinical phase** is defined as the period between when a diagnostic test is able to recognize the disease and the onset of symptoms. In this period the disease may only be identified with secondary prevention (or as an incidental finding). The **critical point** is the moment in the natural history in which treatment of the disease becomes less effective than before: screening aims to identify the disease before and not after this critical point. For screening to be potentially effective, the critical point should occur during the detectable preclinical phase but the test and diagnosis should occur prior to that point, beyond which treatment becomes relatively ineffective [4,5,7].

The principal factors affecting the **cost effectiveness** of a screening test are cost, diagnostic accuracy, prevalence of disease in the sample and the percentage of "localized" tumors of those identified. [6,8].

A screening program can be planned only if a number of conditions are met or at least not disregarded [4,5,7,8]. With regard to the **test**, it should be ethically and psychologically acceptable so that the maximum number of people may respond to enrolment. It should be simple and accessible to all, especially to the targeted population. The test should also clearly have maximum sensitivity: since the prevalence of most diseases for which screening is proposed is <5%, a sensitivity of at least >95% would be needed (if the specificity is <95%, and vice versa), otherwise the true positives would be less than the false positives. With respect to sensitivity there is, nonetheless, the collateral question of overdiagnosis or pseudodisease. In this case the disease is identified, but the efficacy produced is only apparent because the disease is slow and indolent, and when correlated with age is unlikely to cause the death of the subject. From the probabilistic point of view, screening programs tend to markedly increase the detection of the more indolent and slow-growing tumors, whereas it is relatively unlikely they detect the more aggressive and highly malignant forms. The test should also have maximum specificity: the incidence of false negatives, with the associated consequences (further and possibly more invasive examinations, high costs, psychological effects, etc.), should be as low as possible. The identification of other and often trivial asymptomatic findings such as renal cysts, hepatic cysts, gallstones or kidney stones constitutes a negative effect. The test should be selective in the first instance, with a limited number of subjects – presumably all true positives – who move on to the second level. For this to occur, the number of indeterminate results needs to be minimized. The test should have a low level of invasiveness with the lowest level of mortality and morbidity possible: at the time of the test the subjects examined have a relatively low risk of death or severe symptoms deriving from the disease being investigated, so their safety should be especially protected. In this sense US finds favor over techniques such as CT which use ionizing radiation. The test should be relatively simple to perform and interpret. A test which requires elaborate preparation/implementation or which can only be read by a limited number of super-specialists does not lend itself to wide application. Even the length of the examination and the use of healthcare workers should be kept to a minimum. Lastly, the test should keep economic costs as low as possible. The **disease** should have a known natural history. It should be known when the critical point is reached, since the test can only be effective if this is located in the detectable preclinical phase. In this way the optimal interval for performing the test can also be established. The disease should be severe enough to ethically and economically justify the costs and risks of the screening. The failure to identify the disease should have serious consequences and this is applicable to the category of tumors, although with differences from case to case. The disease should not be overly rare otherwise the pretest and post-test probability would be inevitably low. The disease should not be easily curable during the clinical phase, otherwise there would be little need for preclinical identification, and there should be an effective treatment for the disease if it is identified prior to the critical point, otherwise an early diagnosis simply translates into "falling ill earlier". Lastly, the available treatment should not be overly dangerous or harmful, since some of the selected cases are false positives or pseudo-diagnoses. The **patient** should have an adequate life expectancy and other general characteristics of good health such that in the advent of a positive finding he can be eligible for treatment. The patient should be appropriately motivated, to minimize the number of cases lost at follow-up.

Let us now examine the possible applications of US in the screening of the main forms of cancer.

The early diagnosis of **breast** cancer translates into a reduction in mortality of 25–30% with respect to the cases diagnosed at the time of clinical presentation, with identification of smaller lesions more rarely involving the lymph nodes. One area of debate regards the age to begin and end screening and the appropriate interval. The ACS recommends performing an annual mammography from 40 years onwards to an age to be defined on the basis of the estimation of individual risk. The recommendations for younger women include a clinical evaluation every three years between the ages of 20 and 30 years and an annual evaluation between the ages of 30 and 40 years. Recommendations for women with an increased risk (family history, personal history of breast cancer or Hodgkin's lymphoma treated with radiation therapy) include an individual definition for an earlier beginning of mammography, US integration and a shorter interval between examinations. Lastly, women with a genetic predisposition (carriers of the genetic mutation *BRCA1* and *BRCA2*) are recommended to undergo surveillance based above all on MR. The association of US with mammography has significantly increased the percentage of breast cancers detected, especially in young women with denser breasts. The combined sensitivity of the two techniques in the various patient populations is 83–91%. The evidence therefore seems to support the additional use of US in the screening of women (age range 30–40 years) with dense or heterogeneous breasts [9].

Palpation is unable to identify most nodules of the **thyroid** with a diameter <15 mm and therefore is generally not considered viable for screening [10]. Moreover, a Japanese study on 88,160 individuals who underwent screening in a period spanning 16 years suggests that the view is sufficient to select suspicious cases to undergo US. Malignant lesions were encountered in 204 individuals (62 males and 144 females) with a percentage of detection in line with the literature [11]. High-resolution US is indisputably able to identify an elevated number of thyroid nodules, and the technique could be proposed for example in conjunction with US screening of the breast, in part because a correlation between the two malignancies has been proposed, although without a clear mechanism [12]. However, there are numerous practical limitations. The incidence of benign nodules in the population is very high (nodules <10 mm are found by US in up to 70% of normal thyroids). Postmortem findings show that the incidence of carcinoma is very low, at least with regard to clinically apparent forms (1.4–6.1/100,000) compared to the significantly higher incidence of apparently silent tumors (5–35% of individuals). There is a similarity in the imaging appearance between benign and malignant nodules, and in theory all identified nodules >8–10 mm should be subject to FNAC (performing FNAC only on suspicious nodules would subtract from screening a quota of carcinomas with a "benign" US appearance). Lastly, 90% of thyroid carcinomas are made up of papillary (especially "microcarcinomas", i.e. nodules <10 mm) and follicular forms which are often indolent, whereas it is rather unlikely that periodic screening would be able to identify the aggressive forms in an early stage, particularly the highly feared anaplastic carcinoma [12–15]. In essence, a program of US thyroid screening risks making a considerably large number of overdiagnoses, with a very high cost–benefit ratio and rather dubious prognostic benefits [15]. The selection of high-risk individuals (subjects with a family history, subjects exposed to radiation therapy of the neck in pediatric age or exposed to environmental radiation, patients with MEN, etc.) could narrow the application field [10].

Prostate cancer is characterized by low mortality, but given its elevated prevalence in the population it is nonetheless the second-leading cause of cancer death [16]. The ACS suggests screening from 50 years of age (45 years of age if first-degree relatives have a history of prostate cancer diagnosed at a relatively young age) with digital rectal examination and PSA assay (protease produced by normal, adenomatous and especially malignant glandular tissue), together with adequate information regarding the benefits and limitations of early diagnosis and treatment. Indeed, while it is true that the PSA assay is able to bring the diagnosis forward by at least 10 years on average, it is also true that this does not demonstrably increase survival. For the most part this is due to silent carcinomas (>30% of cases), which would not effectively progress and are therefore overdiagnosed due to the screening, and as a result overtreated. In addition, PSA is not specific and its widespread use runs the risk of having a large number of patients undergo biopsy who in fact have no malignancy. In Europe many currently advise against the PSA assay in asymptomatic patients and without clinical indications, due not only to the problem of overdiagnosis, but also to the significant percentage of false positives, the undemonstrated effect on the duration of life and the complications of prostatectomy (incontinence, impotence, etc.) [16]. Even the use of TRUS in asymptomatic patients appears to be rather unconvincing, since the technique is characterized by a relatively low positive predictive value (18–52%). This is due to the problem of unrecognizable isoechoic tumors, benign hypoechoic nodules which produce false positives, and the frequent multifocal nature of the disease [16]. Currently screening may be suggested on a voluntary basis, with periodic check-ups and PSA assay and subsequent evaluation with TRUS and/or biopsy in suspicious cases.

General screening for carcinoma of the **ovary** is currently not recommended, although it is indubitably hoped for in the future, should cost-effective systems become available [17]. An early diagnosis can translate into high survival (>80% for stages I and II). However, the relatively low prevalence of the disease, combined with the not very high specificity of the currently available diagnostic options, discourage mass screening [17–19]. There are, nonetheless, categories of increased risk, such as women with a family history, which require surveillance. The annual gynecologic examination with bimanual rectal-vaginal exploration has limited efficacy since it only detects 30% of masses identifiable with TVUS [20]. Screening can instead be based on CA-125 and/or US with a suprapubic approach but preferably with a transvaginal approach: TVUS is currently the imaging modality with the highest sensitivity for small ovarian tumors. It should, however, be borne in mind that while it is true that >80% of women with ovarian cancer have elevated levels of CA-125 (>35 IU/mL), it is also true that this figure falls to around 50% in cases of stage I and stage II disease [19]. Despite an overall elevated specificity, this tumor marker can give rise to false positives. These include healthy women (1%), subjects with cirrhosis, pancreatitis, first trimester pregnancy, pelvic inflammatory disease or endometriosis, and patients with advanced-stage non-ovarian abdominal malignancies (40%) [17,21]. A study of 22,000 women produced discouraging results: 11 tumors were identified (0.05%), of which seven were already in stage III–IV, and seven women with normal levels of CA-125 subsequently developed ovarian cancer [22]. The use of more sensitive biomarkers is desirable, possibly in combination [19]. With regard to TVUS, prospective studies indicate elevated sensitivity (85–95%) but with 2–5% of false positives [18]. The sequential use of an annual CA-125 assay and TVUS in cases with pathologic levels of the marker appears to be the most rational approach, although still not optimal because it is able to reduce the number of false-positive diagnoses and produces a sensitivity of 79–100% [18]. In women with a family history of ovarian cancer a multimodal evaluation combining clinical, US and laboratory findings is indicated to achieve an early diagnosis. There is undeniably the need for monitoring of women with markedly high risk (as high as 40%), i.e. those women with hereditary non-polypoid colorectal cancer, hereditary breast ovarian cancer syndrome or hereditary site-specific ovarian cancer syndrome. Moreover, in these cases prophylactic ovariectomy tends to be advised. In women with a less marked family history, e.g. with a single first-degree relative with a history of ovarian cancer, in whom the estimated risk is around 7%, surgery seems too radical, so periodic screening beginning at 25–30 years is generally the option chosen. In addition, all of these women develop the possible carcinoma of the ovary at a premenopausal age when the CA-125 assay and TVUS more readily produce false positives. Appropriate counseling of the women at risk regarding the current limitations of prevention is therefore advisable.

The rationale behind the screening for carcinoma of the **endometrium** is given by the advanced stage of disease at the onset of symptoms and, in contrast, the favorable prognosis for cases identified early (stage IA) with a 5-year survival rate of 90% [23]. The identification of precancerous lesions (endometrial hyperplasia and polyps) and endometrial carcinoma could benefit from TVUS, also with CD. An endometrial thickness of <5 mm virtually rules out malignancy. A screening program of 1074 asymptomatic women between 57 and 61 years of age, with an endometrial thickness threshold of >4 mm and a PI<1, showed a sensitivity for carcinoma of 94%, but a specificity of only 48% [24]. This suggests that women with an above-average risk should probably be selected for formulating a rational screening program, possibly in combination with the study of ovarian cancer (which has a peak incidence at a slightly younger age) [25]. Currently, however, screening for endometrial cancer is not considered sufficiently beneficial or justifiable, unless it is carried out in high-risk subjects (e.g. women with hereditary non-polypoid colorectal cancer) with the annual measurement of the endometrial thickness at TVUS [17].

With regard to the **testicle**, there are a number of conditions which constitute risk factors for the development of tumors, such as cryptorchidism (present in the history of 3.5–14.5% of patients diagnosed with testicular cancer, particularly with seminoma) and microlithiasis. US is clearly the technique of choice for surveillance (more so than for the screening) of these individuals, with the premise however that cryptorchidism is a clinical diagnosis whereas microlithiasis – defined as the presence of at least five calcified foci in the testicle – can only constitute an incidental US finding [26]. Since orchiopexy prevents infertility but not the risk of cancer (4–10 times higher than in individuals with normally descended testicles), periodic US monitoring is indicated in patients operated for cryptorchidism [27]. As an alternative, a testicular biopsy can be performed at the age of 18–20 years: if this is positive for a germ-cell intratubular tumor (carcinoma in situ), there is a 50% probability of developing an invasive carcinoma, whereas if the biopsy is negative the patient has a risk of cancer similar to that of others of his age and does not require monitoring [28]. With regard to microlithiasis, which is caused by the deposit of calcium in the seminiferous tubules and has a prevalence of 0.05–0.6% (in focal or diffuse form, either uni- or bilateral), its real weight as a risk factor is debatable. An association with testicular tumors has been hypothesized, in particular with germ-cell tumors, but this has not been confirmed by all studies (Fig. 1.8). Currently it does appear prudent to suggest to patients with an incidental finding of microlithiasis (and probably also with non-microlithiasis testicular calcifications) to undergo an annual US examination as well as performing self-palpation, or at least to discuss the existence of the problem.

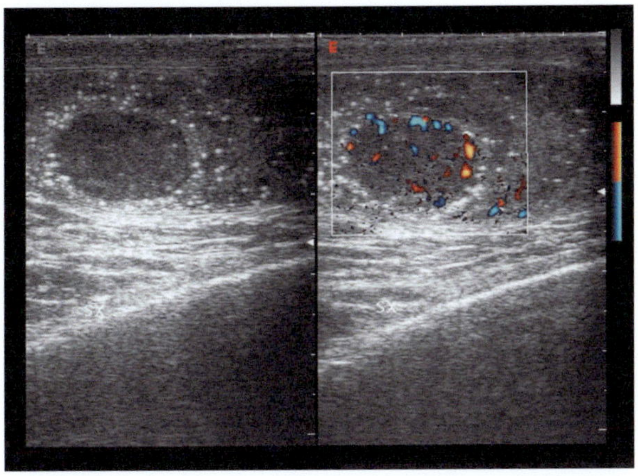

Fig. 1.8 Testicular seminoma associated with microlithiasis. US and PD study shows a relatively homogeneous and well-defined hypoechoic nodule with moderate vasculature within the testicle. Numerous fine calcifications around the lesion and throughout the testicle can also be visualized

The routine use of tumor markers, CT examinations or testicular biopsy in these patients does not appear reasonable [26,29,30]. Beyond these circumstances, the rather low incidence of testicular cancer discourages mass screening, unless reserved for a strict age range (20–30 years).

Hepatocellular carcinoma (HCC) can unquestionably be managed more effectively if it is identified early, in part because the improvements obtained in recent years in the treatment of cirrhosis and HCC itself have enabled an improvement in survival to be achieved in these patients with tumor identified with screening [31–34]. Nonetheless, greater understanding of the natural history of this disease is needed, which has a highly variable doubling time, variable growth rates and variable progression in subjects of different race and with different etiologic factors of hepatitis [32]. Screening is viable in countries with an elevated incidence and, at the same time, adequate healthcare facilities. High-risk subjects need to be selected, especially those with HBV infection (males >40 years, females >50 years, family history of HCC, subjects with cirrhosis), HCV infection (if >40 years), alcohol-induced cirrhosis, genetic hemochromatosis or primary biliary cirrhosis [31,35]. Serum alpha-fetoprotein (AFP) and/or US may be used, although the use of CT or MR has been proposed in the United States [36,37]. Despite these latter modalities being undeniably more accurate, they involve higher costs and greater invasiveness and are relatively unsuitable for the periodic screening needs of countries with a high incidence. In a study simulated on patients aged 50 years with hepatitis C cirrhosis [36], screening for HCC with AFP assay and US produced, in relation to the non-screening option, an increase in the cost-effectiveness ratio of USD 26,689/year, quality of life corrected, an increase of USD 25,232 for screening with AFP assay and CT, and an increase of USD 118,000 for screening with AFP assay and MR. Moreover, no randomized controlled trial has demonstrated a reduction in disease-specific mortality associated with screening for HCC, nor have they clearly defined which is the most cost-effective test, which patients should be included and which interval should be adopted [38]. With regard to the latter, a dynamic CT study is indicated [38] at least every 12 months, with shorter intervals in high-risk subjects, even though CT studies on the growth rate of small HCCs [39] have indicated the need for three-monthly examinations. Annual US screening has identified single lesions in 60% of cases and multiple lesions in 40%. However, only in 30% of cases is the single lesion <3 cm, and only in 23% of cases is it <2 cm and therefore ideal for surgical resection. This suggests the need for more frequent US examinations (2, 3 or even 4 times/year) since the doubling time of HCC is thought to be 2–4 months. Moreover, there are no randomized controlled trials which demonstrate the superiority of the six-month interval over the annual one [31,40]. The mean size of nodules identified with six-monthly screening is smaller than those of HCC identified with longer intervals [35]. In Italy, as in many Asian countries where HCC is particularly widespread, screening is based mainly on three- or six-monthly US, possibly associated with AFP assay. AFP, whose value is not correlated with the size of the lesion but which nonetheless is an important prognostic index, has been found to be absolutely normal (<20 ng/mL) in 31% of cases of HCC identified at US screening, and markedly increased (>400 ng/mL) in only 22–29% of these. The sensitivity is 60% with a threshold of 20 ng/mL but it falls to 22% with a threshold of 200 ng/mL, thus indicating that this marker cannot be used as a single screening test [31,35]. The AFP assay can reduce the number of US false negatives by producing pathologic values in some of these subjects, while at the same time being able to produce a certain increase in false positives [41]. It is not uncommon for the re-evaluation of subjects with negative US and increased AFP to identify small iso-hypoechoic lesion, particularly when deep or superficial, which went unrecognized during an initial US study. US screening has shown extremely variable sensitivity, from 33% to 96%, in different studies in relation to different factors [31,42]. Several prospective and retrospective studies comparing pretransplant US with findings from the explanted liver have shown a rather low sensitivity of 30–50% per patient and 20–45% per lesion, calling into serious question the possible application of US screening [42–44]. Accordingly, the sensitivity appears not to depend on the degree of heterogeneity of the parenchyma, the hepatic volume or the site of the nodule but strictly on the size of the nodule. The conclusions which can be drawn are that the combination US + AFP with six-monthly intervals, while not being especially sensitive and increasing costs with respect to the two tests taken individually, does have a rationale in the monitoring of at-risk patients, considering the relatively low aggressiveness of HCC in most patients. Protocols which instead alternate AFP and US do not have an adequate rationale [31,45]. Since lesions <10 mm are rarely the expression of a HCC, such US findings tend not to require work-up unless they are associated with an increase in AFP, and are simply monitored. Nodules >10 mm have a good probability of being malignant and therefore undergo the work-up of HCC [31,45]. The individual lesions <3 cm identified by screening are hypoechoic in 60% of cases, isoechoic in 24% of cases and hyperechoic in 16% of cases. In addition, 48% show a mosaic appearance and 36% have a peripheral hypoechoic halo [41]. With regard to the site, defined per patient with individual lesions <5 cm, 50% of lesions are located in a posterior segment, 34% in an anterior segment, 11% in a lateral segment and 4.5% in a medial segment [41].

Renal cell carcinoma (RCC) is relatively too uncommon and relatively too little aggressive to justify any form of screening. In particular, small RCCs – those that would probably be identified during screening – on the one hand tend to have a lower grade and extension than symptomatic lesions, and on the other create greater problems for differential diagnosis. Renal malignancies ≤35 mm identified incidentally are in fact slow growing (on average 3.6 mm/year), especially if well defined. Also bearing in mind that during the follow-up of these lesions the identification of metastases is rare, an approach of "wait and see" has been suggested in elderly, run-down or high-surgery-risk subjects, rather than an approach of aggressive surgery (even though it would be rather difficult to convince an elderly subject with a new diagnosis of a small renal tumor to not undergo surgery!) [46]. On the other hand, several studies have reported sensitivity and specificity for US that is far from optimal in the identification of small RCCs [47]. However, a Japanese study reported the findings of US screening performed on 200,000 subjects over a 13-year period. RCC was identified in 0.09% of cases, with T1 lesions accounting for 38% of cases and a constant absence of lymph node involvement and distant metastases in all identified cases, and with effective resection in 98% of cases (cumulative survival at 10 years of 98%) [48,49]. To increase the cost–benefit ratio, the authors of this study underline the importance of exploring not only the kidneys but the entire abdomen. Hypothetically, US screening for RCC could be combined with screening for aneurysms of the abdominal aorta, which is increasingly encouraged now that endoprostheses are available and could be performed in a similar age range, possibly with the selection of male subjects.

To conclude, one must ask whether a US abdominal examination in asymptomatic subjects can have a rationale for the purposes of general oncologic screening and the search for "disease" in the broad sense. With increasing frequency, individuals are encountered who "self-prescribe" periodic examinations (usually annual) with US of the abdomen, pelvis and often the thyroid, on the basis of an often general "family history". There are no scientific arguments in support of this practice so it therefore does not appear to be sustainable. In Japan, where it should be recalled the average build of the individuals is smaller than that of Europeans and still smaller than that of Americans, the results of a general abdominal US screening program have been reported. In an eight-year study performed on over 200,000 subjects, generally resectable malignancies were identified in 0.31% of cases. These included 201 HCCs, 81 gallbladder carcinomas, 57 pancreatic carcinomas and 169 RCCs, with a 5-year cumulative survival rate of 79.5% [48]. In reality, a US examination performed on non-selected asymptomatic individuals has a much higher probability of identifying relatively irrelevant findings (hepatic cysts, renal cysts, gallstones, kidney stones, etc.) than identifying malignancies in an early stage. Most tumors identifiable with transabdominal US, with the exception of HCC (which nonetheless generally has onset in specific categories of individuals), RCC and bladder cancers, are in fact identified in a relatively advanced stage, often beyond the critical point: gallbladder, pancreas, gastrointestinal tract, female reproductive system and prostate. The false negatives relative to tumors present but not yet identifiable with US are added to the false positives, a source of further costs and often additional unnecessary diagnostic or therapeutic procedures. These are the same considerations that have been made with regard to CT screening [2,3,8], which is encumbered by greater costs and a higher level of invasiveness, but which at least has the extenuating characteristic of greater panoramic views and, when performed with intravenous contrast media, greater diagnostic accuracy.

1.4 Ultrasound and Neoangiogenesis

The **acquired properties of cancer** include: self-sufficiency in growth signals (and insensitivity to anti-growth signals), cellular immortalization (apoptosis), proliferation (unlimited potential for replication), invasion, metastasization and neoangiogenesis (sustained formation of vessels) [50]. Neoangiogenesis is the requirement for both tumor growth, which is angiogenesis dependent, and metastasization [51]. Tumor growth beyond 1–3 mm in fact requires a functioning network of blood vessels to support its anabolic and catabolic activity [51–53].

Neoangiogenesis is characterized by an increased number of small vessels – the microcirculation – which develop within the tumor from the activity of host endothelial cells activated and stimulated by tumor growth factors [50,54] (Fig. 1.9). The vasculature of the tumor is typically characterized by an irregular and chaotic architecture without a precise "hierarchy" between the different vascular structures, a prevalence of tortuous and dilated capillaries with few complete arteries and veins, variable vessel branching with the possibility of blind collateral branches, an absence of vasomotor control, immature vessels which are fragile and permeable to macromolecules, arteriovenous fistulas and intermittent or unstable flow with acute vessel collapse and hemorrhage [50,53]. The low flow resistance, due to the absence of vasomotor control and arteriovenous fistulas, is counterbalanced by high interstitial pressure, caused by the increased vessel permeability and consequent diffusion of osmotic substances. The result is areas of different flow resistance [55]. The vascular distribution is heterogeneous, with areas of coexisting low and high vessel density, the latter being particularly present in the peripheral regions of the tumor. In part the network is inefficient in terms of oxygen supply, which explains the tendency for necrosis, especially in the central region [56]. The microvessel density (MVD) is inversely proportional to the tumor volume [57].

The **study of tumor vascularity** is important for a number of reasons. It may confirm the effective presence of a lesion, by negatively or positively increasing the contrast with the surrounding tissue. Since the degree of vascular density is correlated with the probability of a malignant nature of a lesion (although with notable exceptions, e.g. the intensely vascular hepatic FNH), it is also correlated with the degree of activity and the propensity to metastasize of the lesion and therefore correlated with prognosis (although at the same time it may indicate greater responsiveness to systemic treatment). The study can also define the anatomic relations of a lesion with the adjacent structures and especially with the vessels (staging, operability, etc.).

The **degree of microvessel density** can be analyzed with direct or indirect systems. Estimation of the intratumoral microvascular density is the main direct method for evaluating angiogenesis and is performed with immunohistochemical staining using antibodies against various endothelial cell-related antigens [54,56]. The degree of MVD is a prognostic variable independent of the malignancies and it correlates with the probability of metastasization and survival, even

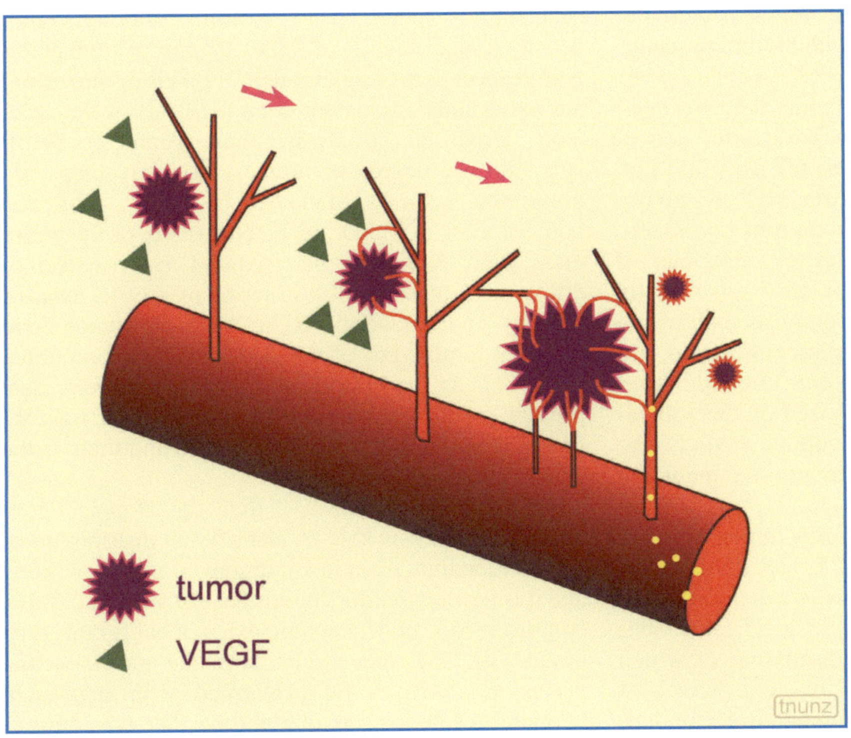

Fig. 1.9 Mechanism underlying angiogenesis. The still small malignancy produces vascular endothelial growth factor (VEGF) which causes the development of new arterioles, which in turn are responsible for further tumor growth

though it is not necessarily related to the rate of tumor growth: a reduction has in fact been measured in animals treated with antiangiogenetic drugs [51]. The vessels of the microcirculation have a very small diameter (2–5 μm) and are only accessible with microscopy: confocal microscopy (resolution ~100 nm), multiphoton microscopy (~100 nm) and electron microscopy (several nm) [53]. These techniques are optimal for the high-resolution evaluation of neovascularization in that they enable calculation of the MVD. However, they do require tumor tissue and therefore a biopsy. In addition they only indicate the MVD at a given location and therefore, in the context of a tumor, numerous central and peripheral samples would be required to reliably define the state of the microcirculation. The estimate of MVD is also a morphologic parameter and does not enable a dynamic functional analysis [50].

The tests for indirectly determining the state of the microcirculation can be divided into two groups: (1) blood angiogenetic factors assay; (2) blood volume and tumor perfusion evaluation with imaging techniques. The latter – some of which are still in the experimental phase or can only be performed in vitro – can be further subdivided into two broad categories: those that indirectly study angiogenesis (perfusion MR, perfusion CT, PET with O^{15}, SPECT, spectral and color Doppler, CEUS, photoacoustic imaging) and those that enable a direct approach, e.g. with contrast media able to bond to the endothelial cells (US with specific microbubbles, MR with specific paramagnetic nanoparticles, PET with tracers bonded to antibodies directed against factors associated with the neocirculation, micro-CT, optical imaging with bioluminescence or fluorescence) [29,58].

The commonly used imaging modalities, however, have a spatial resolution that is inferior to the abovementioned microscopic techniques: CT 100–500 μm, MR 100–500 μm, CEUS 50–100 μm, PET ~4 mm (up to 1.5 mm in the future), US several mm [29,52,59]. CD is able to identify vessels up to a diameter of 40 μm, especially when they are located superficially and the power mode is used. Imaging modalities are therefore unable to resolve the microcirculation, but they do provide important morphofunctional information in vivo. The techniques are based on the equivalence tumor perfusion and blood volume = MVD (the perfusion is the total blood flow to a tissue, including the capillary flow).

Each of the different imaging modalities used for the study of tumor vascularity – CT, MR (dynamic or with other techniques of functional acquisition), PET (with different radiotracers), Doppler and CEUS – has advantages and limitations, the discussion of which goes beyond the possibilities of this text. Which of these will in the future be the technique or techniques for the evaluation of tumor perfusion cannot be safely stated at present. However, the US techniques are in no way inferior in this sense to CT, MR or nuclear medicine [60,61].

Color Doppler is able to obtain a color signal corresponding to small intraparenchymal or intralesional vessels which are not visible in B-mode. Either in baseline or with contrast media, the Doppler techniques in fact provide a good architectural representation of the tumor macrovasculature, at least with regard to the superficial structures and, above all, with high-frequency transducers [59,62]. Power Doppler, which is more sensitive to slow flow and to morphologic detail than color Doppler, is more susceptible to artifacts and does not bring substantial improvements to the study of tumor vascularity [56,59]. The flow in the small vessels (<200 μm) is similar to the movement through the tissues (<1 cm/s) and therefore cannot be identified with Doppler techniques [59]. In order to be detected by Doppler, a vascular signal needs to have a sufficient intensity and velocity: the first can be increased with the use of contrast media (with the disadvantage of increasing artifacts), but the second cannot be altered. The state of large- and medium-diameter vessels identified with Doppler tends to be (but is not necessarily!) correlated with the state of the microcirculation [62,63]. Correlation between color signal density and histologic grade of the tumor vasculature has been experimentally demonstrated [64,65]. The parameters which have been proposed include pulsatility index, resistance index, acceleration index, peak systolic velocity, color density (quantification of the number of colored pixels with respect to the total number of pixels of the lesion) and other indices calculated on the basis of the color maps. Often, but not always, these parameters correlate with the degree of tumor vascularity measured invasively, such as MVD [56,63,64,66]. From the point of view of MVD, the heterogeneity of the tumor mass also explains the frequent coexistence of different Doppler spectra in terms of profile, systolic velocity and, above all, RI in the same tumor or in different tumors but of the same histotype and grade [56]. This is the source of the heterogeneous data present in the literature. Intraobserver and interobserver reproducibility are also limited and there is the problem of deep attenuation.

CEUS is more sensitive than the Doppler techniques, in that it is able to identify the distribution of contrast medium even in conditions of ultraslow flow, and it is less susceptible to motion artifacts [62,67]. US contrast media are to a certain extent ideal for this type of analysis, since they are intravascular and enable the perfusion study to be performed with maximum temporal resolution, i.e. in real time. The resolution is also greater than that of Doppler techniques, with the possibility of direct demonstration of vessels 20–40 μm in diameter (corresponding to the precapillary level) [62,63]. CEUS offers a reproducible estimate of the perfusion, and the signal intensity (echogenicity) is proportional to the concentration of microbubbles in the area of interest. The perfusion curve obtained after injection of the bolus of contrast medium is characterized by an initial rapid and intense increase in signal intensity, a brief maximum and a more-or-less rapid decrease over time [60] (Fig. 1.10). The most widely used technique for quantifying the absolute perfusion parameters or the parameters proportional to the blood flow in that particular area is the destruction–reperfusion technique. When all of the microbubbles in a particular section are destroyed by pulses with an elevated MI, the subsequent filling depends on the new microbubbles which enter the section from the adjacent tissues and can be detected in a nondestructive manner (low MI). While keeping the transducer in a fixed location for the entire time, a sequence of predefined ultrasound pulses is transmitted, with a high-power initial pulse and other less intense pulses aimed at the harmonic stimulation of the new microbubbles entering the section [60,62,68]. The percentage of filling, with administration of contrast medium by both infusion and bolus injection (but in the latter case an initial injection is needed for calibration), follows a curve whose initial increase depends on the mean flow velocity in the ROI and whose maximum peak indicates the vascular volume fraction: the product of these measurements is a proportional measure of the real tissue perfusion [57,60,62,68]. Many US devices are equipped with internal software for automatic quantification of the enhancement as an objective estimate of perfusion. As an alternative, the images can be sent to off-line systems. There are numerous perfusion parameters which can be calculated from the intensity/time curves: peak signal intensity, time to maximum enhancement (time to peak), time to enhancement, area under the curve, positive gradient and duration of enhancement [53,62,69,70]. The enhancement detected with the scansion in real time can even be automatically summed into a single vascular map [71]. For quantitative studies, however, the settings of the device should be standard and should not be modified over time, and the same goes for the injection protocol and acoustic window. In addition, the transmission parameters should be correlated with the concentration of the contrast media in the tissue [60]. CEUS findings correlate experimentally with data obtained with immunohistochemical markers of angiogenesis and also with those obtained with dynamic MR. In a recent series, CEUS patterns and parameters were found to correlate more closely with MVD than VEGF expression [72].

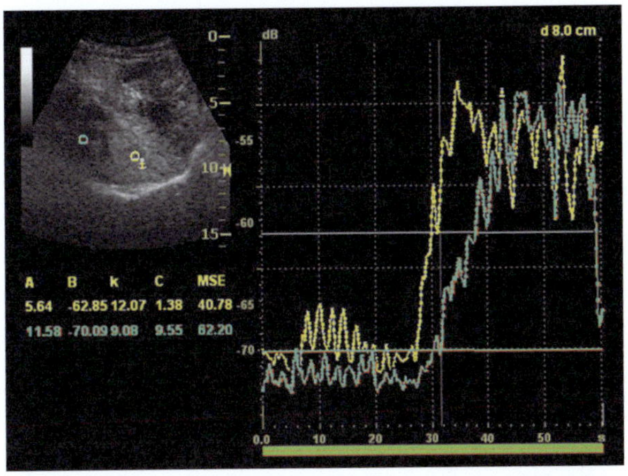

Fig. 1.10 Signal intensity–time curve. Perfusion curves obtained by positioning a yellow ROI on a hypervascular hepatic lesion and a blue ROI on the adjacent normal hepatic parenchyma

In a study on murine neuroblastoma, CEUS, in contrast to PD, was able to distinguish experimental tumors and control tumors based on the different characteristics of the signal intensity at the moment of arrival of the contrast medium [73]. Animal studies have also shown changes in the destruction–reperfusion curves after antiangiogenesis therapy with a reduction in the duration and intensity of the enhancement and an increase in the time required for reperfusion. The regression of functional vascular parameters precedes the reduction in size of the tumor [74]. In addition, an experimental study showed a partial lack in the correlation between CEUS and MR, with the risk of the former underestimating the vascularity of tumors with small and collapsed vessels, due to the greater resistance offered to the microbubbles than to the MR contrast medium [75]. The main limitations of the study of angiogenesis with CEUS are related to the acquisition in a singe layer, recirculation of contrast medium, attenuation in the deep tissues, and dependence on patient build. At the level of the abdomen the patient needs to be able to maintain breath-hold for the entire time required, and the acquisition parameters need to be kept constant. A future outlook is provided by targeted imaging, with microbubbles specifically tailored for the tumors (e.g. with tumor-specific peptides on the surface of the microbubbles) or their vessels (e.g. with antiendothelial monoclonal antibodies on the surface of the microbubbles) [61,76].

1.5 Cancer Staging

In addition to screening, which is a topic in itself, various phases need to be considered when imaging, and in our case US, is used in the diagnosis of the patient with a malignancy. This includes diagnosis or "first" diagnosis (**identification** of the lesion and therefore its topographical position, **characterization** or differential diagnosis of the lesion, in the sense of non-tumor vs. tumor, benign vs. malignant and primary vs. metastatic), **staging** (evaluation of the spread of the disease, not only for the purposes of completing the diagnosis, but also for treatment and prognosis), **treatment planning** (including an evaluation of operability), the **evaluation of response** during and after treatment (both in the short term for the judgment of radicality, the identification of residual tumor and the exclusion of complications, and in the long term for follow-up) and the identification of **recurrence**.

Staging is fundamental because it influences the treatment and especially the prognosis which, in general, worsens in terms of 5-year survival with increasing stage. Accurate staging is crucial in the patient who is a candidate for surgery. In most cases, the treatment of choice for tumors in the initial stages is in fact **resective surgery with radical or curative intent**. According to the protocols, this can be practiced with a more radical or more conservative intent with respect to the anatomic parts surrounding the tumor. In some cases, radical surgery can even be performed in the event of local recurrence, lymph node involvement or the excision of metastases. A crucial factor in all cases is that the anatomic-pathologic evaluation reveals an adequate margin of healthy tissue around the excised mass. In other cases, with locally advanced tumors, **palliative surgery** and/or **cytoreductive surgery** may be performed. Tumor debulking, i.e. the removal of more-or-less large parts of the tumor mass, makes possible an improvement in the effects of systemic or radiation therapy. Included among the tumors that are generally considered inoperable are tumors with an excessive local extension which would not allow en bloc resection except at the price of persistent functional damage, tumors with a local-regional extension so great as to suggest an elevated probability of still occult distant metastases, and tumors associated with distant metastases, with the exception of those that are highly chemosensitive such as testicular cancers. One method for improving the possibility of performing and the effectiveness of "curative" surgery is the use of chemotherapeutic and/or radiotherapeutic treatment either preoperatively (**neoadjuvant**) or postoperatively (**adjuvant**). In this way curative surgery may be able to obtain a result similar to that of radical surgery but without adjuvant treatment, or it may be possible to eradicate (potential) micrometastases after surgical resection, or to re-evaluate a lesion not initially considered for radical surgery (debulking). In fact neoadjuvant treatment aims at obtaining a downstaging of the tumor, i.e. reducing the stage of the disease with the possibility, in the event of a positive response, of then intervening surgically. Lastly, mention should be made of chemotherapy as an initial palliative choice in cases of advanced disease, in the first diagnosis phase or in the presence of recurrence. Most patients in the metastatic phase of disease are treated with chemotherapy to reduce symptoms and prolong life. Defining the stage of disease is important even in the patient who is not a candidate for radical surgery, at least in the first instance, since the evaluation of treatment response will mainly be based on the comparison between the extent of disease before and after treatment [33,77].

Tumor spread occurs in a number of patterns: continuous spread, in relation to the growth of the tumor itself; contiguous spread, along ligaments, vessels, nerves or other structures adjacent to the mass; lymphatic spread, with involvement of the lymphatic vessels and the lymph nodes draining the anatomic region of the mass; hematogenous spread, from the embolization of tumor cells in distant organs; cavitary spread, with the transmission of tumor cells in the fluids of serous cavities; and iatrogenic spread, as a consequence of seeding of tumor cells during medical procedures.

The TNM staging system of solid tumors is a standardized modality for objectively and concisely defining the anatomic extension of a tumor in a given time so as to make possible the evaluation of changes over time. The system combines information regarding the size and/or depth of the primary tumor (T parameter – **local**) with information concerning spread to the lymph nodes (N parameter – **regional**) and metastases (M parameter – **distant**) in a series of categories or stages. The addition of numbers to the T and N components indicates ascending degrees of tumor extension (T0 – no evidence of primary tumor – T1, T2, T3, T4 – worsening local extension; N0 – no evidence of lymph node involvement – N1, N2, N3 – worsening lymph node involvement), whereas for the M parameter there is only the alternative absence (M0) or presence (M1, with possible distinction between different sites). The definition of the T parameter is generally based on the size of the primary tumor and/or its location and/or deep extension (wall of hollow organs) or invasion of adjacent structures. The N parameter is usually defined on the basis of the site of the lymph nodes involved with respect to the tumor, as well as their number, size and/or mobility. It should be noted that the N parameter includes only the lymph node stations considered to be "regional" with respect to the tumor in question, whereas metastases to "extraregional" lymph nodes are a part of distant spread. Lastly, the M parameter considers the organs and structures involved secondarily by distant metastasization, with the possible distinction of different sites [78]. In general, stage 0 corresponds to the earliest form with the most favorable prognosis (i.e. carcinoma in situ), stage I to localized carcinoma, stage II to local and/or limited regional spread, stage III to local-regionally advanced spread and stage IV, with the poorest prognosis, to generalized metastasization [78].

The TNM system is used to formulate treatment decisions, to define prognosis, to stratify patients in clinical studies and to compare the populations and results of different centers. TNM is applied to most solid tumors. Exceptions include melanomas (Clark levels for the "T" parameter), gynecologic tumors (FIGO staging) and lymphomas (Cotswold classification of Hodgkin's lymphoma also extended to non-Hodgkin's lymphomas) [77]. Clearly, each level of staging, both clinical-radiologic and surgical-pathologic, can over- or understage disease spread by assigning a stage respectively higher or lower than the real one. In surgery candidates, therefore, a broad range of information needs to be obtained: type of malignancy, size, histologic grade, presence of lymphatic or vascular permeation, presence of associated carcinoma in situ, extent of local invasion, completeness of the excision and state of regional lymph nodes [77]. It should in fact be borne in mind that the anatomic extension of the disease as defined by the TNM staging system or similar systems is not the only parameter for therapeutic management and prognosis, because other factors, such as the degree of tumor cell differentiation (i.e. the grade) and the presence or absence of certain biomarkers (within the tumor tissue and/or in circulation) are also important. Tumor markers have a more-or-less important and specific role to play in the diagnosis, staging, treatment evaluation and prognosis of many malignancies. The main serum markers are AFP (hepatoblastoma, HCC and nonseminomatous germ cell tumors of the testicle, as well as seminomas and ovarian germ cell tumors), beta-HCG (nonseminomatous germ cell tumors of the testicle, ovarian choriocarcinoma), PSA (prostate cancer), PLAP (seminoma), LDH (melanoma, Hodgkin's lymphoma, germ-cell testicular tumors), CEA (gastrointestinal cancers as well as mucinous ovarian adenocarcinomas), CA15-3 (breast cancer), CA-125 (ovarian cancer, peritoneal mesothelioma, advanced abdominal tumors), CA19-9 (gastrointestinal cancers, especially of the pancreas), calcitonin (medullary carcinoma of the thyroid), thyroglobulin (differentiated thyroid carcinomas) and immunoglobulins or their fragments (myeloma, solitary plasmocytoma). The most important urinary markers are 5-HIAA (carcinoid), vanillylmandelic acid (pheochromocytoma), catecholamine (neuroblastoma) and kappa and lambda chains (myeloma) [77].

1.6 Ultrasound and Response to Treatment

The evaluation of the response to treatment refers to the diagnostic procedures used for the study of patients undergoing treatment for a malignant lesion, with the specific aim of verifying the effectiveness or otherwise of the treatment and the possible side-effects. The demonstration of the type of response to local, regional or systemic therapy is a crucial feature of oncologic imaging. Being able to personalize the treatment protocol is in fact fundamental, as it avoids both hypotreatment, with persistence or worsening of the disease, and hypertreatment, with unnecessary pharmacologic or radiation-induced toxicity. Response to treatment determines the subsequent therapeutic choices: as a general rule, in the event of a complete response treatment is consolidated and then suspended, with partial or stationary response the same therapeutic choice is continued, and in the case of disease progression the patient is offered a second-line treatment.

The different types of treatment (conventional multichemotherapy, hormone therapy, antiangiogenetic agents, radiation therapy) produce effects which, in their diversity, are nonetheless the consequence on the one hand of destructive phenomena and on the other of induced reparative phenomena. From many points of view all of this can be detected with imaging modalities, including US.

In general, hypoechoic lesions tend to become hyperechoic following treatment, particularly due to fibrosis, a phenomenon which is particularly present in cases of lymphoma and sarcoma. Lesions that are already hyperechoic tend to become heterogeneous, with the appearance of hypo-anechoic areas due to liquefactive necrosis. The reduction in vascularity is indubitably one of the most important effects, particularly in light of the description above of neoangiogenesis, and this feature will be covered in more detail later. A typical reparative phenomenon is calcification. Tissue necrosis in fact produces a reduction in pH and releases phospholipids and glycoproteins, thus creating favorable conditions for the precipitation of insoluble calcium salts. This is particularly characteristic of mucoid and papillary tumors: typical examples include the calcification of the peritoneal metastases of papillary serous ovarian carcinomas in cases that are responsive to chemotherapy and the calcification of Hodgkin's disease lesions after radiation therapy. In these cases, the residual mass can be quite large and persistent due to the fibrosis, even when the tumor component is completely inactive. The necrosis can be liquefactive or coagulative and can occur rapidly or progressively according to the treatment modality used. In any case, the US changes are partial and nonspecific: for example, detecting a lymph node treated with radiation therapy or a hepatic nodule treated with PEI on the basis of the echotexture can be challenging. In some malignancies, e.g. soft tissue sarcomas, a positive response to neoadjuvant treatment may be expressed with the formation of a peripheral fibrous pseudocapsule, which better circumscribes the lesion and also facilitates surgical excision. A phenomenon which occasionally occurs in treated lesions is differentiation, as in the case of germ-cell tumors. The differentiation of the tumor tissue produces a series of changes, including a reduction in size, increased margination, an increase in the cystic, adipose and/or calcified components and a decrease in vascularity [79–82]. Even indirect signs, such as the disappearance of retention of the bile ducts or urinary tract, can indicate a response to treatment of a lesion which has reduced its obstructive action on proximal anatomic structures.

Size criteria are in reality the only truly consolidated criteria and certainly the most reliable in clinical practice. The first standard evaluation criteria of response to treatment to be widely adopted were developed by WHO [83]. In this system the measurement of the lesion is bidimensional and is based on the product between the longest diameter and the largest diameter perpendicular to it. The **WHO criteria** include the following categories: (1) complete response: disappearance of all known lesions, confirmed at 4 weeks or more; (2) partial response: reduction of ⩾50% of the sum of the products of all known measurable lesions, in the absence of new lesions, confirmed at 4 weeks or more; (3) disease in progress: increase ⩾25% of the sum of the products of all known measurable lesions, or onset of new lesions; (4) stable disease: size changes not classifiable in the other categories (i.e. reduction <50% or increase <25%), in the absence of new lesions. There are also lesions defined as "non-measurable" by the WHO system, i.e. lesions which can be identified but whose exact size cannot be determined.

A simplified unidimensional estimate was developed in the 1990s by a Canadian-American committee and received immediate and widespread application both in clinical trials and in practice [84,85]. The system involves the measurement of only the longest diameter of the measurable lesions and up to a total of 5 lesions per organ and 10 lesions among the different organs. These lesions, defined as target lesions, are then used as the basis for the classification of response, whereas all the other lesions, defined as non-target lesions, are only evaluated for their presence or absence. This **RECIST system** includes categories which are slightly different from the WHO criteria: (1) complete response: disappearance of all known lesions, target and non-target, and normalization of serum levels of tumor markers, confirmed at 4 weeks or more; (2) partial response: reduction of ⩾30% of the sum of the largest diameters of the target lesions and/or persistence of elevated serum levels of tumor markers, confirmed at 4 weeks or more; (3) disease in progress: increase ⩾20% of the sum of the largest diameters of all target lesions and/or unequivocal progression of known non-target lesions and/or appearance of new lesions; (4) stable disease: size changes not classifiable in other categories (i.e. reduction <30% or increase <20%), in the absence of new lesions.

As can be seen, these are rather complex definitions which should be the domain of the oncologist and not formulated by the US operator, for example at the time of writing the report. Except in special cases, the US operator should only report the measurement of the lesions identified and then indicate a possible "worsening" in terms of the previous presentation, whereas drawing from this a definition of "progression" could prove incorrect (e.g. because afterwards no effective increase ⩾20% of the sum of the diameters of the target lesions occurs).

The definition of a non-target lesion is particularly important. These may be defined as such because they are measurable but small (<20 mm if evaluated with conventional radiologic procedures or <10 mm if evaluated with spiral CT or MR) or because they are non-measurable (bone or cystic lesions, malignant pleural, pericardial or peritoneal effusion, carcinomatous mastitis, pulmonary or cutaneous carcinomatous lymphangitis, leptomeningeal diffusion) [84].

Although the unidimensional measurement of the RECIST system is today the most utilized by oncologists, the US operator should nonetheless continue to indicate the two largest diameters in the report. In addition, in cases of multiple metastases it is crucial that the operator measures at least the five largest lesions in each organ and does not simply provide a generic description of "multiplicity'. The US operator may not be informed regarding which lesions have been defined target lesions and which non-target lesions, so the operator is better off providing an excess of measurements rather than a lack thereof. Current imaging is characterized by multiplanar views, which are intrinsic to US and MR and also adopted by multislice CT. It is therefore possible to accurately define the three largest diameters of the lesions on three orthogonal planes or even calculate the volume of the lesion with 3D acquisitions. In part this involves an abstraction, since the volume can be defined only in lesions with a regular shape or at least well-defined sharp margins. In addition, factors such as the focal zone depth of the ultrasound beam can influence the measurement (the depth of the focal zone would therefore need to be kept constant in serial examinations of a tumor!) [86]. Nonetheless it is rather peculiar, and perhaps debatable, that in the light of the possibility of such sophisticated measurements the WHO criteria are based on a bidimensional evaluation and the RECIST criteria on a unidimensional evaluation.

It should also be noted that the RECIST criteria, which are primarily aimed at making phase II studies on antitumor treatment comparable, and only secondarily at the application in clinical practice, have an extremely radical position with respect to US. In fact, they state that if the primary aim is the objective evaluation of treatment efficacy, US should not be used except in cases of particularly superficial lesions (i.e. lymph nodes, subcutaneous lesions and thyroid nodules) and therefore open to clinical confirmation [84]. This is an extreme position, related to the poor diffusion of US diagnostic imaging in North America and the attitude of preconceived diffidence of many oncologists ascribable to the lower objectivity of US, defined as "necessarily subjective" [84]. In reality, the applicability of US to the cancer patient should be defined case by case, and when the circumstances enable a sufficiently informative US study to be carried out, there is no reason for utilizing more complex modalities. In fact, even though the final evaluation of antitumor treatment in cancer patients is eminently entrusted to the "heavy machines" of PET, CT and MR, US is often used, especially in the evaluation between the various treatment rounds.

There are two fundamental rules for the **response to treatment evaluation**: (1) a "baseline" examination should be available, i.e. reference imaging performed at the beginning of treatment, or for example immediately after surgery for the primary tumor; (2) the same technique or combination of techniques used in the baseline study should also be used in the subsequent phases of evaluation between treatment rounds and restaging until the end of treatment. It would also be desirable that the baseline and follow-up examinations were always performed with the same scanner, the same examination technique (including the scanner settings) and the same operator, although this is clearly difficult to obtain in clinical practice. In surgery patients, the baseline examination for monitoring is clearly the first postoperative examination, since the examination of initial staging can no longer be used. At the beginning the oncologist, ideally in consensus with the radiologist, should define a precise monitoring plan – open to modifications with changes in the findings – which takes into consideration the techniques used, the body volume to include, the target and non-target lesions and the interval between examinations. The timing depends on a number of factors, such as the "time to progression" [87]; at least for phase II studies an evaluation is recommended after each round, i.e. every 6–8 weeks [84]. In subjects treated with chemotherapy the evaluation takes place immediately after the treatment, whereas in patients who undergo radiation therapy or surgery a period of 3 months is indicated to allow for stabilization of the local modifications.

The ultimate goal of cancer treatment is to increase patient survival. In the evaluation of treatment response, however, it is not always possible to wait for an increase in survival, thus creating the need for surrogates [87,88]. The traditional surrogate is given by the progressive reduction in size and subsequent disappearance of the tumor. Despite their differences, the different evaluation systems – WHO and RECIST – are based on the objective demonstration of a measurable reduction in tumor mass. Even volumetric measurements, setting aside the intrinsic difficulties in measuring the size of the lesion (accuracy, shape and margins of the tumor, etc.), is a relatively late index which often requires months to be verified and which does not in itself express the presence or otherwise of viable residual tumor tissue [85,89]. This is particularly true for some types of relatively recently introduced cancer treatments: treatment with new generation drugs (antiangiogenetic and antivascular drugs), percutaneous ablation treatments, transcatheter treatments (embolization, radioembolization, chemotherapy and chemoembolization) and radiation therapy (conventional or stereotactic) [52,85,90] (Fig. 1.11). In all these cases, distinguishing between responders and non-responders solely on the basis of size measurements is often problematic. One of the obstacles to the development of antiangiogenetic drugs is in fact the lack of effective systems for verifying the effects. These drugs produce a stabilization of the disease with a possible "cystic" transformation and then much later a reduction in the size of the lesion. Therefore, in order to evaluate the effects and modulate the dosage other types of information are required [91,92]. In the setting of percutaneous ablation a perilesional safety margin needs to be included in the treatment area, such that immediately after treatment the lesion actually appears to be increased in size. Then there are certain malignancies, such as lymphomas, which are not amenable to an evaluation exclusively based on size. Moreover, as stated above, there are many occasions when measuring the lesion is difficult or impossible: lesions with a significant calcified, necrotic or cystic component, malignant effusion, lesions located in the meninges, pleura or peritoneum, carcinomatous mastitis, pulmonary carcinomatous lymphangitis, diffuse skin lesions, bone lesions (especially if diffuse), micro-

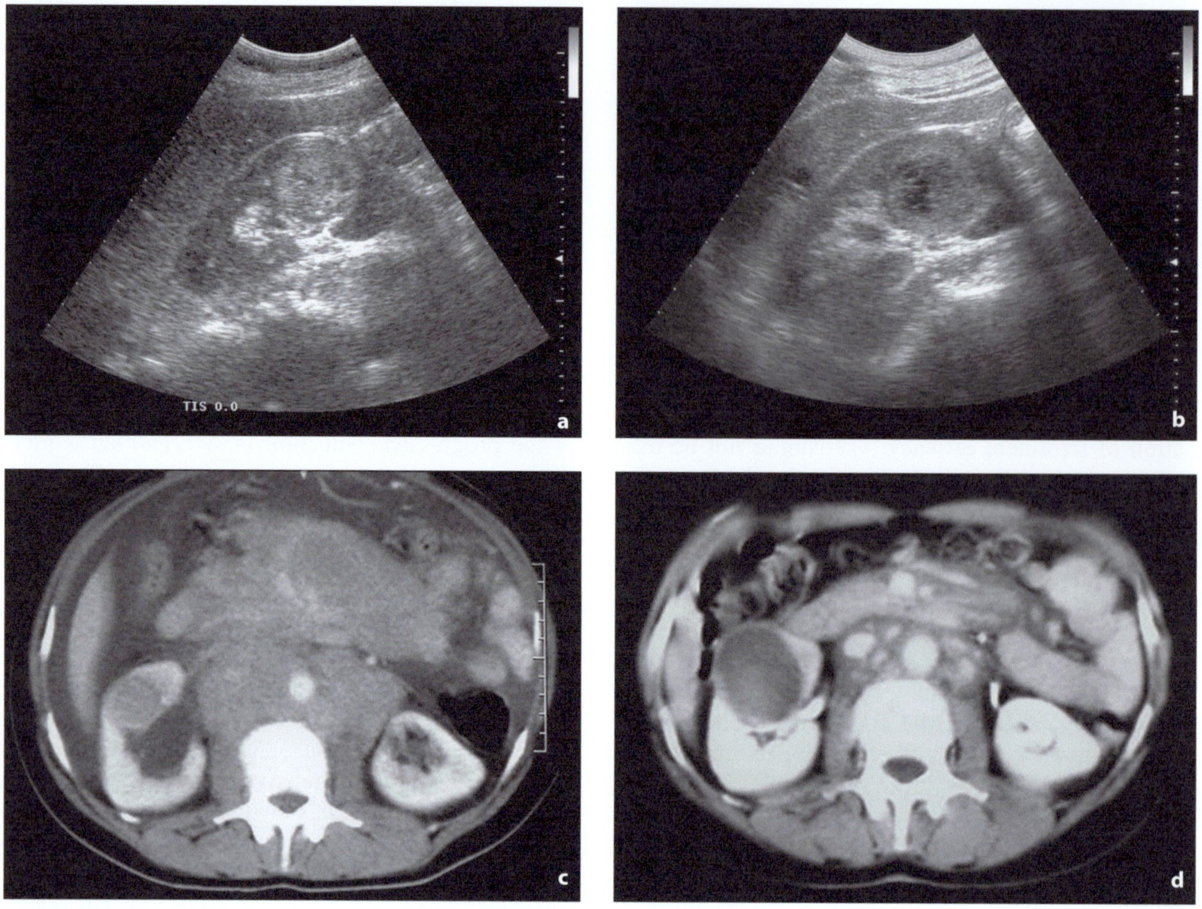

Fig. 1.11a-d Renal and retroperitoneal lymphoma before and after chemotherapy. The pretreatment US study (**a**) shows a heterogeneous echogenic mid-renal nodule. The US study performed after two rounds of chemotherapy (**b**) demonstrates a mild increase in the size of the lesion, which has also developed central hypoechogenicity. The comparison between pretreatment CT (**c**) and post-treatment scans (**d**) confirms the valid response of the right renal lesion, which has developed liquefactive necrosis hypoattenuation. The paradoxical volume increase of the lesion would have been interpreted as disease progression according to the size criteria

nodules (<10 mm or occasionally even <20 mm according to RECIST), multiple macronodules (>10 according to RECIST), etc. [84]. Lastly, it should also be borne in mind that different portions of the tumor mass do not respond in the same way to treatment and that small amounts of active residual tumor tissue may be lodged within necrotic, liquefactive or calcified areas.

Even though phase II studies can be based on size criteria alone [84], and even though there are no valid alternative systems of a **functional** type, there is increasing need for different parameters to associate with lesion size which are able to offer functional information regarding the state of tumor activity, with an evaluation of vascularity, vessel permeability, metabolism, oxygenation, etc. By obtaining early functional information it may be possible to differentiate respondents from non-respondents earlier, and in the case of no or poor response to treatment to modify the protocol without having to wait for the demonstration of poor or no decrease in lesion size at the end of treatment. It is difficult to say which modality among those discussed in the previous section is currently the most appropriate for performing this task, and different sites of primary and secondary tumors will probably require modalities. Functional information can undeniably be obtained with PET (with FDG but also with other radiotracers, and obtaining qualitative data as well as quantitative data with the SUV calculation), with perfusion CT or with various MR techniques. In addition, imaging fusion (e.g. PET-CT) makes possible the simultaneous acquisition of functional and morphologic data.

Although they have been excluded from the evaluation of treatment response according to RECIST except for superficial and palpable lesions [84],

US and its associated techniques are probably set to take new ground, especially in real-time contrast-enhanced perfusion analysis. The **Doppler techniques** have been widely proposed for the evaluation of variations in the degree of tumor vascularity. Numerous criteria have been suggested for the evaluation of treatment response, but to date none have received sufficient standardization and widespread use. They include Doppler signals, flow velocities, the Doppler effect, the acoustic effects recordable with PD, semi-quantitative indices and especially the RI. Spectral analysis is a precise technique for measuring flow, but it is limited to only several vessels chosen arbitrarily by the US operator. PD can indicate the relative vascular volume of the blood flow, whereas it can be more accurate in expressing the degree of perfusion [18]. Doppler techniques are able to evaluate the response not only to conventional chemotherapy and antiangiogenetic drugs but also to percutaneous and transcatheter intra-arterial treatments: the changes to tumor vascularity detected correlate with histologic findings [90,91,93]. A study on the serial changes of superficial lymph nodes in patients with NHL demonstrated a progressive decrease in vascular supply at CD in responsive patients, whereas the RI and PI showed no significant changes. In a recent study, a contrast-enhanced Doppler technique (dynamic flow) proved able to predict the response to the specific treatment of liver metastases from GIST as early as the first day after treatment, with a strong correlation between the reduction in vascularity and tumor response [66].

Clinical experience with **CEUS** is still limited. The effectiveness of CEUS has been demonstrated, albeit only qualitatively, in patients with liver metastases from GIST in the monitoring of response to targeted therapy with imatinib [94]. In liver metastases treated with stereotactic radiation therapy a reduction in the peak lesion signal intensity and a reduction in the lesion intensity/parenchyma intensity ratio in the arterial phase have been demonstrated. The demonstration of both these parameters was better with CEUS than with CT [93]. In liver metastases treated with chemotherapy it was noted that the pretreatment arterial contrast enhancement was greater in the late responders than in the non-responders, whereas during the treatment it decreased only in the responders [60].

1.7 Ultrasound, Follow-up and Recurrence

Cancer follow-up refers to all of the diagnostic procedures used for the study of patients who have been treated for a malignancy but who, in the absence of evidence to the contrary, are free from disease. The aims of follow-up are numerous, and include the early identification and treatment of local-regional recurrence or metastases, identification of metachronous forms (e.g. urothelial tumors, contralateral breast carcinomas, etc.), enhanced understanding of the natural history of malignancies, and psychological support for patients.

Subjects enrolled in clinical trials require particularly thorough monitoring with short intervals. In the remaining cases, which make up the majority, evaluating the effective utility of relatively aggressive follow-up on a case-by-case basis is instead important. This is done under the hypothesis that early diagnosis of disease recurrence can effectively lead to successful treatment with a positive influence on morbidity and mortality. In many cases, for example in patients operated on for colon or lung cancer, the application of the principles of "evidence-based medicine" has produced disappointing results, in that it has failed to demonstrate a significant clinical and statistical impact of follow-up on survival (quality-correlated) [95,96]. Given the overall costs of follow-up, and bearing in mind the instrumental, pharmacologic and radiobiologic invasiveness of the various techniques used for this purpose, it appears clear that a careful selection needs to be made of those patients who can effectively benefit from monitoring and in whom there is an adequate probability of recurrence. Moreover, the most appropriate times (time between one examination and another, time when examinations should be interrupted) and methods (which diagnostic tests to use) for follow-up need to be established.

Tumor **recurrence** refers to the reappearance of disease, identified clinically and/or instrumentally, after a variable length of time following radical surgery or complete response to systemic treatment. This is therefore different to **residual** tumor, where there is a malignant component right from the beginning which has resisted treatment and which can further develop and spread. Recurrence can be at various levels, and this influences the diagnostic procedures, treatment and prognosis. The pattern of "treatment failure" indicates the first identified site of tumor recurrence and it can be at seven levels: in correspondence with T, N or M or their combinations (TN, NM, TM or TNM). T recurrence is clearly due to the presence of residual although microscopic tumor tissue which after a variable period of time grows and becomes recognizable. Conceptually, therefore, this is really residual disease, despite being unrecognizable with the current modalities of diagnostic imaging. A recurrence at the level of the lymph nodes or a distant organ or structure is clearly a case of tumor cells which had migrated from the primary tumor prior to radical treatment and subsequently became manifest macroscopically.

The technique used for the diagnosis of disease recurrence should have high sensitivity for the early identification of recurrence, it should reduce false positives as much as possible and should be able to provide a precise evaluation of the state of the disease for the purposes of correct treatment planning. All of this should occur with the lowest possible level of invasiveness and costs.

1.8 Gray-Scale Ultrasound: Examination Technique

Current US devices are equipped with two – if not more – **multifrequency** transducers. These are chosen on the basis of their frequency as well as their shape and footprint in relation to the area to be explored. It is important to exploit the different frequencies available and to modify them during the examination and vary the position of the focal zone. A variation in the frequency and focus zone, especially during an examination of the breast with a small parts transducer, or of the liver with an abdominal transducer, enables the insonation characteristics to be adapted to the build of the patient, while at the same time performing an optimal exploration of all the superficial and deep portions of the organ. Current transducers have numerous crystals which may be arranged in several rows, with optimization in both transmission and reception. In addition, their large bandwidth allows them to reach a broad range of frequencies.

High-frequency transducers (7–15 MHz) enable a detailed evaluation of superficial structures, but they have a rather restricted FOV (generally 4 cm) and limited tissue penetration. Whenever the study of deeper structures is required, or the effective width of a superficial but voluminous lesion needs to be defined, a lower frequency transducer should be used (2–7 MHz), despite the consequent loss of resolution.

Although very-high-frequency transducers are currently available, the application of **spacer pads** may prove useful in the study of superficial lesions, both in B-mode and CD (Figs. 1.12, 1.13). These are particularly useful for nodulations which alter the skin profile, for example creating a zone of convexity, because they enable the insonation to be adapted to achieve an optimal evaluation of the mass in question.

Study of the area of interest should be conducted as much as possible according to different and combined approaches, with scan planes performed at different angles (Fig. 1.14).

Depending on the circumstances, the operator should seek to use both the "superficial" and "abdominal" transducers available. The use of an **abdominal transducer** during the exploration of **superficial structures** can prove useful in certain circumstances, e.g. to define the exact volume of a large mass whose diameter and deep extension may be difficult to evaluate with a superficial transducer. Furthermore, an abdominal transducer can be used to explore masses which penetrate into or emerge from the deep tissues, below the skeletal or other structures obscuring direct visualization with the surface transducer. This is the case in the evaluation of masses which extend from the jugular into the superior mediastinum or masses in the groin which penetrate into the pelvis (Figs. 1.15, 1.16). A **surface transducer** at the **abdominal** level can be particularly useful – especially in individuals who are more accessible to the study such as pediatric and thin subjects – in numerous applications such as the study of peripheral or capsular hepatic lesions, superficial splenic lesions, malignant infiltration at the

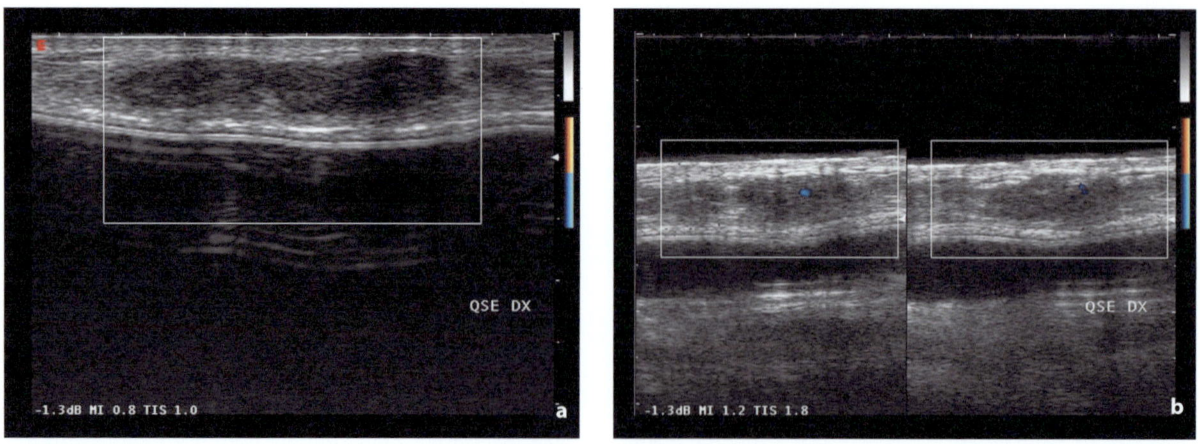

Fig. 1.12a,b Adenosis of the breast, study with spacer. With the same Doppler frequency (7.1 MHz) and the same focal zone, the scan without spacer pad (**a**) is unable to capture the color signals which are instead visible with the spacer (**b**). Patient with prosthesis

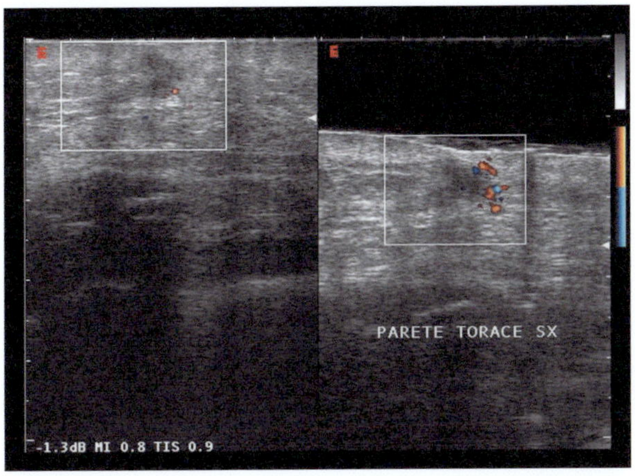

Fig. 1.13 Recurrence of breast carcinoma after radical mastectomy, study with spacer. With the same Doppler frequency (7.1 MHz) and the same focal zone, the use of the spacer pad (*right*) makes possible the capture of the flow signals, which are not identifiable with direct contact (*left*)

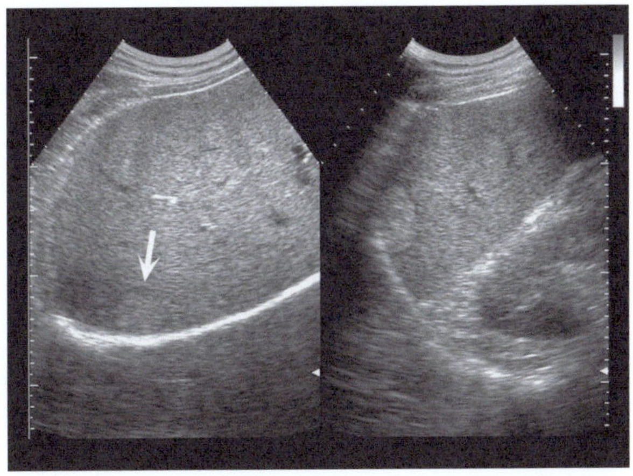

Fig. 1.14 Hepatic hemangioma, intercostal exploration. Subcostal scan (*left*) identifies a moderately echogenic posterior subcapsular lesion (*arrow*), whereas the intercostal scan (*right*) provides good visualization of the hyperechoic lesion

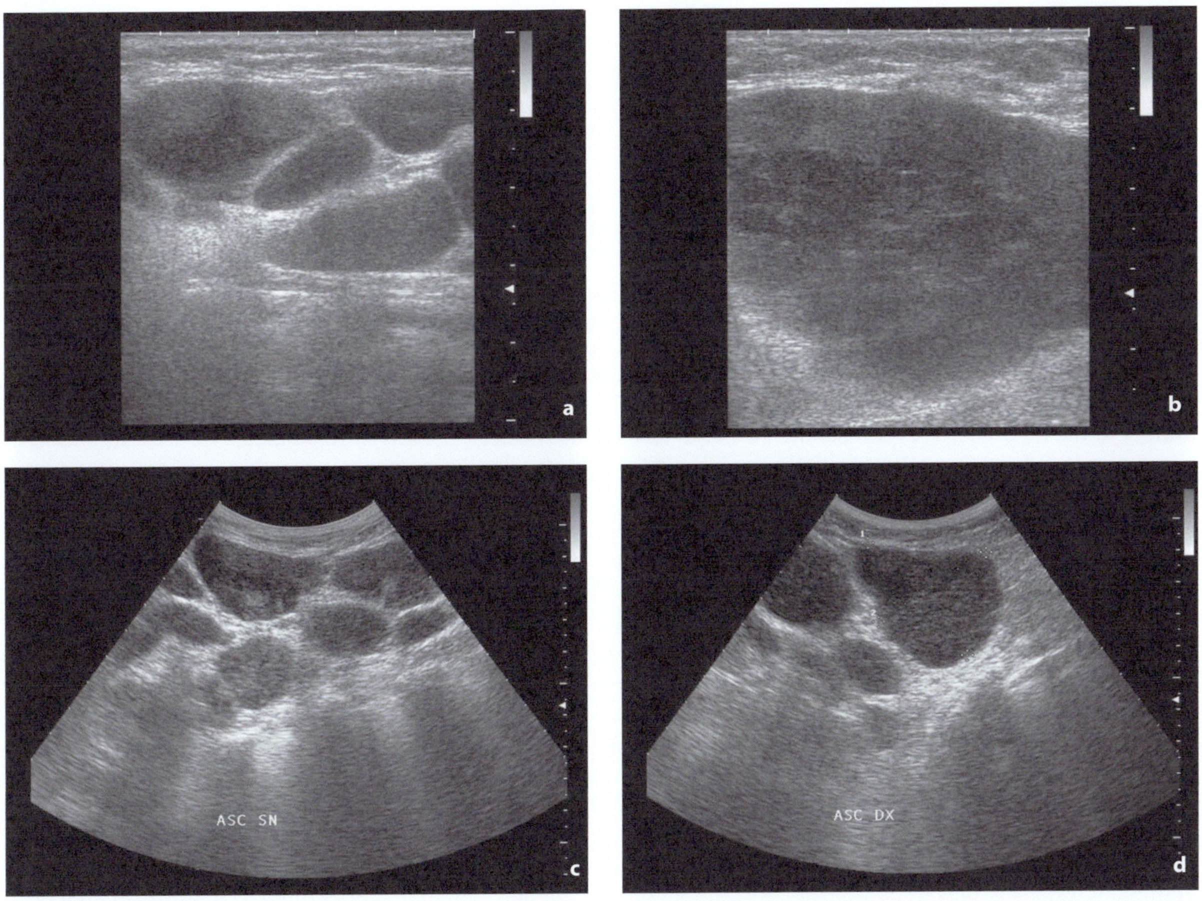

Fig. 1.15a-d Multiple axillary lymphadenopathies from NHL, study with abdominal transducer. High-resolution study (**a**, **b**) identifies multiple large axillary adenopathies, but only the "abdominal" transducer (**c**, **d**) makes possible an overall view of the non-confluent enlarged lymph nodes and measurement of the largest nodes

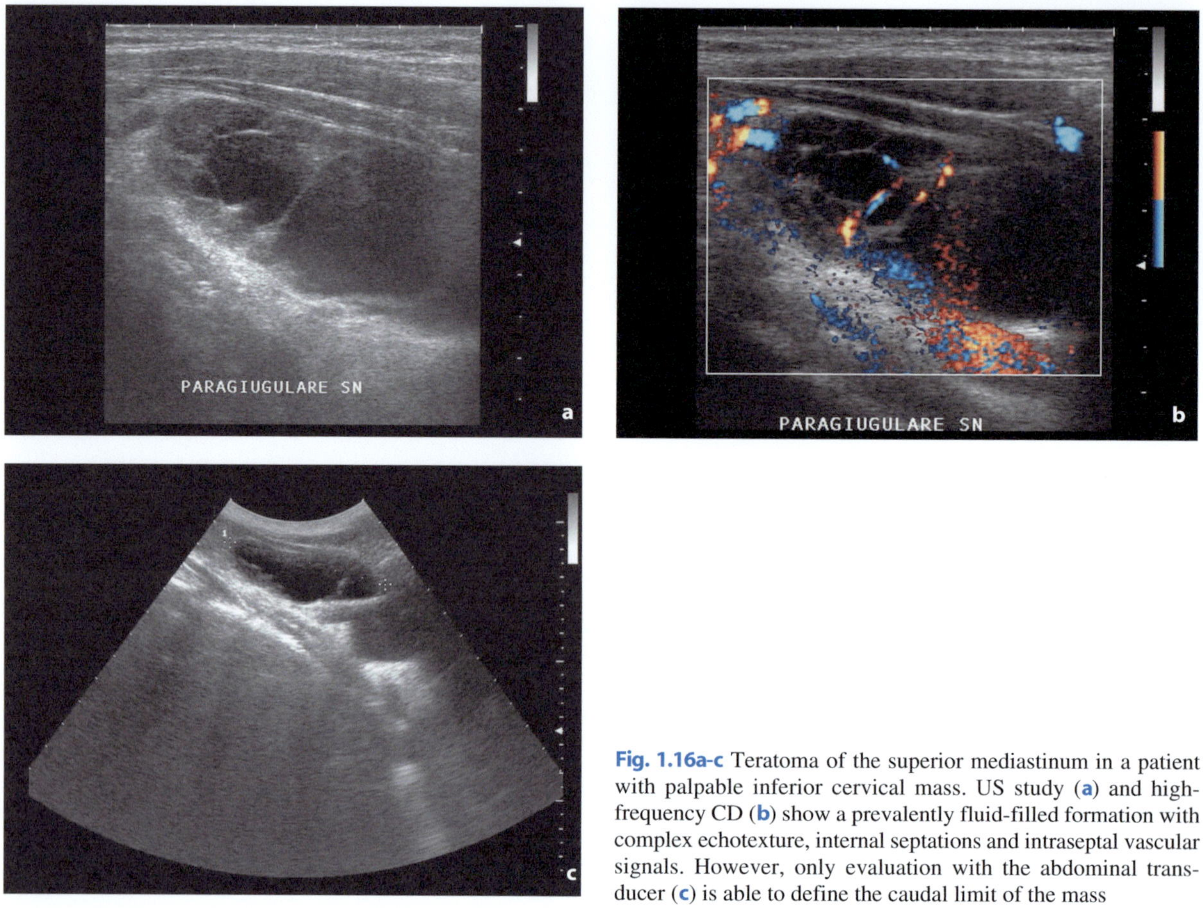

Fig. 1.16a-c Teratoma of the superior mediastinum in a patient with palpable inferior cervical mass. US study (**a**) and high-frequency CD (**b**) show a prevalently fluid-filled formation with complex echotexture, internal septations and intraseptal vascular signals. However, only evaluation with the abdominal transducer (**c**) is able to define the caudal limit of the mass

level of the greater omentum or the peritoneal wall, and tumors of the digestive tract and the abdominal wall itself (Figs. 1.17–1.22, Video 1.2). The study of tumors of the digestive tract can benefit from the technique of **graded compression**. Initially developed for acute diseases and in particular appendicitis [97], the technique involves progressive compression of the pathologic area with a high-resolution transducer, with the aim of reducing the distance between the transducer and the area of interest and displacing intestinal gas overlying the same area, while reducing the echogenicity due to the gas in the lumen of the pathologic bowel loop under investigation. In general, graded compression enables a higher-frequency transducer to be used in the study of structures which are not precisely superficial, such as the deep structures of the neck or a limb.

An important role for the "up close" evaluation of malignant lesions is played by transducers with a non-percutaneous approach: transrectal, transvaginal, transurethral, intravascular, etc. **Transvaginal** US (TVUS) is currently performed with high-resolution microconvex transducers (5 MHz, 6.5 MHz or 7.5 MHz) which are equipped with color- and power-Doppler modality and now also with software for CEUS [98]. **Transrectal** US (TRUS) is performed with linear or convex transducers or a combination of both, i.e. transducers capable of simultaneously providing longitudinal and transverse views. In addition to a CD and PD evaluation, the currently available transducers can also provide a contrast-enhanced analysis. Relatively high frequencies are used – higher than 5 MHz, possibly 7.5 MHz – and the examination is performed with the patient in the left lateral or knee-chest position, the latter being required for biopsy. The study should be preceded by a digital rectal examination to rule out polypoid lesions in the rectum and especially to define which part of the gland – in the case of a prostate study – has the greatest consistency and therefore is the most suspicious. Alternatively, the detailed findings of the urologic examination should be made available. Performing a cleansing enema prior to the examination is also useful for avoiding artifacts.

Intraoperative, **endoscopic** and **laparoscopic** US is finding an increasing number of applications, with increasingly high-frequency and multipurpose trans-

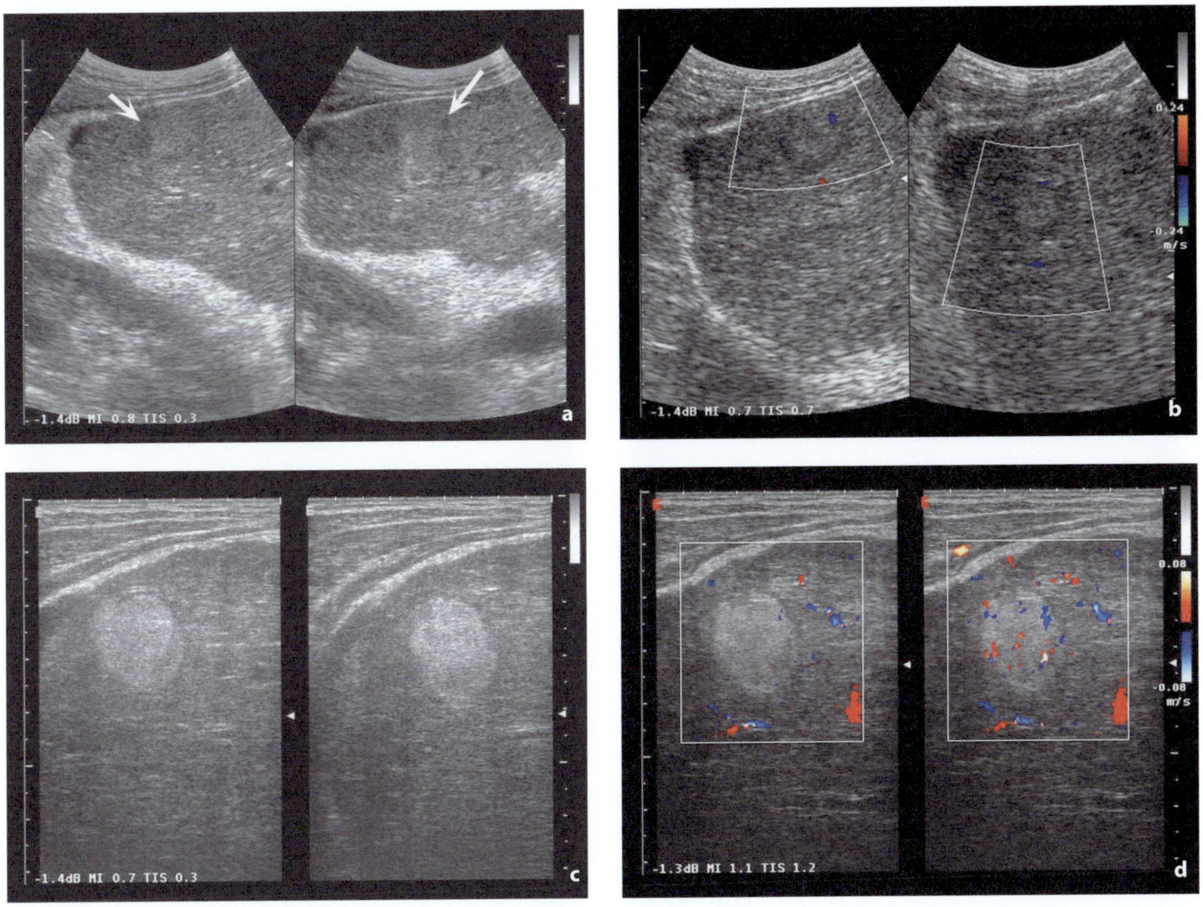

Fig. 1.17a-d HCC, study with superficial transducer. US (**a**) and CD (**b**) study with abdominal transducer has difficulty visualizing the heterogeneous hypoechoic nodular lesion with poor vascular signals located anteriorly at the level of the V hepatic segment (*arrows*). US (**c**) and CD (**d**) evaluation with high-frequency transducer instead provides a good visualization of the echogenic nodule with a peripheral hypoechoic halo and multiple internal arterial vessels

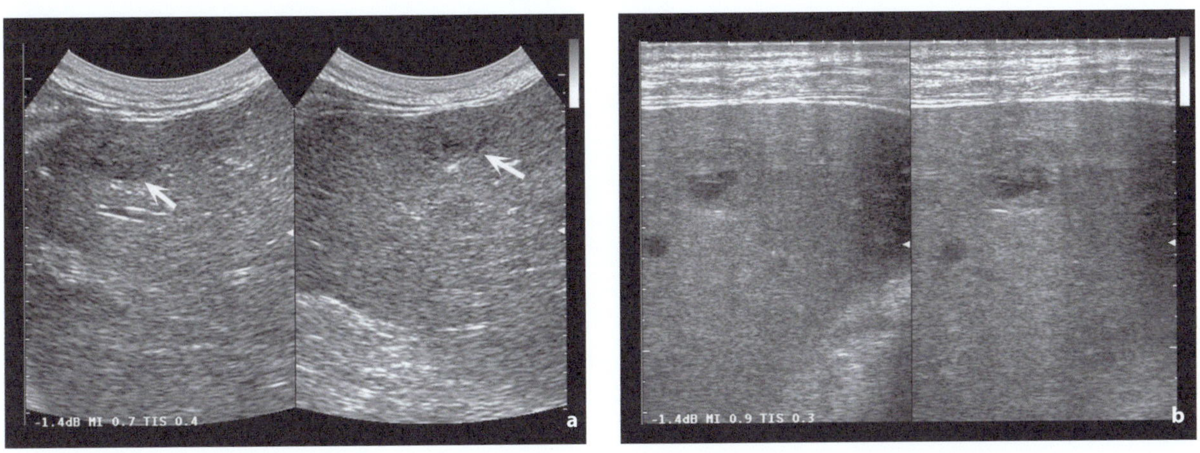

Fig. 1.18a,b Liver metastasis from melanoma, study with surface transducer. The study with the abdominal transducer (**a**) reveals in the close-up images a heterogeneous hypo-isoechoic hepatic lesion (*arrows*). The use of the high-frequency transducer (**b**) provides much better definition of the internal structure of the lesion, characterized by a hypoechoic halo and partial internal necrosis

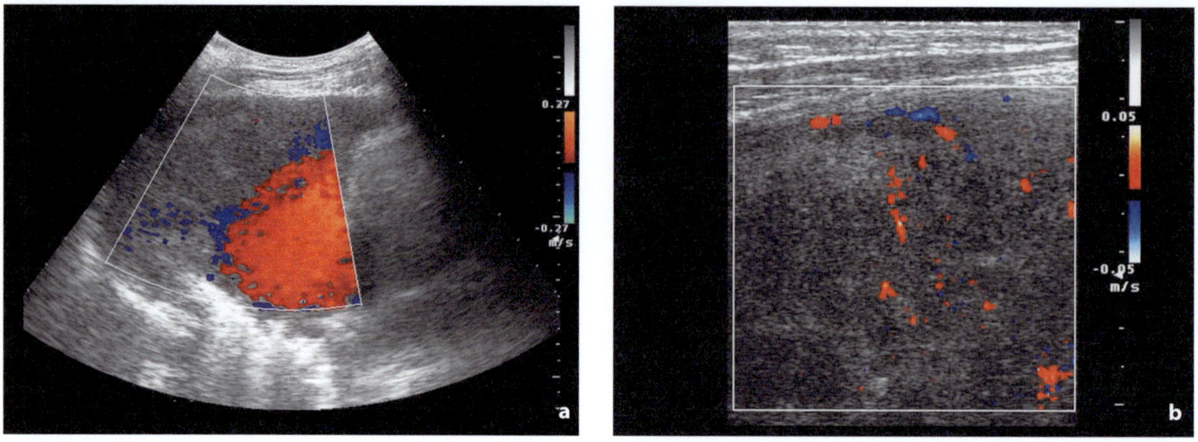

Fig. 1.19a,b Lung cancer, study with surface transducer. The evaluation with abdominal transducer (**a**) of the pulmonary mass attached to the thoracic wall is markedly hampered by the artifacts produced by cardiac pulsatility, the attenuation of which renders optimization for slow flow impossible. The use of a high-frequency transducer (**b**) provides good definition of the moderate vascularity within the superficial portion of the mass

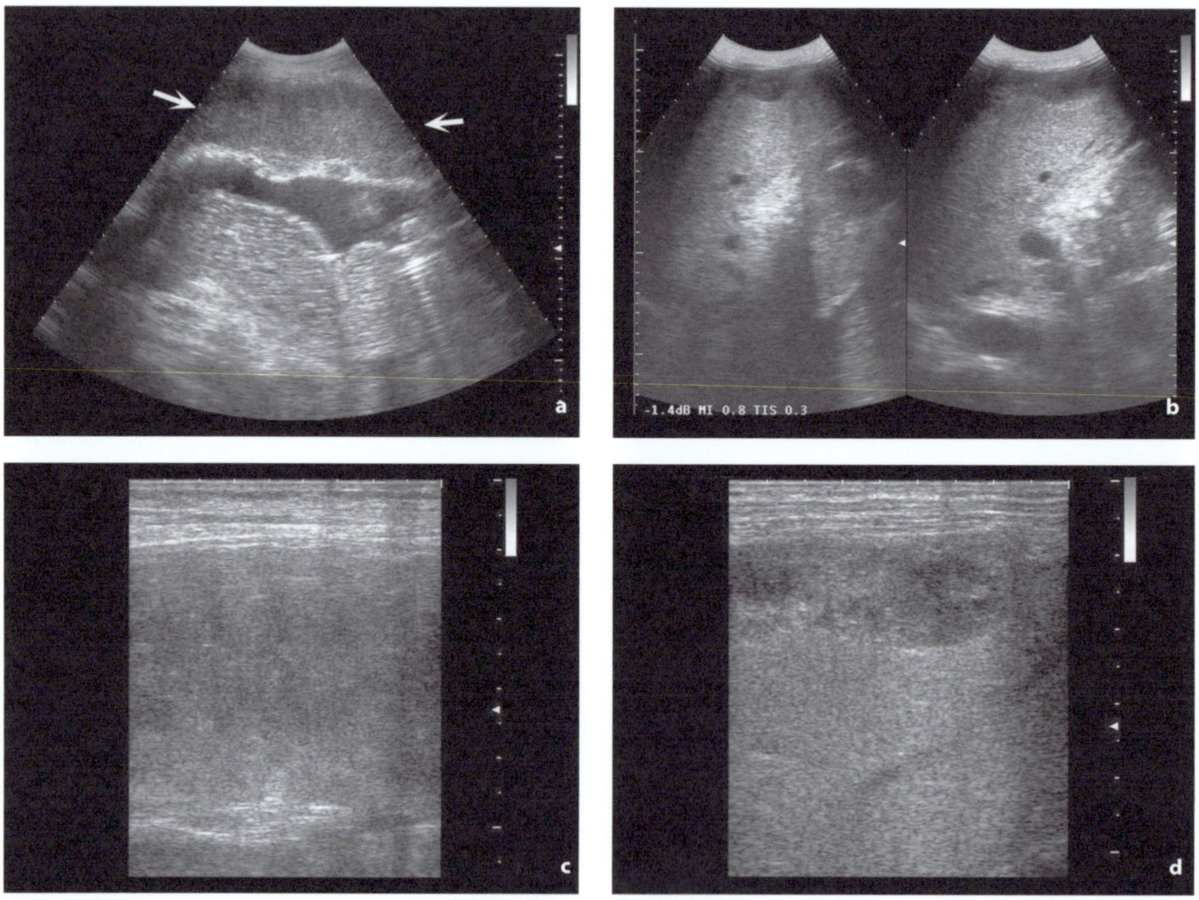

Fig. 1.20a-d Peritoneal carcinosis from ovarian cancer, study with surface transducer. The abdominal study shows significant omental thickening (**a**, *arrows*) associated with peritoneal effusion and dilatation of a deep bowel loop, as well as a poorly defined lesion of the anterior hepatic surface (**b**). Evaluation with a high-frequency transducer provides better definition of the heterogeneous, hypoechoic structure of both the omental involvement (**c**) and the anterior hepatic capsular lesion (**d**)

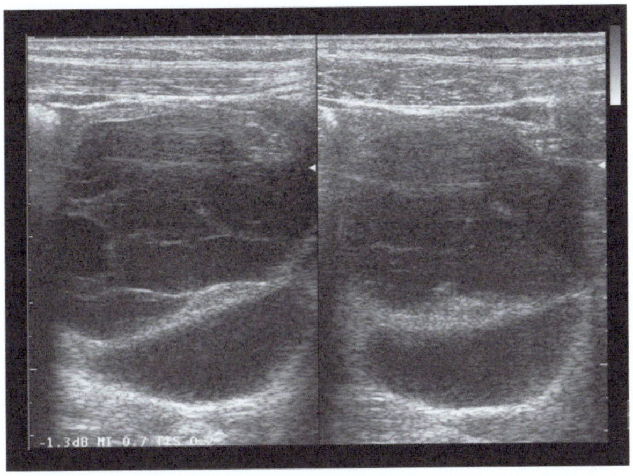

Fig. 1.21 Benign ovarian cyst. Transabdominal study with a surface transducer provides a valid demonstration of the internal septated structure of the cyst, similar to that obtainable with a transvaginal transducer. This is thanks to the slight build of the patient and the superficial position of the cyst

ducers able to obtain CD, CEUS and 3D images, as well as perform interventional procedures (Figs. 1.23, 1.24) [99].

With regard to **equipment settings**, presets can be very useful. These differ not only in terms of the more obvious parameters which the operator may adjust, but also for the less obvious ones, such as power output (MI), which influence ultrasound penetration. Although there are automatic correction systems of the time gain compensation and also the lateral gain (auto optimize control), knowing how to vary the presets according to need is important [100].

The exploration of superficial structures (especially the breast) and abdominal organs (especially the liver) should be done in a dynamic fashion, with a repeated variation of the transmission frequency of the transducer, the gains and the focusing depth, to be certain the different portions of the structure being studied have been explored with the most appropriate settings. In general, the **focus zone(s)** should be placed at the level of or, better still, immediately below the area of interest. The signal coming from the tissues situated at the level of the focal zone of the transducer is in fact more intense than the signal of the tissues that are more superficial or deeper to it [101]. Small cystic formations or calcifications can therefore go unrecognized if they do not fall within the level of the focal zone, where the thickness of the scan is at its thinnest. The possibility of varying the position of the focus zone or the availability of multiple focus zones and transducers with a broad range of frequencies enables optimal exploration of the entire FOV, with greater lateral resolution. However, occasionally multiple

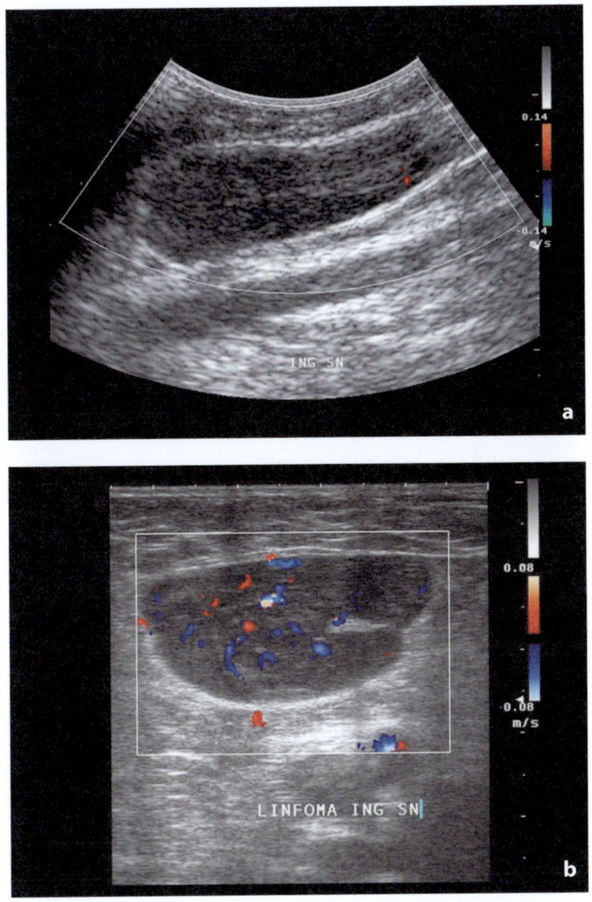

Fig. 1.22a,b Inguinal lymphadenopathy from NHL. Low-frequency study (**a**) is unable to define substantial color signals within the large superficial lymphomatous formation, whereas in high-frequency evaluation (**b**), the abundant vascular structure of the lesion is identifiable

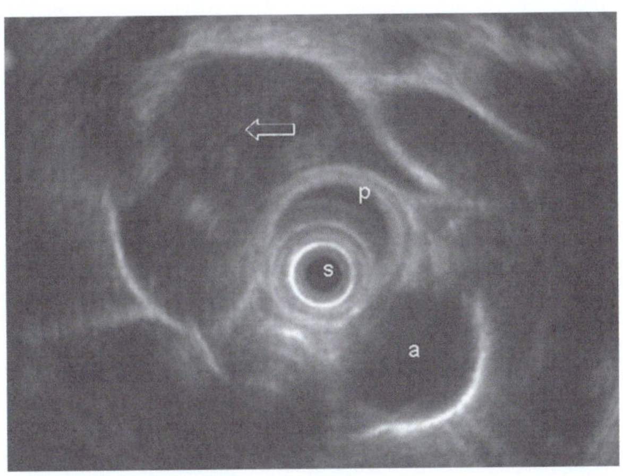

Fig. 1.23 Bronchoalveolar cysts. Radial scan EUS shows irregular hypoechoic area of the mediastinum in relation with the bronchi (*arrow*); *s*, probe; *p*, balloon; *a*, aorta. (Courtesy of Dr. P. Marone, INT Pascale, Italy)

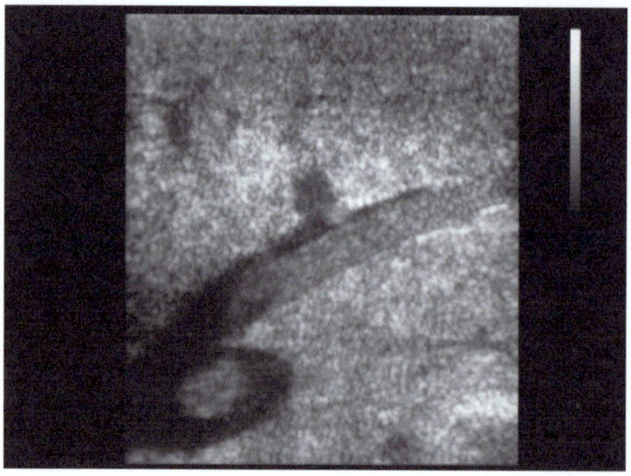

Fig. 1.24 Intraoperative US, intrahepatic venous thrombosis. Thrombotic echogenic centroluminal defect at the level of the middle suprahepatic vein and the inferior vena cava

focus zones are unable to create an effectively uniform transition between the different levels of depth, and a single well-positioned focus zone may be better. Increasing the number of transmit focus zones narrows the beam profile, with improved lateral resolution but decreased temporal resolution.

An excessively low **gray gain** can, for example, cancel out the weakly intense echoes within cystic formations or make a markedly hypoechoic lesion appear anechoic. On the other hand, an excessive gain can create echogenic artifacts within a simple cyst.

The dynamic range is used to improve the echo display, making the low-amplitude echoes distinguishable. Nonetheless, increasing the dynamic range decreases contrast.

Tissue harmonic imaging has been widely used, firstly at the abdominal level and subsequently at the level of superficial structures [102,103]. This option is based on the use not of the first return echo from an insonified tissue (fundamental), but on the subsequent echoes harmonic to the first, and especially the second (second harmonic). The nonlinear high-frequency echoes generated by the propagation of ultrasound in body tissues are exploited to create tissue harmonic imaging. This offers greater spatial and contrast resolution, with increased sharpness of the findings, but not without a certain difficulty in the study of particularly dense and reflective tissues [100,104,105]. An alternative technology to conventional second harmonic imaging is broadband harmonic imaging, which is obtained with pulse or phase inversion and which exploits two paired pulses, of which the second is identical to the first but with inverted phase [106]. With respect to standard US, this option increases the signal-to-noise ratio, improves lateral resolution and the resolution of small contrast differences in tissues, with the attenuation of side-lobe artifacts. In particular, the harmonic pulse inversion modality also manages to obtain superior spatial and contrast resolution [103]. This becomes particularly useful at the abdominal level in the study of obese subjects or in the exploration of areas such as the retroperitoneum or the pelvis. Tissue harmonic imaging is particularly useful in both the superficial and abdominal location for defining the cystic nature of hypo-anechoic masses, in that it is able to more clearly visualize the fluid content. Even the identification of small nodules (e.g. hepatic nodules) can be improved with the technique [100,106].

Like tissue harmonic imaging, the technique of spatial **compound imaging** is an alternative modality for the transmission and reception of ultrasound. It offers superior contrast and greater sharpness of surface structures through scans which incline the ultrasound beam, with the result that the different points of the FOV are evaluated with different incidences. Therefore the direction angle of the transmitted beam can be electronically altered (beam steering) in real time in order to perform multiple partially overlapping scans of the object, and a mean summed image with superior spatial resolution is obtained. The background noise is reduced, as are spurious echoes and other artifacts, thus obtaining images with greater contrast, sharper-appearing lesions and greater definition of the internal architecture and the distortion surrounding the lesions themselves [100,107]. The main applications of the technique are at the level of the superficial structures (Video 1.3). Compound imaging can be combined with tissue harmonic imaging. In this case it has been demonstrated, at least at the level of the abdomen, that more detailed images can be obtained with association of the two techniques. The combined technique proved to be superior than compound imaging alone, which in turn was superior to tissue harmonic imaging alone (the latter being superior to standard US) [108]. It should however be borne in mind that the reduction of artifacts such as acoustic shadowing is not always an advantage: a good example is the value of posterior attenuation in the study of breast nodules [109] (Fig. 1.25). Compound imaging can also be combined with extended FOV and 3D acquisitions.

A narrow FOV carries higher frame rates, with better spatial resolution and particularly better temporal resolution. Enlarging the FOV helps to improve the panoramic view of US. This can be obtained by using trapezoid imaging or extended FOV (EFOV). Trapezoid imaging makes scanning beyond the transducer footprint possible and is especially employed with linear probes. The **panoramic reconstruction** modality

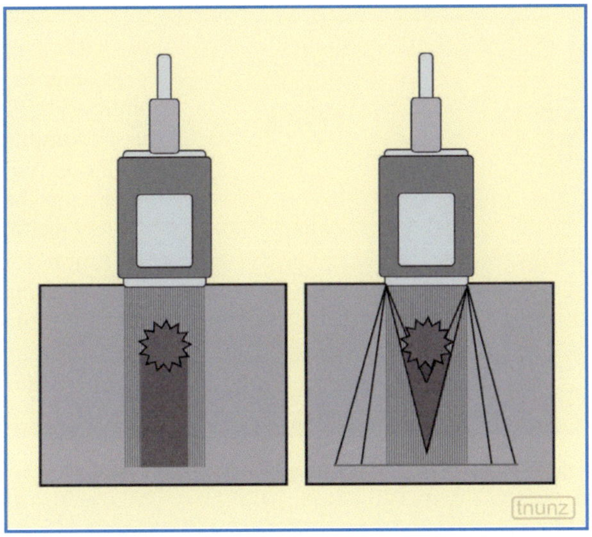

Fig. 1.25 Reduction of posterior attenuation with spatial compound imaging. With conventional imaging there is intense acoustic shadowing whereas with compound imaging the posterior attenuation is triangular in shape and also less marked and less extended in depth

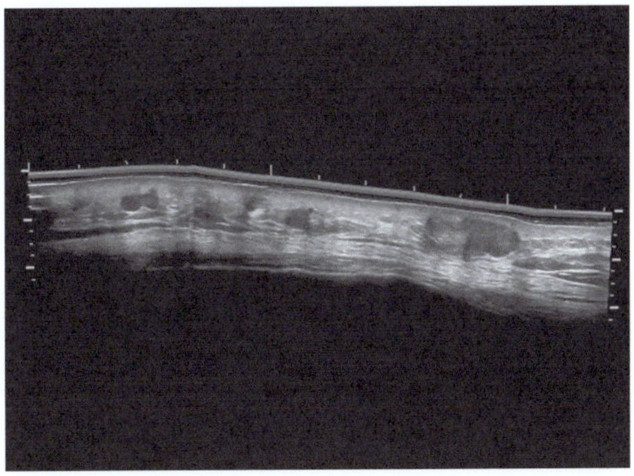

Fig. 1.26 Recurrence of melanoma of the derma, US EFOV. The panoramic study shows numerous heterogeneous hypoechoic subcutaneous nodules in a single image

or EFOV can in part overcome the known panoramic limitations of US with respect to CT and MR. The technique produces 2D and 3D images which are more easily comprehensible for the clinician and can be usefully employed at both the abdominal and superficial level, on the basis of course of the type of transducer utilized [100,110] (Figs. 1.26–1.30). The images, which may be extended as much as several tens of centimeters, are obtained interactively through manual translational movement of the transducer across the skin surface of the patient, with continuous position comparison and without loss of spatial resolution. There are also systems with dedicated transducers equipped with positional sensors. The obtainable images may also be based on tissue harmonic imaging, CD, PD or CEUS and can even be obtained with special transducers such as those for TVUS [111]. The principal advantages with respect to the standard US acquisition are improved definition of the topographic relations between the masses and the adjacent structures, a more accurate estimate of the size and volume of the lesions, especially when these are wide, and a better depiction of extended tubular structures such as vessels, the bile ducts and the ureters, as well as intestinal segments. Identifying very peripheral lesions or alterations with respect to the area of interest is also possible, as is precise measurement of the distance between the two normal or pathologic structures which normally could not be included in a single US FOV. The possibility of comparing a certain US finding in later examinations is increased by EFOV, since the images produced are

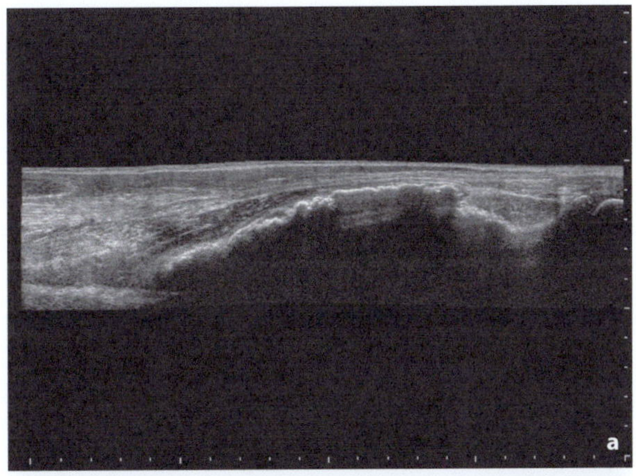

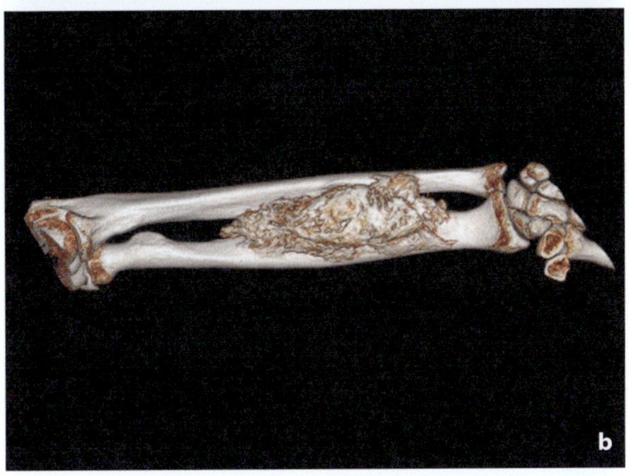

Fig. 1.27a,b Osteosarcoma of the radius. US EFOV scan (**a**) offers good visualization of the irregular bone surface and the action of the mass on the overlying muscle compartment. Correlation with 3D multislice CT reconstruction (**b**)

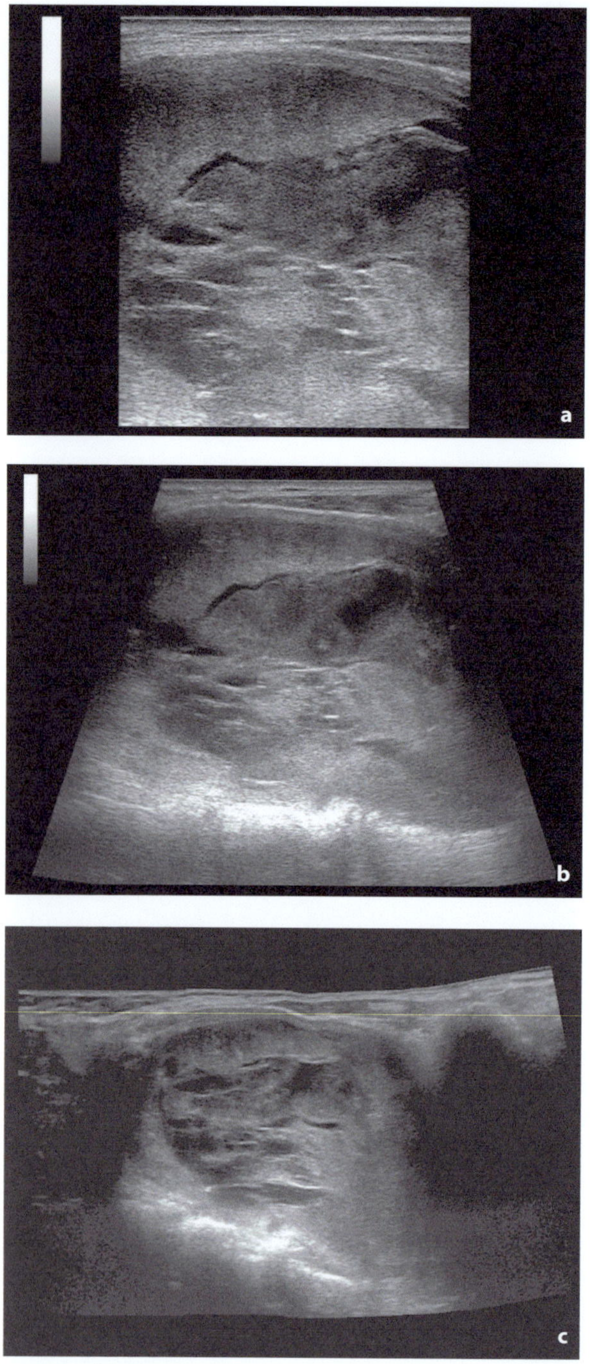

Fig. 1.28a-c Benign thyroid nodule, possibility of longitudinal assessment. The conventional FOV (**a**) scan fails to include the entire mass, whereas the trapezoid scan (**b**) and mostly the EFOV scan (**c**) allow a comprehensive display

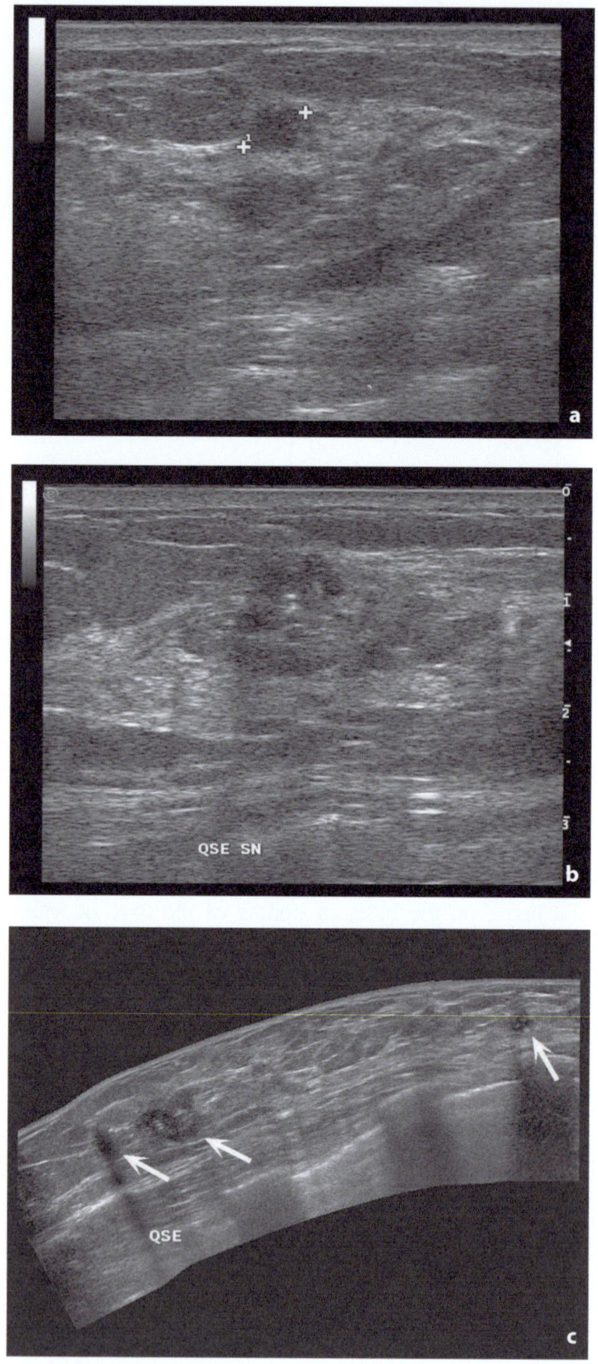

Fig. 1.29a-c Multifocal breast cancer. Two conventional FOV scans (**a**, **b**) identify multiple hypoechoic breast lesions. The EFOV image (**c**) provides an optimal depiction of the spatial relationship between the tumors in the external upper quadrant (*arrows*)

more immediate and comprehensible for the clinician than standard images. It should however be noted that in EFOV there is a proportional reduction in the image size with an increase in the scanned area.

3D US is able to offer a plastic and volumetric depiction of the structures in question (Figs. 1.31–1.33). The technique acquires a series of slices of the region of interest with slightly different orienta-

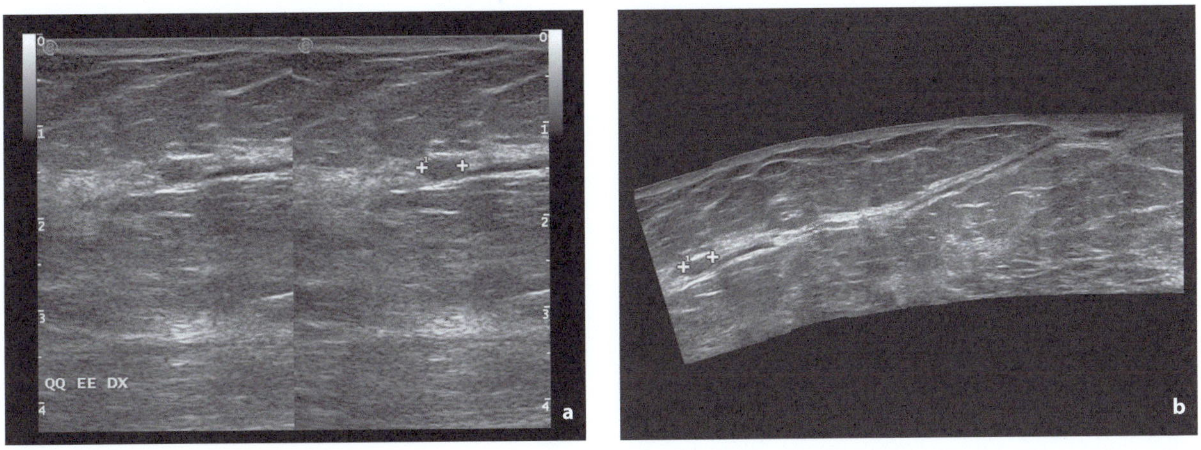

Fig. 1.30a, b Periductal breast nodule in a patient with nipple discharge. The conventional breast scan (**a**) identifies a small hypoechoic nodule adjacent to a dilated duct. The EFOV image (**b**) offers a comprehensive view of the entire dilated duct from the nipple to the nodule (*calipers*)

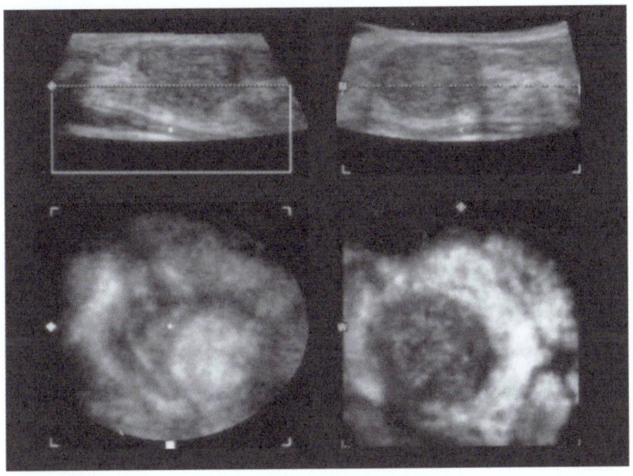

Fig. 1.31 Phyllodes breast tumor, 3D US scan. Multiplanar and 3D images of large heterogeneous hypoechoic breast nodule

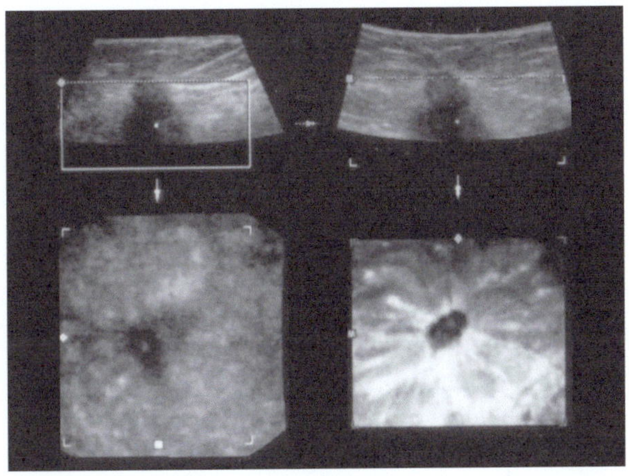

Fig. 1.32 Breast carcinoma, 3D US. Multiplanar and 3D images of the hypoechoic nodule with beam attenuation

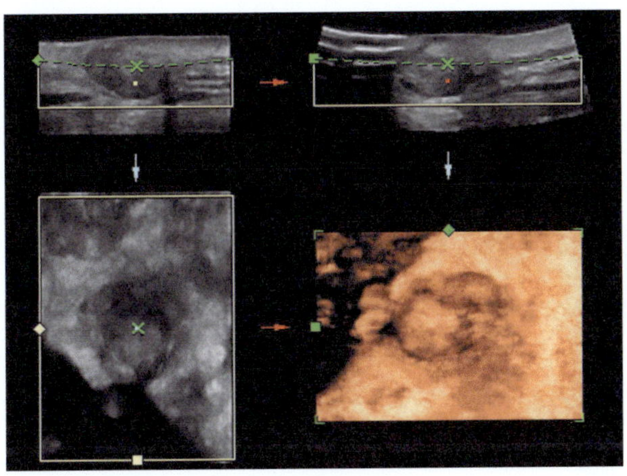

Fig. 1.33 Recurrence of melanoma of the derma, 3D US. Multiplanar and 3D images of large heterogeneous hypoechoic nodule

tions, thus obtaining a series of volume data to be processed which are then depicted as surface, volume or 2D images in the different planes (multiplanar images, including those according to a plane parallel to the skin surface) [112]. Initially the 3D images were produced with mechanical movement of the transducer, but current systems are based on a freehand acquisition with dedicated transducers and systems capable of recording the position and orientation of the transducer in space together with the corresponding US images [113,114]. 4D US refers to a 3D modality with elevated frame rate in which the images are almost in real time and therefore also have the dimension of time [100]. 3D US can also be coupled with tissue harmonic imaging to produce superior image precision and clarity, with CD and PD and the possible separation of venous and arterial flows, and with

CEUS. Interventional procedures can be facilitated by multiplanar views, especially in terms of recognizing the needle.

Elastography is especially used for surface structures and in particular for the breast. The technique measures the elastic properties of normal and pathologic tissues, distinguishing between hypo-anelastic lesions (malignant) and hyperelastic lesions (benign), although there is the possibility of overlap between the two extremes. In practice, the technique evaluates the degree of distortion of tissues under the application of gradual mechanical compression with the transducer, and obtains a high-contrast elastogram superimposed on the B-mode image in which the elastic tissues are color-coded red, the anelastic tissues blue and the intermediate tissues green [115–117].

B-flow is a non-Doppler modality for representing vascular flow, first introduced for high-frequency transducers and then for abdominal transducers. The technique is free from artifacts which often hamper CD or PD exploration and is also independent of the angle of insonation. B-flow offers greater spatial resolution than CD and PD with a higher frame rate and without the need of being circumscribed to a precise area (as with the CD box) [118] (Video 1.4).

1.9 Gray-Scale Ultrasound: Imaging Characteristics

Focal lesions can be characterized at US by a solid or liquid structure. **Solid lesions** are characterized by scattered echoes of varying intensity (level) and can be divided into four categories: (1) solid homogeneous lesions – echoes similar in intensity and dimension, generally fine and uniformly distributed; (2) heterogeneous solid lesions – echoes with differing intensity and dimension, with varied distribution; (3) solid lesions with acoustic shadowing – homogeneous or heterogeneous but with beam attenuation; (4) prevalently solid complex lesions – the prevalently solid and usually heterogeneous portion is associated with minority fluid-filled portions due to cystic components or necrotic-hemorrhagic phenomena (Figs. 1.34–1.36). Then on the basis of the intensity of the echoes, both solid lesions with homogeneous echotexture and those with heterogeneous echotexture can have a hyperechoic, isoechoic or hypoechoic echostructure. Generally speaking, hypoechoic lesions have an elevated "water" component, whereas hyperechoic lesions are characterized by a rich capillary network or a significant stromal component. The greater or lesser echogenicity should be defined as much as possible in relation to the adjacent parenchyma, which constitutes the background of the echoes. However, clearly a mass

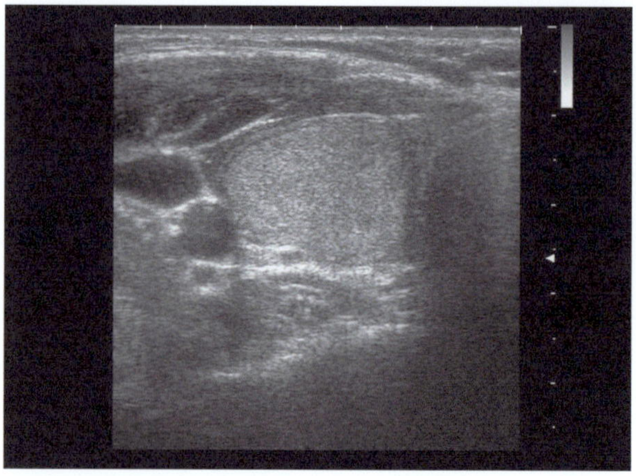

Fig. 1.34 Benign thyroid nodule. Homogeneous hyperechoic nodular formation, with thin peripheral hypoechoic halo

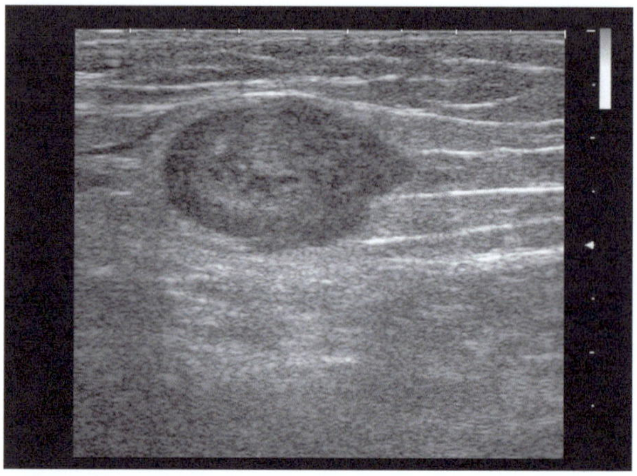

Fig. 1.35 Inguinal metastatic lymphadenopathy from ovarian cancer. Large heterogeneous hypoechoic lymphadenopathy with initial central necrosis and mild perifocal edematous hyperechogenicity

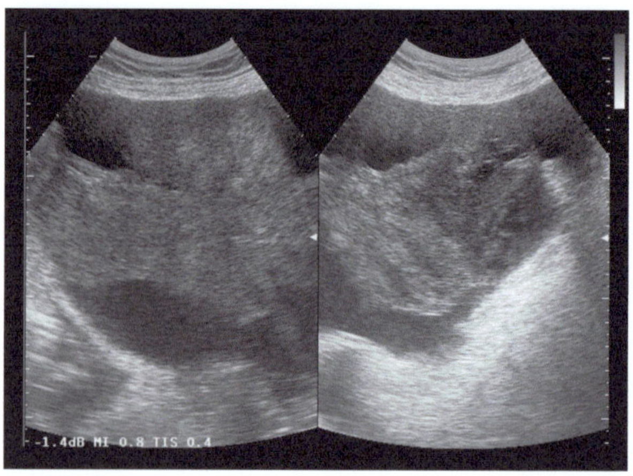

Fig. 1.36 Ovarian cancer. Complex mass with solid and liquid components and microcystic structures

which does not develop within a parenchyma can easily be defined as hypoechoic or hyperechoic in the absolute sense. In addition, the characteristics of the parenchymal "background" can clearly change: lesions which might appear hyperechoic in a normal liver can have a hypoechoic appearance in the setting of steatosis. For the breast the background can be prevalently echogenic, if glandular, or prevalently hypoechoic, if with fatty involution, such that the greater or lesser echogenicity tends to be defined in relation to the subcutaneous fat of the breast [119]. The isoechoic lesion, which produces the same reflection of echoes as the surrounding parenchyma, clearly cannot be recognized as such and can be identified only in the presence of indirect signs such as the outline of an organ or the displacement of surrounding structures.

In general, tumors, and especially epithelial tumors, are hypoechoic, being characterized by elevated cellularity and a limited stromal component and therefore by few interfaces which reflect the ultrasound. Examples include thyroid carcinomas, breast cancers, metastatic or lymphomatous lymph nodes, hepatic nodules and splenic nodules. In lesions from melanoma there is generally marked hyperechogenicity due to the very poor acoustic absorption of melanin. In addition, even benign lesions such as adenomas of the parathyroid can often be markedly hypoechoic as a result of their uniform hypercellularity.

The transmission of the acoustic signal through a lesion and posterior to it, and therefore the posterior echogenicity, can be increased, normal or reduced. **Beam attenuation** (posterior acoustic shadowing) is the expression of the presence of intense reflection of the ultrasound beam resulting from, for example, calcifications, hyalinosis and fibrosis (including tumor stroma). Even a gaseous component can produce a similar effect, either as the only curved echogenic image with posterior attenuation or as individual attenuating nuclei. The posterior shadow may be only mildly visible or markedly apparent to the point of obstructing the visualization of the tissues immediately distal to the lesion or even the deep portion of the lesion itself (Fig. 1.37). When instead the superficial interface of the lesion creates the artifact, the lesion itself can be concealed, especially its anterior portion, as for example in the case of nodules with a calcified shell or the "tip of the iceberg" sign in ovarian teratomas with calcification. Beam attenuation, to the point of producing posterior acoustic shadowing which conceals the deep (non-calcified) portion of a lesion and/or healthy soft tissue immediately distal to this, can in the first instance orient the diagnosis towards malignancy. This posterior attenuation has been investigated particularly in the breast and, according to some authors, can be correlated with hypercellularity, while others suggest it correlates with the type of tissue organization within the tumor [109].

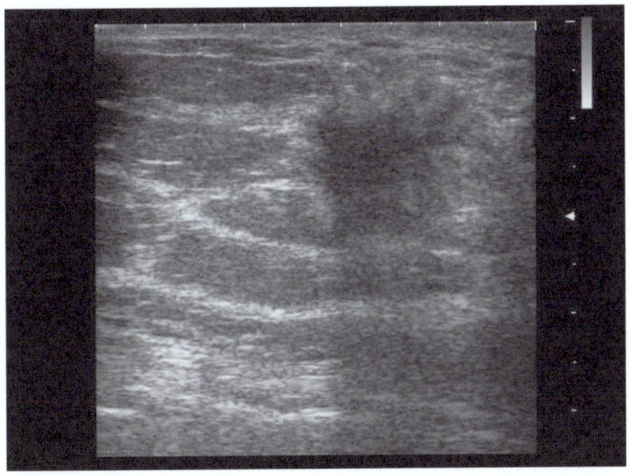

Fig. 1.37 Breast cancer. Heterogeneous hypoechoic nodule with ill-defined margins and acoustic shadowing concealing the deep portion of the lesion itself

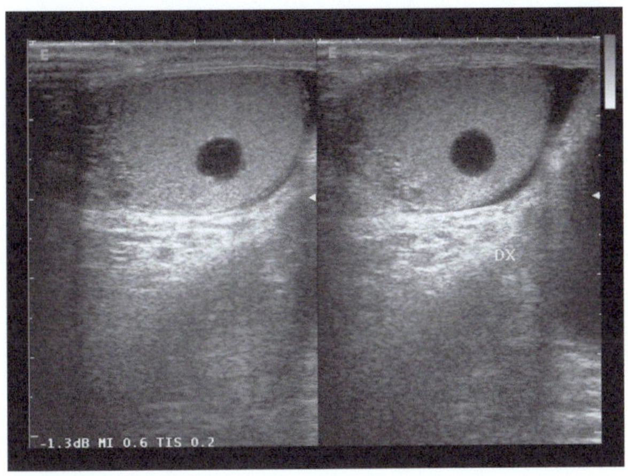

Fig. 1.38 Testicular cyst. Round, unilocular and anechoic formation of the testis

Lesions with a **liquid structure** can also be divided into four categories: (1) simple fluid-filled lesions – homogeneous anechoic, non reflecting; (2) reflective corpuscular lesions – generally dense internal echoes, occasionally mobile with a shift in patient position, also identifiable with optimized gray gain; (3) septated cystic lesions or with parietal polypoid lesions (solid sessile or pedunculated lesions with intraluminal development; (4) prevalently cystic complex lesions – generally corpuscular, with possible septations and internal debris, especially if irregular in thickness or distribution, or with a few solid components (Figs. 1.38–1.44). Septated lesions may have a variable number of internal septations, which may be partial or complete (in the latter case the formation may be

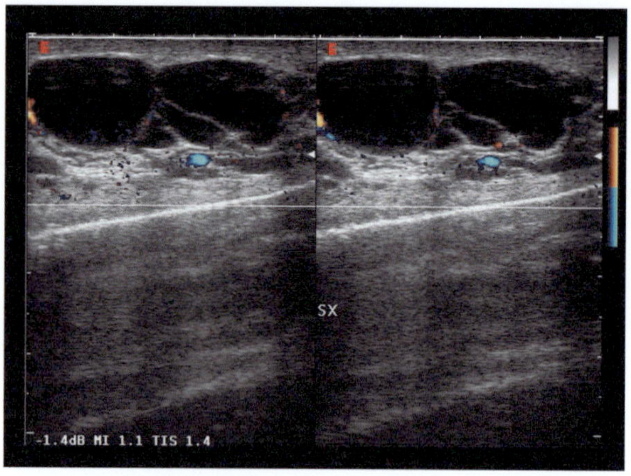

Fig. 1.39 Epididymal cyst. Cystic, lobulated and multilocular formation with the presence of some thin internal septations and vascular signs at directional PD

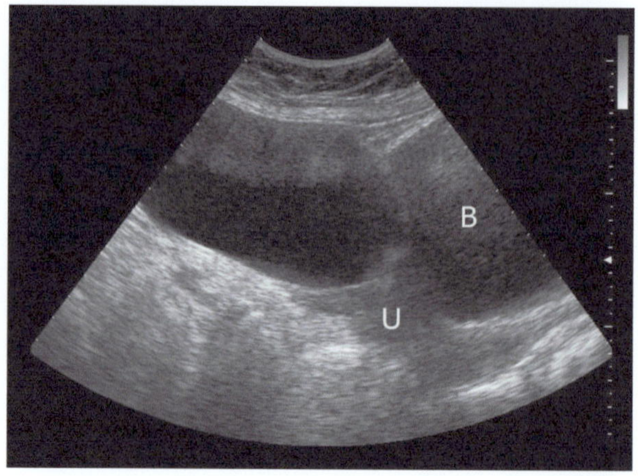

Fig. 1.40 Simple ovarian cyst. Large homogeneous anechoic formation with thin walls and no internal septations. *U*, uterus; *B*, bladder

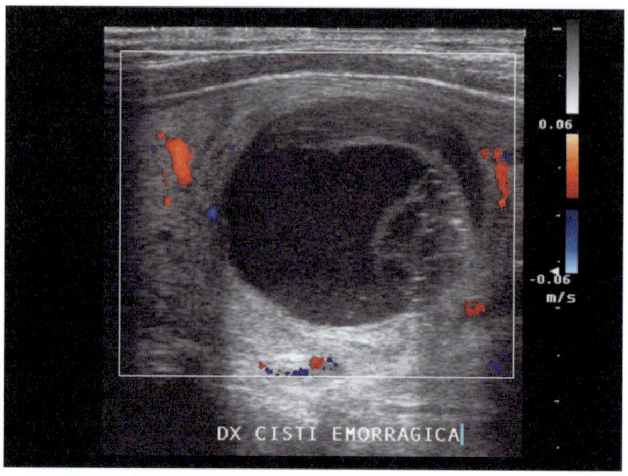

Fig. 1.41 Hemorrhagic cyst of the thyroid. A complex cystic formation can be identified in the thyroid lobe, with echogenic septations and mildly corpuscular content, and no vascular signs at CD

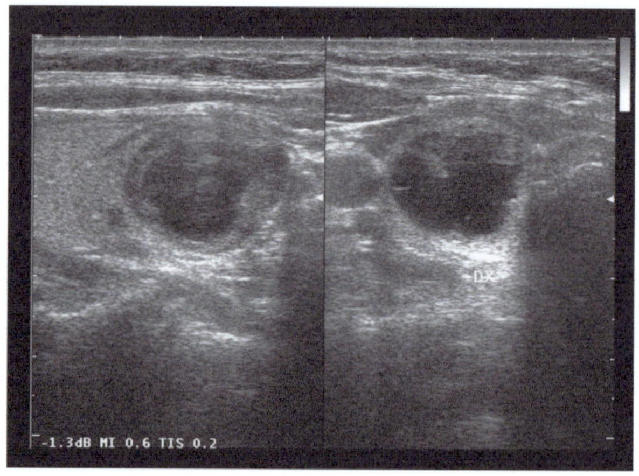

Fig. 1.42 Prevalently cystic colloid thyroid nodule. Nodular formation with significant internal anechoic component and hypoechoic margin varying in thickness

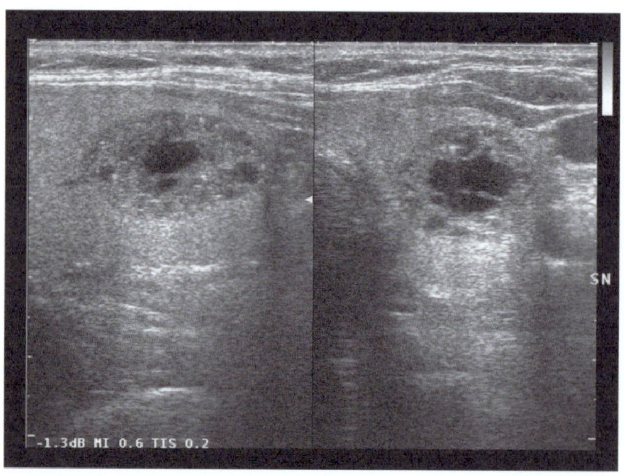

Fig. 1.43 Partially cystic colloid thyroid nodule. Hypo-isoechoic mass with central anechoic area and peripheral anechoic areas. Several small peripheral calcified nuclei are also identifiable

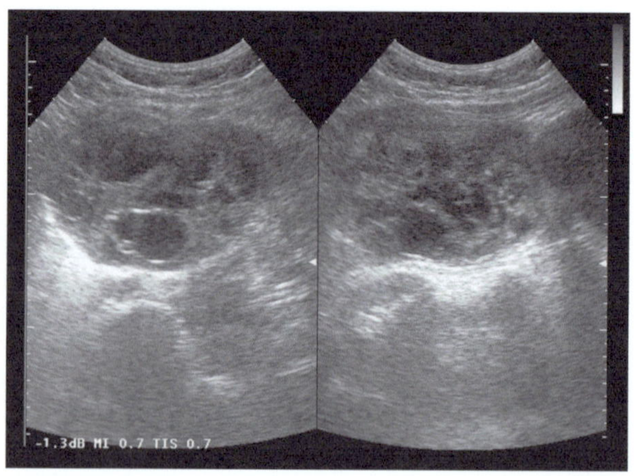

Fig. 1.44 Ovarian endometriotic cyst. Multicystic hypoechoic mass of the right adnexa

described as multilocular) and thin and regular or thick and irregular. All pathologic fluid-filled (cystic) lesions present several more-or-less evident and characteristic artifacts: posterior wall enhancement, i.e. an increase in relative echogenicity of the deep structures of the cyst itself with respect to more lateral structures at the same depth; lateral acoustic shadowing, i.e. two hypoechoic bands tangentially to the two sides of the cyst and directed towards the deep structures. In general, good transmission of the ultrasound beam through a focal lesion, even to the extent of producing **increased through-transmission**, orients the diagnosis towards benignity, especially for superficial structures, although there are some notable exceptions (Fig. 1.45). In the liver, hemangiomas and HCCs are more likely to produce increased through-transmission, which is absent in metastases (unless there is a background of steatosis) [120]. **Lateral acoustic shadowing** can therefore be present, as occurs especially in fluid-filled lesions, or absent, especially in solid lesions.

There are various **characteristics of focal lesions** which need to be considered, both for defining the appearance of the lesion and for writing up the diagnostic report: shape, echostructure, margins, dimensions, number, site and relations with adjacent structures. It should also be borne in mind that in small lesions the morphologic appearance is poorly definable, with a greater overlap between benignity and malignancy than in larger lesions.

The **shape** can be regular or irregular. Lesions with regular shape may be rounded (ratio between the two largest orthogonal diameters <1.5), oval (ratio between 1.5 and 2), elongated (ratio >2) or lobulated (multiple lobulations formed by the confluence of more than one lesion or asymmetrical growth in different directions, with a polycyclic appearance of the margins). A lesion with an irregular shape is instead particularly asymmetrical and therefore cannot be easily attributed to any of the above-mentioned typologies nor can its size be easily determined. The greater the irregularity in shape is, the higher the probability of a malignant nature of the lesion, although this is clearly a generalization.

The **echotexture** can be homogeneous or heterogeneous. The latter, which is also defined as "mixed", can be the result of components with different degrees of anaplasia, histologically different components, irregular divisions in the vascular supply, regressive phenomena (spontaneous or treatment-induced) and possible overlying infection. The complex echostructure illustrated above is the maximum expression of heterogeneity of the echotexture of the lesion, which cannot be classified as hypoechoic, isoechoic or hyperechoic. In absolutely general terms, the greater the heterogeneity of the echotexture is, the higher the probability of a malignant nature of the lesion. Clearly, however, the finding should be evaluated on a case-by-case basis. Necrotic phenomena tend to be hypoechoic or even anechoic, thus they can simulate cystic components. Hemorrhage can be expressed with a different echogenicity according to the time of the bleeding. Adipose components are usually hyperechoic. Cystic areas are anechoic with a homogeneous or more-or-less dense corpuscular content. **Calcifications** can be divided into microcalcifications (punctate echogenic nuclei <1–2 mm with no posterior acoustic shadowing) and macrocalcifications (echogenic nuclei >1–2 mm with posterior acoustic shadowing). The number, whether sporadic or multiple, and the site, whether intralesional, peripheral or with patent "egg-shell" appearance (complete or partial), should also be

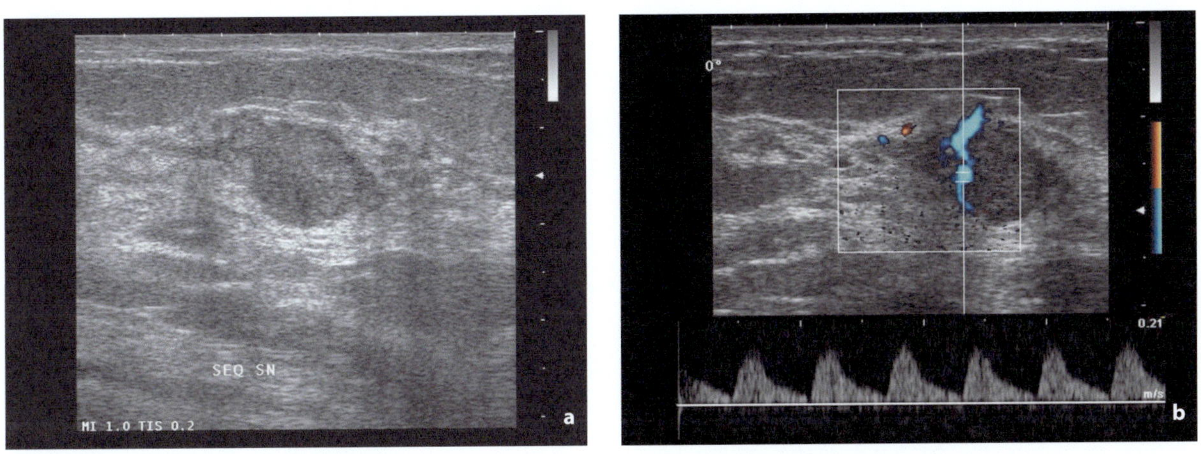

Fig. 1.45a,b Medullary carcinoma of the breast. Hypoechoic and relatively homogeneous oval nodule with well-defined margins and increased through-transmission (**a**). The spectral analysis identifies a relatively elevated resistance spectrum (**b**)

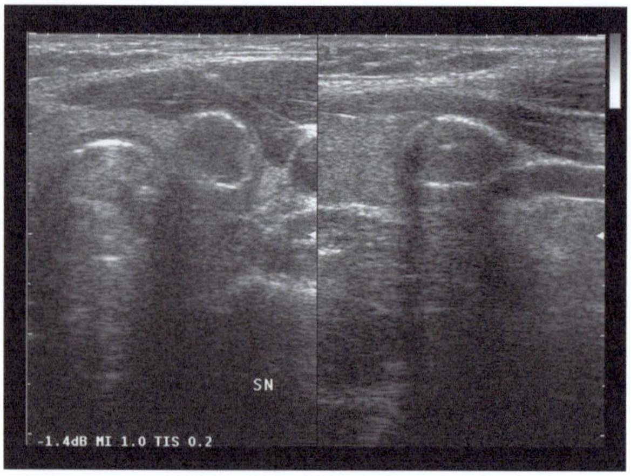

Fig. 1.46 Benign thyroid nodule. Hypoechoic mass with prominent thin and uniform egg-shell calcification, which produces posterior acoustic shadowing

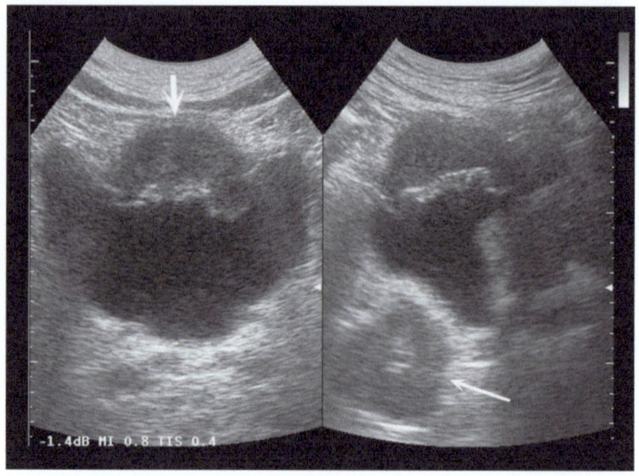

Fig. 1.47 Synchronous tumor, vesical and rectal. Large hypoechoic lesion thickening and distorting the anterior wall of the bladder (*short arrow*). A hypoechoic circumferential thickening of the rectal walls is associated (*long arrow*)

defined. Large central or eccentric calcifications may be found in primary or secondary malignant masses, as well as in benign lesions. Marginal "egg-shell" calcifications are especially found in benign lesions, e.g. in the thyroid (Fig. 1.46). Microcalcifications are typically found in papilliferous carcinomas of the thyroid and of course in breast carcinomas, as well as being an important finding in the testis. In some cases the pervasiveness of the calcifications is so slight as to be barely perceptible if at all with US, which depicts a mild and heterogeneous hyperechogenicity (e.g. in liver metastases from colon cancer).

The **margins** (borders) can be sharp and regular, ill-defined (indistinct), lobulated (both micro- and macrolobulated), angular (sudden variations in the profile) or spiculated (fine bands irradiating around the lesion).

The **dimensions** of the lesions can be measured with the electronic calipers of the device, by searching for the scan plane where the lesion appears at its widest and measuring the longest diameter and the largest perpendicular diameter on this image. The volume of the lesion can then be calculated by measuring the maximum length, width and height of a lesion on two scans obtained on orthogonal planes and applying the ellipsoid formula, by which the measurements are multiplied by 0.524 (an operation which is performed automatically by the software of the US device). Alternatively, the calculation can be based on measurement of the lesion perimeter. However, these are at least in part abstractions, since the measurements can be influenced by a number of factors, including the irregular shape of the lesion or ill-defined and infiltrating margins. Volumetric measurements performed in 3D are more accurate than those in 2D, with less interobserver variability and a greater repeatability. The measurements obtained are less dependent on the dimensions, morphology and echostructure of the lesion [114,121].

The **number** of lesions is important. A distinction needs to be made between solitary lesions and multiple lesions, since generally speaking the latter case is much more suggestive of a malignant and especially secondary nature of non-cystic lesions, although the possibility of multiple benign lesions or multifocal primary tumors cannot be ruled out a priori. The solitary lesion is instead open to all possible etiologies. There is also the possibility of multiple lesions in different organs, which is also initially suggestive of the metastatic nature of non-cystic lesions, although there is still the possibility of synchronous tumors and above all the coexistence between lesions of different types, not only benign and malignant but also neoplastic and non-neoplastic (Fig. 1.47).

The **site** of parenchymal lesions is another important aspect. A distinction needs to be made between intraparenchymal, peripheral (or subcapsular) and capsular (possibly exophytic or pedunculated) lesions, with the evaluation as well of a specific position, e.g. adjacent to a vessel, a duct or the hilum of an organ. With regard to the liver the segmental anatomy is clearly followed, but when writing up the report some anatomic references should also be noted. In the case of particularly large lesions, identifying the source can be challenging due to the involvement of several structures and the consequent difficulty in defining the structure of origin (e.g. gallbladder tumors infiltrating the adjacent parenchyma vs. hepatic tumors infiltrating the gallbladder). In order to identify the organ of origin of a lesion, and thus distinguish invasion from the

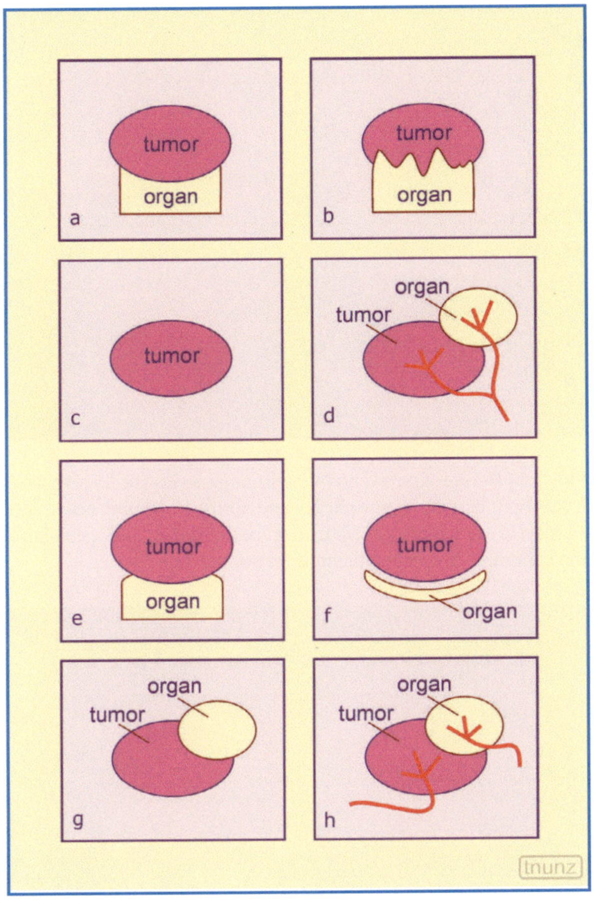

Fig. 1.48 Some useful signs in identifying the organ of origin of a tumor. When the mass arises from the adjacent organ, the edge of the organ will have a beak shape (**a**, beak sign), the organ will be embedded in the tumor (**b**, embedded organ sign), a small organ will become undetectable (**c**, phantom organ sign) and the mass will share its vascular supply with the organ (**d**, prominent feeding artery sign). In contrast, when the mass has merely compressed the organ and not grown from it, the organ will show a dull edge (**e**), the organ will be deformed into a crescent shape (**f**), a small organ will still be detectable (**g**), and the mass will not share its feeding vessels with the organ (**h**)

simple compression of this organ by an extrinsic mass, several signs should be borne in mind. These include a beak-shaped deformity of the organ adjacent to the mass (beak sign), an inability to visualize the organ itself if it is smaller than the mass (phantom organ sign), an absence of a crescent-shaped deformation of the organ (embedded organ sign) and the presence of a common vascular supply between the mass and the organ (prominent feeding artery sign) [122] (Fig. 1.48).

The **orientation** of the lesion with respect to the skin surface, and therefore the transducer, should also be noted. Benign forms of tumors of the breast, thyroid and soft tissue tend to have their long axis parallel to

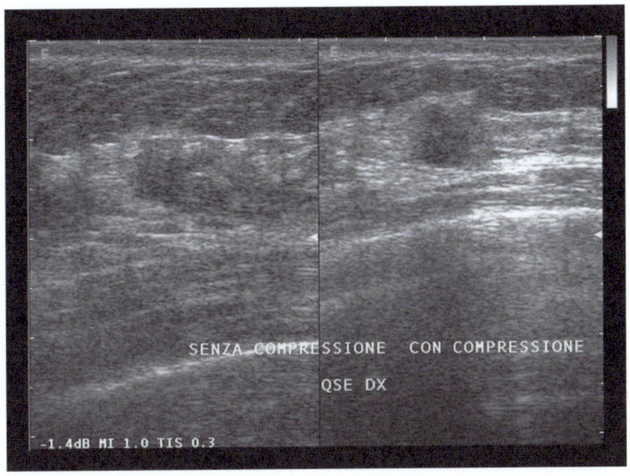

Fig. 1.49 Infiltrative ductal carcinoma, graded compression study. The targeted application of the transducer (*right side*) better depicts the nodular appearance of the poorly defined hypoechoic area

the skin surface, and therefore parallel to the support plane of the transducer, whereas malignant lesions have their long axis perpendicular to the skin (anti-parallel orientation).

Determining the **deformability** or otherwise of surface lesions through compression of the transducer is also important. Compressibility is in fact suggestive of a benign lesion, whereas malignant lesions tend to be less compressible (they tend to be hard and inelastic, also on palpation). Mobility with respect to the adjacent anatomic structures can suggest the absence of invasion. Occasionally variations in compression make identification of isoechoic superficial lesions possible, which are identifiable due to the different compression characteristics with respect to the surrounding tissue (Fig. 1.49). The same result can be achieved by using elastography to test an area with a focal lesion of suspicious nature. Compression with the transducer can help to define the generally hard consistency and tenderness, at least in surface lesions, which are useful elements for differential diagnosis. In the case of neoplastic lesions, the tenderness may be due to rapid growth, infiltration of anatomic structures sensitive to pain and/or compression of adjacent structures. Running the transducer over the skin may also reveal an increased consistency or even a "bump", which may be useful for identifying masses that are not immediately recognizable.

The **transition** between the lesion and healthy parenchyma may be sharp or mediated by a generally thin hypoechoic (e.g. liver) or hyperechoic (e.g. breast) halo. The halo, situated between the lesion and the parenchyma, can have a number of meanings: lesion capsule, adjacent parenchyma compressed by expan-

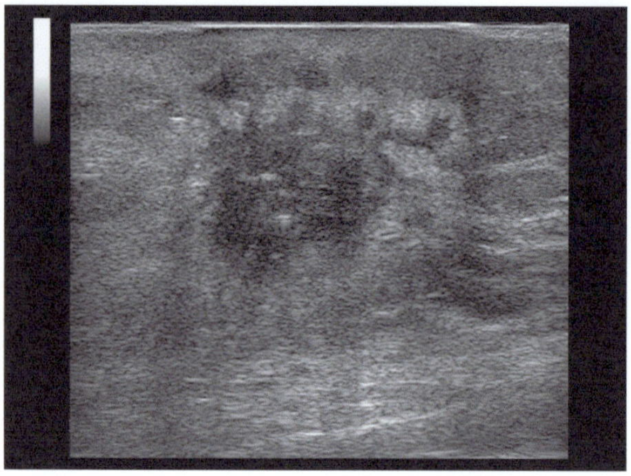

Fig. 1.50 High-grade, invasive ductal carcinoma of the breast, desmoplastic reaction. The large tumor invading the skin shows a thick and irregular hyperechoic border due to fibrotic reaction

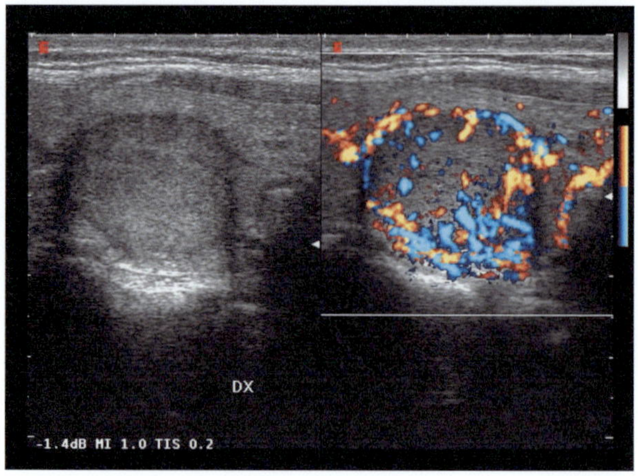

Fig. 1.51 Benign thyroid nodule. Homogeneous iso-hyperechoic mass bounded by a peripheral and uniform hypoechoic halo. Moderate vascularity, especially perinodular and peripheral intranodular, is appreciable at directional PD

sive growth, desmoplastic or inflammatory response of the tissue (Fig. 1.50). A **peripheral hypoechoic halo** can be the expression of perifocal compressive edema, perilesional vessels or a tumor component with active growth. In the thyroid the halo may be seen in both malignant and benign lesions, but it is a finding typical of the latter and in fact when it has a continuous and uniform appearance it is considered a reassuring sign (Fig. 1.51). In the liver, however, a peripheral hypoechoic halo in iso- or hyperechoic lesions was initially thought to be a sign of malignancy and also of particular aggressiveness, as a consequence of compressive atrophy of the normal hepatocytes adjacent to the lesion with persistence only of the sinusoids responsible for the hypoechogenicity. In reality this finding can be identified in HCC, metastases and cholangiocarcinoma, as well as in benign lesions such as hemangiomas, adenomas, FNH, focuses of extramedullary intrahepatic hematopoiesis and fungal microabscesses. This halo is probably due to compressive edema and the tumor growth itself. In any case it should be included in measurements of the size of the lesion (Fig. 1.52, 1.53). A hyperechoic rim is instead often an indicator of benignity. It may be found in the liver in cases of atypical hemangiomas but also in FNH, granulomas or splenosis [123] (Fig. 1.54). It can also be found in hyperplastic nodules and adenomatosis of the parathyroid and breast fibroadenomas.

The type of **growth** of the tumor can be **expansive**, with a well recognizable and measurable formation and overall regular shape, which causes a mass effect on the adjacent structures. In this case indirect signs may be apparent such as displacement/compression of vessels, ducts or other anatomic structures, or focal deformation of the profile of an organ. In the latter case the organ may display a bulge of its surface or a

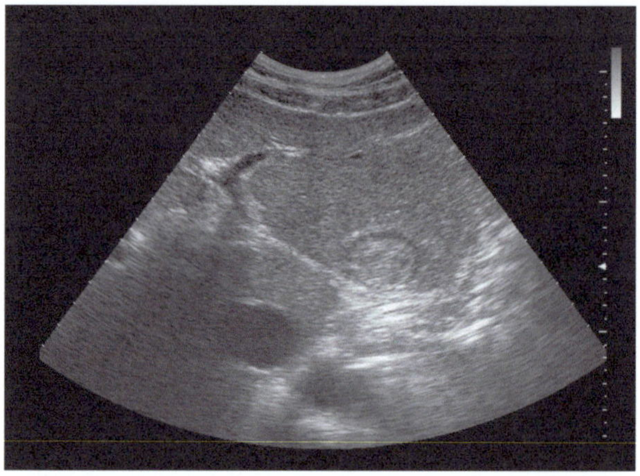

Fig. 1.52 Liver hemangioma, hypoechoic halo. The hyperechoic left lobe lesion shows an evident perifocal hypoechoic halo

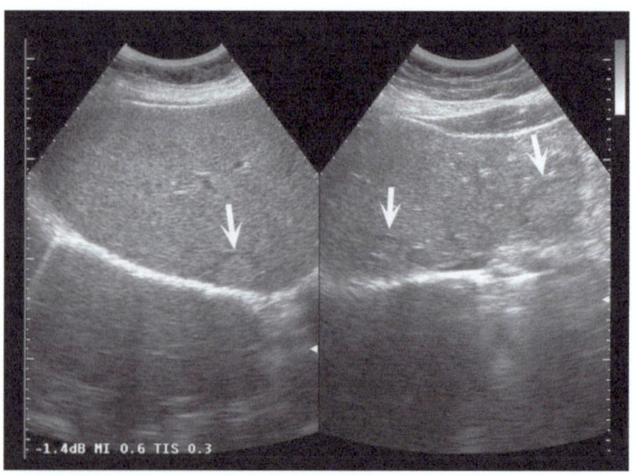

Fig. 1.53 Liver metastasis from lung cancer. The substantially isoechoic lesions are largely identifiable thanks to the presence of a thin peripheral hypoechoic halo (*arrows*)

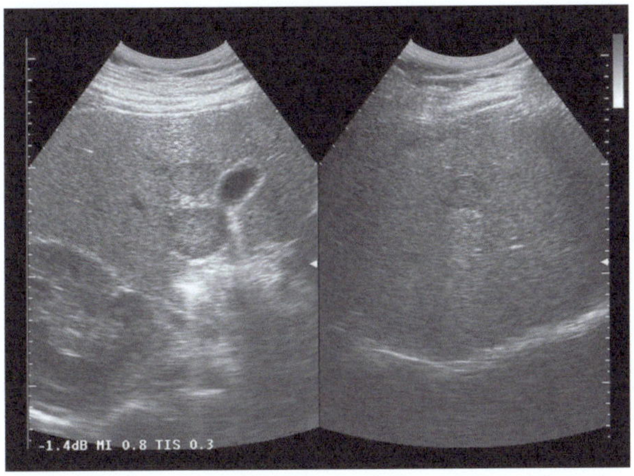

Fig. 1.54 Liver metastases from melanoma. Evidence of three hypoechoic nodules with a vague target appearance due to increased central echogenicity, bounded by a thin hyperechoic rim

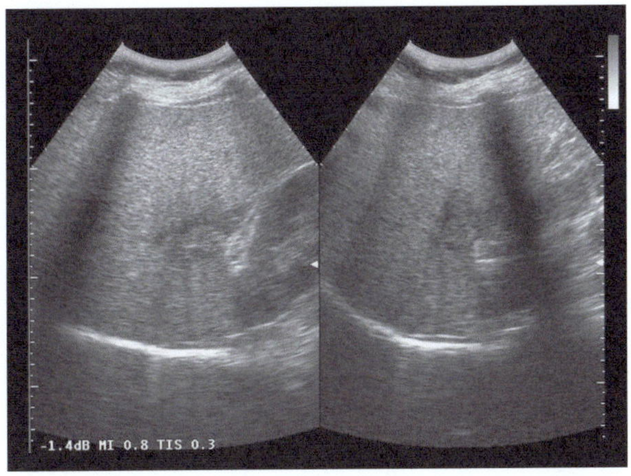

Fig. 1.55 Liver metastases from breast cancer, capsular retraction. Heterogeneous hypoechoic lesion produces a locally concave and retracted appearance of the posterior surface of the right hepatic lobe

lesion which patently protrudes, with exophytic (e.g. HCC) or even pedunculated development (e.g. hepatic FNH). In some organs the compressed perilesional parenchyma is transformed into a pseudocapsule. Alternatively, growth may be **invasive**, with poorly defined tissue which tends to encroach on rather than displace the surrounding structures, such as vessels, and which deforms the organ in a broader sense, without a focal bulge but occasionally with diffuse enlargement which may respect the basic morphology of the organ. When the diffuse structural undermining of the organ is mild, it may go unrecognized. In contrast to expansive lesions, invasive lesions may produce retraction of the surface of an organ. For example, **hepatic capsular retraction**, with a concave distortion of the hepatic contour, may occur in a series of circumstances, on the basis of atrophy, fibrosis or scarring (metastases, HCC, cholangiocarcinoma, epithelioid hemangioendothelioma, large cavernous hemangiomas, percutaneous ablative outcomes, confluent hepatic fibrosis, traumatic or ischemic outcomes, segmental chronic biliary obstruction, etc.), although it is found above all in malignant lesions, with relative specificity [124] (Fig. 1.55).

Various **changes to the surrounding tissues** may occur: compression, distortion, ischemia (even from infiltration or compression of afferent vessels) and dilatation of ducts (e.g. lactiferous or biliary ducts). Lesions which tend to grow without developing fibrous septa, such as lymphomatous lesions, tend to encroach upon adjacent vessels rather than invade them, which instead is common among lesions with a significant stromal component. The presence of **normal intralesional vessels** which cross the area in question suggests either benignity or a malignant lesion with particularly rapid invasive growth. In the latter case, however, it is more likely the vessels show signs of luminal thrombosis or stenosis. A characteristic of malignant lesions or the infiltration of adjacent structures by malignant lesions is the **fixity** with respect to structures which would normally show movement. Examples include reduced respiratory motion in pulmonary tumors invading the chest wall, or the absence of movement of invasive cervical tumors with respect to the act of swallowing.

1.10 Spectral Doppler: Examination Technique and Imaging Characteristics

Duplex Doppler is based on B-mode guide images with the manual placement of an electronic cursor to obtain a pulsed velocity trace. Based on the variation in the Doppler signal (Doppler shift), it is possible to deduce the velocity and direction of the signal in motion, and thus of the blood in the vessels [125].

Spectral Doppler graphically describes the flow velocity (in terms of frequency and distribution) at a given point (sample volume) and a given time, with the values placed on a Cartesian plane where the velocity is depicted on the *y*-axis and time on the *x*-axis. By convention, the negative flows are away from the transducer and are placed below a line known as the baseline, and the positive flows towards the transducer are placed above this line, although they may be inverted by the operator. The position of the baseline can be modified, generally by moving it towards the lower part of the available box and reducing the PRF so that the flowmetry spectrum is given the maximum space available (obviously without producing aliasing artifacts, whereby the maximum velocities, i.e. the systolic peaks, are "chopped off" and carried down to the lower part of the box, below the baseline). The width of the sample volume can be modified and is usually adapted to occupy 50–75% of the diameter of the available vessel, bearing in mind that too wide a sample will suffer from the effects of (arterial) parietal pulsatility and that too central a sample may record mainly the highest velocities, to the detriment of the general profile of the flow in the vessel in question. The line used for the placement of the sample volume can also modify the sampling angle between the incident beam and the direction of flow (θ angle) – this angle should be selected between 30° and 60°, be compatible with the positioning need and be oriented approximately according to the long axis of the vessel. With a cine loop, all the systolic-diastolic cycles can be reviewed from the last "frozen" image, and the flow data can be quantified from the "cleanest" cycles. Clearly, however, these characteristics are only partly applicable in small longitudinal vessels, although the operator should aim to achieve them: the width of the sample volume should be reduced to the minimum possible (usually 1 mm), the gain should be increased until the threshold of artifacts is reached (so as not to lose the minor flows), the PRF should be reduced as much as possible and the θ angle should be set below 60° [112].

The pulsed Doppler spectrum can be used to obtain a variety of information. First of all, if the sampling is performed correctly, the absence of a signal indicates an absence of flow. In the presence of flow, the device is able to automatically indicate the value of maximum flow recorded (peak systolic velocity, V_{max}), the mean velocity (V_m, indicated according to the device as the mean of the maximum velocities or the effective mean value of all the measured velocities) and the diastolic velocity (or end-diastolic velocity, which defines the minimum flow value, V_{min}). In addition, the value of two semiquantitative indices can be automatically obtained, the **resistance index** (RI, given by $(V_{max} - V_{min}) / V_{max}$, which can vary between 0 and 1) and the **pulsatility index** (PI, given by $(V_{max} - V_{min}) / V_m$), which are general indicators of the resistance to flow distal to the sampling point. Under normal conditions, the vasomotor tone of the arteriolar musculature is mainly responsible for flow resistance, whereas in malignancies the scarcity of vessel musculature usually produces low-resistance flows, even though the sole use of semiquantitative indices is rarely able to distinguish between benign and malignant tissue, except for extreme values, as described below [126]. It should also be noted that these semiquantitative indices are influenced by a number of factors: intravascular pressure, peripheral vascular resistance, vessel wall compliance and the area of the cross-section of the vessel. Low values in these indices suggest low-resistance flow, whereas high values indicate high resistance, even though the assumption that RI effectively reflects the resistance variations in the vascular bed distal to the sampling point is controversial [127,128].

Obtaining a good clean spectral trace with a valid representation of at least three systolic-diastolic cycles (from which a mean can be calculated) can be challenging for small vessels such as those within a lesion, for example, in the thyroid, breast or a lymph node (even though the RI and PI values are not dependent on the angle of incidence of the ultrasound beam, with respect to which a small intralesional vessel can clearly have a markedly varied arrangement) [112]. In particular, in the presence of very slow flows, with a systolic velocity <10 cm/s, obtaining reliable semiquantitative indices can be rather difficult. The Doppler flow parameters should also be measured on more than one intralesional vessel, chosen arbitrarily by the operator, who nonetheless will clearly sample those vessels that offer a particularly "bright" or more prominent CD signal than others. The mean of the values obtained should then be calculated, even though for some sites such as the ovary there is a tendency to rely on only one of the recorded samples for the diagnosis, in particular the recording with the most "malignant" values [129]. Also in studies of the breast with multiple samplings of a number of vessels, several authors [130,131] selected the samples which gave the highest RI and PI. In musculoskeletal tumors the ratio between the maximum and the minimum recorded RI on at least five different vessels has been used [132]. Several studies have used only the velocity of the systolic peak, which, with a threshold of 25 cm/s, offers 72% sensitivity and 88% specificity in the diagnosis of malignancy of parathyroid nodules [133], and with a threshold of 16 cm/s offers 83% sensitivity and 92% specificity in the diagnosis of malignancy of adnexal masses with TVUS [134]. Lastly, there is also the possibility of using V_{min} for the purposes of differential diagnosis: one study obtained a 100% positive predictive value for metastasis with end-diastolic velocity <1 cm/s at the level of cervical lymph nodes [135].

After an initial enthusiastic reaction, the findings offered by quantitative spectral data and the semiquantitative indices have produced controversial results. On the one hand, malignant tumors have been found in different organs and structures with different types of acoustic impedance. These include lesions with low RI, probably in relation to the poor vasomotor control of the neocirculation and the presence within it of arteriovenous microfistulas, and lesions with high RI, which is probably an expression of the elevated interstitial pressure, which in turn is dependent on the elevated permeability of the newly formed vessels. On the other hand, there is the problem of establishing threshold values for discriminating between benignity and malignancy. A too stringent cut-off, however, would increase the specificity to the detriment of sensitivity, whereas a less rigorous cut-off would have the opposite effect, reducing the specificity of the differential diagnosis.

Malignancy may be indicated in the presence of both arterial and venous flows, arterial flows with high systolic peak velocity (albeit still in the setting of low flows!), vessels with significantly different flow spectra, turbulent flows, poorly modulated flows and the obliteration of the systolic window. In some sites, such as the ovary, elevated V_{max} values seem to indicate not only malignancy but also the higher-grade form of lesions, therefore correlating with prognosis [128]. RI and PI can be either increased or decreased according to the organ being studied. In soft-tissue tumors there is a broad overlap between benign and malignant lesions, with RI slightly lower in the latter (0.62 on average vs. 0.72 in benign lesions) [129]. Similar results have been reported by a number of studies on breast nodules, with RI equal to 0.62 on average in benign lesions and 0.66 in malignancies [131]. Other studies have obtained different results, with RI>0.99 and PI>4 being very specific for breast cancers [130] (Fig. 1.56).

Spectral data may also have prognostic implications. One study showed markedly better survival for breast cancer patients with V_{max} of internal flow <25 cm/s at spectral analysis than patients with higher intralesional flow velocities [136].

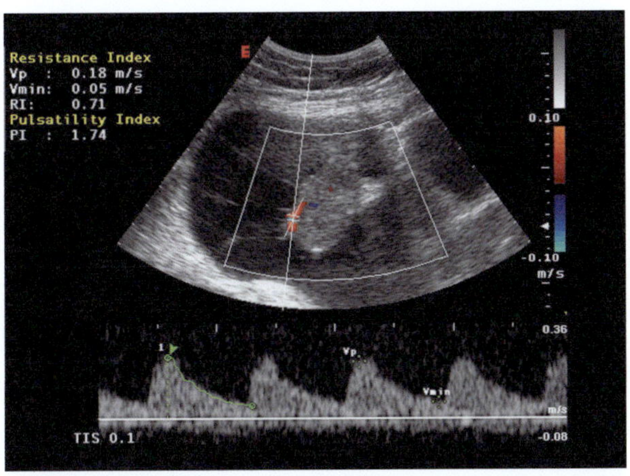

Fig. 1.56 Ovarian cancer, spectral evaluation. Transabdominal recording of the flowmetry trace of the most prominent vessel within the solid component of the complex adnexal mass shows V_{max} equal to 18 cm/s, RI 0.71 and PI 1.74. The θ angle is correctly oriented

1.11 Color Doppler and Power Doppler: Examination Technique

Color Doppler consists of bichromatic color maps which are superimposed over the B-mode images at the points where movement is recorded, and therefore in correspondence to vascular flow. The intensity of the color in terms of the background scale indicates the flow velocity at each point, whereas the color itself indicates the direction of flow. By convention, flows away from the transducer are coded blue, whereas flows towards to the transducer are coded red.

One of the main limits of CD is its poor sensitivity for slow flows, a feature which limits the use of Doppler techniques in the study of focal parenchymal lesions. Although the current devices have achieved a good level of sensitivity, maximizing the ability of the system to detect parenchymal flows is nonetheless particularly important. To do so, numerous parameters need to be taken into account [125]. First of all, the use of PD (see below) is often preferable to CD. The former is in fact more sensitive to slow flows. However, it is also more sensitive to motion artifacts and does not provide information regarding the direction of flow (although there is the possibility of directional PD on some devices) (Figs. 1.57, 1.58). Moreover, the lowest possible **pulse repetition frequency** (PRF) needs to be used. The PRF indicates the number of sound pulses per time unit, and therefore the frequency at which our system interrogates the object – for "slow" objects it is clear that the "interrogations" also need to be similarly slow. A PRF of around 750 MHz is used for superficial tissues, whereas around 1000–1300 MHz is used in the abdomen due to motion artifacts. The **transmit frequency** of the transducer, regardless of the B-mode frequency and generally lower than this, should be appropriately reduced for the study of deep structures and appropriately increased for superficial structures. The **color gain**, which is a parameter independent of B-mode gain, should be increased until the appearance of artifacts, with the typical "colored snowstorm" images, and then reduced just below this threshold in order to maximize the sensitivity of the color while at the same time suppressing artifactual signals – this generally corresponds to a reception sensitivity of around 60%. The **pass filter** (wall filter) should be set at the minimum possible and therefore at the maximum sensitivity. The lowest filter available in the device should be used for superficial tissues, in general 50 Hz, whereas abdominal parenchymas still require at least minimum filtration (around 100 Hz) to avoid excessive motion artifacts. The **color box** should be sized to the area of interest, without excluding portions of this but above all without the inclusion of excessive background tissue, which can be the source of artifacts. Moreover, an excessively wide box reduces the qualitative yield in real time of the system. The compression applied by the transducer on the skin should be optimal, especially for superficial structures. Excessive compression can attenuate or even eliminate vascular signals, particularly in benign lesions, and therefore produce a false interpretation of the images [125] (Figs. 1.59, 1.60). In a manner similar to the spectral analysis, the cine loop function makes a review of all the frames acquired from the last "frozen" image possible and allows documentation of those most representative of the vascular situation and least degraded by artifacts.

Once a map of the vasculature of the area being studied has been obtained and these optimized parameters have been used to maximize the sensitivity of the system for slow flows, the color guide can be used to obtain flowmetry spectra and therefore quantitative and semiquantitative data from the spectrum. Of course to do so the setting of the device should be modified, particularly with an increase in PRF, since the vessels being sought are those with the fastest flows, on which the cursor of the sample volume should be positioned for spectral Doppler.

Power Doppler or color-Doppler energy modality consists of monochromatic maps which are superimposed over the B-mode images at the points where movement is recorded, and therefore corresponding to vascular flow. Visualization of the flow is based on estimation of the integral of the power spectrum. Unlike CD, therefore, PD is not based on the flow velocity, but only on the flow intensity (amplitude of the Doppler

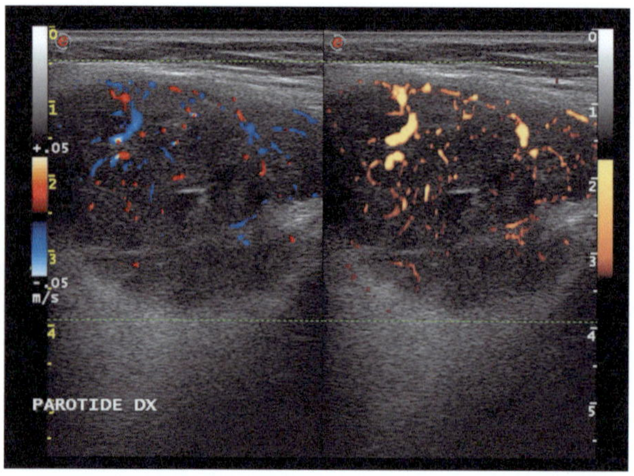

Fig. 1.57 Parotid nodule (Warthin's tumor), comparison between CD and PD. The double display shows greater flow signal on the power-Doppler side (*right*) than on the color-Doppler side (*left*)

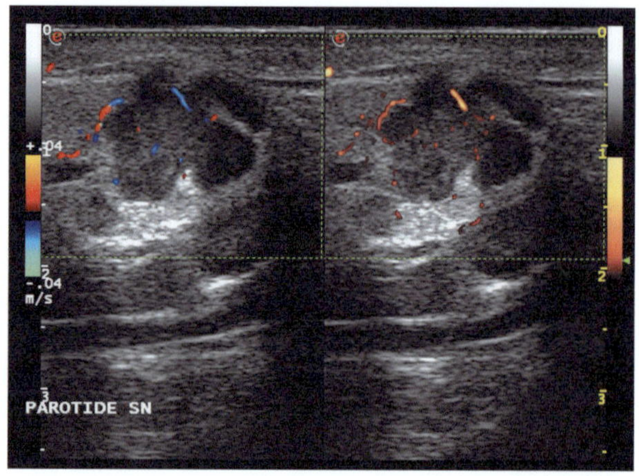

Fig. 1.58 Parotid adenoma, comparison between CD and PD. The double display shows greater flow signal on the power-Doppler side (*right*) than on the color-Doppler side (*left*)

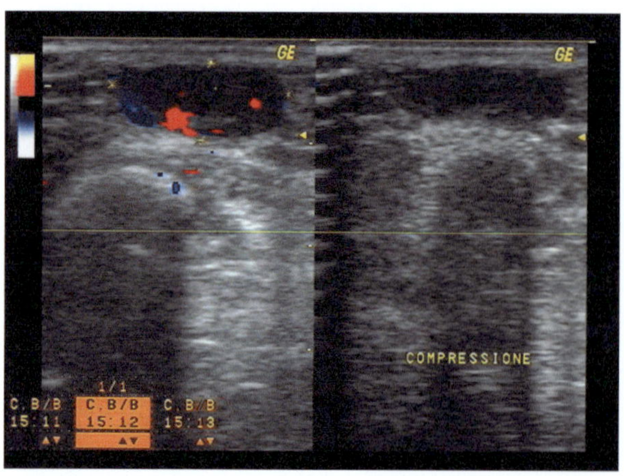

Fig. 1.59 Cutaneous hemangioma, compression study. Hypoechoic subcutaneous mass of the forearm with peripheral venous flows. During compression (*left*) the lesion is deformed and the flows are cancelled

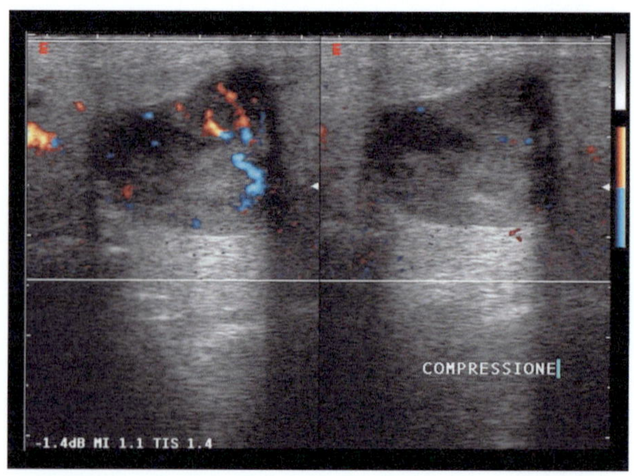

Fig. 1.60 Pleomorphic adenoma of the parotid, compression study. Directional PD image before and after the application of pressure with the transducer (*left*), which cancels the intranodular flow

shift signal) as an indicator of the number of erythrocytes traveling through a vessel. It is therefore more independent of the angle of insonation and more sensitive to slow flows. The intensity of the color with respect to background noise indicates the intensity of the flow without providing information on the velocity of the flow itself and without coding the direction of flow which is a characteristic of CD (although the directional PD modality does exist). Aliasing is not present and there is less dependence on the angle of incidence of the ultrasound beam with respect to CD [39]. In addition, the gain may be increased without the "noise" which fills the CD images obtained with an excessively high gain. The macro-vascular network of the tumor is well demonstrated with 3D PD, which provides excellent information regarding the vascular distribution, variation in vessel diameter, tortuosity and method of subdivision of the vessels themselves. PD is therefore characterized by higher sensitivity to vascular flows, especially slow flows. Nonetheless it does have some important limitations. First of all, the susceptibility to motion artifacts (heart beat, vascular pulsatility, intestinal peristalsis, respiratory motion of the subject, tissue motion) is greater than in CD and this particularly limits abdominal applications due to the presence of real flows, such as in lesions of the left hepatic lobe [137]. In addition, the ability to detect deep signals, which already in CD is lower than in B-mode, is even lower in PD. In the liver, for example, PD is more sensitive than CD in identifying intralesional signals originating from superficial or intermediate nodules, but not for signals from deep lesions and this is particularly evident in conditions which increase beam attenuation such as steatosis or cirrhosis [137] (Fig. 1.61). It should also be borne in mind that PD involves a lower temporal resolution than CD and therefore visualizes vessel pulsatility less immediately. Moreover, since the technique does not demonstrate aliasing it may be less useful in the search for flows to be sampled for spectral analysis [138].

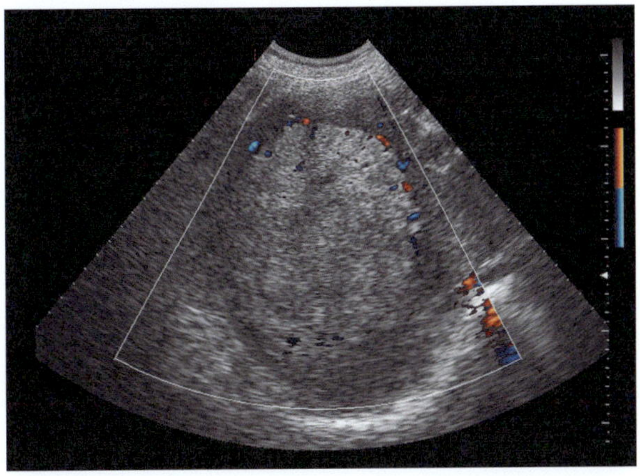

Fig. 1.61 Hepatocellular carcinoma. Large heterogeneous echoic lesion of the right hepatic lobe, with moderate peripheral vascular signals at directional PD in the superficial portion. The poor flow signals originating from the deep portion of the mass are attributable to the poor penetration of the signal

One of the possibilities for attenuating some of the limitations to the sensitivity of CD and PD is the use of sonographic contrast media, which increase the intensity of the signal and prove particularly useful for the identification of slow flows (Figs. 1.62, 1.63). However, the contrast media also increase the artifacts associated with the Doppler techniques and in particular the blooming artifact. To avoid this artifact, a slow administration of the contrast medium is required, thus foregoing the possibility of a dynamic study just at the most important moment, i.e. when the contrast medium itself arrives at the target area. However, although the use of contrast media is currently associated

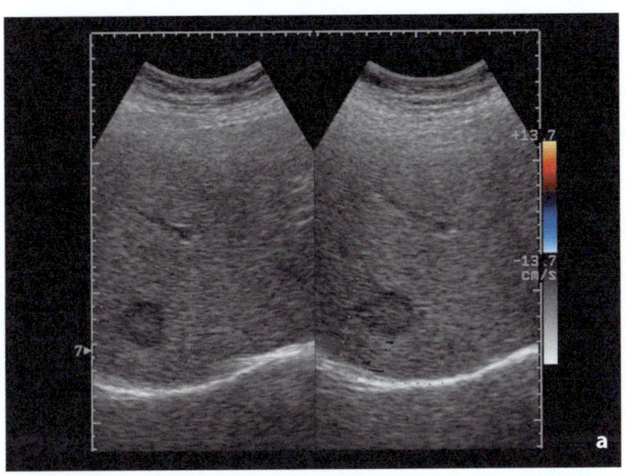

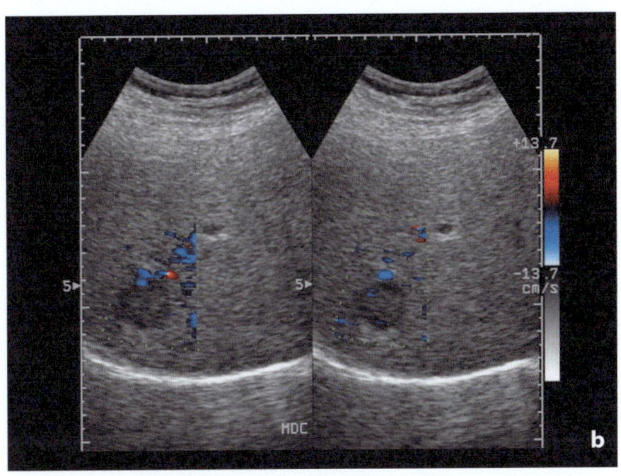

Fig. 1.62a,b Hepatocellular carcinoma, before (**a**) and after (**b**) injection of contrast medium. The baseline CD study fails to show flow signals, whereas the contrast-enhanced study identifies an afferent arteriole and several intranodular arterial vessels

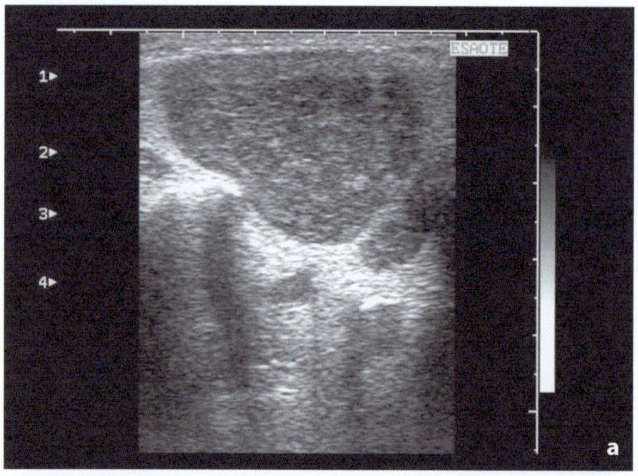

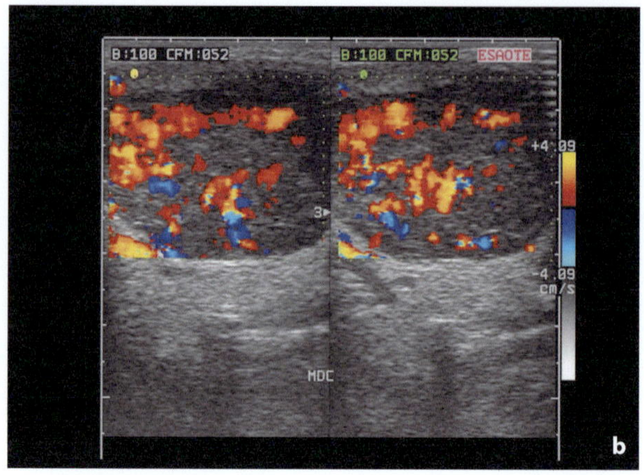

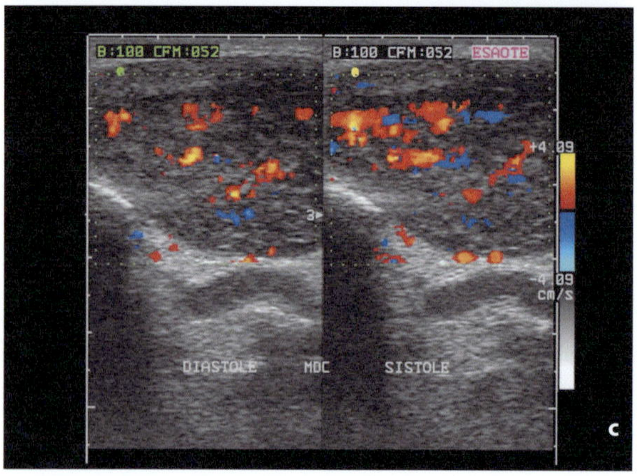

Fig. 1.63a-c Pleomorphic adenoma of the parotid. Well-defined relatively homogeneous hypoechoic nodule (**a**). Contrast-enhanced CD study (**b**, **c**) shows intense arterial pulsing (difference between systole and diastole intranodular vascularity)

particularly with CEUS, it can be useful to perform a Doppler study in the area of interest in the late phase, when the blooming effect of the contrast medium is reduced.

From the point of view of CD, the use of contrast media offers the possibility of utilizing a higher frame rate, because a lower number of pulses per scan line than in baseline can be used to achieve the same sensitivity. Alternatively, a higher transmit frequency of the transducer can be used, thus increasing the resolution between the contrast-enhanced examination and baseline. Still today, therefore, contrast media can be used to "save" a nondiagnostic CD study, although this indication is becoming increasingly more limited with respect to gray-scale contrast enhancement [139].

1.12 Color Doppler and Power Doppler: Imaging Characteristics

Doppler techniques are able to obtain a valid representation of the vascularity of tissues and their alterations, within certain limits (Video 1.5). The vascularity of a lesion can be absent (avascularity, at least within the resolution limits of the technique) or present. When present it may be arterial, venous or mixed, with a possible arterial or venous prevalence. Arterial and venous vessels can be distinguished with the color evaluation, since the former are pulsed flows and the latter continuous, a feature which is more readily evident on CD than PD, although confirmation should come from spectral analysis (bearing in mind that low-resistance arterial flows can mimic venous flows). The vascular structures may be distributed prevalently at the perilesional or intralesional level, and when intralesional they may be central, peripheral or diffuse. In general, the presence of intralesional signals, especially if central or diffuse, is suggestive of malignancy, whereas prevalently perilesional or peripheral intralesional vessels are more typical of benign lesions. The presence of perinodular vessels can facilitate visualization of a poorly identifiable lesion, e.g. if isoechoic (Fig. 1.64). The afference can be peduncular, with a vascular pole from which the various intralesional branches progressively emerge, or peripheral (capsular), with multiple small branches penetrating the nodule at different points. Whereas peripheral

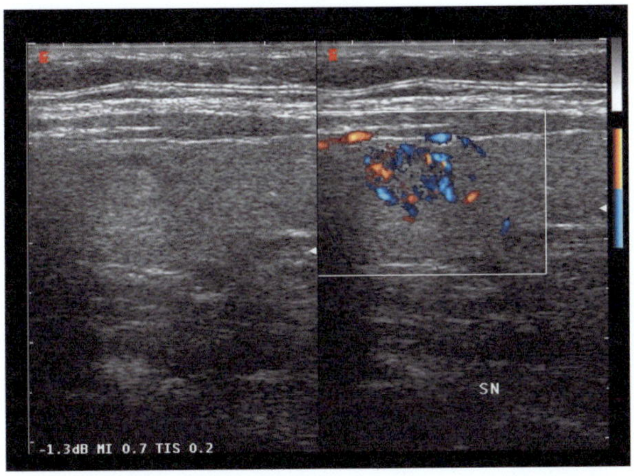

Fig. 1.64 Benign thyroid nodule, CD study for identification. The US study poorly visualizes the mildly hyperechoic nodulation, which instead is made apparent by the perinodular and peripheral intranodular flow shown with directional PD

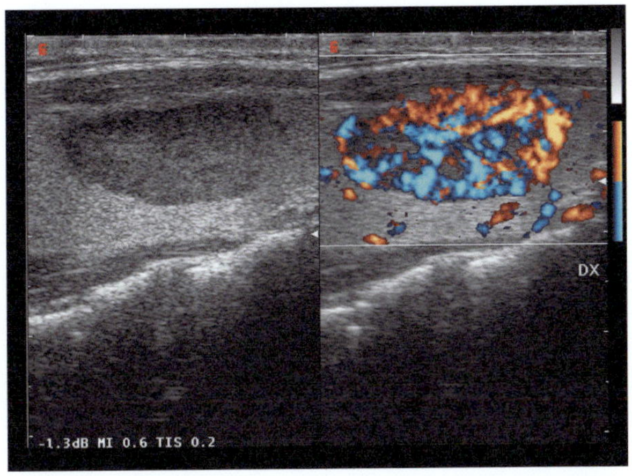

Fig. 1.65 Adenomatous nodule of the thyroid. Intense and diffuse hypervascularity of the nodule on directional PD in comparison with the surrounding parenchyma

vascularization suggests benignity in a nodule of the salivary gland, the presence of multiple afferent vessels penetrating the capsule is a characteristic of metastatic lymphadenopathy. There may also be multiple vascular poles, especially in malignant lesions. When adequately identifiable, the internal vessels of a lesion can have a homogeneous or irregular and anarchic distribution, with areas of greater or lesser vascularity.

In some cases the vessels transit a certain area of altered echogenicity undisturbed, i.e. without signs of a "mass effect". This, together with the absence of intralesional hypervascularity, suggests the benignity of the finding, as is the case in areas of focal steatosis or in areas of the liver that are free from fat infiltration [126].

In general, the greater the vascularity of a lesion, the higher the probability that it is malignant, although there are exception in both senses (Figs. 1.65, 1.66). The applications Doppler techniques have in this sense undergone particular development. With the first generations of ultrasound devices equipped with CD functions, the finding of intralesional flows was considered in itself suspicious of malignancy or at least sufficient to suggest further examinations. For example, the finding was considered important for suggesting the malignancy of a thyroid or breast nodule, or for suspecting the metastatic nature of a superficial lymphadenopathy. However, with the current devices the sensitivity for slow flows has increased considerably, and therefore most solid lesions show color signs (as indeed they should!). The debate has therefore become more complex, having shifted from a situation of "present-absent" to one of a more complex qualitative and possibly quantitative analysis.

The **degree of vascularity** should be related to the

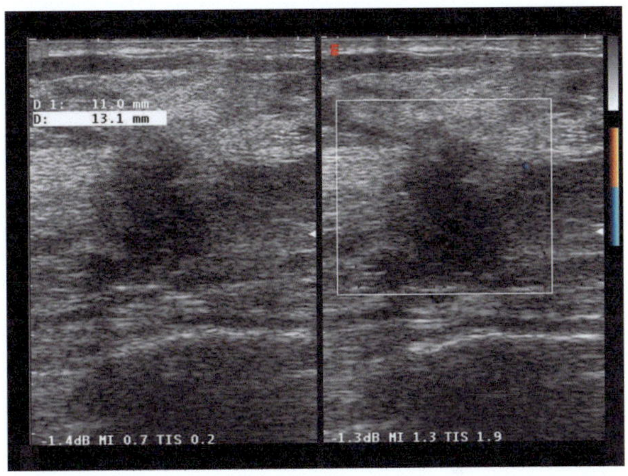

Fig. 1.66 Hypovascular invasive ductal carcinoma. Lobulated, heterogeneous hypoechoic lesion with irregular margins, antiparallel position and posterior shadowing. The nodule nonetheless displays poor vascular signals

parenchymal context. A lesion can be hyper-, iso- or hypovascular in relation to the adjacent parenchyma and not in an absolute sense, even when it is decidedly vascular, as for example the thyroid parenchyma of a young subject. A lesion, therefore, is hypervascular not when it shows a moderate number of flow signals, but when these are greater in density with respect to the normal perilesional tissue. Alternatively, a lesion can be avascular when even a minimal flow signal is absent. The "historical" problem of this type of evaluation, however, is diagnostic subjectivity, for which even in the scientific field the diagnosis is often based on graduation scales of the finding and is of limited practical reliability. More quantitative systems include those either in the scanner or on PC, which are based on a count of the number of colored pixels. For example, commercially available software can be used to define a vascularity index, which is obtained from the difference between the total number of pixels and the number of colored pixels, divided by the total number of pixels and multiplied by 100 [140]. Alternatively, postprocessing techniques can be used to eliminate the gray-scale background in order to isolate and quantify the color signal [141]. A further possibility involves creating wash-in and wash-out curves, i.e. curves constructed from data sampled from a ROI which represent the inflow and outflow of contrast medium over a given time [142].

In addition to the hypervascularity in itself as an expression of neoangiogenesis, there are other features of the nodular vasculature which should be evaluated and which can be **suggestive of malignancy**. These include the presence of not only perifocal but also intrafocal vessels, the presence of central vessels (identifiable only at the center or penetrating, with a course from the periphery to the center), the presence of multiple vascular poles distant from each other, the presence of both afferent (arterial) and efferent (venous) vessels, an irregular distribution of the vessels with poorly vascular zones and highly vascular and chaotic zones, the coexistence of vessels with different diameters (without a hierarchical subdivision of the vessels in increasingly smaller branches), the existence of wide vessels (generally venous lakes), the stenosis (aliasing!) and sudden variations in diameter ("jumps"), a tortuous and angulated course of the vessels (rather than delicately curved and regular), the presence of vessels which on two planes connect to form an auto loop, the presence of blind vessels and aneurysms, the trifurcation of vessels (presence of three branches dividing simultaneously from a single proximal vessel), the diffusion of vessels not from the vascular pole to the center and then branching to the periphery but from outside the lesion to the periphery and then to the center through multiple afferent vessels, and the presence of bidirectional or variable flow in the same vessel with a mosaic appearance (arteriovenous fistulas) [131,132,143] (Fig.1.67). Many of the characteristics described above can be identified in adequately large lesions (>10–15 mm), in which there may also be other morphostructural criteria suggestive of malignancy. For subcentimeter lesions the possibility of identifying suspicious CD elements is lower. Even in totally or prevalently necrotic lesions, even when malignant, CD is not able to supply significant additional information and may even be misleading. It should also be noted that the Doppler techniques, even when combined with tissue harmonic imaging, are unable to identify the presence and characteristics of the microcirculation proper of the lesion and that their imaging characteristics are limited to the analysis of vascular macrostructure. The main role of CD is to provide additional information for the US characterization of focal lesions. However, CD can to a certain extent be useful during the identification phase, especially with regard to hypoechoic or anechoic lesions. The contiguity of lesions with the vessels "opacified" by the color signal can in fact facilitate identification and distinction from the vascular images themselves. In addition, lesions which are significantly more or less vascular than the surrounding parenchyma can be identified precisely due to the contrast with the color signal of the surrounding parenchyma [144]. This is clearly the case for the liver as well as other parenchymas such as the thyroid. Occasionally a nodular mass which is isoechoic or at any rate poorly distinguishable from the parenchymal background (possibly heterogeneous) can be confirmed with CD, which highlights the perinodular and intranodular peripheral vessels, thus making the lesion itself more apparent.

The hypervascularity of a lesion can also have a **prognostic significance** for the tumor, being a predictor for a higher grade or increased probability of lymph node involvement and metastasis, although not all studies have confirmed this. One study, for example, recorded a markedly better survival among women with breast cancer with V_{max} of internal flow <25 cm/s at spectral analysis than women with higher intralesional flow velocities [136]. An evident disorganization of the vascular structures correlates with a high grade of lesion anaplasia [126,138].

In some cases the type of vascularity can be exploited not only for distinguishing benignity/malignancy, but also for characterizing the different types of lesions. In the liver in particular, several

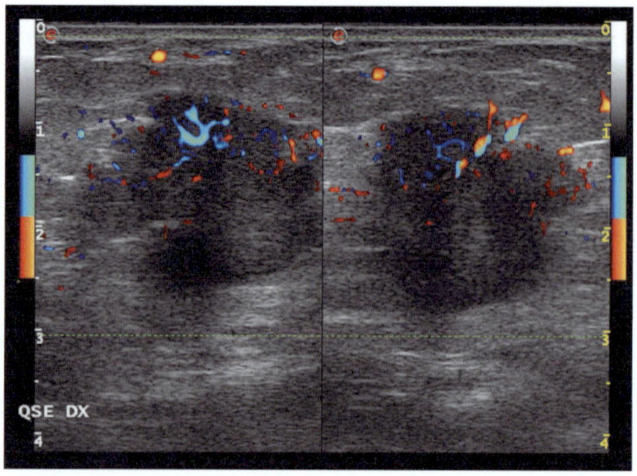

Fig. 1.67 Breast cancer, anarchic vascular distribution. The size and course of the intranodular vessels is chaotic, with U-shaped vessels and bidirectional flow

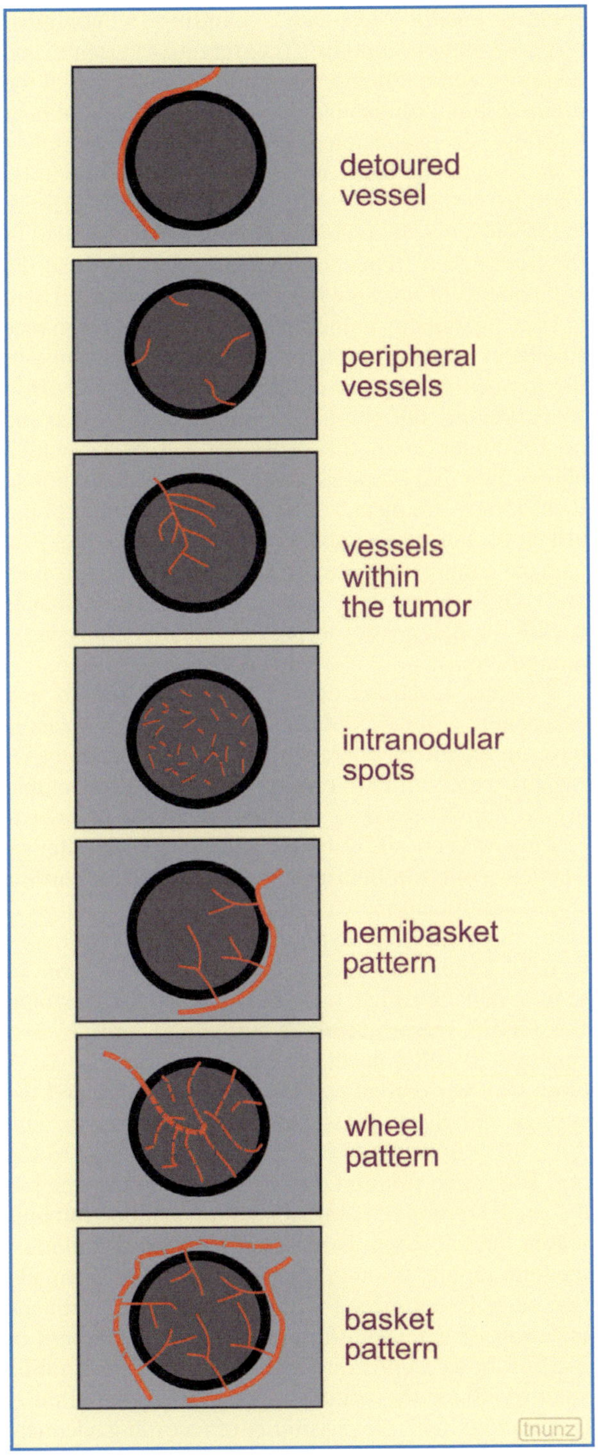

Fig. 1.68 Main CD patterns of focal hepatic lesions. The patterns include prevalently peripheral vessels (metastases but also HCC and possibly hemangiomas), a vascular displacement (metastases but also benign lesions with expansive growth), intratumoral vessels (HCC and metastases), FNH if with central disposition and cartwheel branching, isolated spots of flow (HCC and metastases) and a uni- or bipolar basket pattern (HCC)

patterns have been described which despite not being specific for any lesion can provide additional information. The pattern of detouring found especially in metastases is characterized by the displacement of a vessel due to lesion growth such that the vessel displays a crescent-shaped path. The spokewheel appearance is typical of FNH and is characterized by the presence of a central artery from which arterial "spokes" irradiate towards the periphery. The "basket" pattern, which is found especially in HCC, is characterized by a hypertrophic afferent vessel which, having reached the nodule, gives off a series of peri- and intralesional branches. The presence of arterial branches within the lesion (vessels within the tumor pattern) in the form of punctate or short linear signals, is nonspecific but most commonly found in HCC [145] (Fig. 1.68).

False flow images can be due to a number of causes, both in terms of the settings of the device and the possible presence of artifacts intrinsic to the CD technique, which, however, can, to a certain extent, be attenuated with an appropriate adjustment of the scanner itself. False flows can be found as the result of an overamplification of the Doppler signal, adjacent structures in motion (cardiovascular pulsatility, respiratory motion, intestinal peristalsis), a priority of the color codified at an excessively low level (appearance of signals within effusion or cystic formations), vibration phenomena (tissue surrounding stenoses or arteriovenous fistulas), a mirror artifact (at the level of a vessel, such as the intercostal or subclavian arteries, adjacent to a highly reflective interface such as the aerated lung or even when the insonation angle is perpendicular to the vessel) or a comet-tail or twinkling artifact (at the level of calcifications) [101] (Fig. 1.69).

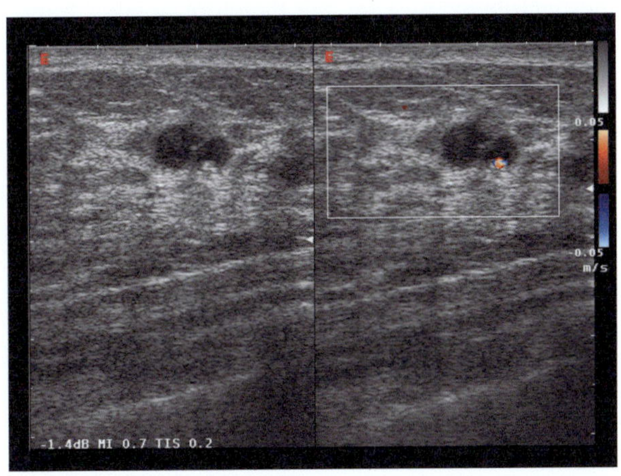

Fig. 1.69 Breast fibroadenoma, twinkling artifact. The small intranodular calcification produces a color signal which simulates the presence of CD flow

1.13 Contrast-Enhanced Ultrasound: Examination Technique

US contrast media are substances able to modify the acoustic impedance of the body tissues they permeate and therefore produce a change in the way they reflect US pulses, which is increased by 20–30 dB. Since the ultrasound reflectivity of circulating erythrocytes is very low, a small volume of microbubbles (several mL) is enough to markedly increase the signal originating from the tissues. The unique aspect of US contrast media is that they are modified by the process – the ultrasound – used to study them. In addition, the various contrast media, which each have a different chemical make-up, present different pharmacokinetics and behavior with respect to ultrasound. They have different resonance and microbubble destruction thresholds for different **mechanical index** (MI) values. US contrast media are therefore much more different from one another than is the case with radiologic iodinated contrast media, and it is therefore possible for them to have a different output when coupled with this or that CEUS system or in different applications. In general, given its elevated compliance, a microbubble contracts when the external pressure increases (the effect of the ultrasound beam) and expands when it decreases. When doing so, the microbubble resonates. It is on the discrimination between this resonance and the ordinary tissue echoes that CEUS is based [146–148].

The first generation of US contrast media included agents such as Levovist, and were mainly employed to intensify the CD signal. However, in part due to the rapid increase in the sensitivity of Doppler systems, this use came to a rapid end. The **first-generation** contrast media are characterized by the air content of the microbubbles. They are therefore notably fragile and their contrast effect can be exploited only for a limited number of acquisitions. The first gray-scale CEUS systems to be developed were in fact intermittent, with an elevated ultrasound beam intensity (MI>0.2). With these systems, also known as "destructive" or "static", the ultrasound beam causes rupture of the microbubbles and records the signal emitted. The contrast medium microbubbles have a weak harmonic response such that to obtain a contrast-enhanced signal the "sacrifice" of the bubbles themselves is required.

With the advent of **second-generation** contrast media such as SonoVue, Definity and Optison, containing gas other than air (low solubility and high stability), the use of continuous CEUS systems has become possible, i.e. systems in which the acquisition occurs in real time [148]. In these systems with a low MI (<0.2) the first-generation contrast media suffer no substantial effects, whereas the second-generation contrast media "resonate", emitting a nonlinear response without rupturing (conservative systems) and therefore without being "used up" by the action of the interrogating ultrasound beam. In the nonlinear response, the expansion of the insonified microbubble is much greater than the contraction and therefore, when the reflected signal is analyzed in the domain of the frequencies, it contains not only the component of the transmitted frequency (fundamental) but also the components of multiple frequencies (harmonic). There is the fortunate coincidence that the resonance frequency of the microbubbles is within the range of the frequencies used in clinical practice (2–13 MHz). In particular, the resonance frequency of SonoVue microbubbles is in the order of 2–3 MHz, which allows their diagnostic use, especially at the abdominal level (study frequency 3.5–5 MHz). The maximum effect of the microbubbles occurs during the first passage through the major circulation, although they are able to recirculate, with a contrast effect that is useful for diagnostic purposes and lasts for several minutes.

Adverse reactions can be clearly linked to any component of the product, although US contrast media have an excellent tolerance profile, without hepatic, renal or cerebral toxicity [149,150]. SonoVue should not be administered to children, pregnant or breast-feeding women and subjects with a specific allergy. Medical **contraindications** include right-left cardiac shunt, significant increase in arterial pulmonary pressure, noncontrolled hypertension, adult respiratory distress syndrome, recent myocardial infarction or severe noncontrolled tachyarrhythmia. To **perform the CEUS examination**, a peripheral vein is first cannulated with a needle cannula of at least 20 G. A three-way tap is then applied to the cannula, and the syringe with the contrast medium and the syringe with 5–10 mL saline solution are in turn connected to the tap. The saline solution is used both to ensure none of the small amount of contrast medium solution remains within the injector apparatus and to flush the contrast medium rapidly through the venous system. Normally the study is performed with a rapid bolus, with the injection of a few milliliters of contrast medium in 1–2 s, followed immediately by the injection of saline solution. Since the volume is very small, the circulation is rapid, with the possibility of recording adequate findings of very fast arterial perfusion (high temporal resolution). After the bolus administration the duration of the effect is 5–7 min, whereas it is much longer in the case of slow infusion (obtaining a stable enhancement with an infusion rate >30 mL/h).

The majority of experimental contrast media are totally, or for the most part, of the intravascular type (blood pool), i.e. able to persist in the vascular system and recirculate without diffusing in the interstitium (unlike CT and MR contrast media). It has, however, been seen that both SonoVue and above all Levovist have a post-vascular parenchymal phase that is useful for diagnostic purposes. In addition, **tissue-specific contrast media** (hepatic-splenic specific) are being developed, the possible availability of which could provide further indications for CEUS [151,152]. Unlike tissues, the contrast media respond to incident ultrasound in a manner that is dependent on the amplitude of the ultrasound waves. With increasing MI, there is first (<30 kPa, i.e. MI<0.05) a response of linear reflection (fundamental) which is proportional to the incident frequency, with the possibility of conventional US images, or, in the case of CD images, with enhanced color signal. With greater energy levels (40–100 kPa, i.e. MI 0.06–0.2), if the frequency of the ultrasound waves is similar to the resonance frequency of the microbubbles of the contrast medium, the microbubbles will resonate (nonlinear or asymmetric oscillation), reflecting a series of harmonic echoes to the transducer (and in particular the preferred second harmonic, i.e. double the frequency of the transmitted ultrasound). With still higher energy levels (>500 kPa, i.e. MI>0.5) the microbubbles oscillate to the point of rupture, making possible the detection of a transitory but very wide signal produced by the rupture. In essence, the higher the energy level of the ultrasound is, the greater will be the nonlinearity of the response [139,153].

Nearly all **real time CEUS systems** exploit harmonic imaging [102,154]. With high MI systems the harmonic signals of both the tissues and the contrast medium are detected, although the former are constant and the latter only present when the microbubbles rupture. With low MI systems, the tissue harmonic signal is instead constantly minimized in favor of the contrast signal. Clearly, since the range of frequencies is very wide, the transducers used in CEUS are very different from those used in conventional US (fundamental), i.e. broadband transducers. However, the need to restrict the reception frequency bandwidth around the frequency of the second harmonic leads to an inevitable degradation in the quality of images obtained with CEUS, i.e. a loss of spatial resolution (in favor of a clear increase in contrast resolution). Since real-time systems use a lower MI and therefore stimulate the microbubbles less, the images produced will display lower contrast resolution (for the same concentration of microbubbles) than those produced with destructive systems, although this is adequately offset by the possibility of continuous image acquisition.

CEUS study in real time, which is the most widespread in clinical practice, makes use of both abdominal and superficial transducers, in both cases with a low transmit frequency. The focal zone is generally placed at 2/3 of the depth. When the focal area of interest is however already definable, the focus zone is placed immediately deep to this area. Moreover, the focal zone can be shifted to different study areas during the examination [102,154]. The gain which is generally used is medium-low and also the superficial portion of the gain-time compensation curve is set to a minimum (but only with abdominal transducers). The amplification is minimized in order to just visualize, prior to the arrival of the contrast medium, the most echoic interfaces such as the diaphragm, the vessel walls and the walls of hollow viscera like the gallbladder. Immediately after the injection of contrast medium the US exploration is performed for several minutes until the progressive extinction of the enhancement. When the contrast medium arrives in the parenchyma through the arterial vessels, the signal originating from the tissues is practically absent. The transducer is then positioned at the desired site to await the arrival of the contrast medium, which enhances first the major arteries, then the minor arteries and lastly the parenchyma with venous structures.

While intermittent systems require a systematic exploration of the various portions of the organ of interest, such as the liver, gradually shifting the transducer the whole time and without the possibility of returning to an area already examined because it would no longer be enhanced, with continuous acquisition systems a free scan of the entire parenchyma is possible, with an evaluation of the different areas from different possible approaches (ascending subcostal, epigastric, intercostals, etc.) and in the desired manner and time. Nonetheless, the examination should be performed with a slow movement of the transducer over the subject's skin and a systematic exploration of the entire organ of interest. During the examination breath-holding may be necessary or shallow calm breathing. The latter is clearly preferable when it enables an adequate exploration, but for deep-seated lesions inspiration is required. In this case the pauses in the acquisition can be used, for example between one videoclip and the next, to allow the patient to breathe freely. In the arterial phase, having the patient perform a hyperventilation in the first seconds after the injection is advisable, and then having them perform a deep and as prolonged as possible inspiration at about 10 s after injection of the contrast medium.

The use of contrast media usually occurs in a targeted manner at the level of a defined anatomic structure. When a more panoramic study is required, as in the case of certain cancers (e.g. patients with lymphoma), it should be borne in mind that the kidneys display the most intense enhancement but also the most transitory. In this sense the pancreas also displays transitory enhancement. The liver, which is nourished to a large extent by the portal venous return, displays a later and more persistent enhancement. The enhancement of the spleen is initially heterogeneous (and can simulate focality), but then becomes more intense, homogeneous and persistent. In these cases using the sequence kidneys-liver-spleen with a single injection is advisable, or subdividing the volume of contrast medium or shifting repeatedly and alternatively from one organ to another (e.g. from the liver to the spleen and vice versa in a patient with lymphoma).

Periodically and without interrupting video archiving, the operator may perform a number of **flashes** of increased MI in order to attenuate the enhancement of an area for several seconds and then evaluate the reperfusion carried out by the new enhanced blood in arrival. Immediately after having performed a flash, the operator should not shift the transducer from the area of interest. Flashes modify the tissue enhancement curve, causing a certain number of additional peaks but also causing a slightly faster fall in the curve itself associated with the destruction of a fraction of the microbubbles. The usefulness of the practice lies in the possibility of re-evaluating an area that has been poorly investigated in the first passage of contrast material. For example, when one nodule in the right hepatic lobe and another in the left hepatic lobe are identified during the baseline US study, the operator may choose to study one during the initial passage, then bring the transducer to the second nodule, perform a flash and analyze the enhancement characteristics of the latter. In addition, the operator may occasionally exit the contrast-specific module to return to the fundamental modality and examine the area of interest again [153].

Similar to what occurs in the Doppler techniques, applying excessive pressure to the skin surface should be avoided in the study of superficial structures, since this can noticeably attenuate lesion enhancement and therefore be a source of diagnostic misinterpretation.

Real-time acquisition appears to be particularly advantageous with respect to the intermittent technique in patients who are unable to maintain prolonged breath-holding and in patients in whom the site of the lesion is still unknown after the baseline study. However, it should also be noted that with many systems the exploration of deep structures can be challenging (to obviate this problem the MI can be increased towards the end of the examination once the intermediate and superficial parenchymal portions have already been adequately explored).

1.14 Contrast-Enhanced Ultrasound: Imaging Characteristics

As stated above, the first use of US contrast media was to increase the sensitivity of the scanner for slow flows. The systems of the time in fact had a limited sensitivity in the study of parenchymas and their focal lesions, and the use of contrast media effectively increased that sensitivity. However, even with contrast media CD has evident limitations, especially with regard to the possibility of only studying vessels of a particular diameter and the presence of artifacts which hinder exploration. The contrast media in fact increase the sensitivity not only for slow flows of diagnostic interest, but also for those which disturb the observer, such as those originating from the heart chambers during a study of the liver. In addition, when injected in bolus form, the contrast media produce a blooming artifact, characterized by an abundance of extravascular signal which masks the appearance of interest. This induces a slower administration of the contrast medium and the trade-off of foregoing the arterial phase, which is an extremely important moment for diagnostic purposes [155].

With regard to **spectral analysis**, the contrast medium produces an intensification of the gray-scale of the spectrum. However, with regard to the acoustics, this produces a "scratchy" sound which is graphically represented by line artifacts – spikes – on the trace (Fig. 1.70). This is due to rupture of the microbubbles or a macroaggregation of the bubbles themselves. Therefore, in order to avoid this distortion of the spectral information, the spectral analysis should be performed on a vessel of interest before the administration of contrast medium and not after [155].

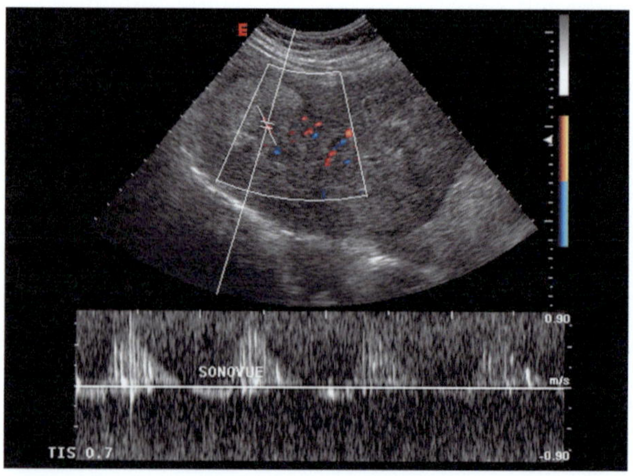

Fig. 1.70 HCC, microbubble spectral artifacts. The presence of circulating contrast medium causes a "dirty" appearance of the flowmetry trace, characterized above all by thin vertical bands (spikes)

Even though **color Doppler** is able to detect as a color signal vessels which are not identifiable per se at US, there is a limit beyond which the technique is no longer able to identify vascular structures. Where this limit lies depends on two factors: the frequency of the Doppler shift and the intensity of the echo. In order to be identified with CD (i.e. that a Doppler shift greater than the shift of tissue motion is perceived), a flow needs to be sufficiently intense and sufficiently fast. Contrast media are able to increase the former by as much as 100 times (in practice with an increase in the signal-to-noise ratio), but they are unable to resolve the latter. At the parenchymal level, in fact, the tissues move at the same speed as the blood contained in their small vessels, and are therefore associated with a Doppler shift similar to that of the vascular one. High frequencies would be required, but these cannot be used for deep parenchyma. In addition, the baseline amplitude of the tissue echo is some 10,000 times greater than that of the blood echo. Therefore the need soon became apparent to "return" to gray-scale US (CEUS), with destructive and nondestructive systems. In the former, with high MI, the microbubbles disappear as acoustic reflectors and emit an intense albeit short-lived nonlinear echo. The nondestructive systems, with low MI, are also known as perfusion US since they enable a real-time evaluation of the circulation of the microbubbles [102,154].

Real time CEUS can be used to perform not only a morphologic analysis but also a perfusion evaluation of the organs and their focal lesions. It has in fact carved out for itself a frontline role in the detection of liver metastases, in the characterization of incidentally discovered focal hepatic lesions or during tumor staging and follow-up and in the evaluation of hepatic lesions treated with interventional procedures [156–161]. At the level of the liver, which is characterized by a double circulation with around 25% originating from the hepatic artery and around 75% from the portal vein, there are **different phases of contrast medium diffusion** which have a certain amount of overlap associated with the recirculation of contrast medium and whether the operator performs any flashes. There is an early phase of arterial-dependent enhancement which begins around 15 s after the peripheral injection and ends after around 40 s. At this point there is the supply of contrast medium from the portal system, with a significant enhancement of the organ (portal-sinusoidal phase) for around 4–5 min. The possibility of detecting hepatic lesions clearly depends on the contrast gradient with respect to the background parenchyma. Hypervascular lesions are especially evident during the arterial phase, when they appear hyperechoic against the still poorly echoic background parenchyma (Fig. 1.71). Hypovascular lesions are instead identifiable above all in the parenchymal phase, when they appear evident as hypoechoic defects in the echoic parenchyma. in this sense it should be pointed out that the imaging characteristics of the lesion are not significantly influenced by the echogenicity of the background parenchyma as it appears in baseline, and therefore, for example in the setting of a fatty liver, the appearance of focal hepatic lesions is the same as seen in a healthy liver. Knowledge of the vascular models of the focal hepatic lesions, even provided by multiphase CT and MR studies, enables an effective characterization in real time, and therefore the possibility of observing the progression of the enhancement in a truly dynamic way (Fig. 1.72).

The **main CEUS patterns** in the liver are ring

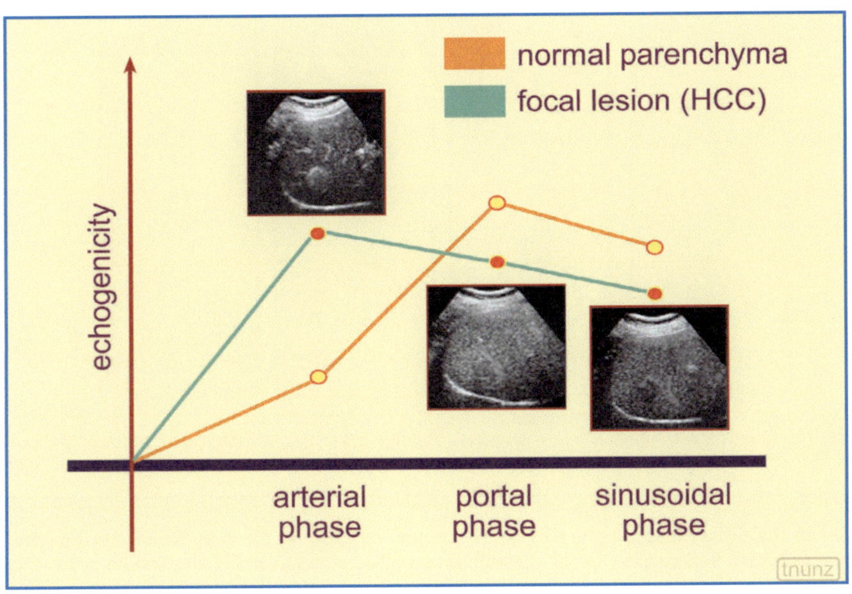

Fig. 1.71 Comparison between the enhancement curves of a hepatic lesion (*HCC*) and the healthy hepatic parenchyma. The lesion is most recognizable in the arterial phase, when there is the maximum enhancement gradient and therefore the maximum echogenicity [158]

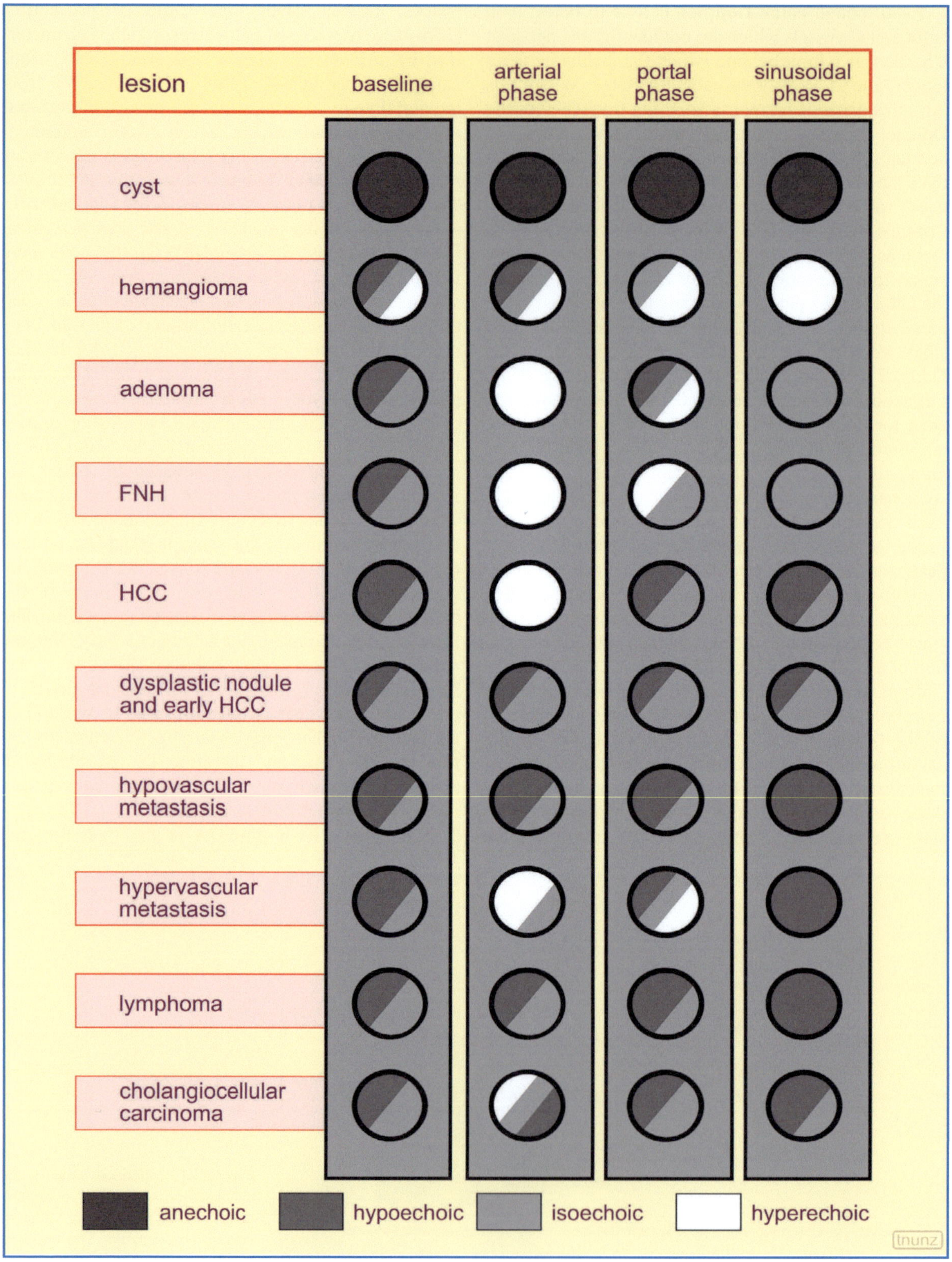

Fig. 1.72 Echogenicity of hepatic lesions in the different phases of CEUS. Tendential variation in the echogenicity of the main hepatic focal lesions: benign lesions tend to be iso-hyperechoic in the parenchymal phase, whereas malignant lesions tend to be hypoechoic

enhancement (more-or-less thick, regular and continuous ring of peripheral arterial enhancement), globular enhancement (peripheral hyperechoic areas, with centripetal development with the passing of seconds), diffuse enhancement (homogeneous or heterogeneous), spokewheel enhancement (rapid enhancement of a central area which branches towards the periphery) [153] (Figs. 1.73–1.77, Video 1.6). In the portal-sinusoidal phase, in absolutely general terms, the benign lesions tend to become (or to remain) iso- or hyperechoic, whereas a hypoechogenicity in this phase is suggestive of malignancy. A hypoechoic lesion in the portal-sinusoidal phase should be considered malignant until demonstrated otherwise, whereas a hyper- or isoechoic lesion in this phase is highly likely to be benign, or at least not metastatic [158]. The appearance of HCC is more complex, because the lesion can be hypoechoic in the portal-sinusoidal phase especially when small. In the cirrhotic liver, however, arterial hypervascularity with portal hypovascularity, and for lesions >2 cm arterial hypervascularity with any behaviour in the later phase, are indicative of malignancy [162]. The correlation with CT and MR is considerable in the arterial phase, whereas, given the intravascular nature of US contrast media, CEUS differs in the portal phase, taking on distinctive imaging characteristics [163]. It is nonetheless clear that CEUS resolves only some of the problems of conventional US – lesions which, due to their depth or overlying structures causing artifacts (e.g. intestinal gas), are little accessible or completely inaccessible at US are just as inaccessible at CEUS.

The **extrahepatic applications** of CEUS, which could provide additional information in the study of the kidneys, pancreas, spleen and other abdominal structures, are less codified. Even less defined are the superficial applications for which there are technical limitations which hamper the quality of the images obtained. Whereas the study of these structures normally takes place with high-frequency transducers which offer excellent spatial resolution, study performed with CEUS software needs to be conducted with lower frequencies which are closer to the typical resonance frequencies of currently available contrast media [162,164,165] (Video 1.7). In general, however, CEUS is able to identify even mild forms of vascularity within solid components of lesions or lesion septations or walls with a sensitivity greater than Doppler systems such as contrast-enhanced PD [98,166]. In particular, a significant indicator of malignancy is given by the presence of vascularity in the venous phase for which the lesion, still hypoechoic with respect to the surrounding parenchyma, appears teaming with internal echoes which are observable above all in real time, with an overall "salt and pepper" appearance (Fig. 1.78).

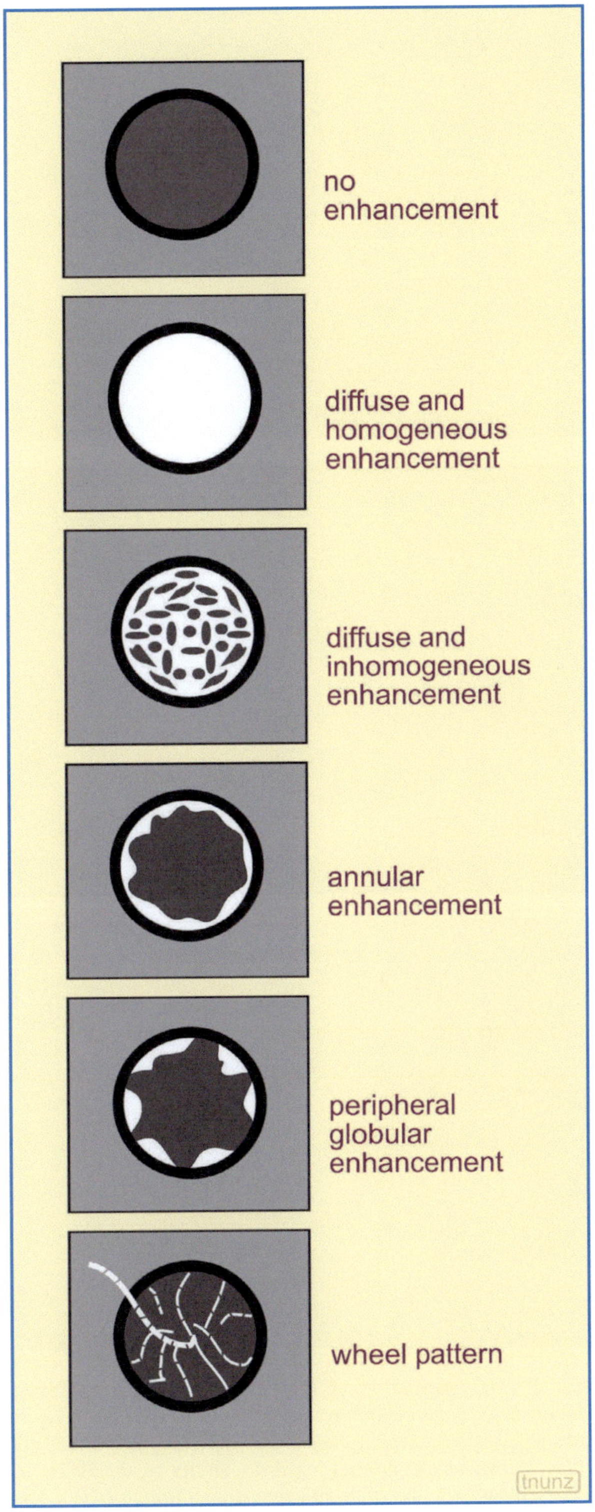

Fig. 1.73 Main CEUS patterns of hepatic lesions. Enhancement can be absent (e.g. cysts), diffuse homogeneous (e.g. adenoma and HCC), diffuse heterogeneous (e.g. HCC and metastases), ring-shaped (e.g. metastases), globular (hemangiomas) or wheel pattern (FNH). Modified from [158]

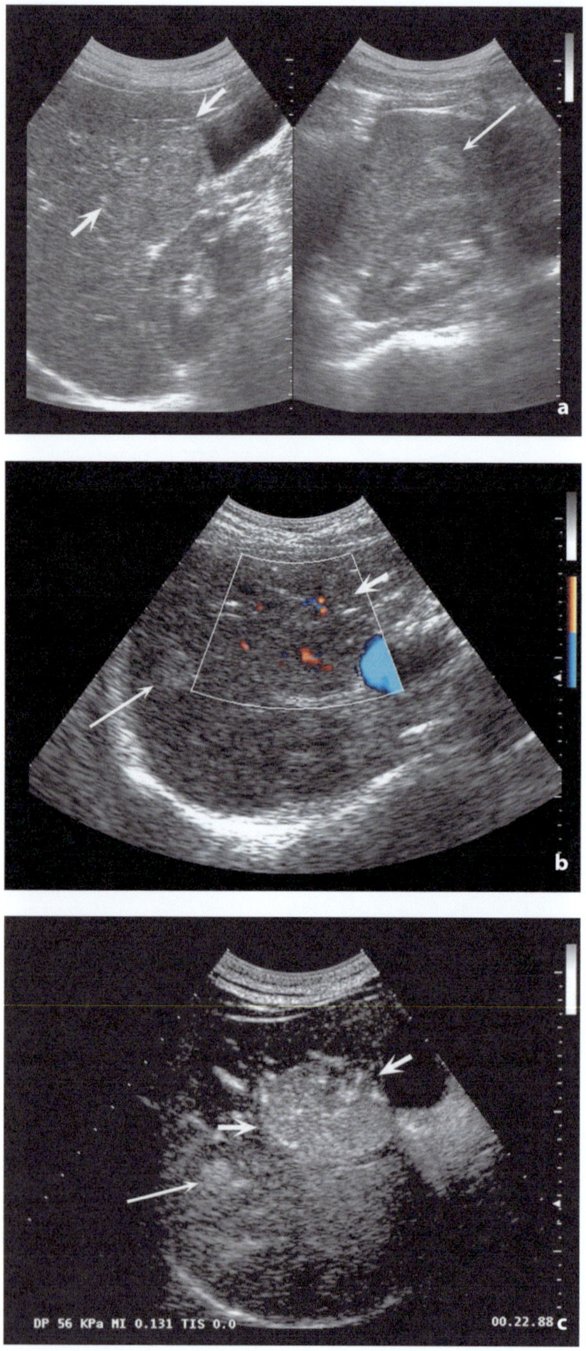

Fig. 1.74a-c Association of FNH and hepatic hemangioma. Hyperechoic angiomatous patch (**a**, *long arrow*) and area of substantial isoechogenicity (*short arrows*). The directional PD study shows central arterial hypervascularity of the FNH (**b**, *short arrow*) with the adjacent hemangioma (*long arrow*). The CEUS scan in the arterial phase (**c**) shows the vascularity of both the hemangioma (*long arrow*) and the FNH (*short arrows*), the latter with a pseudocapsular appearance and internal arterial vessels

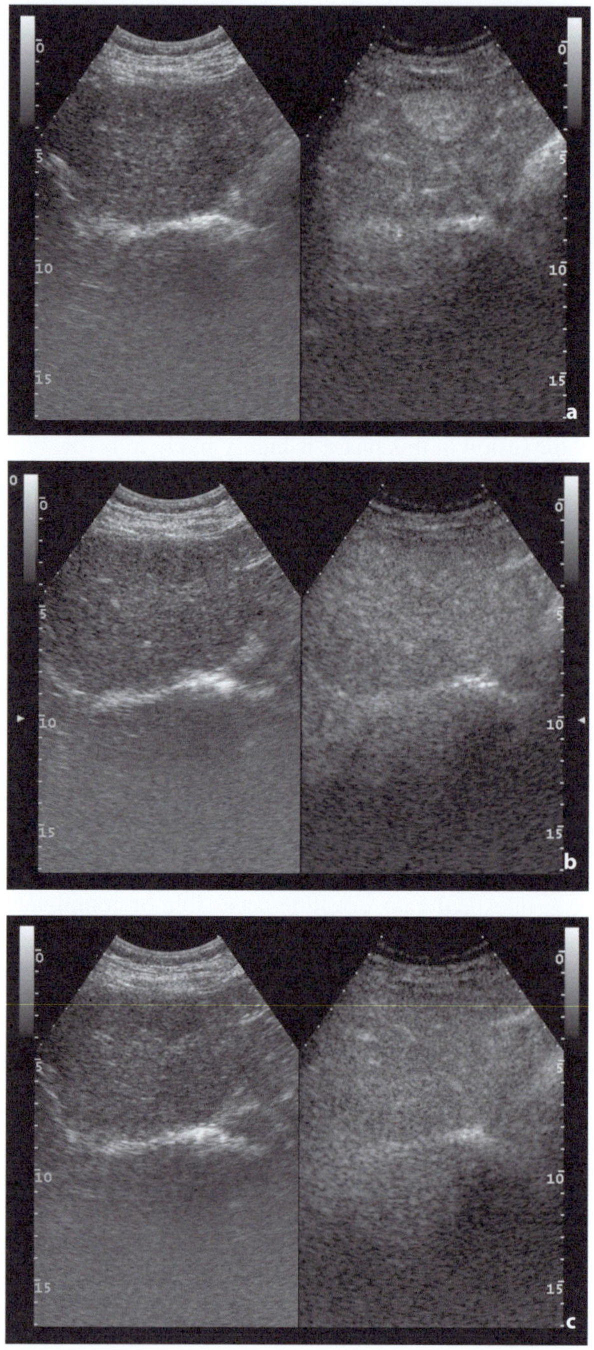

Fig. 1.75a-c FNH, CEUS appearance. The near-isoechoic liver lesion becomes intensely and homogeneously hyperechoic in the arterial phase of contrast enhancement (**a**, *right side of the double display image*). The lesion is isoechoic to the surrounding parenchyma on the portal phase scan (**b**, *right side*) and on the sinusoidal phase scan (**c**, *right side*)

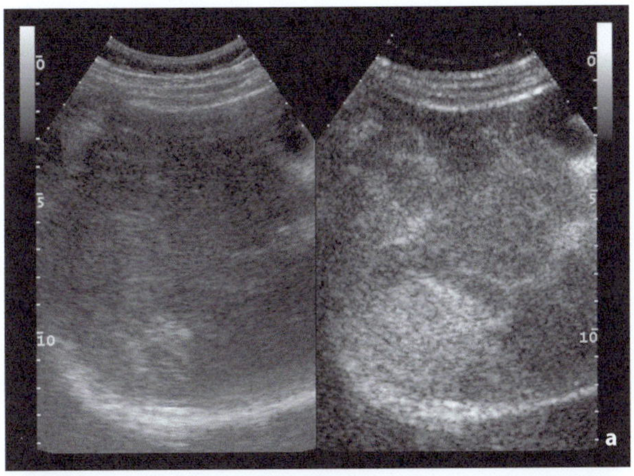

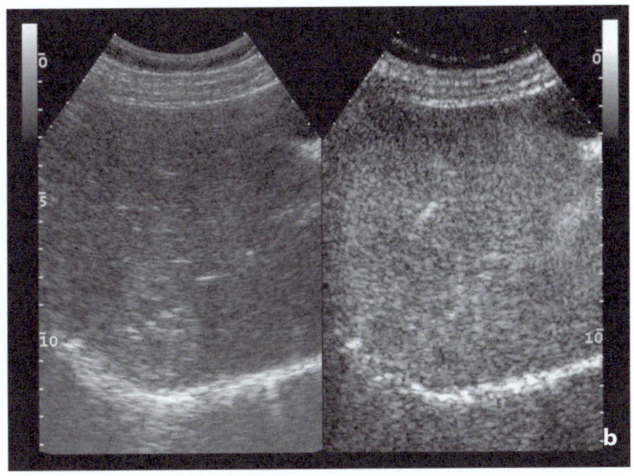

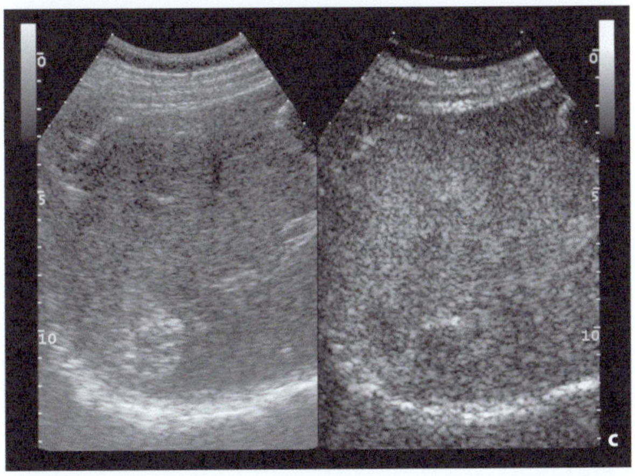

Fig. 1.76a-c HCC, CEUS appearance. The heterogeneous liver lesion becomes intensely and homogeneously hyperechoic after contrast injection (**a**, *right side of the double display image*). The lesion is near-isoechoic to the surrounding parenchyma on the portal phase scan (**b**, *right side*) and is inhomogeneously hypoechoic on the sinusoidal phase scan (**c**, *right side*)

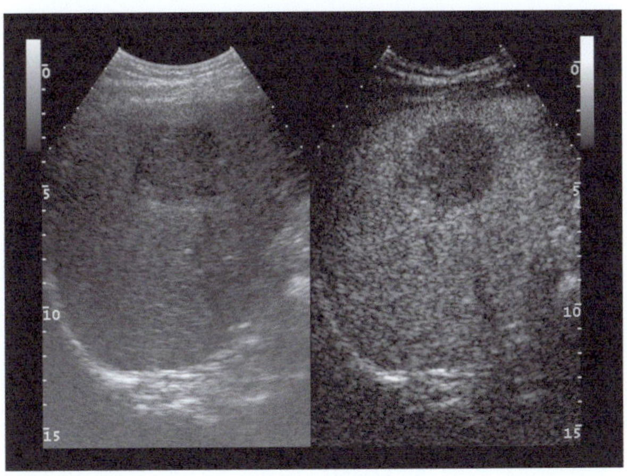

Fig. 1.77 Liver metastasis from lung cancer, CEUS appearance. The double display scans shows on the left the fundamental mode appearance of the hypoechoic lesion and on the right the simultaneous contrast-enhanced portal-phase showing the hypoechoic, dotted appearance typical of malignant (metastatic) lesions

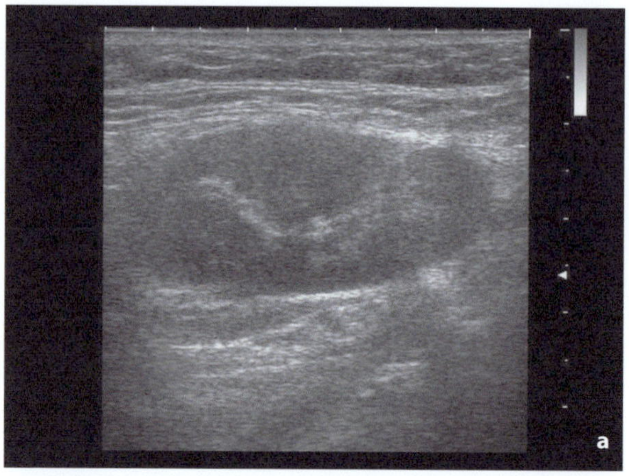

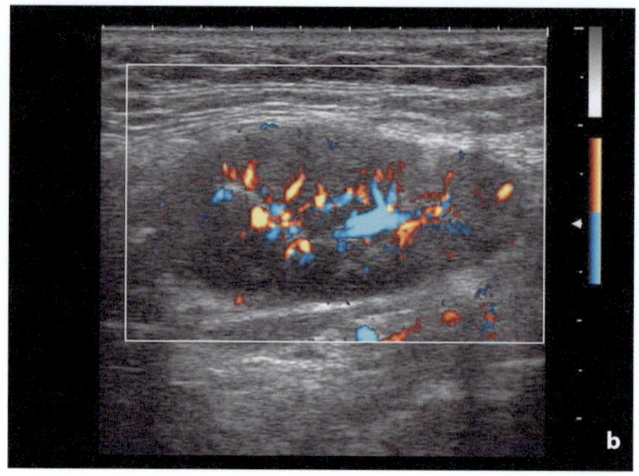

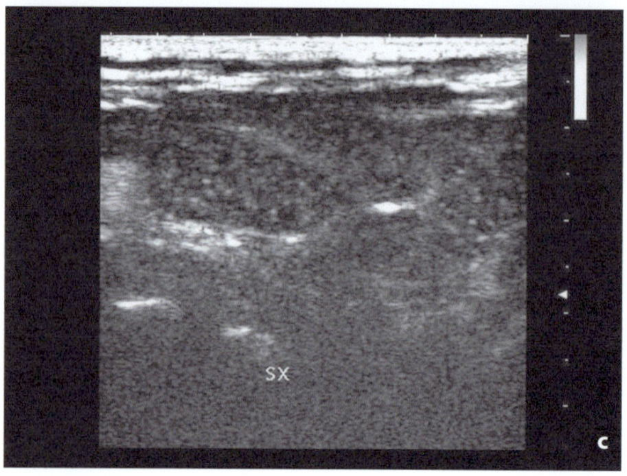

Fig. 1.78a-c Cervical lymphadenopathy from follicular lymphoma. Conspicuous lymph node with the hilum still visible but with marked cortical thickening (**a**). Directional PD shows relatively symmetrical central vascularity (**b**). CEUS highlights the typical "salt and pepper" appearance, with internal echogenic nuclei indicative of the lymph node "microcirculation" (**c**)

References

1. Belton AL et al (2003) Tumour size measurement in an oncology clinical trial: comparison between off-site and on-site measurements. Clin Radiol 58:311-314
2. Catalano O et al (2004) Ethical, deontologic, social, and economic reflections on screening with helical CT. Part I: general aspects. Radiol Med 108:299-309
3. Catalano O et al (2004) Ethic, deontologic, social, and economic reflections on screening with helical CT. Part II: specific aspects. Radiol Med 108:310-319
4. Black WC et al (1997) Screening for disease. AJR Am J Roentgenol 168:3-11
5. Herman CR et al (2002) Screening for preclinical disease. Test and disease characteristics. AJR Am J Roentgenol 179:825-831
6. Stanley RJ (2001) Inhert dangers in radiologic screening. AJR Am J Roentgenol 177:989-992
7. Obuchowski NA et al (2001) Ten criteria for effective screening: their application to multislice CT screening for pulmonary and colorectal cancers. AJR Am J Roentgenol 176:1357-1362
8. Baker SR (2003) Abdominal CT screening: inflated promises, serious concerns. AJR Am J Roentgenol 180:27-30
9. Berg WA (2004) Supplemental screening sonography in dense breasts. Radiol Clin North Am 42:845-851
10. Eden K et al (2001) Screening high-risk populations for thyroid cancer. Med Pediatr 36:583-591
11. Suehiro F (2006) Thyroid cancer detected by mass screening over a period of 16 years at a health care center in Japan. Surg Today 36:947-953
12. Park JS et al (2006) Sonographic screening for thyroid cancer in females undergoing breast sonography. AJR Am J Roentgenol 186:1025-1028
13. Kane RA et al (2003) Ultrasound of the thyroid and parathyroid glands. Controversies in the diagnosis of thyroid cancer. Ultrasound Q 19:177-178
14. Mihmanli I et al (2006) Concurrent routine breast and thyroid sonography for detection of thyroid tumors (letter). AJR Am J Roentgenol 187:W448
15. Miki H et al (1998) Value of mass screening for thyroid cancer. World J Surg 22:99-102
16. Clements R (2001) Ultrasound of prostate cancer. Eur Radiol 11:2119-2125
17. Sharma A et al (2006) Screening for gynaecological cancers. Eur J Surg Oncol 32:818-824
18. Ascher SM et al (2002) Cancer of the adnexal organs. In: Bragg DG et al (eds) Oncologic imaging. WB Saunders Company, Philadelphia, 549-574
19. Hensley ML et al (2004) Cancer screening: how good is good enough? J Clin Oncol 22:4037-4039
20. De Priest PD et al (1992) Transvaginal ultrasound screening for ovarian cancer. Clin Obstet Gynecol 35:40-44
21. Jeong et al (2000) Imaging evaluation of ovarian masses. Radiographics 20:1445-1470
22. Jacobs I et al (1993) Prevalence screening for ovarian

cancer in postmenopausal women by CA-125 measurement and ultrasonography. BMJ 306:1030-1034
23. Valenzano M et al (2001) The role of transvaginal ultrasound and sonohysterography in the diagnosis and staging of endometrial adenocarcinoma. Radiol Med 101:365-370
24. Vuento MH et al (1999) Screening for endometrial cancer in asymptomatic postmenopausal women with conventional and color Doppler sonography. Br J Obstet Gynaecol 106:14-20
25. Fleischer AC (1997) Transvaginal sonography of endometrial cancer. In: Fleischer AC et al (eds) Ultrasound and the endometrium. Parthenon Publishing Group, New York, 69-74
26. Kim B et al (2003) Testicular microlithiasis: clinical significance and review of the literature. Eur Radiol 13:2567-2576
27. de Leval J et al (1993) Testis tumor: the problem of the undescended testis. J Belge Radiol 76:100-101
28. Giwercman A et al (1989) Prevalence of carcinoma in situ and other histopatological abnormalities in the testes of men with a history of cryptorchidism. J Urol 142:998-1002
29. Miller FN et al (2007) Testicular calcification and microlithiasis: association with primary intra-testicular malignancy in 3,477 patients. Eur Radiol 17:363-369
30. Rashid HH et al (2004) Testicular microlithiasis: a review and its association with testicular cancer. Urol Oncol 22:285-289
31. Bruix J et al (2005) Management of hepatocellular carcinoma. Hepatology 42:1208-1236
32. Colombo M (2005) Natural history of hepatocellular carcinoma. Cancer Imaging 5:85-88
33. Rockall TA et al (2004) Multidisciplinary treatment for cancer: surgery, chemotherapy and radiotherapy. In: Husband JE et al (eds) Imaging in oncology. Taylor & Francis, London, 43-65
34. Sangiovanni A et al (2004) Increased survival of cirrhotic patients with a hepatocellular carcinoma detected during surveillance. Gastroenterology 126:1005-1014
35. Ren F-Y et al (2006) Efficacy of ultrasonography and alpha-fetoprotein on early detection of hepatocellular carcinoma. World J Gastroenterol 12:4656-4659
36. Arguedas MR et al (2003) Screening for hepatocellular carcinoma in patients with hepatitis C cirrhosis: a cost-utility analysis. Am J Gastroenterol 98:679-690
37. Peterson MS et al (2000) Pretransplantation surveillance for possible hepatocellular carcinoma in patients with cirrhosis: epidemiology and CT-based tumor detection rate in 430 cases with surgical-pathologic correlation. Radiology 217:743-749
38. Federle MP (2002) Use of radiologic techniques to screen for hepatocellular carcinoma. J Clin Gastroenterol 35(5 Suppl 2):92-100
39. Kubota K et al (2003) Growth rate of primary single hepatocellular carcinoma: determining optimal screening interval with contrast enhanced computed tomography. Dig Dis Sci 48:581-586
40. Majima Y (1984) Growth rate of hepatocellular carcinoma by ultrasonography and its clinical significance. Acta Hepatol Jpn 25:754-765
41. Hirata K et al (1997) Mass screening for hepatocellular carcinoma by ultrasonography. In: Gandolfi L et al (eds), Current trends in digestive ultrasonography, Karger, Basel, 17-27
42. Bennett GL et al (2002) Sonographic detection of hepatocellular carcinoma and dysplastic nodules in cirrhosis: correlation of pretransplantation sonography and liver explant pathology in 200 patients. AJR Am J Roentgenol 179:75-80
43. Dodd GD et al (1992) Detection of malignant tumors in end-stage cirrhosis livers: efficacy of sonography as a screening technique. AJR Am J Roentgenol 159:727-733
44. Liu WC et al (2003) Poor sensitivity of sonography in detection of hepatocellular carcinoma in advanced liver cirrhosis: accuracy of pretransplantation sonography in 118 patients. Eur Radiol 13:1693-1698
45. Bruix J et al (2001) Clinical management of hepatocellular carcinoma. Conclusions of the Barcelona-2000 EASL conference. European Association for the Study of the Liver. J Hepatol 35:4214-30
46. Bosniak MA et al (1995) Small renal parenchymal neoplasms: further observations on growth. Radiology 197:589-597
47. Jamis-Dow CA et al (1996) Small (≤3-cm) renal masses: detection with CT versus US and pathologic correlation. Radiology 198:785-788
48. Mihara S et al (1998) Efficacy of ultrasonic mass survey for abdominal cancer. J Med Syst 22:55-62
49. Mihara S et al (1999) Early detection of renal cell carcinoma by ultrasonographic screening. Based on the results of 13 years screening in Japan. Ultrasound Med Biol 25:1033-1039
50. Jeswani T et al (2005) Imaging tumour angiogenesis. Cancer Imaging 5:131-138
51. Nishida T (2005) Angiogenesis, which is essential for cancer growth, is a diagnostic and therapeutic target. J Gastroenterol 40:320-321
52. Kelland LR (2005) Targeting established tumor vasculature: a novel approach to cancer treatment. Curr Cancer Ther Rev 1:1-9
53. Rehman S et al (2005) Molecular imaging of antiangiogenic agents. Oncologist 10:92-103
54. Cuenod CA et al (2006) Tumor angiogenesis: pathophysiology and implications for contrast-enhanced MRI and CT assessment. Abdom Imaging 31:188-193
55. Cosgrove D (2003) Angiogenesis imaging - ultrasound. Br J Radiol 76:S43-S49
56. Anderson H et al (2001) Measuring changes in human tumour vasculature in response to therapy using functional imaging techniques. Br J Cancer 85:1085-1093
57. Forsberg F et al (2002) Comparing contrast-enhanced ultrasound to immunohistochemical markers of angiogenesis in a human melanoma xenograft model: preliminary results. Ultrasound Med Biol 28:445-451
58. Provenzale JM (2007) Imaging of angiogenesis: clinical techniques and novel imaging methods. AJR Am J Roentgenol 188:11-23
59. Ferrara KW et al (2000) Evaluation of tumor angiogenesis with US: imaging, Doppler, and contrast agents. Acad Radiol 7:824-839
60. Delorme S et al (2006) Contrast-enhanced ultrasound for examining tumor biology. Cancer Imaging 6:148-152
61. Kruskal JB et al (2006) Will improved assessment of response to antiangiogenic therapies be achieved with contrast-enhanced gray-scale US? Radiology 240:1-2
62. Cosgrove D (2003) Angiogenesis imaging–ultrasound. Br J Radiol 76:S43-S49

63. Blomley MJ et al (1998) Liver vascular transit time analyzed with dynamic hepatic venography with bolus injections of a US contrast agent: early experience in seven patients with metastases. Radiology 209:862-866
64. Donnelly EF et al (2001) Quantified power Doppler US of tumor blood flow correlates with microscopic quantification of tumor blood vessels. Radiology 219:166-170
65. Schroeder RJ et al (2001) Tumor vascularization in experimental melanomas: correlation between unenhanced and contrast enhanced power Doppler imaging and histological grading. Ultrasound Med Biol 27:761-771
66. Lassau N et al (2006a) Gastrointestinal stromal tumors treated with Imatinib: monitoring response with contrast-enhanced sonography. AJR Am J Roentgenol 187:1267-1273
67. Lucidarme O et al (2004) Angiogenesis model for ultrasound contrast research: exploratory study. Acad Radiol 11:4-12
68. Pollard RE et al (2002) Contrast-assisted destruction-replenishment ultrasound for the assessment of tumor microvasculature in a rate model. Technol Cancer Res Treat 1:459-470
69. Fleischer AC et al (2008) Contrast-enhanced transvaginal sonography of benign versus malignant ovarian masses: preliminary findings. J Ultrasound Med 27:1011-1018
70. Li J et al (2005) Time-intensity-based quantification of vascularity with single-level dynamic contrast-enhanced ultrasonography. A pilot animal study. J Ultrasound Med 24:975-983
71. Rubaltelli L et al (2007) Automated quantitative evaluation of lymph node perfusion on contrast-enhanced sonography. AJR Am J Roentgenol 188:977-983
72. Du J et al (2008) Correlation of real-time gray scale contrast-enhanced ultrasonography with microvessel density and vascular endothelial growth factor expression for assessment of angiogenesis in breast lesions. J Ultrasound Med 27:821-831
73. McCarville MB et al (2006) Angiogenesis inhibitors in a murine neuroblastoma model: quantitative assessment of intratumoral blood flow with contrast-enhanced gray-scale US. Radiology 240:73-81
74. Krix M et al (2003) Sensitive noninvasive monitoring of tumor perfusion during antiangiogenic therapy by intermittent bolus-contrast power Doppler sonography. Cancer Res 63:8264-8270
75. Galiè M et al (2005) Tumor vessel compression hinders perfusion of ultrasonographic contrast agents. Neoplasia 7:528-536
76. Lindner JR (2004) Molecular imaging with contrast ultrasound and targeted microbubbles. J Nucl Cardiol 11:215-221
77. Neal AJ (2004) Staging of cancer. In: Husband JE et al (eds) Imaging in oncology. Taylor & Francis, London, 31-41
78. Wittekind Ch et al (2005) TNM atlas. Springer-Verlag Berlin.
79. Ferrozzi F et al (2002) Structural changes induced by antineoplastic therapies: keys to evaluate tumor response to treatment. Eur Radiol 12:928-937
80. Husband JE (1996) Monitoring tumor response. Eur Radiol 6:775-785
81. Lagalla R et al (1998b) Monitoring treatment response with color and power Doppler. Eur J Radiol 28:149-156
82. MacVicar D et al (1997) Assessment of response following treatment for malignant disease. Br J Radiol 70:41-49
83. Miller AB et al (1981) Reporting results of cancer treatment. Cancer 47:207-214
84. Therasse P et al (2000) New guidelines to evaluate the response to treatment in solid tumors. J Natl Cancer Inst 92:205-216
85. Therasse P et al (2006) RECIST revisited: a review of validation studies on tumour assessment. Eur J Cancer 42:1031-1039
86. Park SH et al (2004) Volumetric tumor measurement using three-dimensional ultrasound: in vitro phantom study on measurement accuracy under various scanning condition. Ultrasound Med Biol 30:27-34
87. Bellomi M et al (2004) Evaluation of the response to therapy of neoplastic lesions. Radiol Med 107:450-458
88. Ollivier L et al (2002) Monitoring tumor response. Cancer Imaging 3:5-6
89. Prasad SR et al (2003a) Radiological evaluation of oncologic treatment response: current update. Cancer Imaging 3:93-95
90. Catalano O et al (1999) Hepatocellular carcinoma treated with chemoembolization: assessment with contrast-enhanced Doppler ultrasonography. Cardiovasc Intervent Radiol 22:486-492
91. Gee MS et al (2001) Doppler ultrasound imaging detects changes in tumor perfusion during antivascular therapy associated with vascular anatomic alterations. Cancer Res 61:2974-2982
92. Miller JC et al (2005) Imaging angiogenesis: applications and potential for drug development. J Natl Cancer Inst 97:172-187
93. De Giorgi U et al (2005) Effect of angiosonography to monitor response during Imatinib treatment in patients with metastatic gastrointestinal stromal tumors. Clin Cancer Res 11:6171-6176
94. Krix M (2005) Quantification of enhancement in contrast ultrasound: a tool for monitoring of therapies in liver metastases. Eur Radiol 15(Suppl 5):104-108
95. Giovagnoni A et al (2005) Evidence Based Medicine (EBM) and Evidence Based Radiology (EBR) in the follow-up of the patients after surgery for lung and colon-rectal carcinoma. Radiol Med 109:345-357
96. Liberati A et al (1997) Assessing the effectiveness of follow-up care for colorectal cancer: a great conceptual and methodological challenge for clinical oncology. Ann Oncol 8:1059-1062
97. Puylaert JB (1986) Acute appendicitis: US evaluation using graded compression. Radiology 158:355-360
98. Testa AC et al (2005) The use of contrasted transvaginal sonography in the diagnosis of gynecologic diseases. A preliminary study. J Ultrasound Med 24:1267-1278
99. Menzel J et al (2000) Gastrointestinal miniprobe sonography: the current status. Am J Gastroenterol 95:605-616
100. Harvey CJ et al (2002) Advances in ultrasound. Clin Radiol 57:157-177
101. Madrazo BL et al (2000) Doppler imaging. In: Shirkhoda A (ed) Variants and pitfalls in body imaging. Lippincott Williams & Wilkins, Philadelphia, 455-473
102. Lencioni R et al (2002) Tissue harmonic and contrast-specific imaging: back to gray scale in ultrasound. Eur Radiol 12:151-165
103. Szopinski KT et al (2003) Tissue harmonic imaging. Utility in breast sonography. J Ultrasound Med 22:479-487

104. Cha JH et al (2007) Characterization of benign and malignant solid breast masses: comparison of conventional US and tissue harmonic imaging. Radiology 242:63-69
105. Desser TS et al (2000) Native tissue harmonic imaging: basic principles and clinical applications. Ultrasound Q 16:40-48
106. Rosenthal SJ et al (2001) Phase inversion tissue harmonic sonographic imaging: a clinical utility study. AJR Am J Roentgenol 176:1393-1398
107. Entrekin RR et al (2001) Real-time spatial compound imaging: application to breast, vascular, and musculoskeletal ultrasound. Semin Ultrasound CT MR 22:50-64
108. Oktar SÖ et al (2003) Comparison of conventional sonography, real-time compound sonography, tissue harmonic sonography, and tissue harmonic compound sonography of abdominal and pelvic lesions. AJR Am J Roentgenol 181:1341-1347
109. Mehta TS (2003) Current uses of ultrasound in the evaluation of the breast. Radiol Clin North Am 41:841-856
110. Kim SE et al (2003) Extended field-of-view sonography. Advantages in abdominal applications. J Ultrasound Med 22:385-394
111. Henrich W et al (2002) Transvaginal and transabdominal extended field-of-view (EFOV) and power Doppler EFOV sonography in gynecology. Advantages and applications. J Ultrasound Med 21:1137-1144
112. Ying M et al (2006) Reliability of 3-D ultrasound measurements of cervical lymph node volume. Ultrasound Med Biol 32:995-1001
113. Bega G et al (2003) Three-dimensional ultrasonography in gynecology. Technical aspects and clinical applications. J Ultrasound Med 22:1249-1269
114. Lyshchik A et al (2004) Three-dimensional ultrasonography for volume measurement of thyroid nodules in children. J Ultrasound Med 23:247-254
115. Alam F et al (2008) Accuracy of sonographic elastography in the differential diagnosis of enlarged cervical lymph nodes: comparison with conventional B-mode sonography. AJR Am J Roentgenol 191:604 -610
116. Giuseppetti GM et al (2005) Elastosonography in the diagnosis of the nodular breast lesions: preliminary report. Radiol Med 110:69-76
117. Zhi H et al (2007) Comparison of ultrasound elastography, mammography, and sonography in the diagnosis of solid breast lesions. J Ultrasound Med 26:807-815
118. Wachsberg RH (2003) B-flow, a non-Doppler technology for flow mapping: early experience in the abdomen. Ultrasound Q 19:114-122
119. Youk JK et al (2005) Focal fibrosis of the breast diagnosed by a sonographically guided core biopsy of nonpalpable lesions. Imaging findings and clinical relevance. J Ultrasound Med 24:1377-1384
120. Konno K et al (2001) Liver tumors in fatty liver: difficulty in ultrasonographic interpretation. Abdom Imaging 26:487-491
121. Riccabona M et al (1995) Distance and volume measurement using three-dimensional ultrasonography. J Ultrasound Med 14:881-886
122. Nishino M et al (2003) Primary retroperitoneal neoplasms: CT and MR imaging findings with anatomic and pathologic diagnostic clues. Radiographics 23:45-57
123. Moody AR et al (1993) Atypical hepatic hemangioma: a suggestive sonographic morphology. Radiology 188:413-417
124. Blachar A et al (2002) Hepatic capsular retraction: spectrum of benign and malignant etiologies. Abdom Imaging 27:690-699
125. Middleton WD (1998) Color Doppler. Image interpretation and optimization. Ultrasound Q 14:194-208
126. Taylor KJ (1995) Pulse Doppler and color flow of tumors. In: Taylor KJW et al (eds) Clinical applications of Doppler ultrasound. Raven Press, New York, 355-366
127. Grenier N et al (2001) Interpretation of Doppler signals. Eur Radiol 11:1295-1307
128. Hata K et al (2002) Prognostic significance of ultrasound derived peak systolic velocity in epithelial ovarian cancer. Ultrasound Obstet Gynecol 20:186-191
129. Kaushik S et al (2003) Spectral Doppler sonography of musculoskeletal soft tissue masses. J Ultrasound Med 22:1333-1336
130. del Cura JL et al (2005) The use of unenhanced Doppler sonography in the evaluation of solid breast lesions. AJR Am J Roentgenol 184:1788-1794
131. Özdemir A et al (2001) Differential diagnosis of solid breast lesions. J Ultrasound Med 20:1091-1101
132. Bodner G et al (2002) Differentiation of malignant and benign musculoskeletal tumors: combined color and power Doppler US and spectral wave analysis. Radiology 223:410-416
133. Schick S et al (1998) Differentiation of benign and malignant tumors of the parotid gland: value of pulsed Doppler and color Doppler sonography. Eur Radiol 8:1462-1467
134. Hata K et al (1995) Intratumoral peak systolic velocity as a new possible predictor for detection of adnexal malignancy. Am J Obstet Gynecol 172:1496-1500
135. Brnić Z et al (2003) Usefulness of Doppler waveform analysis in differential diagnosis of cervical lymphadenopathy. Eur Radiol 13:175-180
136. Peters-Engl C et al (1999) Tumor flow in malignant breast tumors measured by Doppler ultrasound: an independent predictor of survival. Breast Cancer Res Treat 54:65-71
137. Kubota K et al (2000) Evaluation of the intratumoral vasculature of hepatocellular carcinoma by power Doppler sonography: advantages and disadvantages versus conventional color Doppler sonography. Abdom Imaging 25:172-178
138. Schroeder RJ et al (2003) Role of power Doppler techniques and ultrasound contrast enhancement in the differential diagnosis of focal breast lesions. Eur Radiol 13:68-79
139. Quaia E (2005) Contrast media in ultrasonography. Basic principles and clinical applications. Springer, Berlin
140. Wilson WD et al (2006) Sonographic quantification of ovarian tumor vascularity. J Ultrasound Med 25:1577-1581
141. Epstein E et al (2002) An algorithm including results of gray-scale and power Doppler ultrasound examination to predict endometrial malignancy in women with postmenopausal bleeding. Ultrasound Obstet Gynecol 20:370-376
142. De Marchi A et al (2002) A preliminary experience in the study of soft tissue superficial masses: color Doppler US and wash-in and wash-out curves with contrast media compared to histological results. Radiol Med 104:451-458
143. Numata K et al (1997) Use of hepatic tumor index on color Doppler sonography for differentiating large hepatic

tumors. AJR Am J Roentgenol 168:991-995
144. Jeffrey RB et al (1995) Sonography of the abdomen. Raven Press, New York
145. Tanaka S et al (1990) Color-Doppler imaging of liver tumors. AJR Am J Roentgenol 154:509-514
146. Bartolozzi C et al (2001) Contrast-specific ultrasound imaging of focal liver lesions. Prologue to a promising future. Eur Radiol 11(Suppl 3):13-14
147. Harvey CJ et al (2001) Developments in ultrasound contrast media. Eur Radiol 11:675-689
148. Liu J-B et al (2008) Contrast-enhanced ultrasound imaging. In: McGahan JP et al (eds) Diagnostic ultrasound, II edition. Informa Healthcare, New York, 39-62
149. Correas J-M et al (2001) Ultrasound contrast agents: properties, principles of action, tolerance, and artifacts. Eur Radiol 11:1316-1328
150. Piscaglia F et al (2006) The safety of SonoVue® in abdominal applications: retrospective analysis of 23188 investigations. Ultrasound Med Biol 32:1369-1375
151. Forsberg F et al (1999) Tissue-specific US contrast agent for evaluation of hepatic and splenic parenchyma. Radiology 210:125-132
152. Numata K et al (2008) Ablation therapy guided by contrast-enhanced sonography with sonazoid for hepatocellular carcinoma lesions not detected by conventional sonography. J Ultrasound Med 27:395-406
153. Catalano O et al (2007b) Terminology for contrast-enhanced sonography: a practical glossary. J Ultrasound Med 26:717–730
154. Bauer A et al (2002) Ultrasound imaging with SonoVue: low mechanical index real-time imaging. Acad Radiol 9(Suppl 1):282-284
155. Forsberg F et al (1994) Artifacts in ultrasonic contrast agent studies. J Ultrasound Med 13:357-365
156. Chami L et al (2007) Benefits of contrast-enhanced sonography for the detection of liver lesions: comparison with histologic findings. AJR Am J Roentgenol 190:683-690
157. Claudon M et al (2008) Guidelines and good clinical practice recommendations for contrast enhanced ultrasound (CEUS) - update 2008. Ultraschall Med 29:28-44
158. Catalano O et al (2005a) Real-time harmonic contrast material-specific US of focal liver lesions. Radiographics 25:333-349
159. Isozaki T et al (2003) Differential diagnosis of hepatic tumors by using contrast enhancement patterns at US. Radiology 229:798-805
160. Minami Y et al (2004) Treatment of hepatocellular carcinoma with radiofrequency ablation: usefulness of contrast harmonic sonography for lesions poorly defined with B-mode sonography. AJR Am J Roentgenol 183:153-156
161. Solbiati L et al (1997) Hepatic metastases: percutaneous radiofrequency ablation with cooled-tip electrodes. Radiology 205:367-373
162. Quaia E et al (2007) Diagnostic value of hepatocellular nodule vascularity after microbubble injection for characterizing malignancy in patients with cirrhosis. AJR Am J Roentgenol 189:1474-1483
163. Burns PN et al (2007) Focal liver masses: enhancement patterns of contrast-enhanced images–concordance of US scans with CT scans and MR images. Radiology 242:162-174
164. Catalano O et al (2006a) Contrast-enhanced sonography of the spleen. Semin Ultrasound CT and MRI 27:426-433
165. Thorelius L (2003) Contrast-enhanced ultrasound: beyond the liver. Eur Radiol 13(Suppl 3):91-108
166. Robbin ML et al (2003) Renal imaging with ultrasound contrast: current status. Radiol Clin North Am 41:963-978

2 Superficial Soft Tissues

2.1 Skin Tumors

The study of primary and secondary skin lesions requires high- or very high-frequency transducers (>13 MHz, better if >16 MHz), multifrequency transducers when available and the possible use of spacers. The availability of matrix array transducers can also be of significant use. In high-resolution study, the different layers of the skin can be identified: the epidermis appears hyperechoic (0.3–0.6 mm thick), the dermis echogenic although less so than the epidermis, with hypo-anechoic areas in its deep portion (1–4 mm thick), the subcutaneous layer with hypoechoic adipose lobules and thin (5–20 mm) echogenic fibrous shoots in between and the echogenic superficial fascia which separates the cutaneous tissue from the underlying muscle [1].

Skin lesions should be evaluated in multiple scan planes, taking care not to apply excessive compression with the transducer. Although US is unable to distinguish with certainty between benign and malignant skin lesions, it does play an important role in the noninvasive definition of lesion thickness, which constitutes an important element for the treatment planning of melanomas in particular. Malignant skin lesions generally appear with irregular margins, heterogeneous echotexture with possible necrotic hypo-anechoic areas and intralesional vascular signals indicating neoangiogenesis. High-resolution US has demonstrated sensitivity and specificity of 100% in differentiating between melanomas/nevi and other lesions, and sensitivity of 100% but specificity of 32% in the distinction between melanomas and nonmelanomatous lesions [2,3].

Epitheliomas display a heterogeneous hypoechoic structure, occasionally with fibrosclerotic echogenic components or hypo-anechoic areas (Fig. 2.1). In the spinocellular form in particular the deep margin of the lesion may be irregular due to infiltration. On CD images basal cell carcinoma shows at the most a slight peripheral vascular signal, whereas spinocellular carcinoma usually displays mixed flows, both central and peripheral, which constitutes a significant indicator of malignancy (sensitivity 88%, specificity 63%) [4]. In addition to melanoma, described below, other skin tumors and pseudotumoral skin lesions should be included in the differential diagnosis: sebaceous cysts, pilomatrixomas, nevi, hemangiomas, vascular anomalies, lymphomas, foreign body granulomas, Kaposi sarcoma and tissue scarring [1].

Malignant melanoma is a relatively frequent tumor whose incidence, although varying in different geographical regions, has nonetheless undergone a rapid increase in recent decades (Figs. 2.2, 2.3). On US images the lesion appears oval-shaped or elongated and relatively hypoechoic with the echogenic epidermal surface conserved (except in the ulcerated or verrucous forms) [1,3] (Fig. 2.4). The deep margin of melanoma is generally sharp, occasionally with

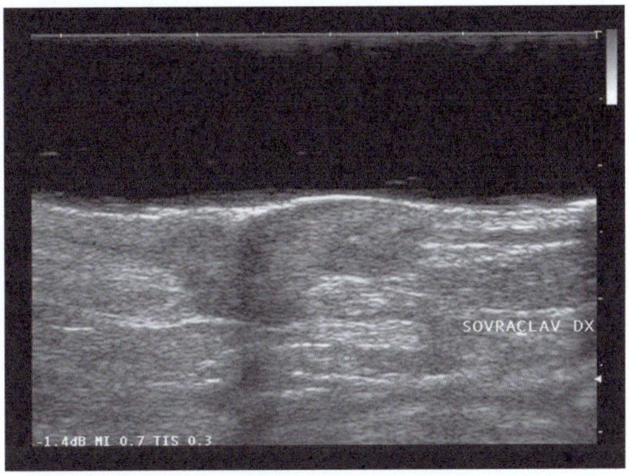

Fig. 2.1 Epithelioma. Hypoechoic, marked thickening of the soft tissue at the base of the neck

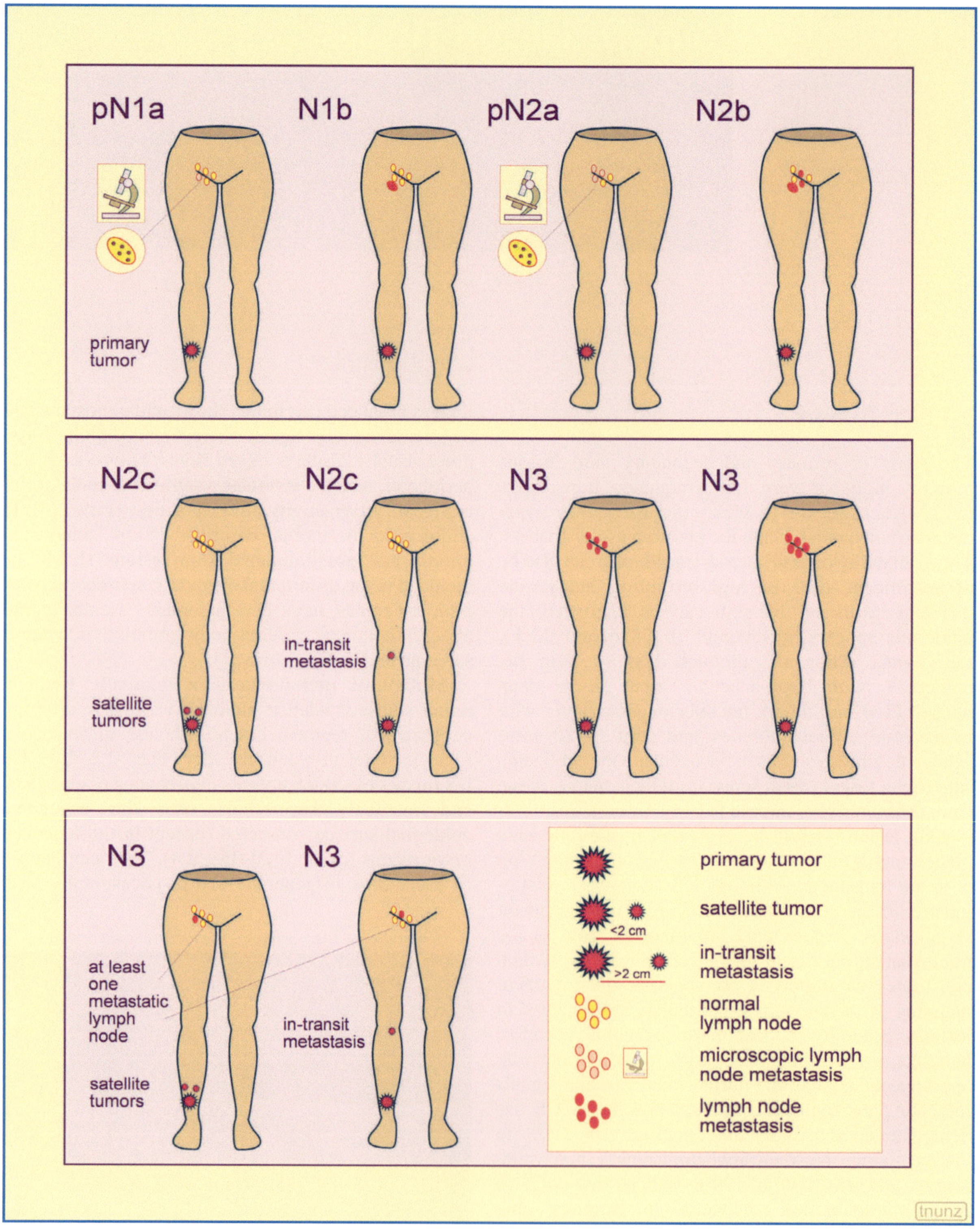

Fig. 2.2 TNM staging system for malignant cutaneous melanoma. Adapted from [5]

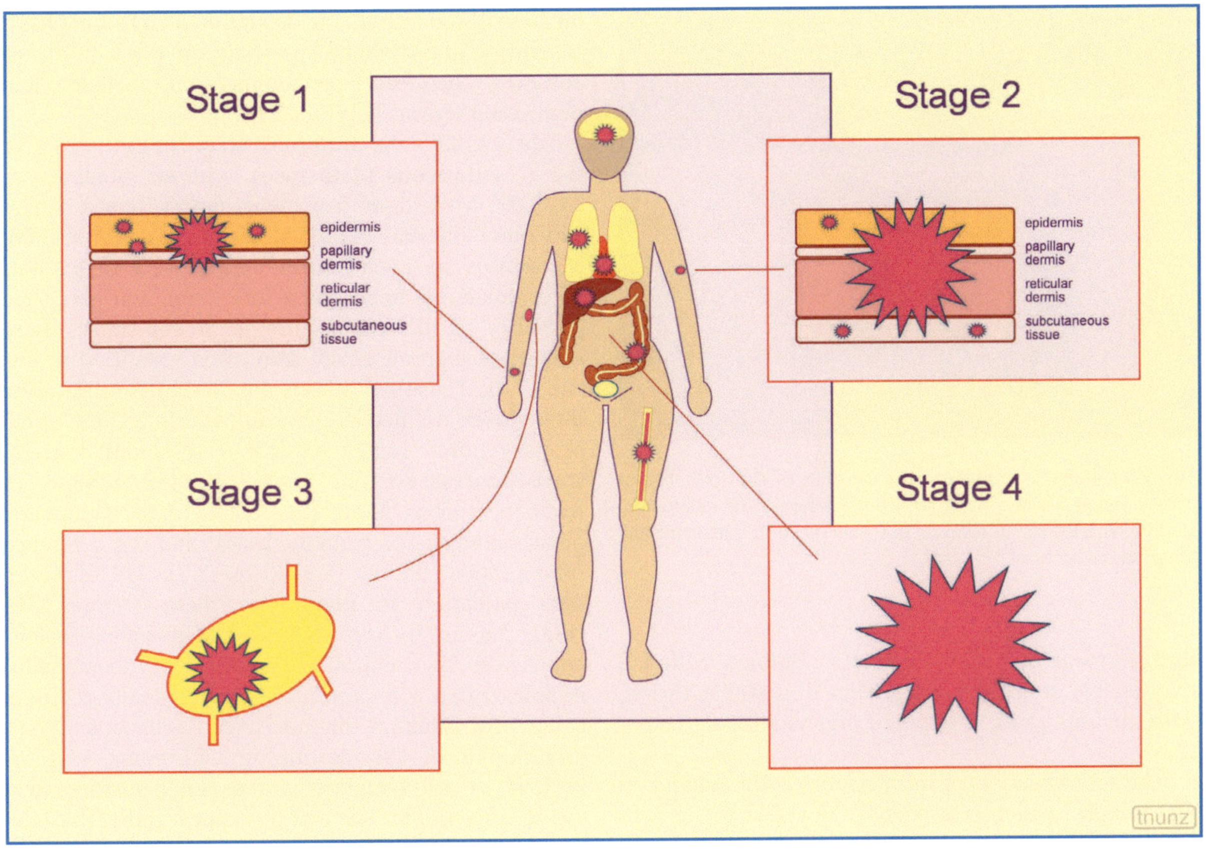

Fig. 2.3 Grouped stages for malignant melanoma

enhanced through-transmission. At this level there may be an inflammatory-reactive infiltrate which also appears hypoechoic and is therefore indistinguishable from the lesion itself, even when the lesion thickness is measured. Similar overestimations of the size of the lesion may be induced by hypoechoic hair follicles. Measurement of the thickness of the melanoma is in fact a crucial parameter in the management and formulation of the prognosis of the disease. The thickness measured histologically (Breslow index, which includes four classes) correlates with the probability of lymph node metastasis (2–5% per lesion <0.76 mm thick but 62% for lesions >4 mm), as well as the risk of distant metastases (2–5% for lesions <0.76 mm thick but 72% for lesions >4 mm). The **thickness of the melanoma** measured at US does not directly correspond with the histologic measurement, due to the loss of tension and dehydration that the excised material undergoes and the histologic ability to distinguish between tumor and reactive tissue. Nonetheless the vertical US thickness correlates with the Breslow index (up to 96% correlation coefficient) and can therefore have marked practical impact. Normally the

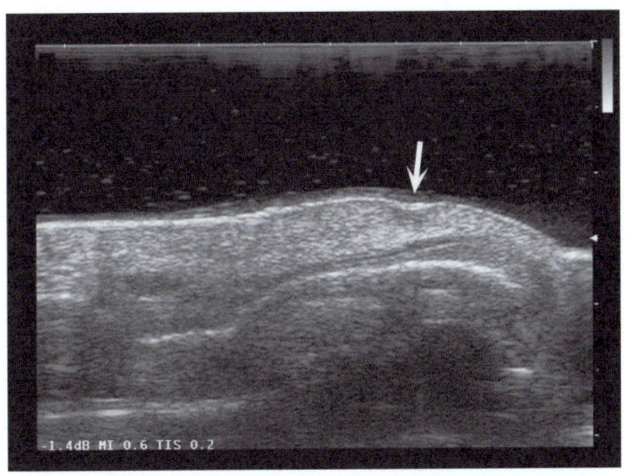

Fig. 2.4 Melanoma of the nose. Hypoechoic lesion with ulcerated surface (*arrow*) corresponding to the nasal ala

lesion suspected to be melanoma is resected, the thickness is measured and then the resection margins may be broadened and investigations may be carried out on the "sentinel lymph node" (Fig. 2.5). The preoperative

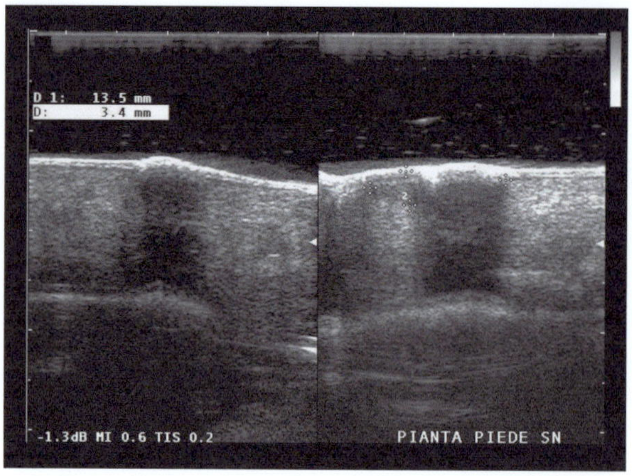

Fig. 2.5 Cutaneous melanoma of the sole of the foot. Hypoechoic lesion 3.4 mm thick with posterior acoustic shadowing studied with the use of a spacer and visualized in transverse and longitudinal sections

measurement of tumor thickness obtained with US may enable surgical management in a single sitting, with obvious gains in terms of organization and costs [2,6].

The identification of intralesional color signals on **CD** images, which is especially possible for lesions >2 mm thick, may also be of considerable importance, being correlated with the Breslow index and therefore survival. In a study on five-year recurrence rate, the most significant indicators proved to be the Breslow index, the presence of tumor ulceration, the state of the lymph nodes, the US thickness and the presence of neoangiogenesis at CD [1,6]. Flows are identified above all in lesions with larger vessels and greater microvascular density and can be found especially at the base of the lesion. The detection of CD signal has a sensitivity of 34% but a specificity of 100% in differentiating between melanomas and other skin pigmented lesions [2] (Fig. 2.6).

Melanoma is the third most frequent tumor to give rise to **cutaneous metastases**, with an incidence of 24–32%. Metastases from lung cancer, breast cancer and other internal malignancies are not uncommon. Metastases are even encountered in 10% of patients with melanoma undergoing follow-up, and given the partiality of melanomas for the lower limbs, these cutaneous metastases are also often identified at this site [7,8]. These metastases are classified as **satellite metastases**, defined as occurring within 2–3 cm of the primary tumor (or of its scar if resected), and **in-transit metastases**, i.e. lesions located at >2–3 cm from the tumor, along the course of the lymphatic ducts between the primary lesion and the reference lymph node station [8,9] (Fig. 2.7). US is better than palpation in identifying these lesions [10] (Figs. 2.8–2.10). Both satellite and in-transit lesions appear on US images as hypoechoic subcutaneous nodules, often with particularly low and almost absent echoes (differential diagnosis with sebaceous cysts, granulomas of various etiology, fibromas, neurofibromas, B-cell lymphomas and small postoperative cystic collections). The margins appear rather irregular or plainly polycyclic, the size is generally <20 mm, and enhanced through-transmission is possible (70% of cases) [7,11–13]. Only 6% of cases, in contrast, display a hyperechoic structure [7,11,13]. These lesions can be solitary or multiple, typically distributed in a line along the same lymphatic vessel, with the largest lesion situated closest to the surgical scar [8]. The location along a lymphatic vessel can occasionally be deduced by the presence of two thin hypoechoic

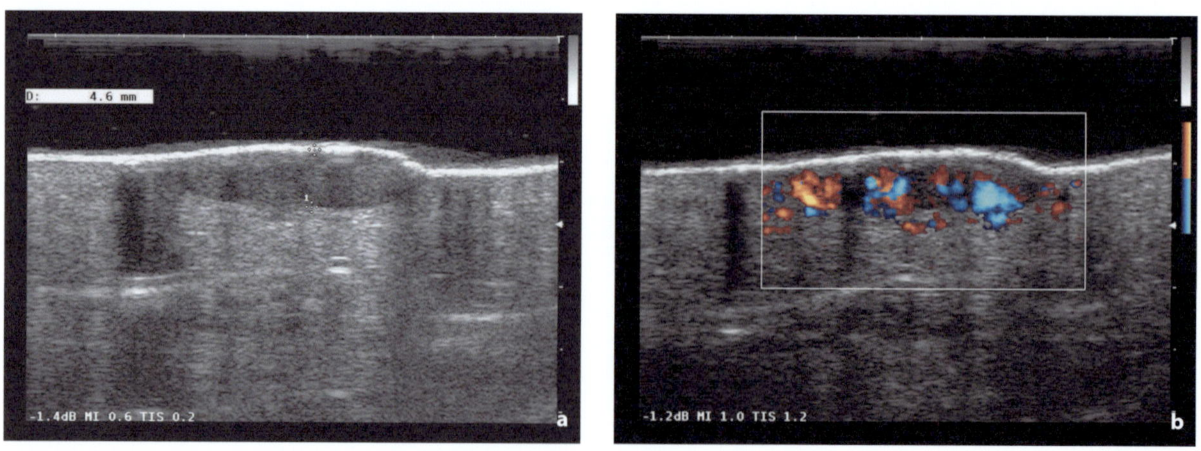

Fig. 2.6a,b Melanoma developing from congenital nevus of the foot. Marked hypoechoic oval-shaped thickening (**a**) which appears characterized by diffuse and intense hypervascularity at directional PD (**b**)

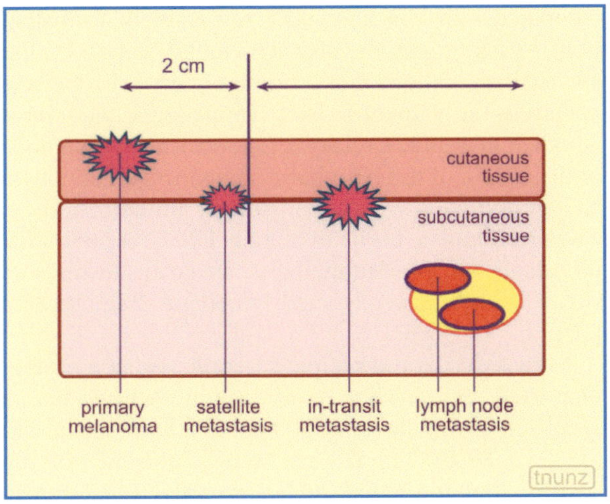

Fig. 2.7 Locoregional spread of malignant cutaneous melanoma. Satellite lesions are within 2 cm of the primary tumor. In-transit lesions are located more than 2 cm from the melanoma

bands visible on the two sides opposite the subcutaneous nodule, which is an expression of the collector full of lymph and/or tumor cells. Vascular signals on **CD** images are found in 70% of metastatic lesions, especially in the larger masses (100% of those >11 mm) [7,14]. At times, the signals are of limited extent, in the form of a single vascular pole, while at others they display a highly vascular lesion with multiple vascular poles and various intranodular vessels. At any rate the vascularity is decidedly useful for the purposes of differential diagnosis, since benign subcutaneous lesions generally show no color signal. Confirmation can be given by FNAC with 23 G needles, with two samples taken for each nodule [8,15].

Periodic US **follow-up** of patients operated on for malignant melanoma performed six-monthly or annually (or even every three months in at-risk patients) should include the excision site [covering an area of some 10 cm surrounding the site, especially in the direction of the reference lymph node station(s)], for the purposes of identifying recurrences in the surgical scar, as well as satellite and in-transit nodules [16] (Fig. 2.11). As stated above, the finding of hypoechoic nodules with vascular signals is highly suspicious of tumor recurrence. CD is particularly useful for distinguishing recurrences in the scar from avascular scar tissue. Follow-up should also include an exploration of the reference lymph node stations. This usually involves the inguinal regions of both sides for melanomas of the lower limbs, the axillary lymph nodes for melanomas of the upper limbs, the axillary, supraclavicular and cervical lymph nodes for melanomas of the head and neck and axillary and

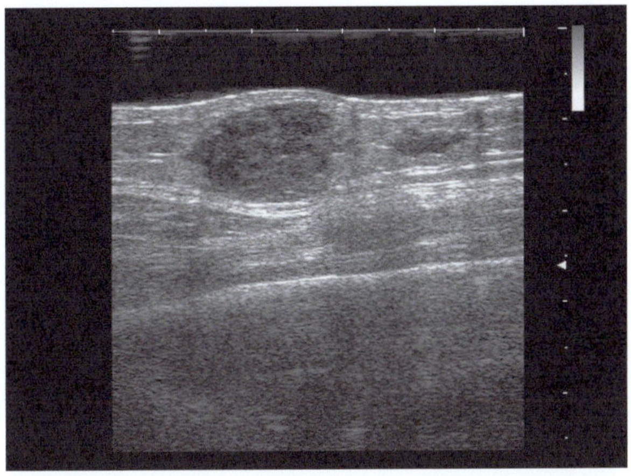

Fig. 2.8 Subcutaneous metastasis of the thigh from melanoma. Two hypoechoic subcutaneous nodules can be identified

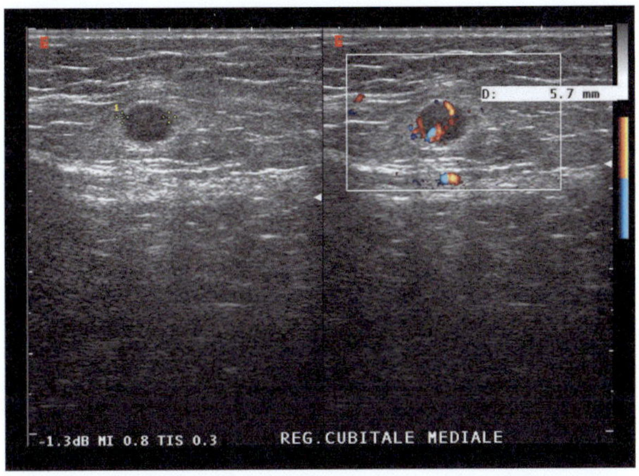

Fig. 2.9 Subcutaneous in-transit metastasis from melanoma at the level of the elbow in patient having undergone repeated operations for melanoma of the hand. Small markedly hypoechoic nodule with color signals at directional PD

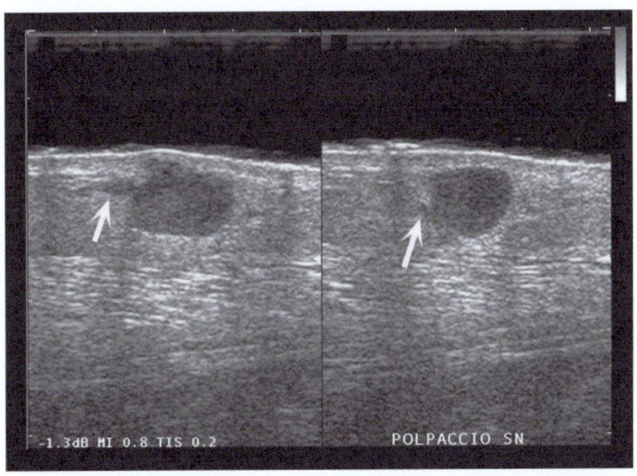

Fig. 2.10 In-transit metastasis of the calf from melanoma of the ankle. Hypoechoic subcutaneous lesion with thin marginal ramifications (arrows) indicative of the lymphatic duct being the site of the tumor spread

inguinal (and possibly also supraclavicular and cervical) lymph nodes for melanomas of the trunk. Indubitably US monitoring is superior to clinical follow-up, with a sensitivity of 89% and specificity of 100% for the identification of lymph node metastases compared with 71% and 100%, respectively, for palpation. In particular, the supraclavicular, subclavicular and axillary stations most commonly give rise to false negatives at palpation [17]. In patients who have already undergone excision of the sentinel lymph node or dissection of the lymphatic compartment, the physical examination can be particularly limited. In these cases it should be borne in mind at US exploration that metastatic lymphadenopathies can be in an unusual site, outside of the expected lymphatic drainage area [10].

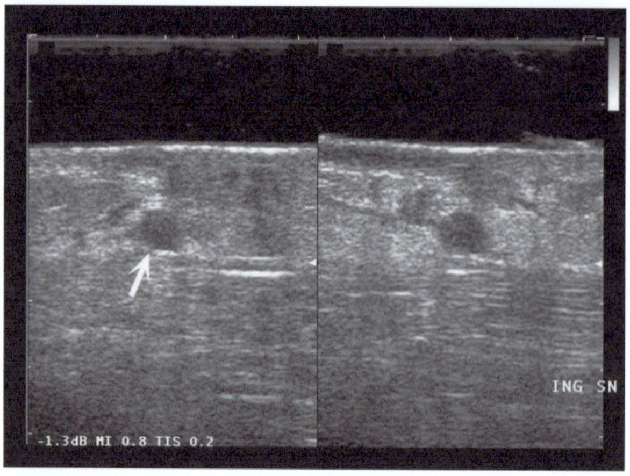

Fig. 2.11 Recurrence of melanoma after inguinal lymph node resection. Postoperative remodeling of the inguinal region, where a hypoechoic nodule of disease recurrence (arrow) can be identified

Metastases to the regional **lymph nodes** are often identified at physical examination, which has a specificity similar to US but a lower sensitivity (71% vs. 89%) [11]. US can be helpful in identifying small pathologic lymph nodes or partial nodal metastases, and in guiding a FNAC of the suspicious lymph nodes. CD, possibly with the use of contrast medium, can facilitate the distinction from fluid collections (hematomas, seromas, lymphoceles) and demonstrate the vascular structures of the lymph node, thus assisting differential diagnosis between reactive lymph nodes with hilar vascularity and metastatic lymph nodes with capsular vascularity [18] (Figs. 2.12, 2.13).

The search for distant metastases is performed in

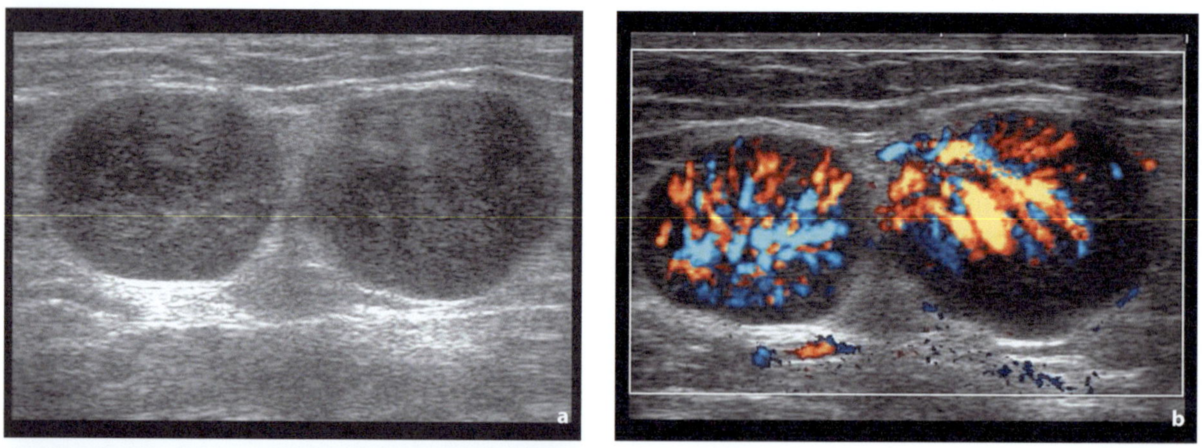

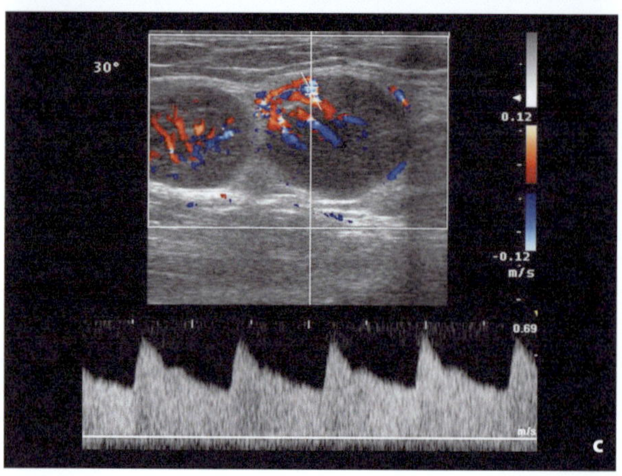

Fig. 2.12 a-c Inguinal lymph node metastasis from melanoma. Two enlarged, rounded, hypoechoic lymph nodes with regular margins (**a**) and marked hypervascularity at directional PD (**b**) and spectral Doppler indicating low resistance but high systolic velocities (V_{max} 61 cm/s) (**c**)

cases of stage IIB or above. For stages I and IIA, an US evaluation of the superficial and hepatic lymph node stations, possibly associated with a plain chest film, may be enough, since the use of the "heavy machines" is not justified in terms of costs/benefits. Patients with melanoma who have metastatic disease are in the minority; moreover diagnostic work-up and chemotherapy have only a limited impact on overall survival. In general CT is used for staging and monitoring. More recently, PET with FDG has proven accurate in the evaluation of metastatic melanoma, and more sensitive than CT [11]. US only plays an ancillary role in these cases.

Identifying all of the sites of deep tumor spread is crucial, which often are rather atypical compared with the hematogenous spread patterns of other tumors (Figs. 2.14–2.16). Abdominal parenchymal metastases more commonly involve the liver, although splenic and renal involvement is not rare [19]. **Liver** metastases in most cases have a micronodular distribution in the form of multiple more-or-less homogeneous hypoechoic areas which are usually quite evident and circumscribed with respect to the parenchymal background. In other cases the lesions are macronodular or occasionally with mass appearance. Calcifications and hemorrhagic foci are possible. CD study usually reveals poor vascular signals, whereas at CEUS the metastases may appear as hypervascular or hypovas-

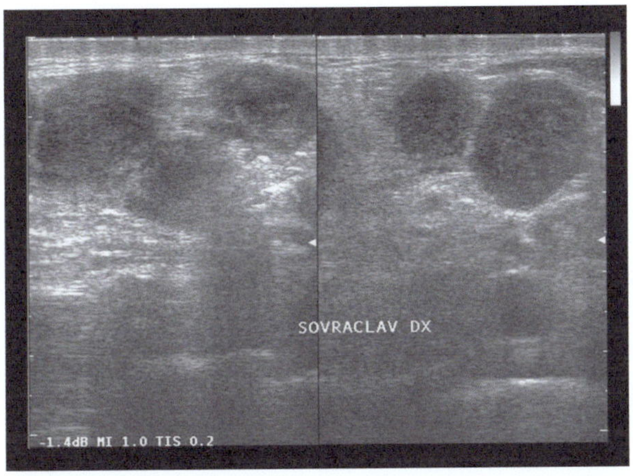

Fig. 2.13 Supraclavicular lymph node metastasis from melanoma. Multiple enlarged heterogeneous hypoechoic lymph nodes

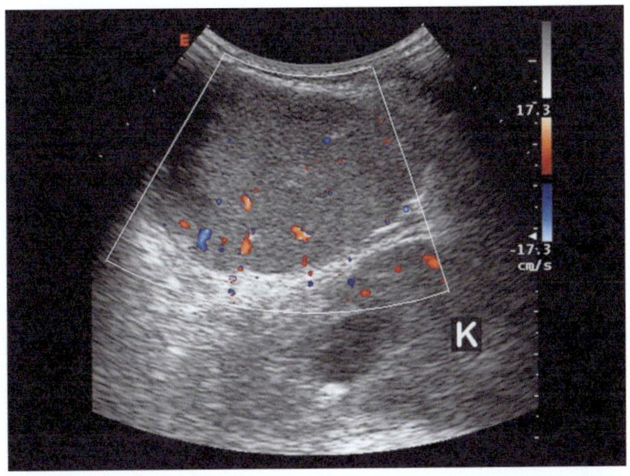

Fig. 2.14 Lumbar metastasis from melanoma. Large hypoechoic mass with relatively homogeneous echotexture and vascular signals at CD. *K*, kidney

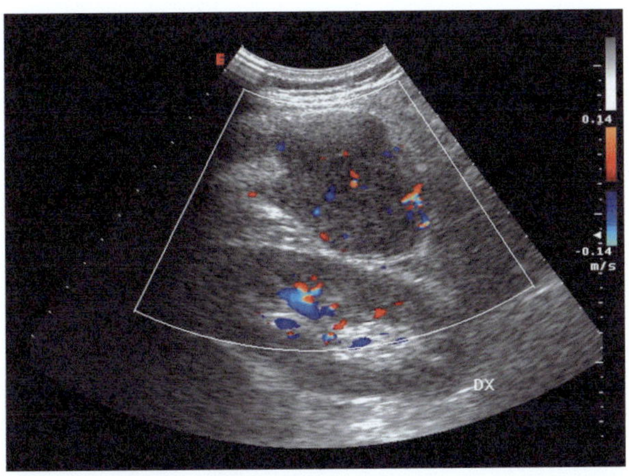

Fig. 2.15 Lumbar recurrence of melanoma in patient operated on for cutaneous lesion resection at that level two years earlier. Large and deep lumbar mass with hypoechoic appearance and heterogeneous echotexture, which is separable from the kidney. CD displays vascularity

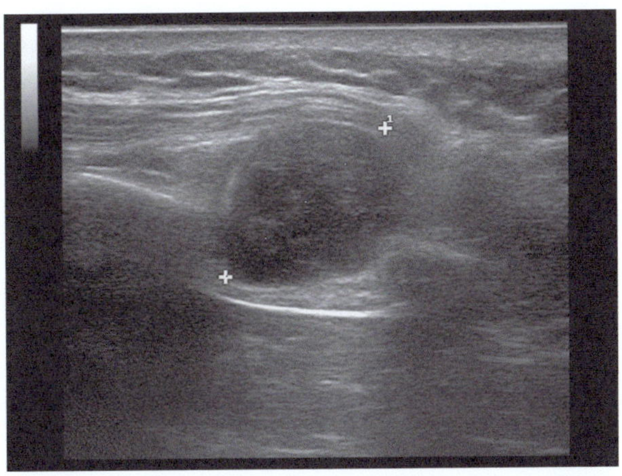

Fig. 2.16 Chest wall metastasis. Intercostal hypoecoic nodule

cular in the different phases of hepatic enhancement (Figs. 2.17–2.19).

Gallbladder metastases (comprising half of all metastases in this organ) account for up to 20% of all postmortem findings. They present as polypoid intraluminal projections and are often multiple and varying in size (generally >10 mm) with signs of vascularity at CD and CEUS. Although their appearance is hyperechoic, the absence of acoustic shadowing and mobility of the lesion with shifting patient position makes their differential diagnosis with calculi relatively easy [20].

Splenic metastases are found in 34% of patients who die as a result of metastatic melanoma, and usually have the same characteristics as liver metastases (Figs. 2.20, 2.21).

Renal metastases may be located within the parenchyma, with a tendency to widen the cortical-medullary thickness, or located peripherally or even markedly protrude into the perirenal fat to the point of suggesting a retroperitoneal rather than renal origin. The typical presentation is multiple small cortical lesions with heterogeneous hypoechoic appearance [11] (Fig. 2.22).

Nodulations in the **suprarenal glands** are possible (up to 50% of patients with metastatic melanoma) and in typical cases are unilateral with a mass appearance (mean diameter 4 cm) and heterogeneous hypoechoic structure [11] (Fig. 2.23).

Peritoneal metastases have an appearance of moderate nodulations or present with diffuse infiltration similar to carcinosis. Metastases may also be

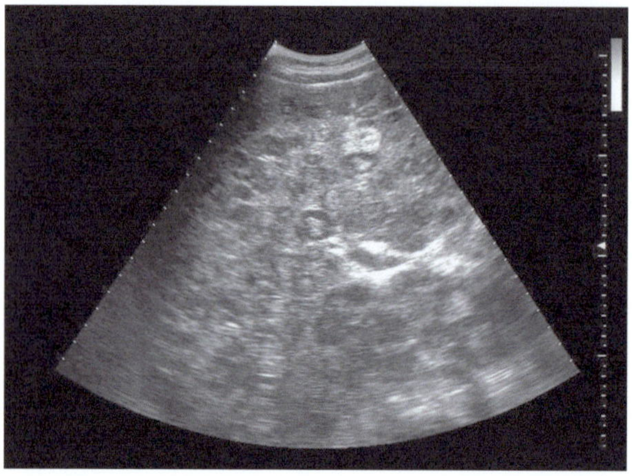

Fig. 2.17 Liver metastasis from melanoma. Numerous hypoechoic or target micronodular lesions

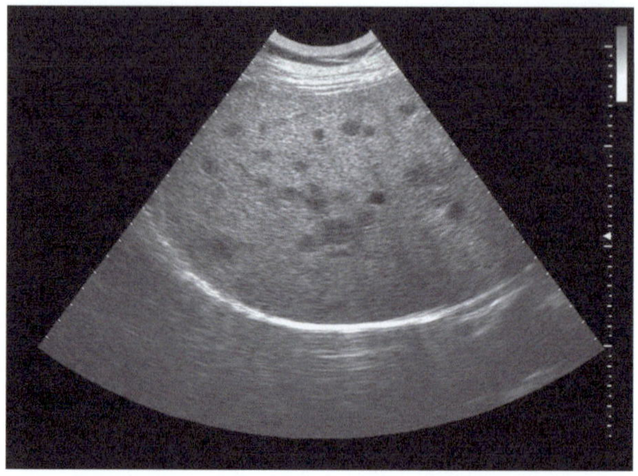

Fig. 2.18 Liver metastasis from melanoma. Diffuse hypoechoic miliary or micronodular lesions in a fatty liver

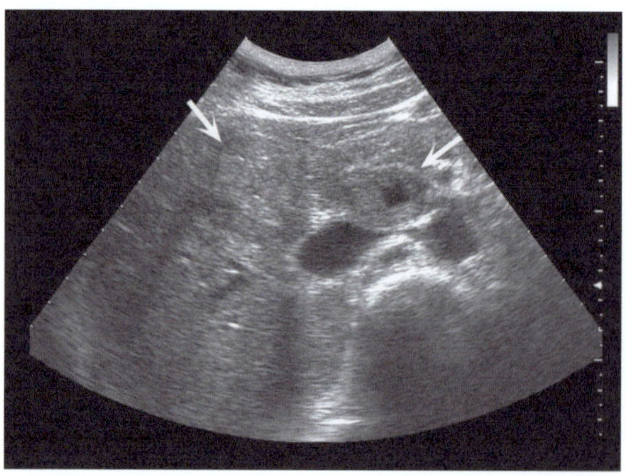

Fig. 2.19 Lymph node and liver metastases from melanoma. Heterogeneous echogenic lesion of the liver (*long arrow*) associated with an enlarged lymph node with a liquefactive anechoic center located in the portal-caval space (*short arrow*)

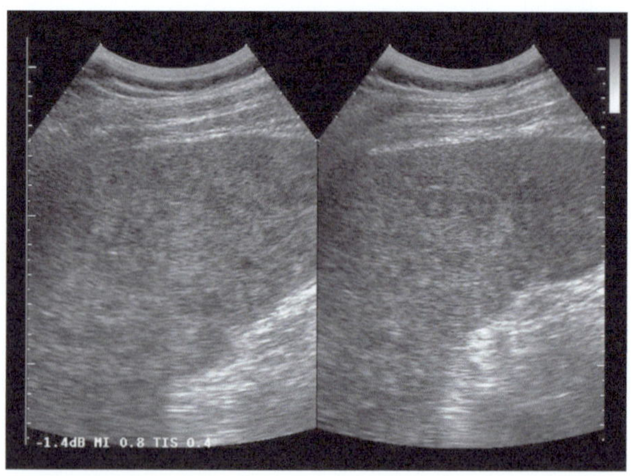

Fig. 2.20 Splenic metastasis from melanoma. Diffuse miliary and micronodular lesions with a hypoechoic or target appearance

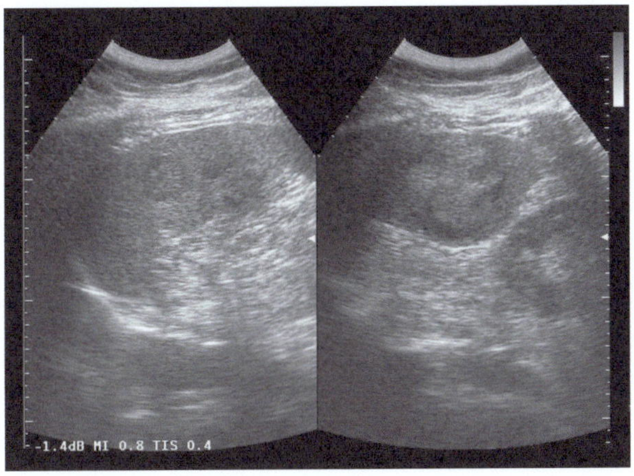

Fig. 2.21 Splenic metastasis from melanoma. Multiple heterogeneous lesions varying in size within the splenic parenchyma

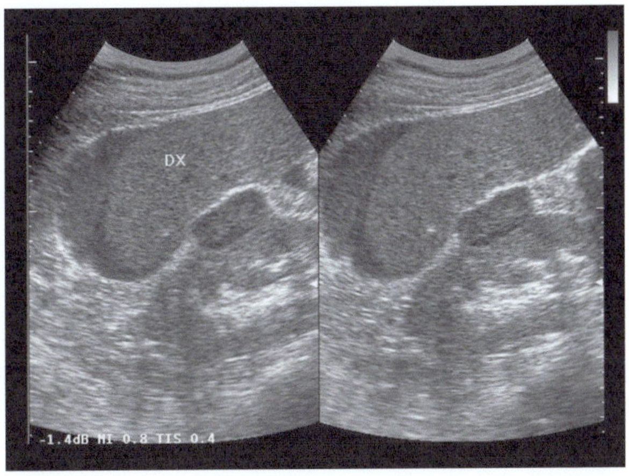

Fig. 2.22 Perirenal metastases from melanoma. Hypoechoic nodulation of the right renal profile. Perihepatic peritoneal effusion with corpuscular and heterogeneous appearance is associate

found in the deep muscles (diaphragm, psoas, etc.) and the abdominal-pelvic **lymph nodes** (Figs. 2.24, 2.25).

Ovarian metastases appear as large, lobulated, relatively well-circumscribed and prevalently solid or cystic masses that are difficult to differentiate from primary carcinomas [11] (Fig. 2.26, Video 2.1).

With regard to the **intestines**, melanoma is the leading cause of metastases. Postmortem studies have reported metastases in the small bowel of 58% of subjects who died from melanoma, even though this location was symptomatic in only 9% of cases. Metastases to the small bowel have been identified in 33% of patients with metastatic melanoma and in 2–5% of all patients with malignant melanoma [21]. The metastases usually appear as multiple submucosal lesions varying in size and often with mesenteric involvement [22] (Fig. 2.27). These small lesions are difficult to identify with US, even with the use of a high-frequency transducer and distention of the bowel loops with oral contrast medium. Instead the study may more readily identify larger, lobulated lesions with exophytic development and ulceration, or central necrosis tending to create a target appearance. US can play a role above all in identifying direct and indirect signs of complications such as intestinal occlusion and intussusception. The latter is generally enteroenteric and often multiple and transitory (Video 2.2).

Metastases to the **breast** may be found in both sexes and can be single or multiple, usually appearing as irregularly shaped hypoechoic nodules with heterogeneous echotexture and moderate vascular signals at CD.

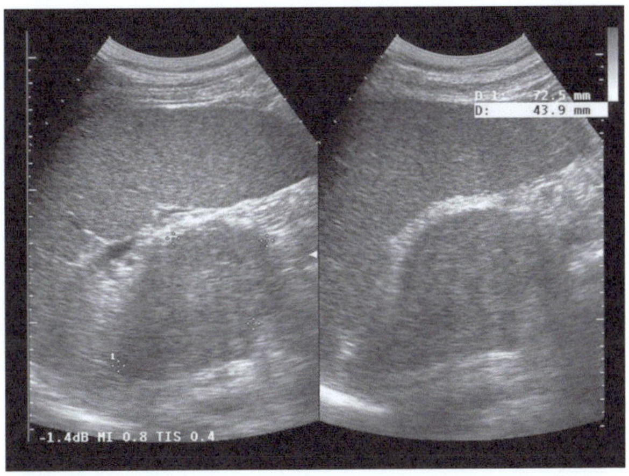

Fig. 2.23 Suprarenal metastasis from melanoma. Homogeneous hypoechoic mass of the left suprarenal gland

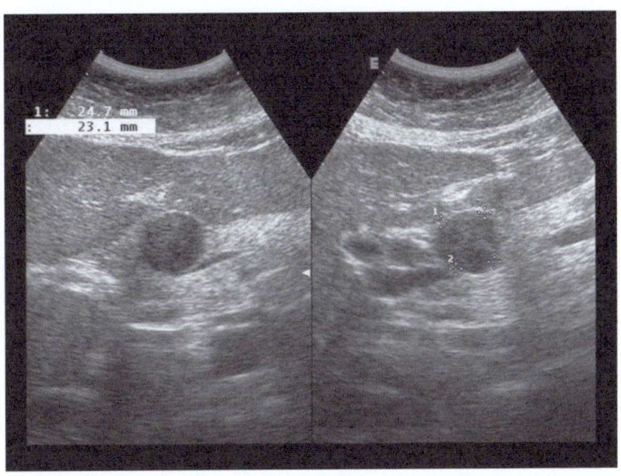

Fig. 2.24 Abdominal lymph node metastasis from melanoma. Rounded hypoechoic lymphadenopathy between the hepatic hilum and the head of the pancreas

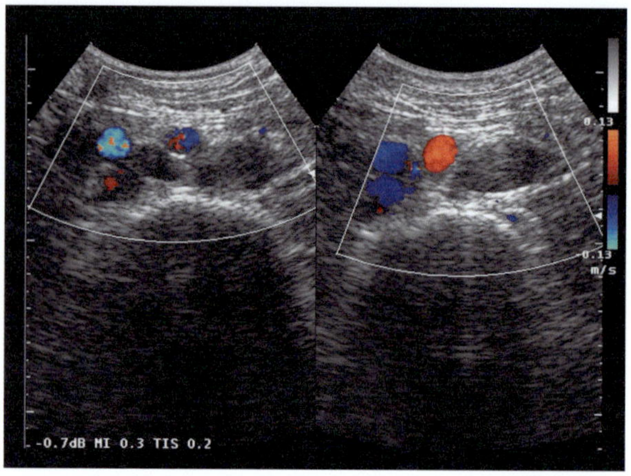

Fig. 2.25 Lumbar lymph node metastasis from melanoma. Multiple enlarged hypoechoic lymph nodes located between the retroperitoneal vessels, the latter being visualized at CD

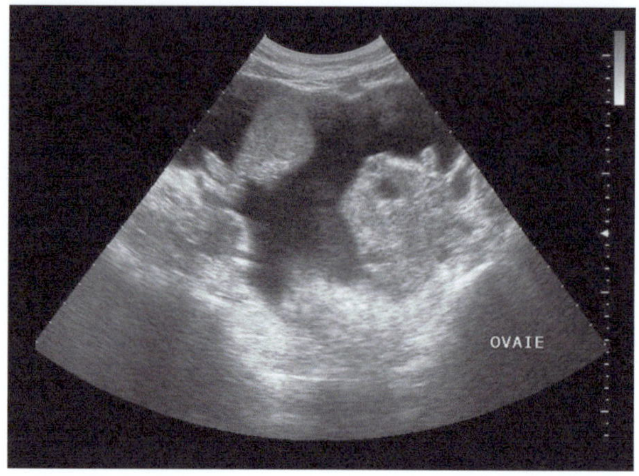

Fig. 2.26 Ovarian metastases from melanoma. Solid bilateral adnexal nodulations. Abundant peritoneal effusion is also identifiable

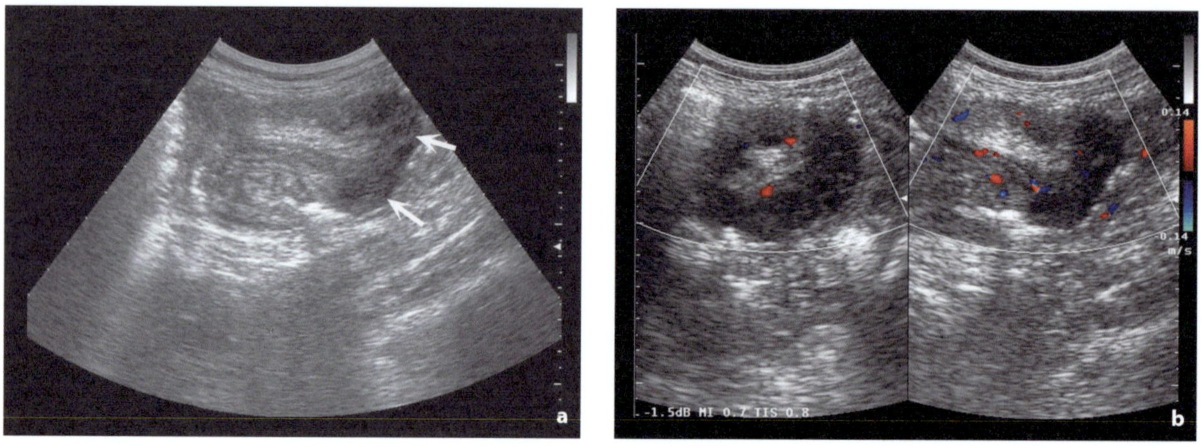

Fig. 2.27a,b Ileal metastases from melanoma, with consequent intestinal intussusception. The longitudinal section shows the hypoechoic parietal melanomatous lesions (**a**, *arrows*) and the echogenic invaginated mesentery. CD shows the persistent vascularity of the invaginating and invaginated intestinal wall (**b**)

2.2 Superficial Lymphadenopathy

Physical examination still plays an important role in the identification of superficial lymphadenopathies. Often, however, enlarged lymph nodes are clinically nonpalpable, even when superficial. This occurs in 20–50% of cases in the neck and 1–8% in axillary nodes, especially in the lymphomatous forms which tend to be less "hard" than metastatic forms. There is also the problem of specificity of the physical examination. Whereas in some sites such as the supraclavicular station the simple palpability of a lymph node is highly suspicious of a pathologic nature, in most other stations the normal lymph nodes are usually palpable.

The US differential diagnosis includes "normal" lymph nodes, "normal" lymph nodes with fibrous-fatty involution, reactive lymph nodes, lymphadenitis (acute, subacute and chronic), lymphomatous lymphadenopathies and metastatic lymphadenopathies. In addition to patient history and fundamental clinical findings, characterization of the lymph nodes should evaluate the following US parameters: size, shape, echostructure, margins and appearance of the perinodal environment. In reality there are no absolute **criteria of lymph node normality**. The simple **identification** of a lymph node has practically no intrinsic significance. In the past a superficial lymph node was thought to be pathologic for the simple fact of it being visualized at US. However, with current devices and small parts transducers this is far from being true. In the neck, "normal" lymph nodes are found in 19–23% of subjects at the submandibular level, in 15–16% in the parotid region (especially preauricular), in 18–19% in the high laterocervical region and in 35–37% at the level of the posterior triangle [23]. Even in the axillary and inguinal regions normal lymph nodes can be identified in most subjects. The only site where only pathologic lymph nodes can be identified is probably the supraclavicular fossa. The number of identifiable normal lymph nodes, at least in the cervical region, is markedly higher in young subjects than the elderly, such that the visualization of numerous lymph nodes in an elderly subject can be an element of suspicion, regardless of the other morphologic characteristics.

Similar considerations apply for the **size**. It was once thought that a lymph node with a maximum diameter greater than 5, 8 or 10 mm was pathologic, but this was simply because the resolution of the devices of the time was unable to identify adipose tissue metaplasia in lymph nodes often greater than 3–4 cm [24]. In reality a precise size threshold cannot be defined, because in some sites (e.g. the suprahyoid and particularly the submandibular regions), "normal" lymph nodes can reach sizes of up to 20 mm as a response to chronic irritative phenomena (caries, pharyngitis, etc.), rendering them comparable to reactive lymph nodes. Moreover in pediatric and young subjects a hyperplastic appearance is common, whereas in the elderly the fibrotic evolution of the lymph node itself tends to ensure that the dimensions are generally more contained. A lymph node may therefore be enlarged but without tumor involvement, or in contrast small but with non-macroscopic tumor foci within. In general, however, a greater (longitudinal) diameter of 20–25 mm and above all a lesser (transverse) diameter of 10 mm (being undoubtedly more reliable than the longitudinal diameter) are today considered the upper limits of "the norm", although with regard to cervical lymph nodes threshold values of 8 mm or even 5 mm are used [23]. More than the absolute diameter, for some time emphasis has been placed on the ratio between the longitudinal diameter and the transverse diameter ("roundness index"), i.e. the **shape**. A ratio of >2, i.e. an oval or markedly elongated shape, is generally indicative of normality or at least benignity, whereas a ratio of <1.5, i.e. a rounded shape, is suggestive of malignancy and in particular metastasis [25]. There are however exceptions: normal submandibular lymph nodes and lymph nodes in pediatric patients with a current inflammation, for example, are very often rounded [24].

The confluence of a number of enlarged lymph nodes is clearly indicative of their pathologic nature without being particularly specific. Often lymph nodes with fibrous-fatty involution have a bilobar appearance which clearly should not be confused with the fusion of two adjacent lymph nodes. Even from the point of view of **echostructure** there are no absolute criteria (Fig. 2.28), since the normal lymph node does not always display an echogenic internal structure defined as the **central "hilum"**, in communication with the perinodal fat. This echogenic structure is caused by the lymphatic sinuses, i.e. the most internal portion of the lymph node medulla, where the sinuses filled with lymph create multiple interfaces [24,26]. The width can vary from a thin echogenic central band to a very wide echogenic area which leaves only a thin shell of cortex at the periphery. The position may be central or eccentric, toward the anatomic hilum, i.e. towards the

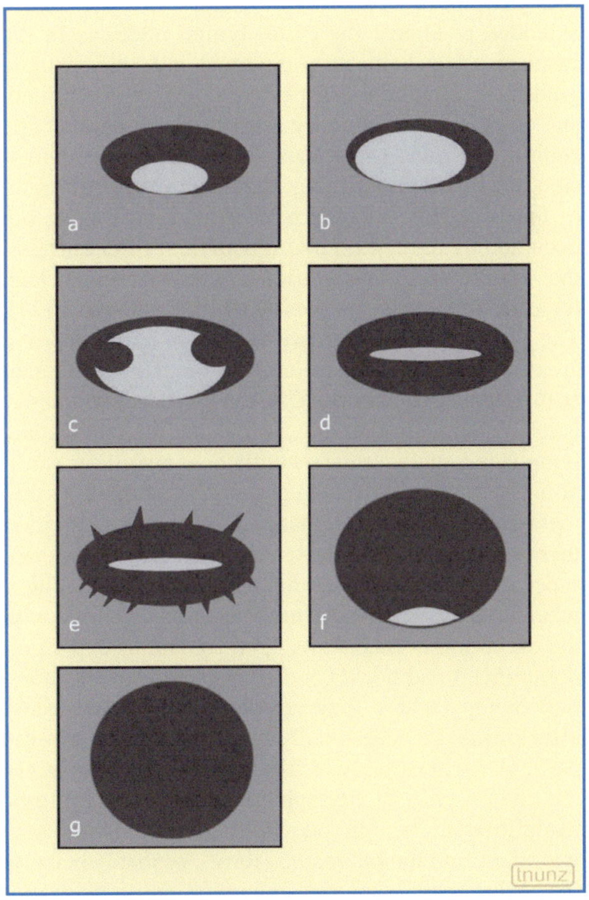

Fig. 2.28a-g Superficial lymph node morphostructural alterations. **a** Eccentric cortical thickening with wide echogenic hilum and oval shape. **b** Asymmetric eccentric cortical thickening with wide echogenic hilum and oval shape. **c** Eccentric cortical thickening with hypoechoic areas in the wide echogenic hilum and oval shape. **d** Concentric cortical thickening with reduction in the width of the echogenic hilum and oval shape. **e** Concentric cortical thickening with reduction in the width of the hilum, perinodal infiltration and oval shape. **f** Marked reduction and displacement of the echogenic hilum and round shape. **g** Absence of the echogenic hilum and round shape

entrance point of the vascular peduncle (at CD). The echogenic hilum can be normal, enlarged, displaced, reduced or absent. Conservation of the central hilum is suggestive of benignity, particularly if surrounded by a layer of symmetrical cortex. Its loss, in contrast, is suspicious of malignancy, especially metastatic. However, these are not absolute criteria, since an echogenic hilum can be identified in 5–28% of malignant lymph nodes and it may be absent in normal lymph nodes, especially if <5 mm where the interfaces of the medulla cannot be identified. It has also been demonstrated that the incidence of visualization of the hilum, at least at the cervical level, increases with age, so its absence especially in the young cannot constitute an absolute criterion of disease [24,26]. Between the two extremes of an absent hilum and the hilum extended to almost the entire lymph node, as in the case of adipose metaplasia, there are intermediate grades with the hilum displaced, interrupted, thinned, etc. A marked asymmetry with displacement of the central hilum is instead pathologic, being the expression of a diffuse thickening of the cortex or infiltration of the nodal tissue in the half of the lymph node not occupied by the central hilum. **Cortical thickening** of the lymph node is significant when asymmetrical, focal or at any rate marked (more than double) [24]. The presence of **calcifications**, liquefactive necrotic areas or markedly cystic areas should be evaluated at the level of the cortex. Calcifications are characteristic of granulomatous lymphadenitis, metastatic lymphadenopathy from medullary or papillary carcinoma of the thyroid, and in general lymphomatous and metastatic lymphadenopathy following radiation therapy or chemotherapy. **Liquefactive areas** are especially found in inflammatory lymphadenopathies, whereas they are infrequent in metastatic forms, with the exception of metastasis from squamous cell carcinoma (head and neck!) and forms treated with radiation therapy where they are common. **Pseudocystic alterations** are occasionally found in lymphomas but particularly in metastases from papillary carcinoma of the thyroid [24]. The lymph node **margins** tend to be ill-defined in benign adenopathies and sharper in metastatic and lymphomatous forms, probably because the replacement of normal lymphoid tissue by malignant tissue produces a more marked variation in acoustic impedance with respect to the adjacent tissues [27]. The identification of **extranodal spread** of the malignancy is often challenging, unless there are signs of adherence or invasion of adjacent structures such as muscles, veins or arteries. This is nonetheless an important parameter, given its considerable influence on prognosis [28]. Irregularities of the margins or the presence of hypoechoic areas or bands in the perinodal adipose tissue may be a sign of spread. However, these findings are identifiable only in some cases when the surrounding fat is particularly echogenic. A prominent thickening of the adipose tissue associated with reduced compressibility with the transducer is typical of acute lymphadenitis.

The **CD and PD appearance** of normal lymph nodes has been described particularly in the neck. Normal lymph nodes, with the exception of those <5 mm which may appear avascular (especially in the elderly and in the neck, in the posterior cervical triangle), display exclusively central vascularity, i.e. situated at the center of the lymph node when this does not have a central hyperechogenicity, or located centrally or eccentrically but within the echogenic "hilar" band. Peripheral vessels at the capsule are absent [24]. The concept of the "hilum" in B-mode and CD in fact may not necessarily correspond, and the latter may identify a hilum where the former does not [23,26]. In general a vessel can be seen penetrating the lymph node hilum which adopts a central position within the lymph node, following its long axis and possibly giving off lateral branches which are usually arranged symmetrically at the sides of the main branch. Pathologic lymph nodes tend to be more vascular than normal ones, with the presence of extrahilar vessels, i.e. with color signals which do not correspond with the signal of the central vessel (Fig. 2.29). This tends to be the case regardless of the size of the lymph node (and therefore even for normal-sized lymph nodes), and above all for metastatic lymph nodes, less so for lymphomatous lymph nodes and still less for benign lymphadenopathies [29]. In general there are four CD lymph node patterns: hilar, punctate (single spots or scattered segments), peripheral (capsular) and mixed (combination of two of the previous patterns) [30]. Variations may also be identified on the basis of the number of recognizable vessels and their distribution, such that eight subtypes may be noted, the first four of which are suggestive of benignity and the last four of malignancy: (1) hilar vessel which exceeds the margin of the lymph node; (2) longitudinal vessel parallel to the nodal long axis or the skin; (3) peripheral branches originating from the longitudinal branch; (4) central punctate signals; (5) curved course of the vessel due to displacement; (6) one or more central vessels with an angle >30° to the skin or the nodal long axis; (7) avascular area in the context of a hypervascular lymph node; (8) two or more vessels not originating from the hilar or longitudinal vessels [32]. A peripheral pattern, where the color signals are detected around the hilum and especially at the periphery, is particularly anomalous. In the typical forms multiple vascular poles can be seen penetrating the lymph node from its margins and are distributed asymmetrically within the node. The peripheral vascular pattern of metastatic lymph

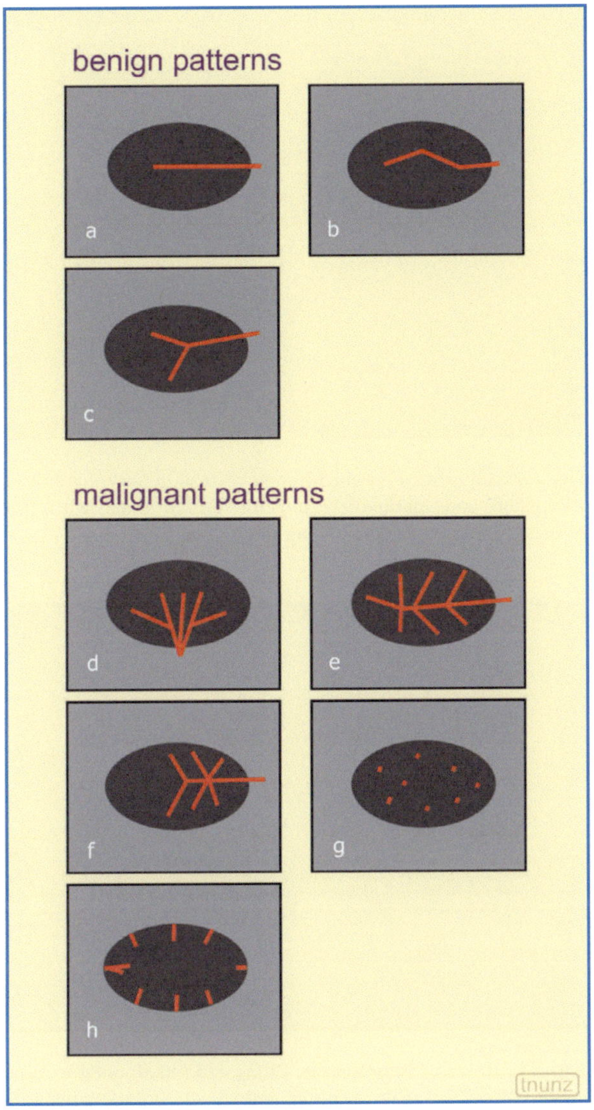

Fig. 2.29a–h Main CD patterns of superficial lymphadenopathies. In the benign forms a single central vessel prevails which may be rectilinear (**a**), angulated (**b**) and/or with branching (**c**). The malignant forms may present an eccentric branching vessel (**d**), a central diffusely branched vessel (**e**), but above all a branching vessel which fails to reach a portion of the node (**f**), or single internal spots (**g**) or multiple capsular peripheral vessels (**h**). Modified from [31]

nodes is explained by the method with which the tumor cells spread, reaching the lymph node through the afferent lymphatic vessels which perforate the nodal capsule precisely from the convex margin [24]. In lymphomas, where the cellular spread occurs from within the lymph node towards the cortex, large hypertrophic hilar vessels may be seen, and although peripheral vessels are possible, especially in the high-grade forms, they are much less frequent than in metastases [24,33]. In the malignant lymph node the central vessels may persist, but with evident displacement of the main vessel or its branches or with a vascular defect in a part of the node, or they may be replaced by multiple vascular poles which reach the periphery of the lymph node from the capsule. These CD patterns have been used to obtain a sensitivity of 96% and a specificity of 77% in malignant-reactive differentiation, with high interobserver reproducibility [34]. PD has been shown to be more sensitive than CD in identifying intralesional vessels and in classifying the patterns, but its use has led to an increased incidence of false-positive results, without an overall diagnostic impact greater than CD [32]. US contrast media can improve demonstration of the vascularity of superficial lymph nodes, making the identification even of dividing branches and small arterioles possible, and therefore facilitating identification of the abovementioned patterns [18,35].

Spectral Doppler findings may vary slightly on the basis of the lymph node station in question. In the neck, a region which has been extensively studied in this sense, the submental and submandibular lymph nodes generally have the highest vascularity: the former have an RI higher than those of other stations, whereas the latter have an RI below the average. No differences in the vascularity and RI between the two sexes have been found, whereas an increase in vascular resistance has been shown with increasing age. Metastatic lymph nodes display higher values of the semiquantitative indices than benign lymph nodes, regardless of the size of the node itself, whereas lymphomatous nodes usually have an intermediate characteristic, with a frequent overlap in terms of non-neoplastic lymph nodes (therefore the contribution of spectral analysis is definitely inferior to that of CD, unless very "extreme" cut-offs are used, thus producing low sensitivity). There is no agreement regarding the threshold values to be used [24]. A PI >1.3–1.6 and an RI >0.72–0.8 in any intranodal vessel is at any rate suggestive of metastasis, or at least malignancy of the lymph node [29,36,37]. An additional characteristic of metastatic lymph nodes is their ability to show heterogeneous traces in different vessels, some with low and others with high resistance [37]. The difficultly of sampling a good spectral trace in small-diameter vessels should also be borne in mind.

Preliminary data with **CEUS** in superficial reactive lymph nodes have shown intense and constant enhancement in lymphomatous lymph nodes, intense but heterogeneous enhancement in non-necrotic and inflamed metastatic lymph nodes with clear perfusion defects, especially in the arterial phase where a punctate appearance can be identified, and an overall hypoperfusion or nonperfusion in metastatic necrotic lymph nodes [24].

The preliminary findings with **elastography** seem to increase specificity. Alam and coworkers identified five patterns, ranging from pattern 1 (absent or very small hard area) to pattern 5 (a hard area occupying the entire lymph node). Considering patterns 3–5 as metastatic, sensitivity and specificity in assessing enlarged cervical lymph nodes was respectively 98% and 59% for US, while sensitivity and specificity moved respectively to 92% and 94% when adding elastography [38].

Lymph nodes with adipose metaplasia and fat deposition in the medulla can reach considerable dimensions, even 4–5 cm. They are characterized by a very wide "central hilum" which leaves only a thin hypoechoic cortical shell. They are commonly found in the groin, particularly in the elderly or subjects with venous problems, and are relatively frequent in the axillary region. They are occasionally labeled "reactive", but the two conditions should not be equated. Whereas the reactive lymph node should be indicated for its presence and size in the report, the same is not required for lymph nodes with fatty involution (Fig. 2.30).

Hyperplastic or **reactive lymph nodes** should not be confused with the previous description, nor with lymphadenitis (Figs. 2.31–2.33). They have sharp margins and homogeneous echotexture, without calcifications or necrotic areas. In the neck comparison with the thyroid parenchyma, being more echogenic than nodal tissue, may be useful. The vascular appearance at CD is typically intense or very intense as in the case of reactive lymphadenopathies found in AIDS patients, although a central pattern is also possible [30].

Acute lymphadenitis tends to produce a marked enlargement of the lymph nodes, which may become confluent and hypoechoic but may retain their oval shape. CD shows intense hyperemia with conserved intranodal vascular structures, with mild edematous attenuation of the perinodal fat being a common finding. Spectral analysis of cervical lymphadenitis has a positive predictive value of 100% for RI <0.5 and PI <0.6 [36] (Figs. 2.34, 2.35).

In **tubercular lymphadenitis** multiple spots may be observed due to dystrophic calcifications or hyalinosis, as well as hyperechoic areas of adipose metaplasia and hypo-anechoic zones of central necrosis. Immediately below the capsule a thin characteristic peripheral echogenic layer may be found [39]. The lymph nodes tend to fuse, creating hypoechoic clusters with posterior acoustic shadowing.

Superficial adenopathies are a frequent finding in **lymphomas**. Some 60–80% of subjects with Hodgkin's lymphoma initially present with a cervical adenopathy, whereas 6–20% have axillary adenopathy

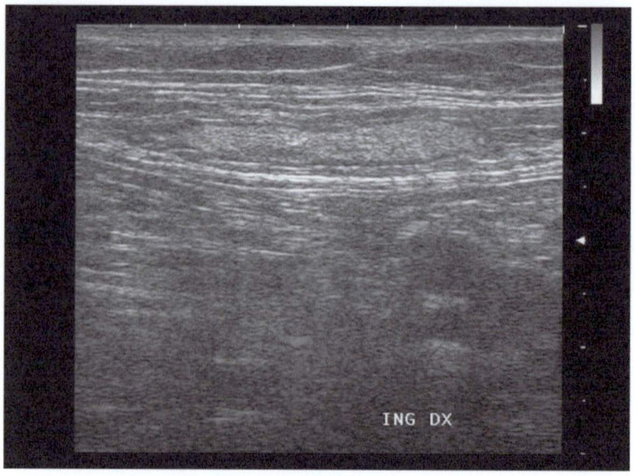

Fig. 2.30 Superficial inguinal lymph node with fatty involution. Elongated and markedly echogenic lymph node with thin residual shell of cortex in the periphery

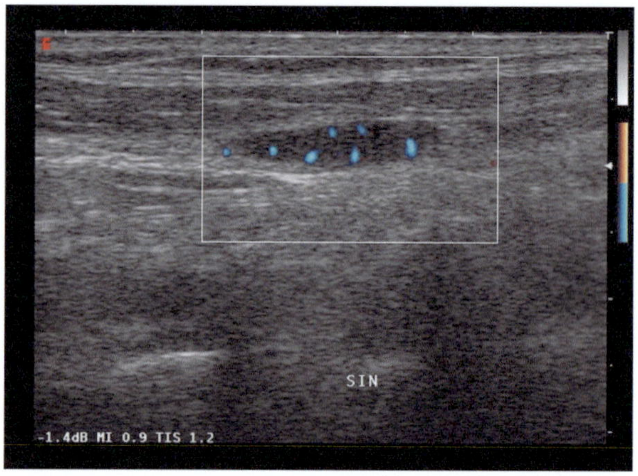

Fig. 2.31 Reactive lymph node. Elongated lymph node with no central hilum and multiple peripheral vessels at directional PD

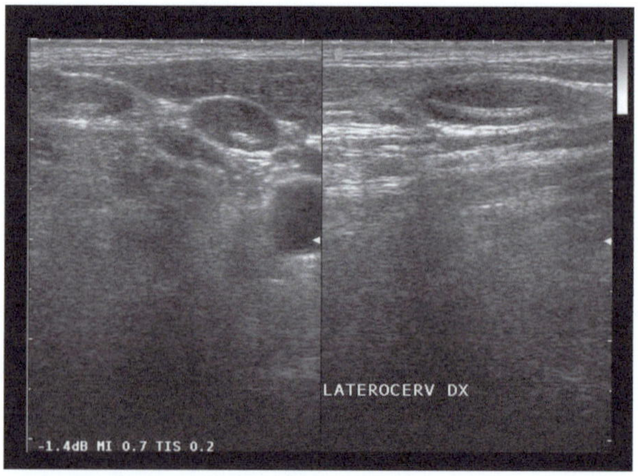

Fig. 2.32 Reactive laterocervical lymph node. Oval lymph node with thin "echogenic hilum"

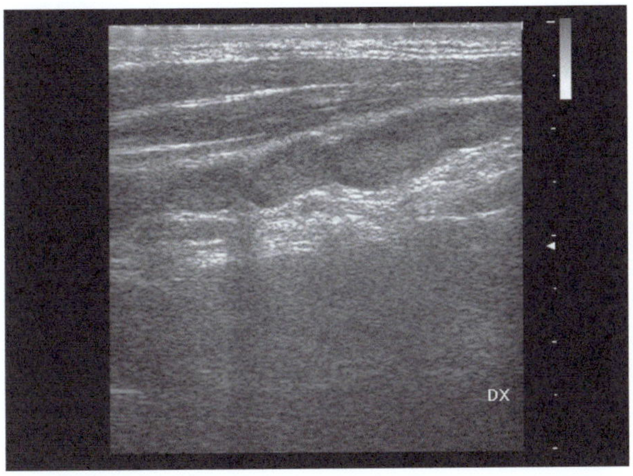

Fig. 2.33 Reactive laterocervical lymph node. Multiple oval/elongated lymph nodes with no "echogenic hilum" (homogeneous hypoechogenicity)

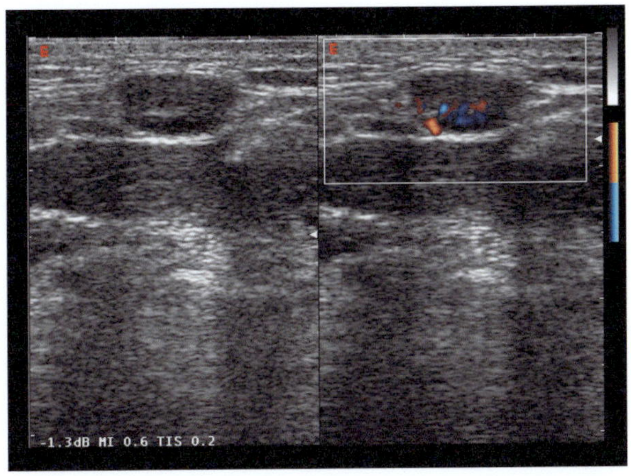

Fig. 2.34 Submental lymphadenitis. Lymph node with thin "echogenic hilum" and conserved vascular structure at directional PD

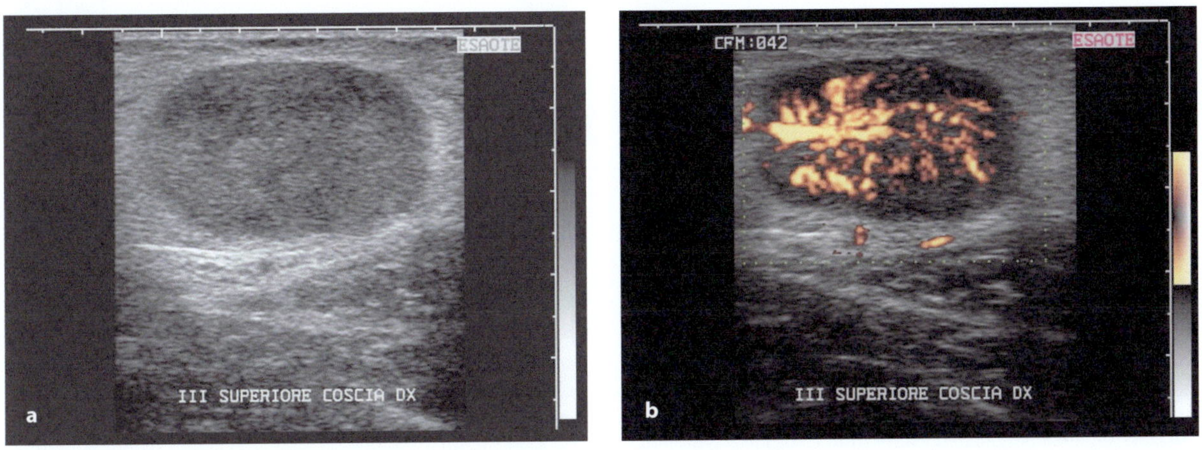

Fig. 2.35a,b Pediatric acute lymphadenitis of the inguinal-crural region. Large relatively homogeneous and hypoechoic lymphadenopathy with well-defined margins and edematous thickening of the surrounding adipose tissue (a). Hyperemic vasculature but with regular and symmetrical vessel distribution at PD (b)

[40]. The lymphadenopathies appear rounded with lobulated margins and generally marked hypoechogenicity, tending to be greater than that in hyperplastic forms and occasionally pseudocystic. Calcifications are rare in nontreated forms (Figs. 2.36–2.41). The size is variable, ranging from several millimeters to a number of centimeters. Particularly large nodes may be found in NHL, especially if high grade, more so than in Hodgkin's lymphoma. However, even small but multiple lymph nodes situated close together or tending to confluence are a frequent finding [40]. During radiation or systemic therapy the nodal echogenicity tends to increase, which is a sign of fibrotic evolution. The vascular network often appears conserved, with a vascular supply at CD generally of the hilar type, not unlike the appearance of the normal or hyperplastic lymph node [33]. Findings usually include a moderate or even intense vascular supply, with color signals at both the center and the periphery, whereas a patently capsular pattern is rare and identifiable only in high-grade lymphomas. The presence of a "hilar" vascular supply does, however, make the differential diagnosis more challenging than it is for metastatic lymphadenopathies [30,33]. Most lymphomatous processes are slow growing and therefore do not produce the subversion of the US and CD characteristics of the lymph node seen in cases of metastases. Indeed, based solely on the US and CD data described above, distinction between lymphomatous lymph nodes and lymphadenitis is often difficult and requires clinical evaluation, monitoring and possibly biopsy.

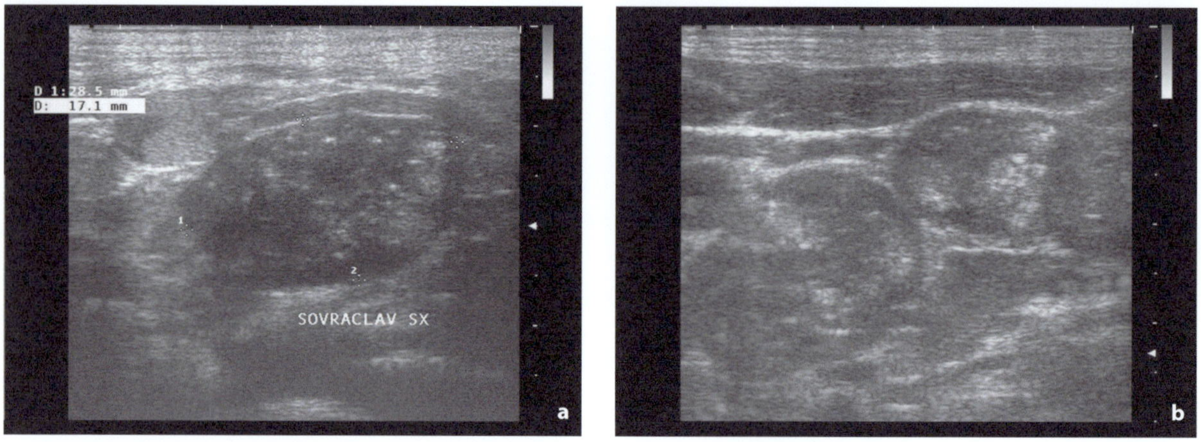

Fig. 2.36a,b Cervical and supraclavicular lymphadenopathies from NHL. Enlarged lymph nodes with multiple calcifications

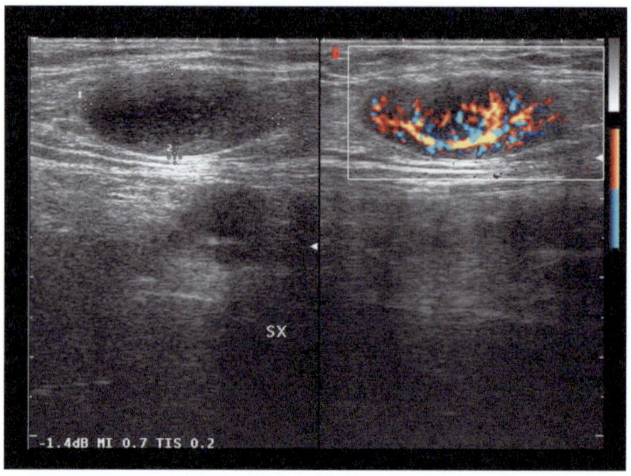

Fig. 2.37 Inguinal lymphadenopathy from Hodgkin's lymphoma. Oval-shaped hypoechoic lymph node with no central echogenic hilum and intense but symmetrical vascular supply at directional PD

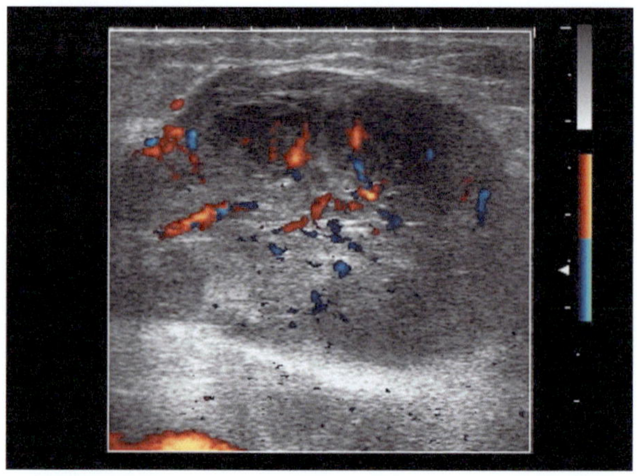

Fig. 2.38 Inguinal lymphoma. Heterogeneous lymph node mass of the groin with vascular signals at directional PD

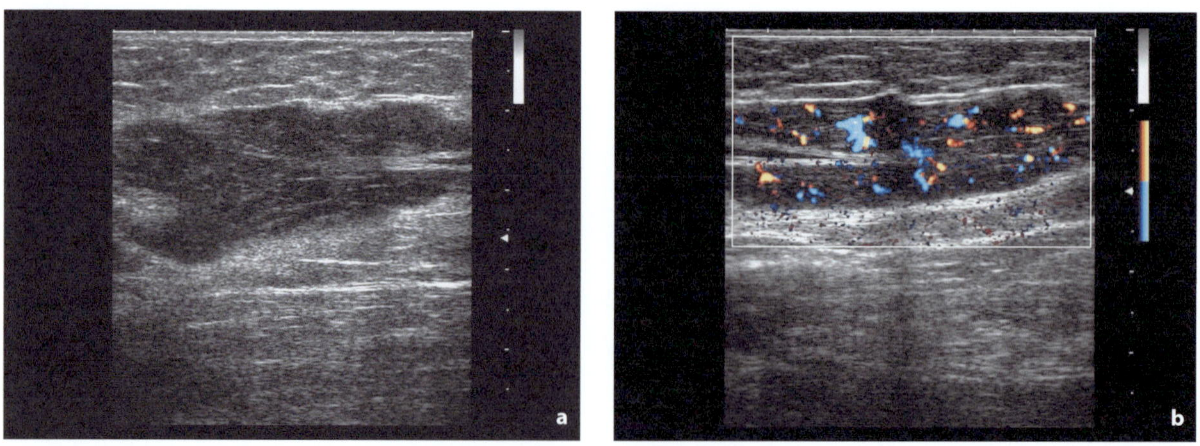

Fig. 2.39a,b Low-grade inguinal lymphoma, negative PET. Large hypoechoic nodule (**a**) with moderate internal vascular supply at directional PD (**b**)

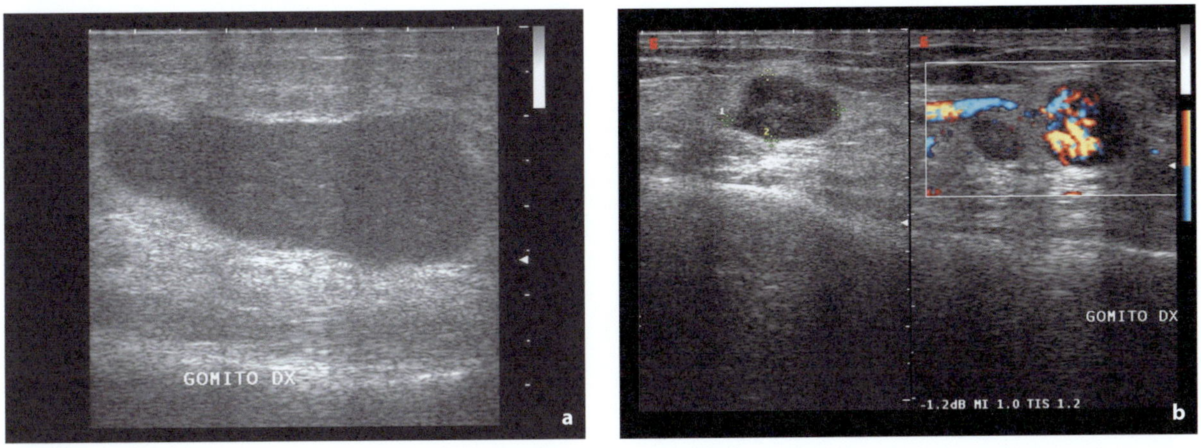

Fig. 2.40a,b Lymphoma of the elbow. Multiple enlarged lymph nodes with hypervascular appearance at directional PD

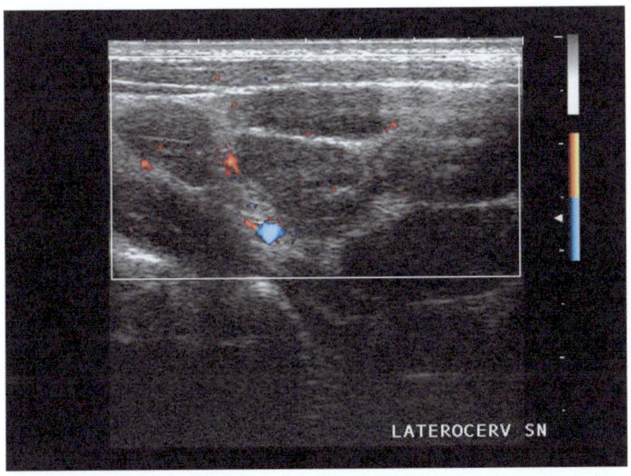

Fig. 2.41 Inactive laterocervical lymphoma (negative PET) post-treatment. Persistence of several small non-confluent hypoechoic lymph nodes with no significant residual vascular signals at directional PD

In **metastatic lymph nodes** the hypoechoic appearance is rather sharp and more marked than in hyperplastic forms. Internal liquefactive-necrotic phenomena with broad hypovascular areas at CD can be identified in lymphadenopathies from squamous cell carcinoma, whereas in metastases from papillary carcinoma of the thyroid patently cystic internal areas appearing avascular at CD may be found. In general, metastatic lymph nodes rarely appear with no vascular signal and usually reveal a more-or-less intense vascular supply [30]. Microcalcifications (<2 mm) can be found in metastases from papillary and medullary carcinoma of the thyroid or in other metastases following treatment (Figs. 2.42–2.50, Videos 2.3, 2.4).

A particular problem is posed by the **sentinel lymph node**. This is the lymph node where the primary tumor drains directly and which may already

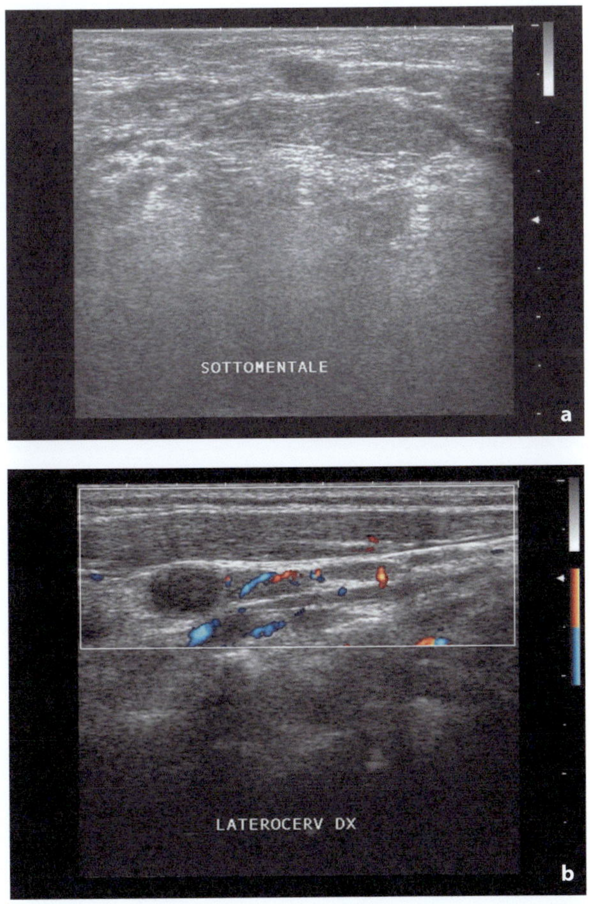

Fig. 2.42a,b Cervical lymphadenopathies from parotid carcinoma. Small but highly suspicious lymph nodes due to their rounded shape and heterogeneous hypoechoic structure with no central hilum, located in the submental (**a**) and laterocervical (**b**) regions

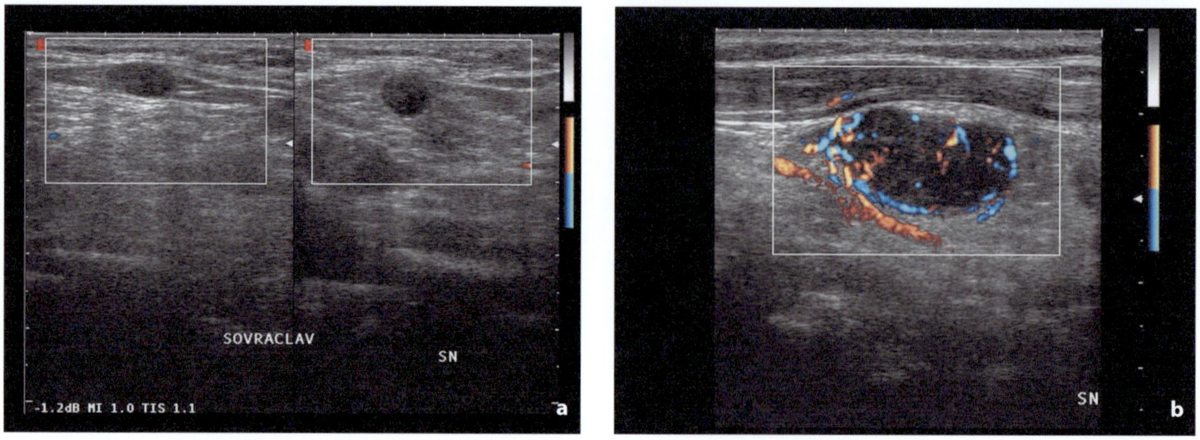

Fig. 2.43a,b Supraclavicular metastases from lung cancer. Two lymph node nodules, the smaller with no vascular signals (**a**) and the larger with diffuse and irregular hypervascularity, especially capsular (**b**), at directional PD

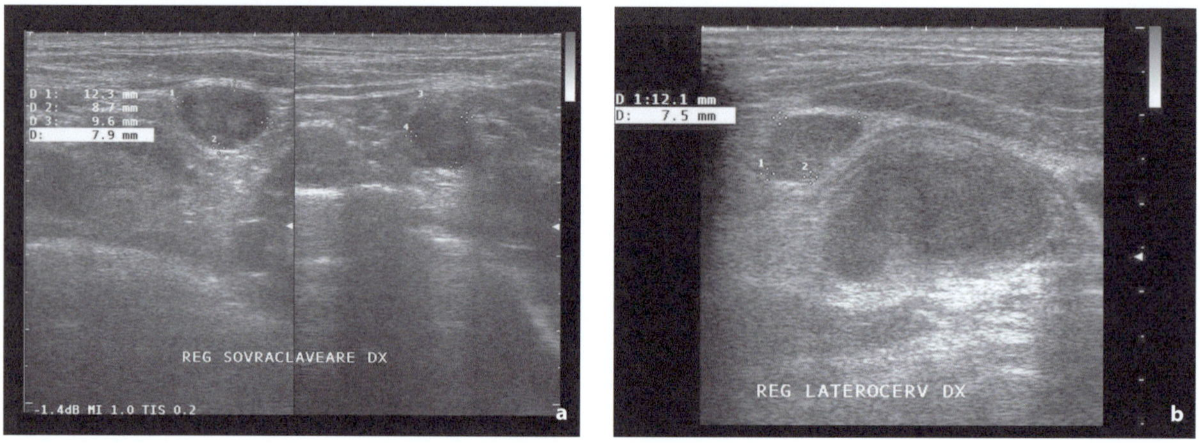

Fig. 2.44a,b Supraclavicular (**a**) and laterocervical (**b**) metastatic lymphadenopathies from lung cancer. Round and relatively homogeneous hypoechoic lymph nodes

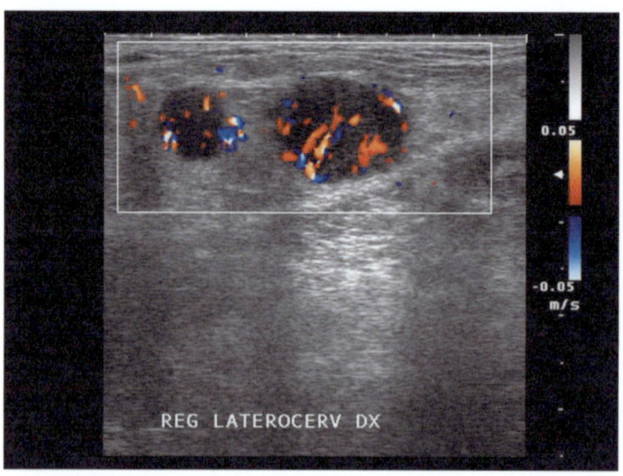

Fig. 2.45 Laterocervical metastatic lymphadenopathies from breast cancer. Two adjacent round and relatively homogeneous hypoechoic lymph nodes with multiple afferent vessels from the periphery, at CD

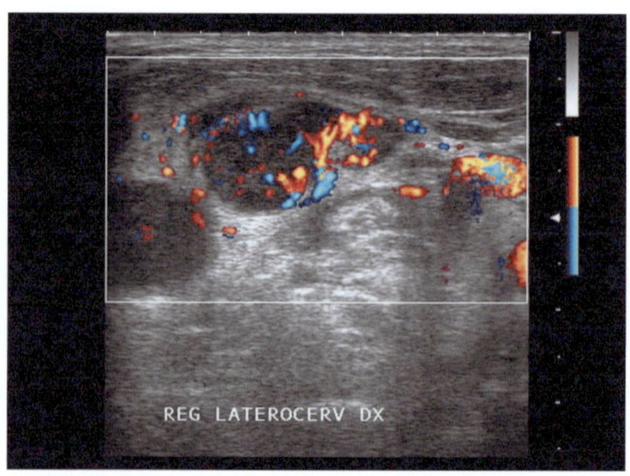

Fig. 2.46 Laterocervical metastatic lymphadenopathies from breast cancer. Two adjacent rounded and relatively homogeneous hypoechoic nodules with multiple hilar but also capsular vessels shown at directional PD

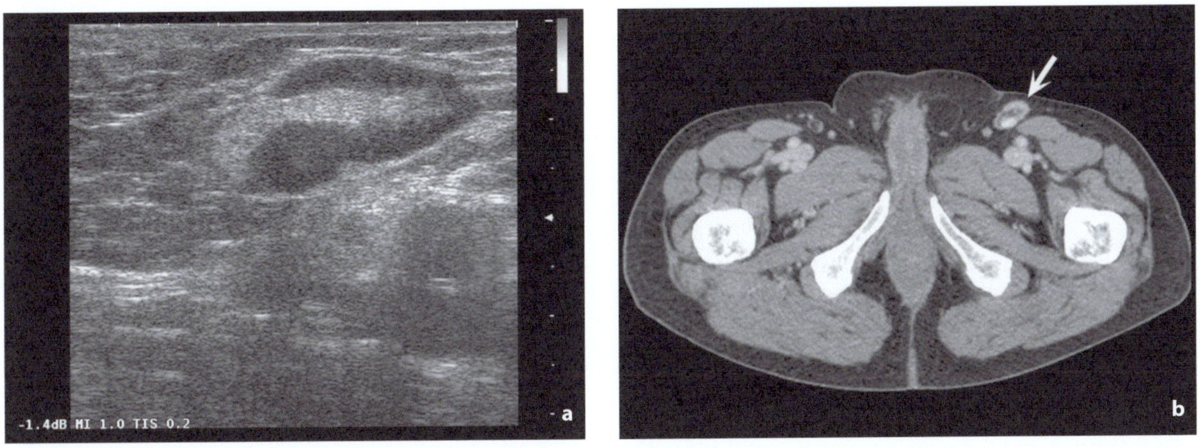

Fig. 2.47a,b Superficial inguinal metastatic lymphadenopathies from sarcoma of the leg. Lymph node with notably thickened and asymmetric cortex shown at US (a) and CT (b, *arrow*)

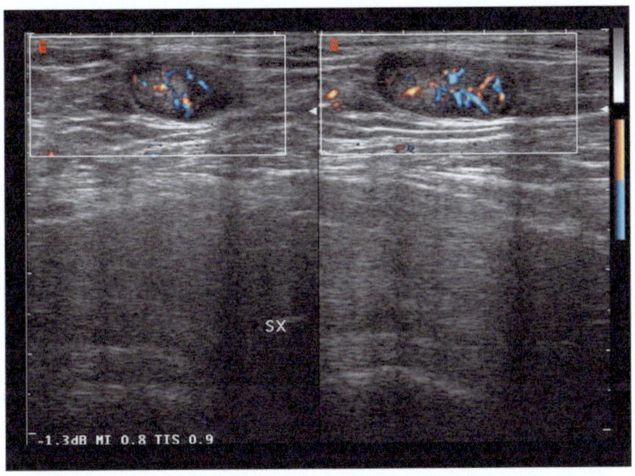

Fig. 2.48 Partial lymph node metastasis from melanoma. Asymmetric cortical thickening, which appears as a relatively hypovascular area of the lymph node at directional PD

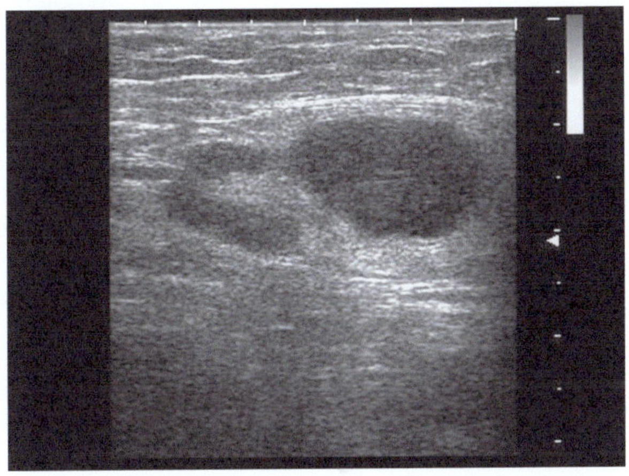

Fig. 2.49 Partial metastatic axillary lymphadenopathy from breast cancer. The lymph node with reactive appearance shows a large internal eccentric nodule

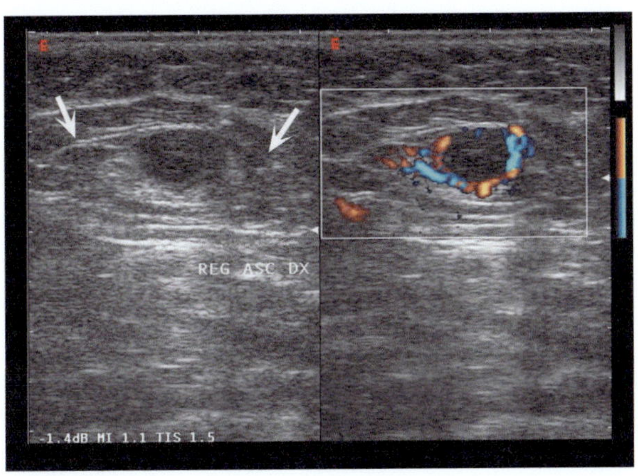

Fig. 2.50 Partial metastatic axillary lymphadenopathy from breast cancer. The lymph node with reactive-free appearance (*arrows*) show a markedly hypoechoic internal eccentric nodule which at directional PD corresponds to a vascular defect of the lymph node

be the site of neoplastic colonization or may still be healthy [41] (Fig. 2.51). There is therefore a need to distinguish between two subsequent occurrences – first, identify the site of the sentinel lymph node, and then determine whether it is normal or pathologic, which is crucial for the purposes of staging. As a general rule, only in the presence of a positive sentinel lymph node is it necessary to dissect the regional lymph node station hosting it. A sentinel lymph node procedure which returns a negative finding means a lymph node dissection that is most probably unnecessary can be avoided (98% negative predictive value for lymphatic diffusion of breast cancer). Overtreatment of these patients can therefore be avoided, especially considering the morbidity of lymphadenectomy and the early and late complications particularly for the limb that is afferent to the regional lymph nodes in question. For example, 60–70% of cases of women with breast cancer (80% of T1 and 65% of T2) have no axillary lymph node involvement at the time of diagnosis and therefore do not require axillary dissection [42,43]. The state of the sentinel lymph node can also be used to indicate adjuvant treatment [44].

In cases of **breast cancer**, this procedure is generally reserved for subjects with T1 and T2 disease, since locally more advanced forms have an elevated probability of axillary metastases, thus suggesting direct lymph node dissection. In addition, there is no agreement in the literature regarding the "negative" impact on survival of axillary lymphadenectomy, so the need for a preoperative demonstration of the effective involvement of the nodes appears vital [45]. The use of the sentinel lymph node procedure is also the subject of controversy, since 1–15% of cases with a negative sentinel node biopsy present metastatic involvement of the axillary lymph nodes [45]. In **melanomas**, particularly of the trunk, the site of the sentinel lymph node is challenging to predict on the basis of anatomic knowledge alone. Albeit in rare cases, it may even be located in deep sites such as the internal mammary chain, the mediastinum or the retroperitoneum. In addition, in 5% of cases the sentinel lymph node can be aberrant, i.e. found outside a lymph node basin, for example epitrochlear, popliteal or retroareolar [44,46]. The lesions that benefit most from the sentinel lymph node procedure are stage II melanomas. The technique has also been proposed for squamous cell tumors of the head and neck, thyroid carcinomas and carcinomas of the penis and vulva [47].

The **search for the sentinel lymph node** was initially performed with India ink [41], which also enables visualization of the lymphatic collectors draining to the lymph node basin and is based on intraoperative identification of the ink-stained lymph node. Currently the search can be performed with lymphoscintigraphy (generally involving the perilesional injection of human serum albumin labeled with Tc^{99m}), preoperatively (gamma camera) or intraoperatively (gamma-sensitive transducers or Geiger counters), which markedly increase the accuracy of the procedure even though it does complicate it in terms of organization and costs. More recently, several animal and clinical studies have been carried out with the use of US contrast media (25% albumin or Sonazoid tissue-specific contrast medium) as lymphatic tracers. The preliminary results are encouraging but require verification [48–50]. In any event, the ink or radiotracer or contrast medium is injected into the perilesional or retroareolar area, the area is massaged and then the diffusion along a lymphatic vessel to a lymph node is studied.

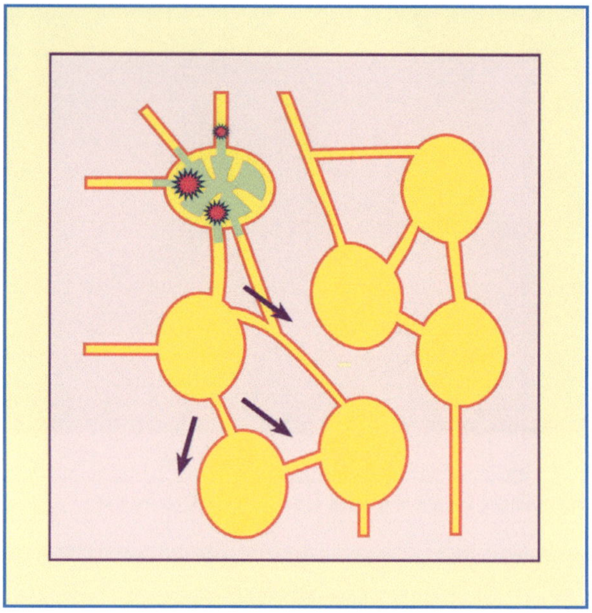

Fig. 2.51 Sentinel lymph node. The sentinel lymph node is the first of the regional lymph nodes to be reached. If the sentinel lymph node is negative at post-excision histopathologic analysis, involvement of other nodes is rare

US evaluation of the lymph node basin which is the site of a sentinel lymph node is usually not enough to define, and especially to rule out with certainty, the involvement of metastatic disease. In the case of melanoma, US has demonstrated a sensitivity of 79% and specificity of 72% on the basis of morphologic findings, and a sensitivity of 82% and specificity of 72% when associated with CD data [13] (Figs. 2.52, 2.53). While a lymph node with a US and CD appearance of metastasis is almost always confirmed as malignant after excision, the same cannot be said for lymph nodes with a normal appearance. In fact tumor deposits <5 mm are identified in 79% of lymph nodes with confirmed metastases from melanoma but with a negative US lymph node study [51]. An alternative is offered by FNAC or core biopsy for the evaluation of lymph nodes that are deemed suspicious at US. Positive cytologic or histologic findings make it possible to forego the sentinel lymph node procedure and proceed directly with lymph node dissection [43]. The sentinel lymph node procedure does in fact have its costs, as well as its organizational problems related in part to its multidisciplinary nature. The sonographer needs to perform a patient and meticulous exploration of the lymph node station(s) of the case in order to identify patently malignant lymph nodes or detect those that are suspicious, indeterminate or simply nonspecific

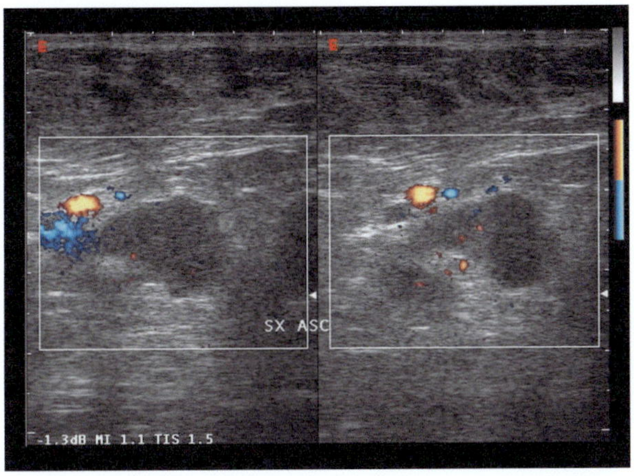

Fig. 2.52 Partial metastatic axillary lymph node from breast cancer. The lymph node with reactive appearance displays a hypoechoic internal eccentric nodule with multiple vessels arising from both the hilum and the capsule shown at directional PD

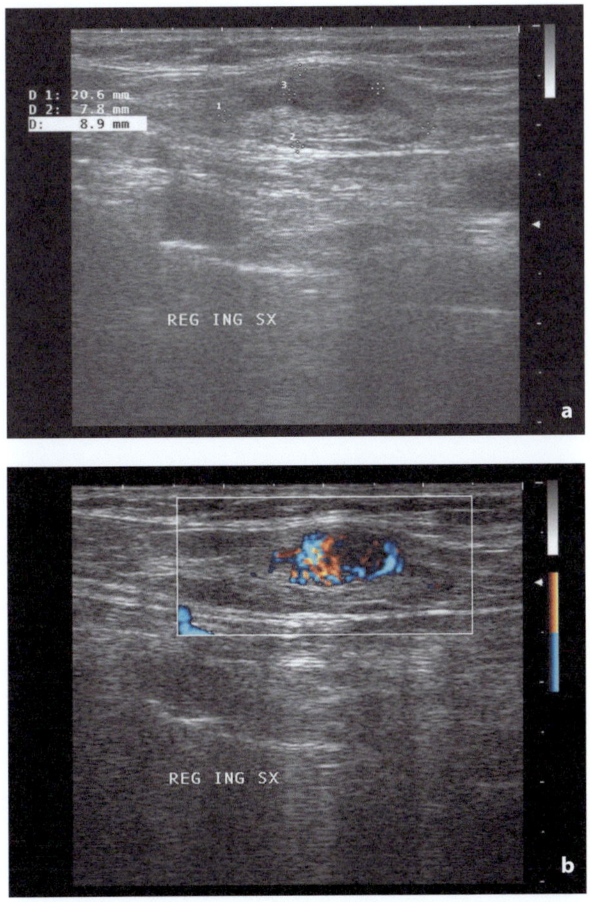

Fig. 2.53a,b Partial metastatic inguinal lymphadenopathy from melanoma. The lymph node with reactive appearance displays a large hypoechoic internal eccentric nodule (**a**) with hypervascular appearance at directional PD (**b**)

and therefore candidates for targeted FNAC or core biopsy. Conceptually the sentinel lymph node procedure could be used in select cases which are still negative (because negative findings at US and FNAC do not rule out micrometastatic involvement) [13,52]. Cases which are positive for metastatic involvement can immediately be scheduled, as stated above, for dissection of the lymph node basin in question.

2.3 Palpable Superficial Masses

Only 1% of **soft tissue tumors** are malignant, so in the presence of a palpable mass or even a documented solid formation the first hypothesis should be that it is almost always a benign lesion. However, the first problem is precisely an initial underestimation of sarcomas and therefore a possible delayed diagnosis. The first level modality in the study of superficial masses, and often conclusive in the case of benign lesions, is high-resolution US, which is able to define a wide range of tumors and non-neoplastic lesions that may give rise to a "palpable mass" (Figs. 2.54–2.59). The referred mass may be the result of no focal lesion at all or the result of an absolutely benign lesion.

Soft tissue lesions may arise from the skin (epidermis and derma), the subcutaneous adipose tissue or the fascia overlying the muscles and deep tissues. Skin masses include dermatofibrosarcoma protuberans (6% of all soft tissue sarcomas), peripheral nerve sheath tumor (also subcutaneous), liposarcoma (rarely), skin appendage lesions (epidermal inclusion cyst, pilomatrixoma, cystadenoma, cylindroma and syringoma), nonmelanomatous metastases, myeloma nodules (also subcutaneous), lymphoma (also subcutaneous), and myxoma (more frequently subcutaneous). The most frequent subcutaneous masses are lipomas, hemangiomas, lymphangiomas, peripheral nerve sheath tumors, malignant fibrous histiocytomas (more frequently deeper), liposarcomas (majority), epithelioid sarcomas, melanoma metastases, myelomas, myxomas, and lymphomas. A fascial origin is typical of nodular fasciitis and fibromatosis [53].

Lipoma is the most common mesenchymal tumor (16%) and has the following histologic variants: classic lipoma (solitary or multiple), fibrolipoma, angiolipoma, infiltrating lipoma, hibernoma, pleomorphic lipoma and lipoblastoma (solitary or multiple) [54]. It has an oval or patently elongated (discoid) appearance, with the long axis parallel to the skin (width/depth

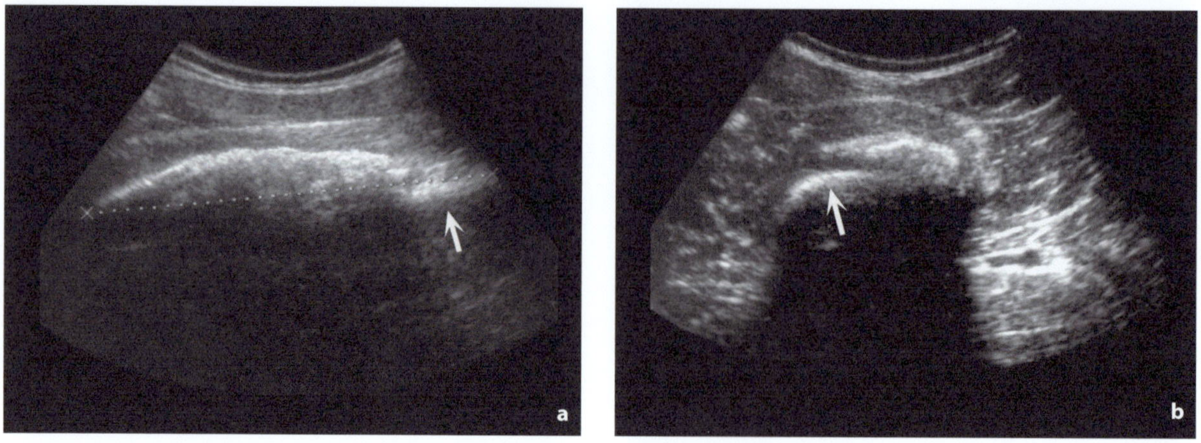

Fig. 2.54a,b Myositis ossificans of the thigh. Large calcified mass deep in the anterior compartment of the thigh (*calipers*), immediately above the femur (*arrow*)

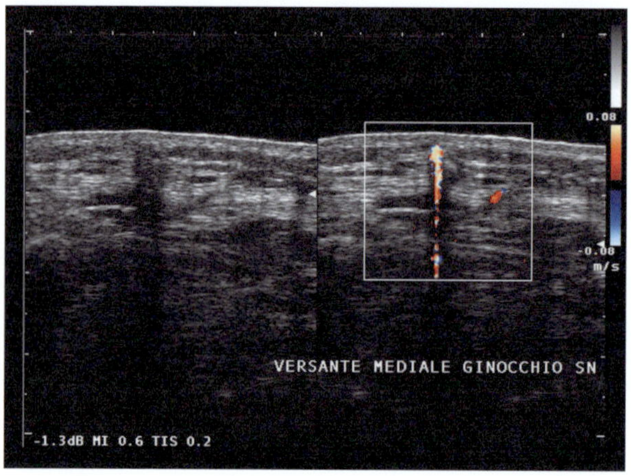

Fig. 2.55 Foreign body granuloma of the leg. Subcutaneous hypoechoic mass with irregular margins. CD identifies the foreign body (metal sliver) thanks to an evident sparkling artifact

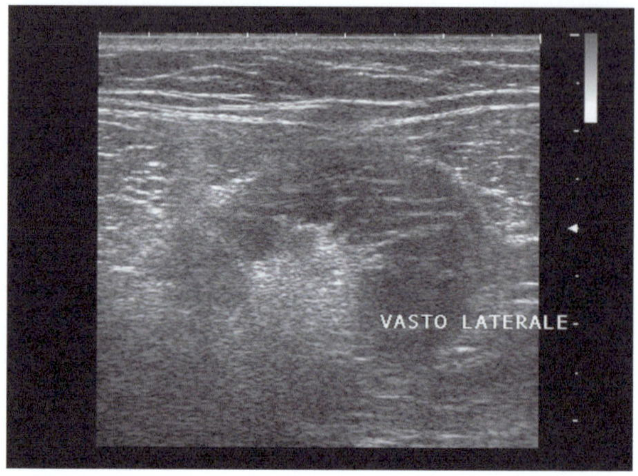

Fig. 2.56 Post-traumatic muscle scar at the level of the thigh. Large echogenic scar in relation with the vastus lateralis muscle

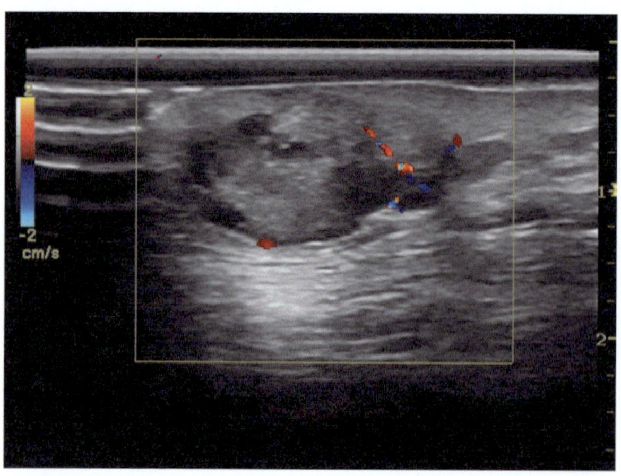

Fig. 2.57 Recurrence of melanoma of the derma. Subcutaneous lobulated hypoechoic nodule with vascular signals at CD

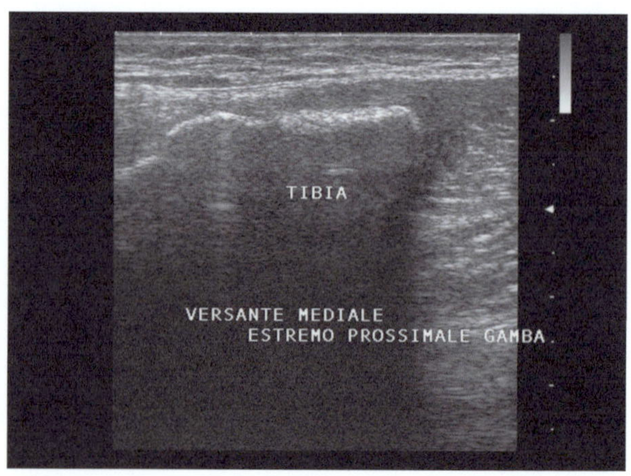

Fig. 2.58 Osteochondroma of the leg. A bony spur on the tibial surface with thin superficial hypoechoic lining and posterior acoustic shadowing

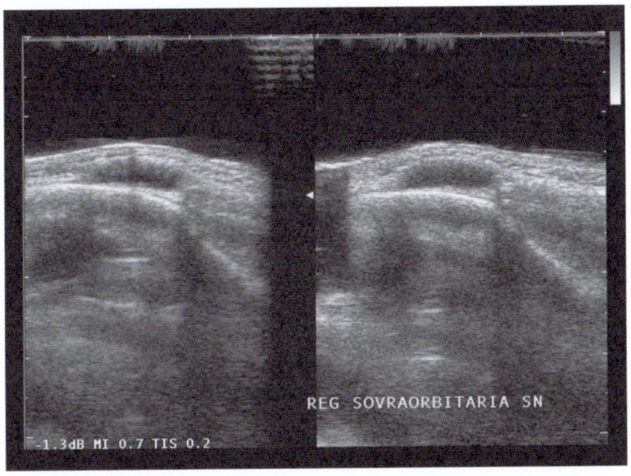

Fig. 2.59 Subcutaneous epidermoid cyst of the forehead in a pediatric patient. Homogeneous hypoechoic mass at the supraorbital level

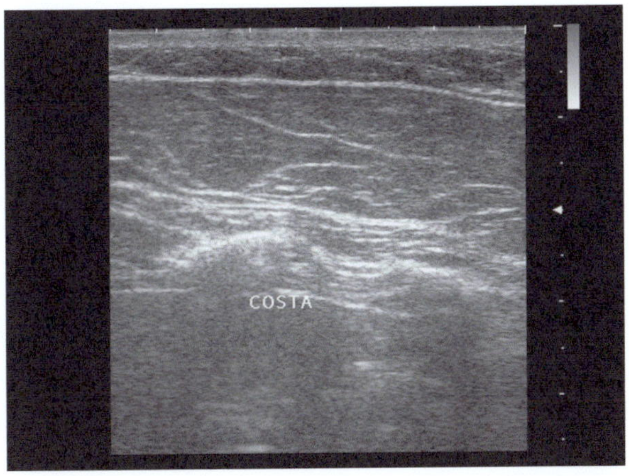

Fig. 2.60 Lipoma of the thoracic wall. An elongated mass can be identified above the muscle and costal plane appearing isoechoic to the subcutaneous fat

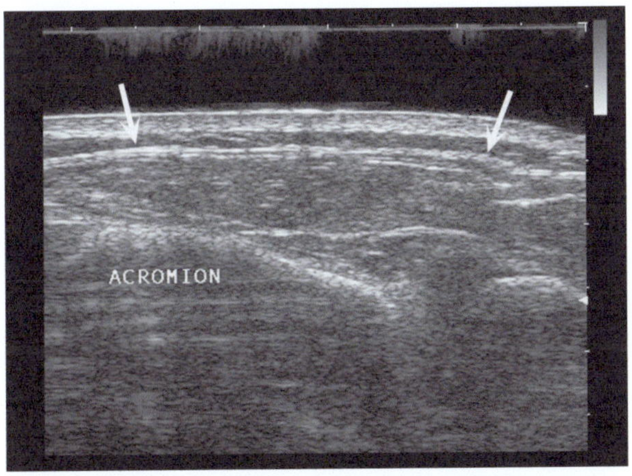

Fig. 2.61 Lipoma of the shoulder. Elongated echogenic lesion (*arrows*) located superficially at the acromioclavicular joint and separable from it

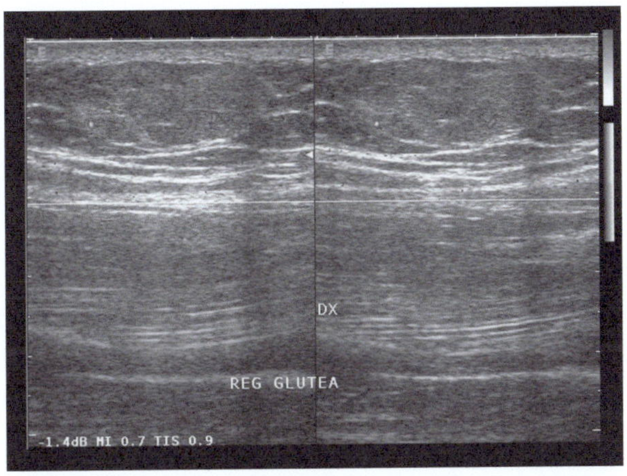

Fig. 2.62 Fibrolipoma of the gluteus. Mildly hyperechoic and slightly heterogeneous subcutaneous mass with sporadic vascular signals at directional PD

ratio around 3:1). Lipomas are predominantly found in the superior half of the body (but only 1 in 4 cases in the head and neck) located in the subcutaneous tissue or occasionally at the level of the muscle (suprafascial site in 70% of cases). The echotexture of lipomas is homogeneous in around 2/3 of cases and heterogeneous in the remaining 1/3, with internal hyperechoic bands oriented towards the long axis of the nodule being a common finding. The margins are well defined in 60% of cases, particularly the more superficial lesions, and ill-defined in the remaining generally deep cases. The echostructure of lipomas is hyperechoic in 29% of cases, hypoechoic in 29%, isoechoic in 20% and mixed in 20%. CD is able to demonstrate sporadic peripheral color signals, generally in the form of a single vessel with a regular course, whereas CEUS displays no variations in the various circulation phases of the contrast medium. In the event that significant color signals or contrast enhancement are detected, a biopsy – possibly targeted to the vascular area – is required to rule out a well-differentiated liposarcoma [55,56] (Figs. 2.60–2.63).

Lobulated **hemangiomas** can be markedly hypoechoic, weakly hypoechoic and occasionally hyperechoic. In addition, they may have a homogeneous, heterogeneous or multilocular appearance. In the latter case, identifying the lesion can be challenging, especially when intramuscular. Characteristics include relatively echogenic phleboliths with posterior acoustic shadowing. Compression with the transducer can significantly reduce the size of the lesion and lead to disappearance of anechoic areas corresponding to

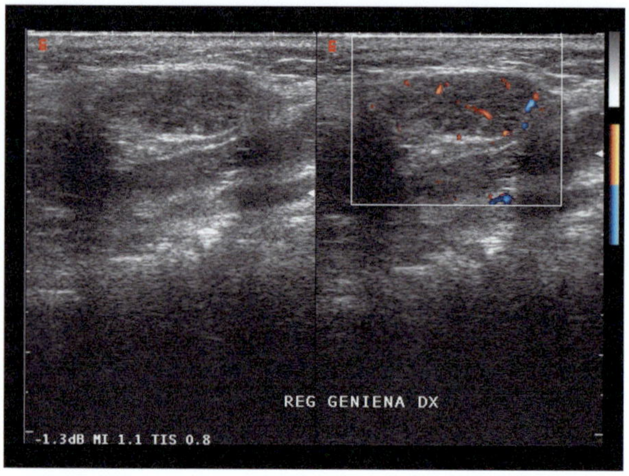

Fig. 2.63 Fibrolipoma of the cheek. Hypoechoic and mildly heterogeneous well-defined mass with some vascular signals at directional PD

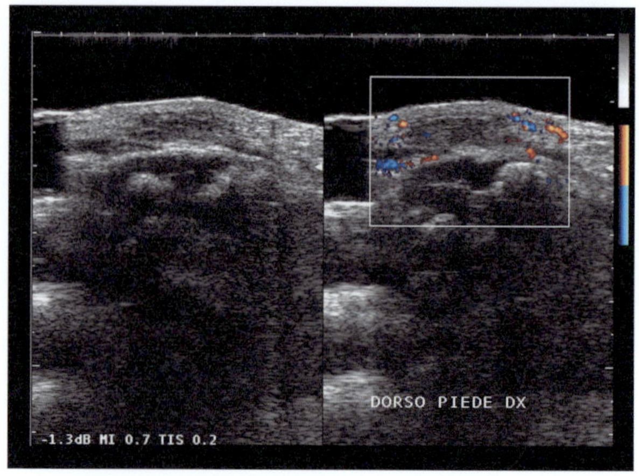

Fig. 2.64 Hemangioma of the foot. Heterogeneous hypoechoic mass with few vascular signals at directional PD

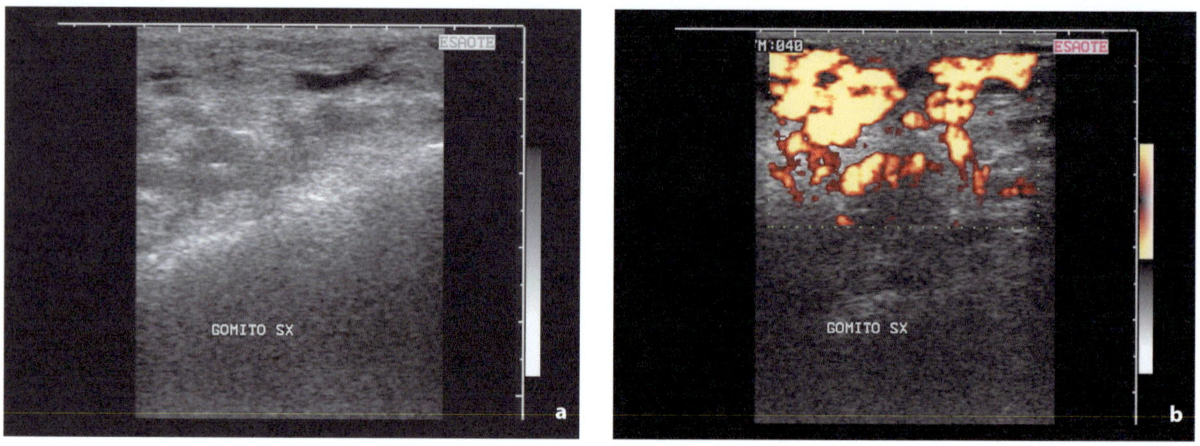

Fig. 2.65a,b Hemangioma of the elbow. Heterogeneous hypoechoic ill-defined mass (**a**) with diffuse vascular pools at PD (**b**)

vascular spaces. The CD signal is variable from hypovascular to hypervascular forms, and compression notably reduces flow [56] (Figs. 2.64–2.68).

Lymphangiomas are found for the most part in infants and prevalently in the head, neck or the upper chest, especially in the axillary region. At US they appear as hypoechoic masses with generally well-defined margins and are usually multilocular with thin septations and possible solid components [57,58].

Bursitis is found in para-articular anatomic regions where the synovial bursae are located. The lesion has a cystic appearance with a thin marked wall and homogeneous internal content or septations and papillary-like projections. CD is able to demonstrate signals in the wall, the septations and the papillary formations, although these findings are not indicative of malignancy. It would be rather unlikely for fluid collections such as abscesses and hematomas to display papillary projections and internal vascular signals, whereas soft tissue sarcomas never have a patently cystic appearance and always display some solid portion [59].

Myxomas are rare and possibly painful benign tumors generally found at the intramuscular level (82%). They are prevalent among females (50%) and middle-to-advanced aged subjects and are principally found in the thigh. They are partially compressible and at US appear oval, well-defined, heterogeneous and hypoechoic with possible cystic areas and often with enhanced through-transmission. The accumulation of perilesional fat often produces a more-or-less complete echogenic perilesional halo and a triangular echogenic area at one or both poles. The latter finding makes

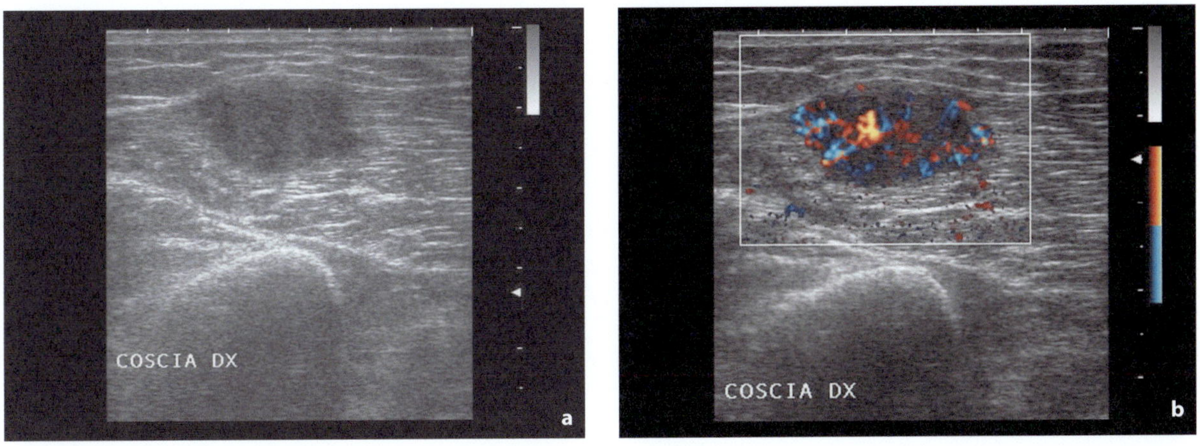

Fig. 2.66a,b Hemangioma of the thigh. Hypoechoic mass within the vastus medialis muscle (**a**). Diffuse vascular signals, especially in the periphery, at directional PD (**b**)

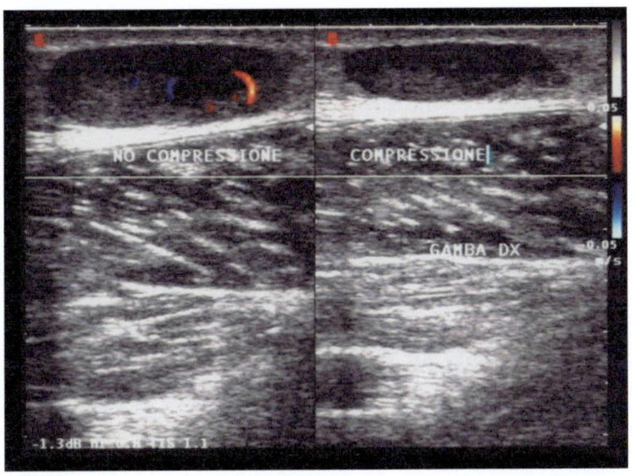

Fig. 2.67 Subcutaneous hemangioma of the leg, compression study. Oval hypoechoic formation with several internal vessels at CD which are completely cancelled with pressure from the transducer (*right side*)

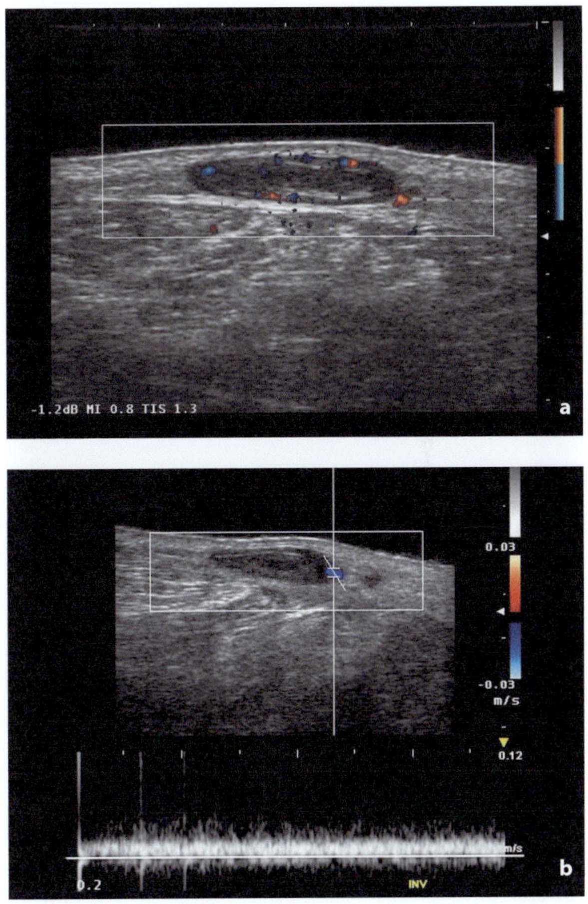

Fig. 2.68a,b Venous hemangioma of the leg. Well-defined hypoechoic formation with some flow signals at directional PD (**a**) and venous flow at the paranodular level (**b**)

differential diagnosis with neurogenic tumors challenging (see below) although, unlike these, myxomas are hypovascular and are not found in continuation with a nerve [56,60] (Fig. 2.69).

Desmoids are fibrous lesions which develop from muscular aponeurosis. They generally appear as ill-defined hypoechoic masses with possible posterior acoustic shadowing and moderate vascular signals at CD (Fig. 2.70).

Nodular fasciitis is an autolimiting reactive process consisting of proliferating fibroblasts and myxoid stroma. Its peak incidence is in the third and fourth decade of life, appearing as a rapidly growing and possibly painful mass located in the subcutaneous layer – in a muscle or the superficial fascia – prevalently in the upper extremities (volar forearms). At US

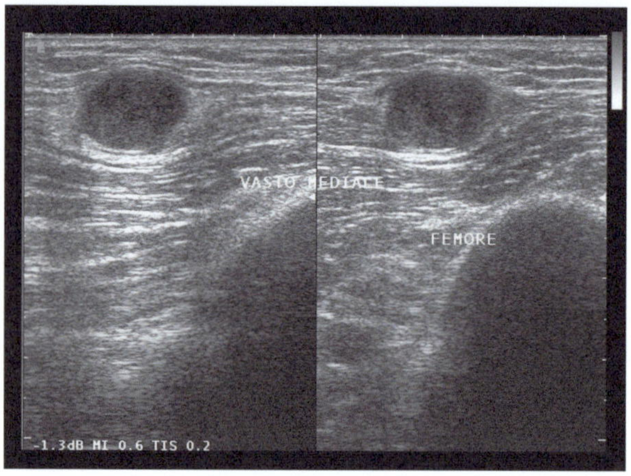

Fig. 2.69 Myxoma of the thigh. Hypoechoic formation with oblong echogenic shell in correspondence with the belly of the vastus medialis muscle

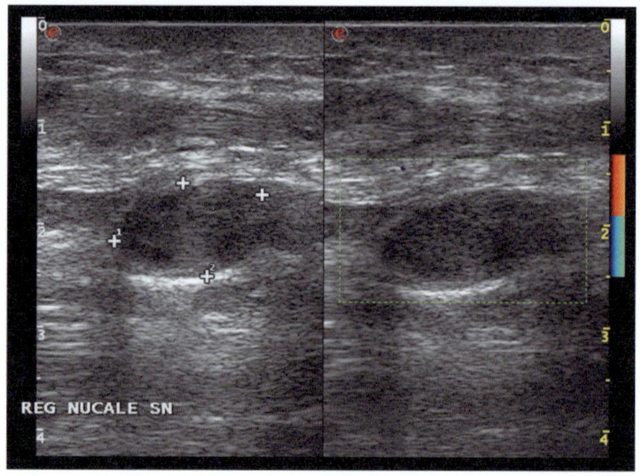

Fig. 2.70 Dermoid. Oval, hypoechoic nodule within the soft tissues of the back of the neck

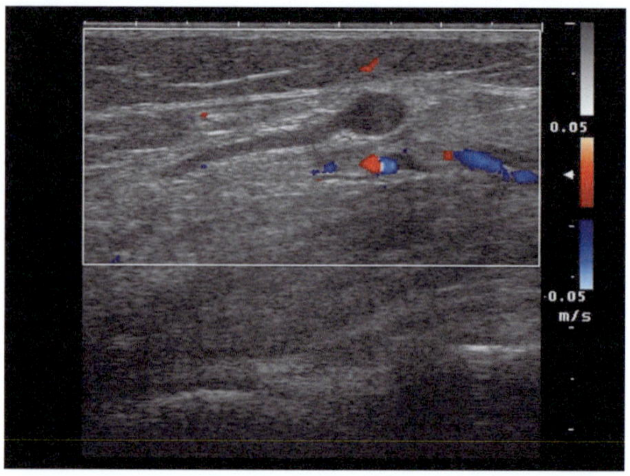

Fig. 2.71 Neuroma from amputation. Bulbous hypoechoic mass at the distal end of a nerve in the thigh of a patient operated on for sarcoma

it appears as an oval or lobulated hypoechoic nodule with heterogeneous echotexture, possible peripheral and central arterial vascular signals at CD and occasionally also microcalcifications [61].

Neurogenic "tumors" include neuromas, neurofibromas (benign and malignant schwannomas), intraneural ganglia, Morton's neuroma (sole of the foot) and post-traumatic neuromas (including those from nerve amputation following surgical resection) (Fig. 2.71). The malignant form consists of a malignant tumor of the peripheral nerve sheaths [62]. Peripheral neurologic symptoms are generally present as well as hypotrophy of the muscles that depend on the diseased nerve. At US the lesion appears oriented along the main axis of the nerve and may appear to extend proximally and distally in a fibrillar echogenic band corresponding to the nerve itself. In addition the lesion displaces the surrounding echogenic fat with the creation of a pseudocapsular image. Schwannomas – the most important neurogenic tumor – are prevalently found on the head, trunk and extremities, are often eccentric to the nerve and appear as oval and well-defined masses with homogeneous hypoechoic echostructure and increased through-transmission. The internal structure may present hyperechoic or cystic-like areas [63]. Neurofibromas are less well-defined and appear lobulated and often spindle-shaped, being elongated along the longitudinal axis of the nerve. Occasionally an internal hyperechoic halo may be revealed which is practically pathognomonic [64] (Figs 2.72, 2.73). During active and passive maneuvers of flexion and extension, neurogenic tumors show little mobility with respect to the surrounding musculotendinous structures [56]. CD shows internal hypervascularity, which is more marked in schwannomas, and the closeness of the neurovascular bundle [62]. Malignant forms generally reach a significant size (>5 cm) and have irregular and infiltrating margins and a heterogeneous internal structure with hypo-anechoic necrotic areas (Figs. 2.74, 2.75, Video 2.5). In the event of FNAC or biopsy the patient feels a painful jolt, which constitutes further diagnostic confirmation.

Skin and hematogenous subcutaneous **metastases** are relatively rare (5–10% of cancer patients) and, excluding melanomas, they originate from breast, lung, renal and gastrointestinal tract cancers (Fig. 2.76). Secondary lesions from melanoma are typically found in the subcutaneous tissue, whereas the others are skin lesions. When small, these lesions tend to be rounded, and then they progressively take on an irregular shape. Occasionally calcifications may be

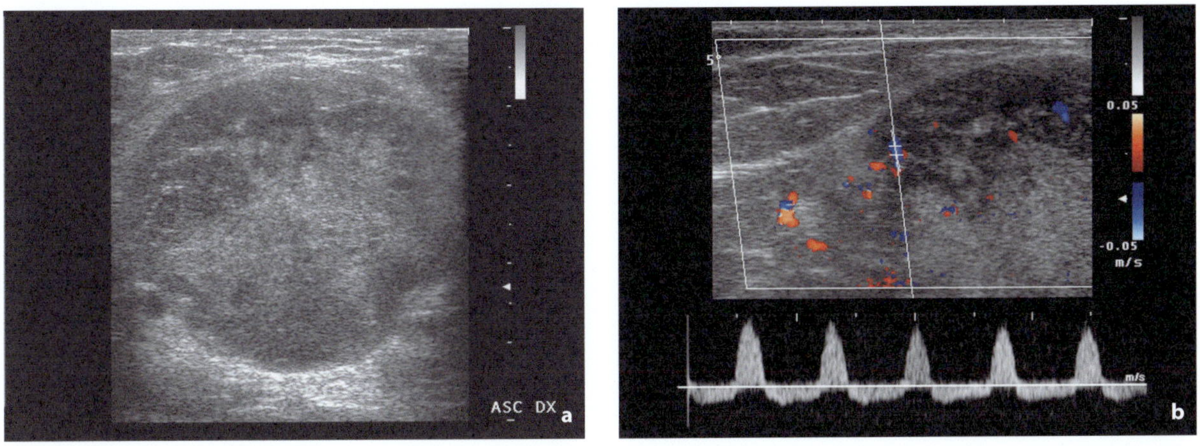

Fig. 2.72a,b Axillary schwannoma (median nerve). Oval macrolobulated nodule with heterogeneous hypoechoic appearance and increased internal echogenicity (**a**). Spectral analysis shows low-velocity flows (V_{max} 13 cm/s) with inversion of flow during diastole (**b**)

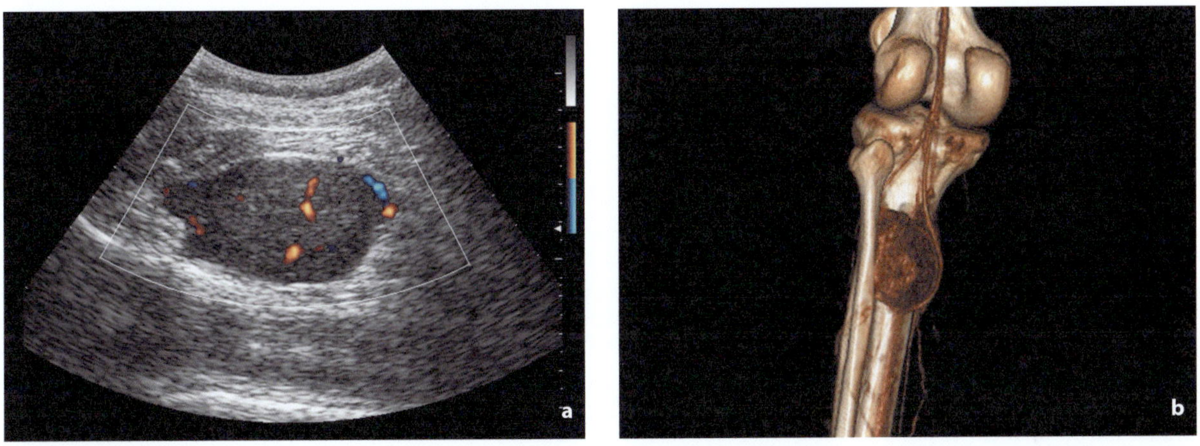

Fig. 2.73a,b Neurinoma of the leg. A lobulated mass with relatively homogeneous hypoechoic appearance and moderately vascular at directional PD can be identified in the proximal third of the leg (**a**). 3D CT reconstruction shows the displacement of the vascular structures adjacent to the mass (**b**)

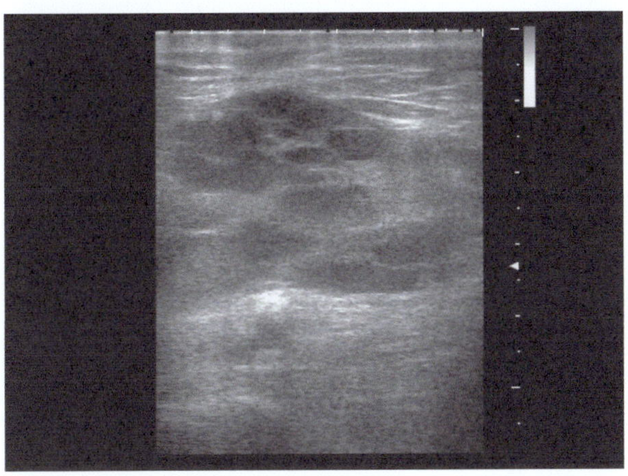

Fig. 2.74 Malignant schwannoma of the leg. Large mass with heterogeneous hypoechoic appearance and broad necrotic-hemorrhagic anechoic areas

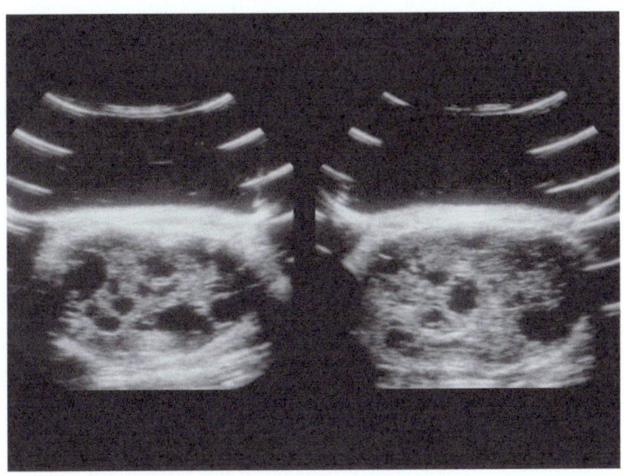

Fig. 2.75 Malignant schwannoma of the forearm. Large mass with heterogeneous hypoechoic appearance and multiple anechoic areas

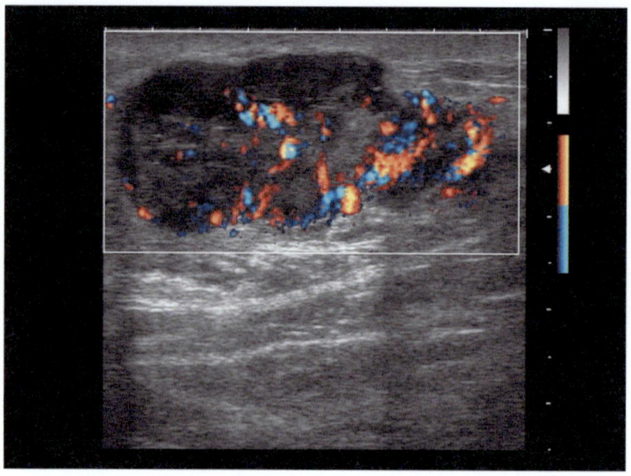

Fig. 2.76 Subcutaneous metastasis of the abdominal wall from lung cancer. Large hypoechoic nodule with moderate and irregular vascular signals at directional PD

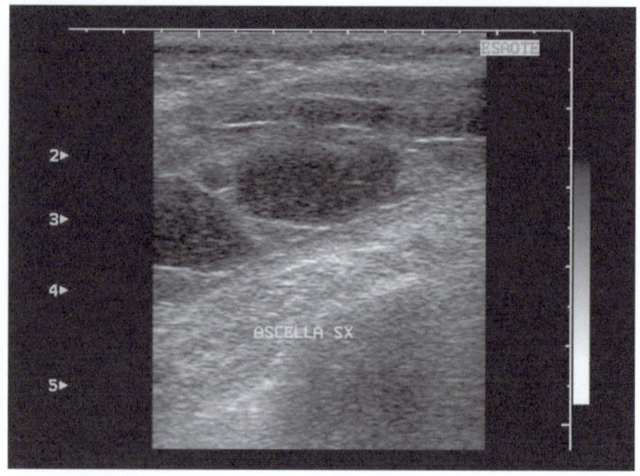

Fig. 2.77 Post-surgical axillary seroma. Hypoechoic, multilocular collection after axillary lymphadenectomy

associated, especially in lesions from gastrointestinal tumors.

Extranodal **lymphomatous** lesions of the superficial tissues are rather infrequent. Skin lesions are often hypervascular, although with a relatively evenly distributed vascularity. In the muscles a diffuse hypoechoic infiltrate may be seen, or better defined nodules with heterogeneous hypoechoic appearance and a variable degree of vascularity at CD [56].

Axillary masses include lymphadenopathies, skin alterations (sebaceous cysts, hydradenitis suppurativa, etc.), mesenchymal tumors (especially lipomas, but also lymphangiomas, neurinomas, etc.), accessory breast tissue or focal lesions thereof, vascular anomalies (aneurysms, etc.) and fluid collections [57] (Fig. 2.77). An "accessory breast" is found in a generally evident manner in 5–6% of women, and when the nipple or areola are absent it may be difficult to diagnose as it merges with other axillary expanses. This ectopic breast tissue may give rise to a focal lesion, albeit rarely, such as fibrocystic changes, milk cysts, fibroadenomas, phyllodes tumors or carcinomas [57,65] (Figs. 2.78, 2.79).

The **axillary lymph nodes** drain the upper limb, the thoracoabdominal wall to the navel and the breast. Modern US devices are able to identify the axillary lymph nodes or a part of them in most subjects. The finding of a lymph node with fatty involution, even of moderate size, is also frequent [66]. The most significant causes of axillary lymphadenopathies are lymphomas and metastases from breast cancer (occasionally occult) or from other tumors such as melanoma (Figs. 2.80–2.85). However, there are also benign forms, such as occur in acute and chronic inflammation, granulomatosis, connective tissue disease or immunodeficiencies (Fig. 2.86). A

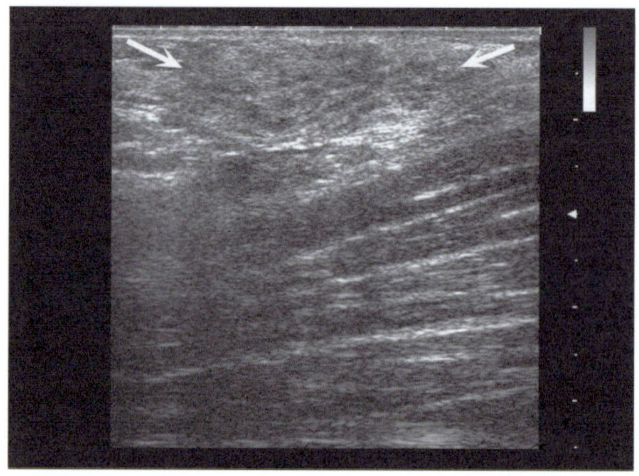

Fig. 2.78 Ectopic breast. Supernumerary glandular breast tissue in the axillary region (*arrows*)

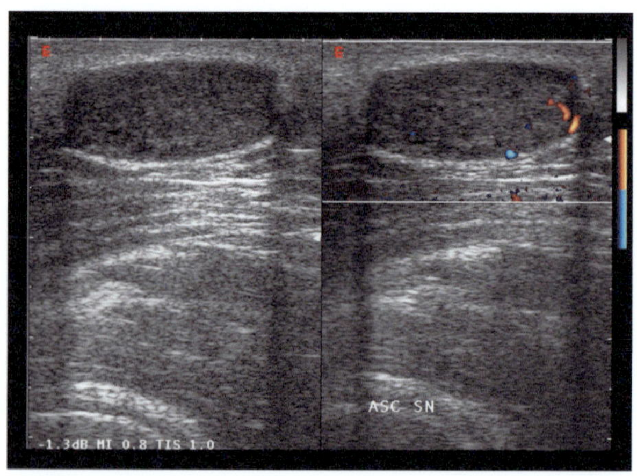

Fig. 2.79 Ectopic breast fibroadenoma. Well-defined nodule with homogeneous hypoechoic appearance and minimal color signals at directional PD arising in the axillary region from ectopic tissue

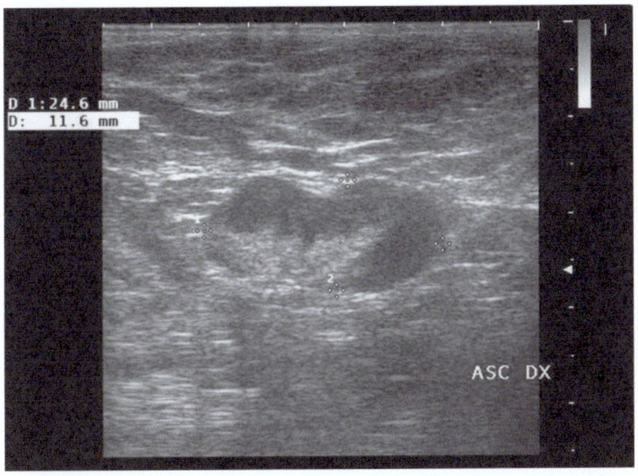

Fig. 2.80 Metastatic axillary lymphadenopathy from breast cancer. Moderately sized (25 mm) oval lymph node with the hilum conserved, but with marked and asymmetric cortical thickening

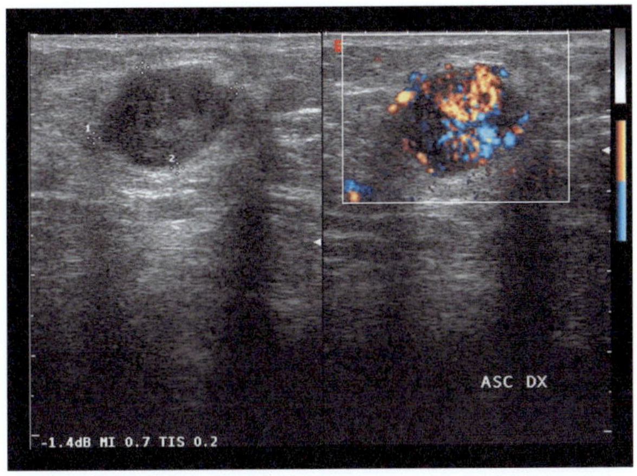

Fig. 2.81 Metastatic axillary lymphadenopathy from lung cancer. Rounded lymph node with a heterogeneous hypoechoic appearance, enhanced through-transmission and multiple vascular poles and marked asymmetric hypervascularity at directional PD

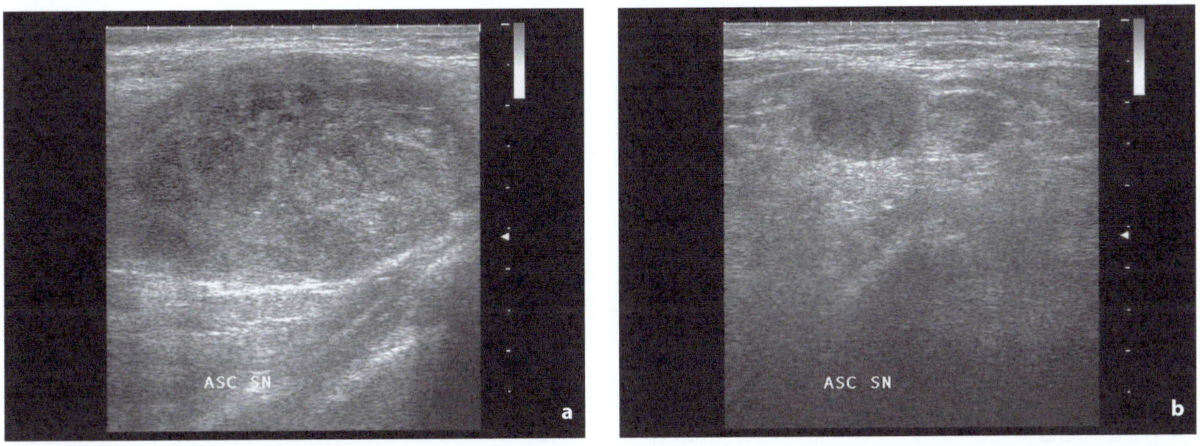

Fig. 2.82a,b Metastatic axillary lymphadenopathy from melanoma. Significantly enlarged lymph node with heterogeneous hypoechoic appearance (**a**). Two additional lymph nodes are associated, the smaller appearing with partial conservation of the central echogenic hilum (**b**)

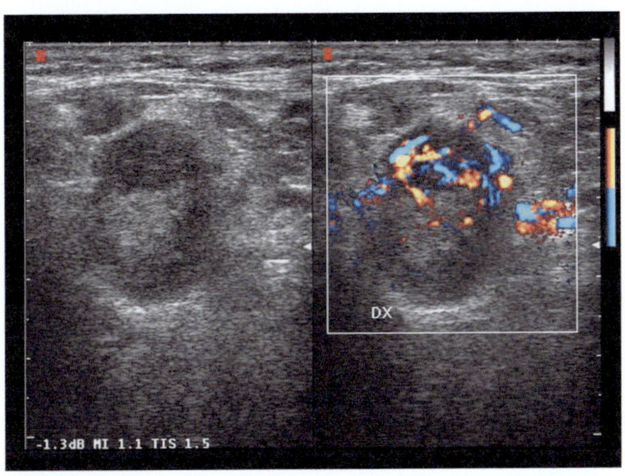

Fig. 2.83 Metastatic axillary lymphadenopathy from melanoma. Heterogeneous lymph node with hypoechoic superficial portion and hypervascularity at directional PD and more echogenic and less vascular deep portion

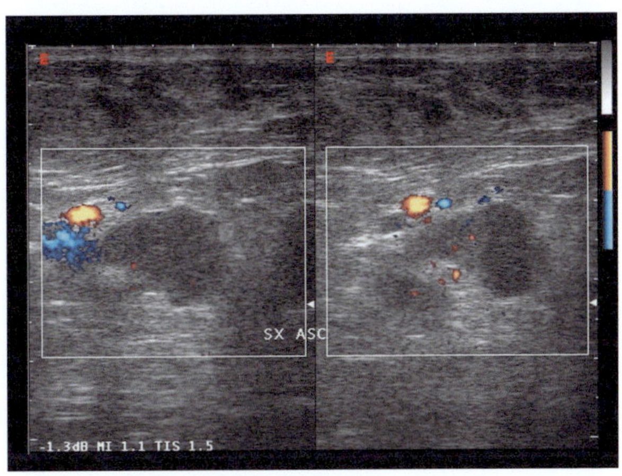

Fig. 2.84 Partial axillary lymph node metastasis of unknown origin (CUP syndrome). Heterogeneous hypoechoic lymph node with eccentrically thickened cortex which appears hypovascular with respect to the hilar signals at directional PD

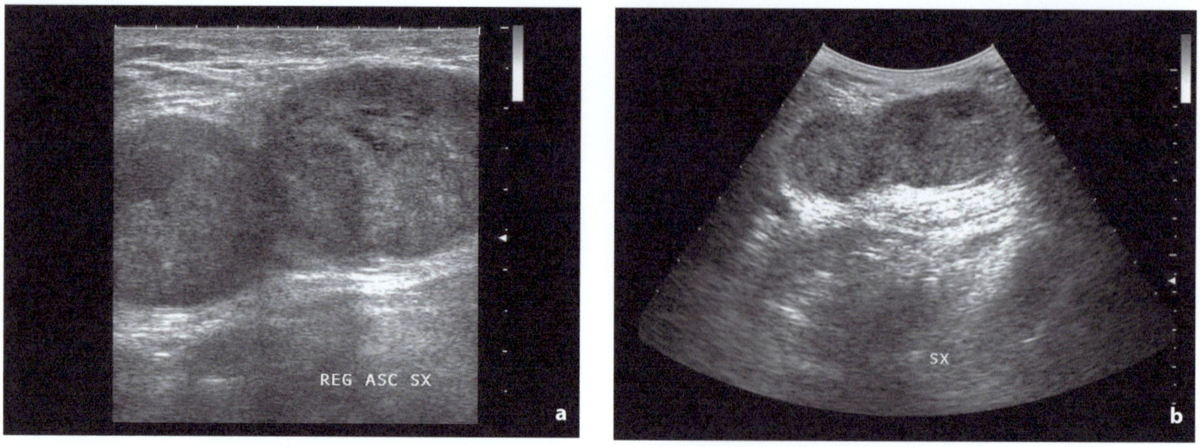

Fig. 2.85a,b Metastatic axillary lymphadenopathy from melanoma. Two enlarged confluent lymph nodes with heterogeneous hypoechoic appearance (**a**). Study with the abdominal transducer (**b**) provides an overall view of the lesion and makes its measurement possible

particular form is lymphadenopathy from silicon in women with implants [57,66]. The finding of enlarged lymph nodes in the axillary and subaxillary region during a mammography is relatively frequent. If this occurs in the absence of visible breast alterations and especially in the presence of a "clear breast", a US evaluation of the axillary region may not be required, especially if there are no clinical indications for suspicion or the nodes are not even palpable and at mammography they have an adipose appearance. However, if the breast cannot be completely explored with mammography due to preponderant glandular or fibroglandular components and if the lymph nodes have a dense appearance, US evaluation is required. In a study [67] on 30 consecutive patients with isolated enlarged axillary lymph nodes at mammography, US study demonstrated pathologic lymph nodes in as many as 20 cases and the definitive diagnosis was a tumor (breast carcinoma, lymphoma or other neoplasm) in 10. In two other studies the incidence of malignancy of enlarged lymph nodes identified incidentally at screening or routine mammography was 45–52% [68,69]. These high values are likely due to the inclusion criteria and in particular to what is precisely meant by "abnormal lymph nodes at mammography". Our personal experience is different: in the large majority of cases only enlarged lymph nodes with an appearance of fatty involution are encountered, or no enlarged lymph node can be found even after a thorough high-resolution US study. At any rate, US is effective in the evaluation of this mammographic finding, being able to effectively identify cases with the real presence of anomalous lymph nodes, characterize their nature and guide FNAC [67]. A false image of axillary nodulation capable of mimicking a

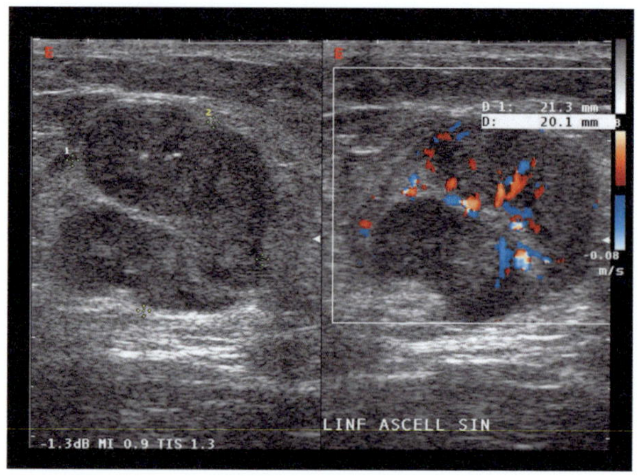

Fig. 2.86 Axillary lymphadenitis. Enlarged hypoechoic lymph node (calipers) with mild hilar vascular supply at CD

hypoechoic lymph node is given by venous vascular anomalies and in particular small saccular aneurysms or varicosities of the subclavian vein. The awareness of this possibility and its demonstration with CD are important, especially for avoiding their puncture [70].

Inguinal masses can be of various kinds: hernias, lymphadenopathies, uterine leiomyomas, endometriosis, desmoids, soft tissue or spermatic cord tumors (lipomas, inclusion cysts, lymphangiomas, liposarcomas, synovial sarcomas, mesotheliomas, etc.), cysts of the round ligament, fluid collections, masses of vascular origin (varices of the round ligament, aneurysm, pseudoaneurysms, etc.), bursitis, undescended testicle or masses of bony origin [71–74]

(Figs. 2.87–2.92). Indubitably the US appearances of these lesions tend to overlap, but clinical findings associated with morphostructural data make their characterization possible.

Masses of the superficial and deep inguinal **lymph nodes**, or also of the crural lymph nodes or of Scarpa's triangle, in the oncologic setting are linked to lymphomas or metastases. The latter may be due to melanomas or skin epitheliomas of the lower limbs (but also of the trunk), to other types of tumors of the lower limbs and pelvis, to malignancies of the external genitalia (vagina, vulva, penis) or of the lower third of the rectum or anus, or to deep abdominal-pelvic tumors (colon, rectum, cervix, endometrium, ovary, etc.) [72,73,75] (Figs 2.93–2.97). US can be used for the preliminary examination of lymph nodes in subjects scheduled for inguinal-femoral dissection (unilateral or bilateral), a procedure which can undoubtedly create significant problems for the patient, with the possibility of lymphedema and consequences for the venous region. In a study with patients with squamous cell carcinoma of the vulva, for example, US was in agreement with postoperative lymph node histology in 92% of cases and with the FNAC performed on the largest or most abnormal lymph node in 90% of cases. The two tests combined were able to correctly classify 95% of the examined inguinal regions [76].

Inguinal **hernias** (direct or indirect), or more rarely femoral hernias, may be congenital or acquired and constitute the most frequent cause of a palpable inguinal mass. They can be easily identified and

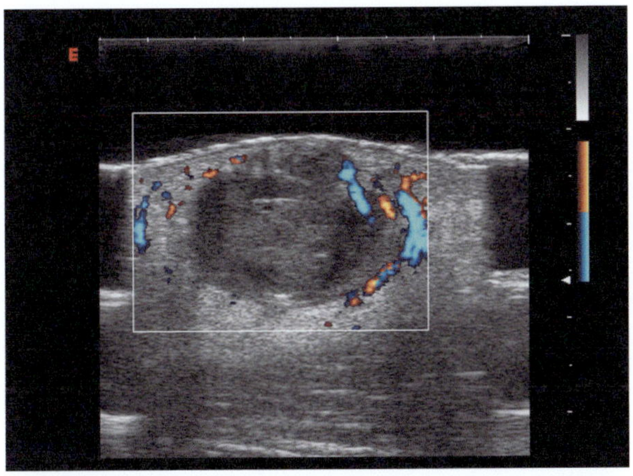

Fig. 2.87 Abscessed inguinal cyst. PD scan with pad showing densely corpuscular cyst with surrounding hyperemia. No internal flow signal is identifiable

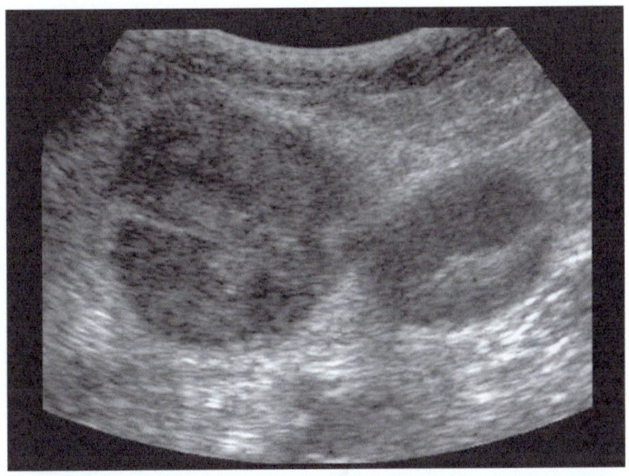

Fig. 2.88 Acute inguinal lymphadenitis. Two large hypoechoic lymph nodes with thin echogenic central residual hilum and edematous thickening of the surrounding fat

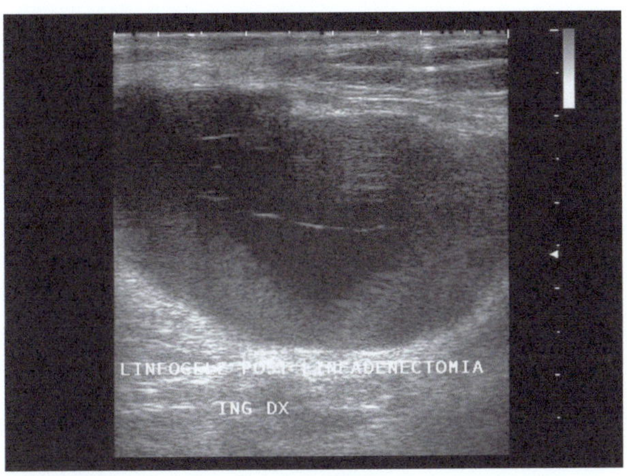

Fig. 2.89 Inguinal lymphocele after lymphadenectomy due to positive sentinel lymph node. Large heterogeneous fluid collection

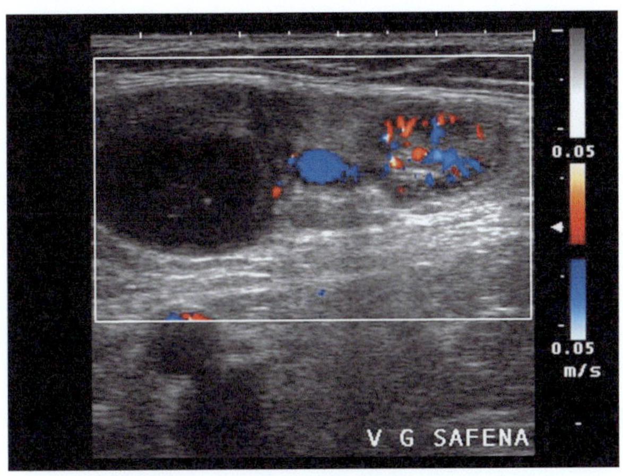

Fig. 2.90 Inguinal lymphocele after lymphadenectomy. CD shows a mildly heterogeneous fluid collection adjacent to the great saphenous vein and a lymphomatous lymphadenopathy

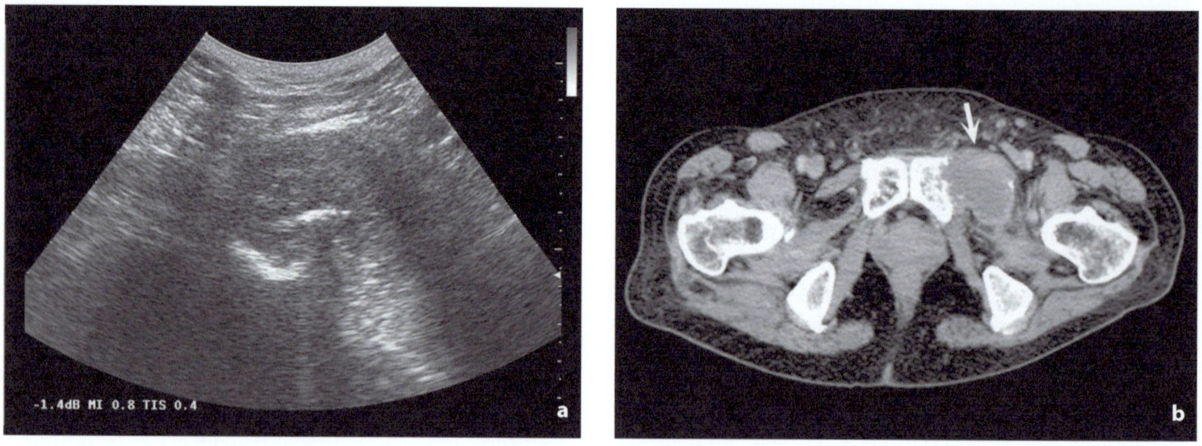

Fig. 2.91a,b Metastasis of the iliopubic eminence from lung cancer. US study of a patient with newly diagnosed lung cancer and inguinal soreness shows a hypoechoic mass incorporating the interrupted bony structures (**a**). CT scan confirms the mass protruding into the deep soft tissue of the inguinal region (**b**, *arrow*)

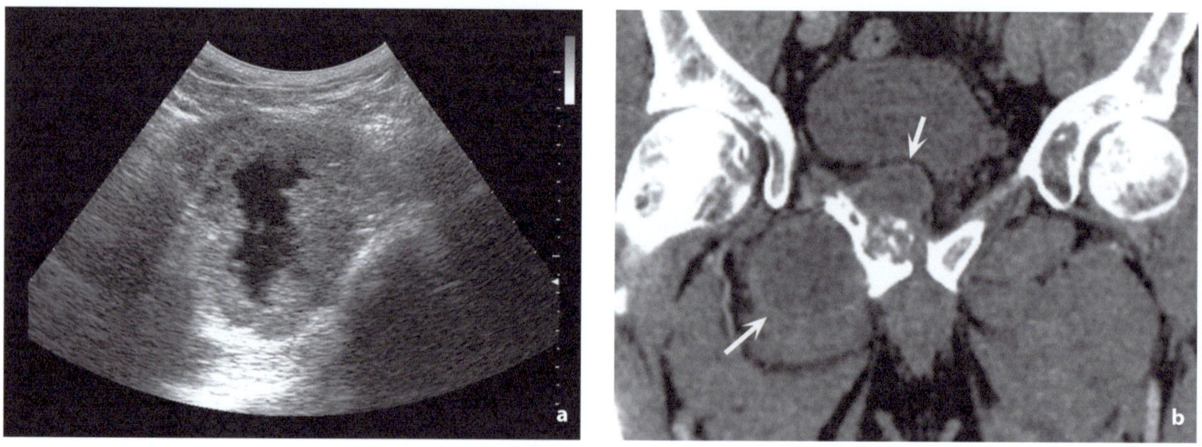

Fig. 2.92a,b Pubic chondrosarcoma. Large mass with necrotic center at the level of the pubis (**a**). Unenhanced coronal CT reconstruction (**b**, *arrows*) better shows the osteolysis and the endo- and exophytic bilobar conformation of the mass but less well defines the apparently homogeneous internal structure

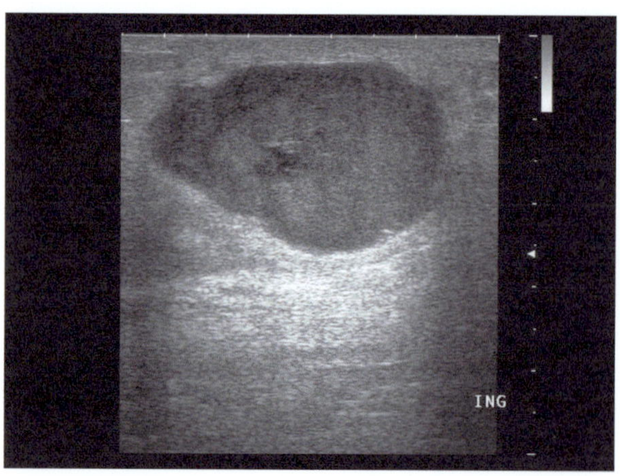

Fig. 2.93 Metastatic inguinal lymphadenopathy from melanoma. Large lymphadenopathy with heterogeneous hypoechoic appearance and initial central anechoic necrosis

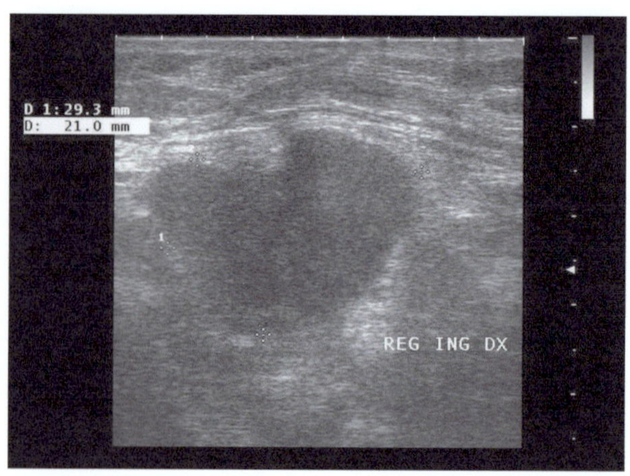

Fig. 2.94 Metastatic inguinal lymphadenopathy as clinical presentation of carcinoid of the cecum. Large (29 mm) lymphadenopathy with heterogeneous hypoechoic appearance

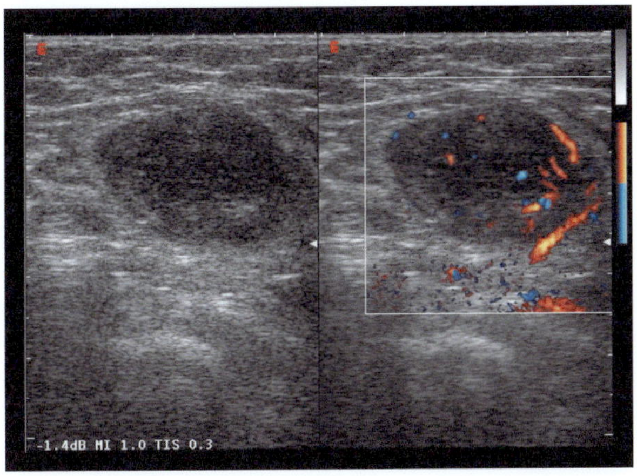

Fig. 2.95 Metastatic inguinal lymphadenopathy from cervical cancer. Heterogeneous hypoechoic lymphadenopathy with tendency to central liquefaction and asymmetric vascularity at directional PD

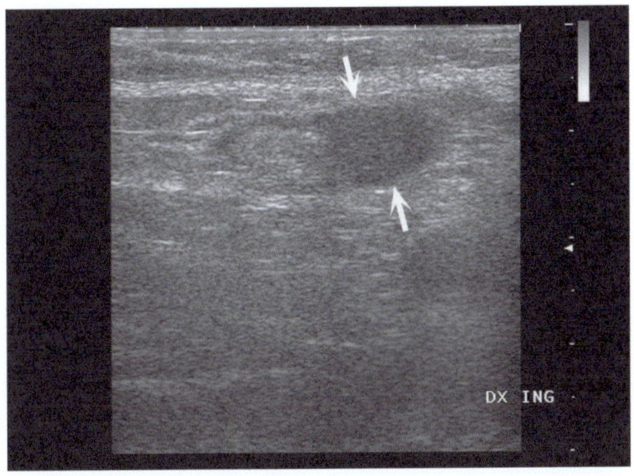

Fig. 2.96 Metastatic inguinal lymphadenopathy from penile squamous cell carcinoma. Partial lymph node involvement with broad eccentric hypoechoic area (*arrows*)

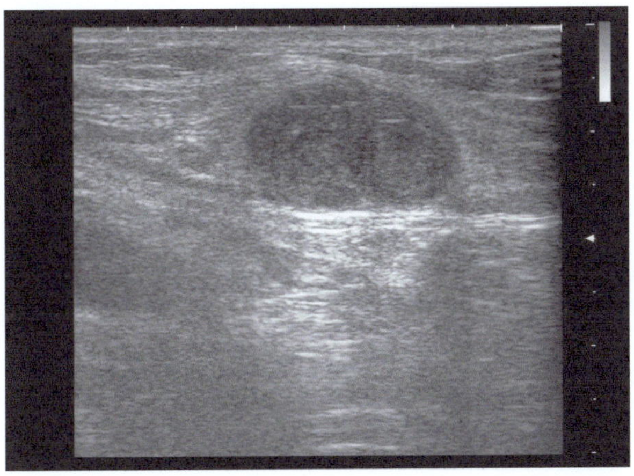

Fig. 2.97 Metastatic inguinal lymphadenopathy from melanoma of the leg. Large heterogeneous hypoechoic lymphadenopathy. Mild perinodular hyperechogenicity from edema

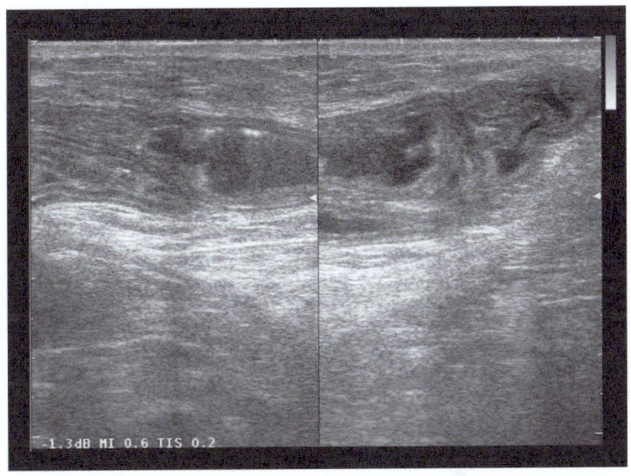

Fig. 2.98 Inguinal hernia involving the ileum. Mass with characteristic stratification of the intestinal wall and intraluminal presence of liquid material and areas of gas

classified by US as elongated formations and are often traceable right up to the internal inguinal ring. Regardless of the identification or otherwise of intestinal segments (Fig. 2.98), the simple excursion of the pseudomass with functional maneuvers is sufficiently diagnostic [77].

Undescended testicles may be found at any point along the inguinal canal, but are generally located in the medial third. They tend to be reduced in size, oval with a homogeneous hypoechoic appearance but with no evidence of a hilum (unlike lymph nodes). A **retractile testicle** may reascend temporarily into the medial portion of the canal [73,74].

Inflammatory processes can arise from superficial soft tissue or from the hip joint, and develop into diffuse cellulitis, circumscribed abscessed collections or synovial proliferations (e.g. from osteochondroma) [78]. A well-defined mass filled with more-or-less dense fluid may be the manifestation of **iliopectineal bursitis**, associated for example with rheumatic disease [73] (Fig. 2.99).

Hematomas are formed for the most part as a consequence of interventional vascular procedures or penetrating traumas. **Arteriovenous fistulas** and **pseudoaneurysms** often have onset after catheterization of the femoral artery. They appear as pulsating masses which can be easily identified at CD, which also enables their distinction from simple hematomas and provides orientation for treatment. The well-defined fluid-filled mass may appear pulsating and may display the movement of fine luminal corpuscles. CD shows turbulent flow and possible parietal

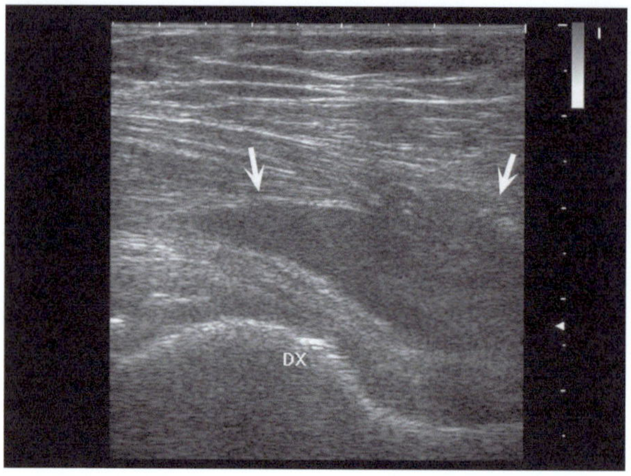

Fig. 2.99 Iliopectineal bursitis in patient with rheumatoid arthritis. Well-defined anechoic mass located immediately anterior to the coxofemoral joint (*arrows*)

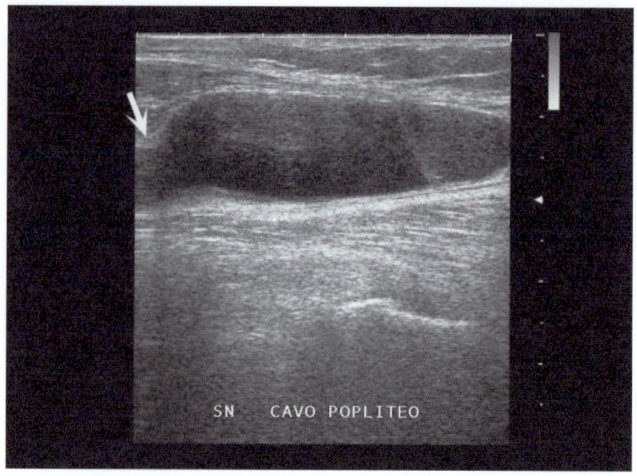

Fig. 2.100 Popliteal cyst. Cystic distension of the gastrocnemius-semimembranosus bursa, which appears as a well-defined relatively homogeneous anechoic mass with a neck (*arrow*) communicating with the joint space

thrombotic components [77]. **True aneurysms**, which are much rarer in this site, have a similar appearance. **Varicocele** may extend in the inguinal canal, displaying multiple collectors with venous flow which are accentuated during the Valsalva maneuver. Varices of the great saphenous vein can have a similar appearance at this level [73,77].

Lipomas of the spermatic cord and the inguinal canal are the most frequent extranodal tumor. They appear spindle-shaped, well-defined and moderately echogenic. Epidermoid cysts appear as hypoechoic masses with internal echoes due to detritus. Tumors of the ductus deferens are very rare [73,75,79].

Masses of the popliteal fossa are generally palpable, at least above a certain size, and are not uncommon clinical findings. The most frequent cause is **popliteal cyst**, i.e. the cystic distension of the gastrocnemius-semimembranosus bursa, which is frequent especially in middle-aged and elderly women with degenerative problems of the knee or in subjects with rheumatoid arthritis. The cysts appear as an oval or more commonly elongated mass situated posterior to the medial femoral condyle and in communication with the knee joint by way of a slit-like opening. The walls are thin but recognizable and the content can be anechoic, finely corpuscular or markedly corpuscular in the event of suppuration. Intraluminal calcified nuclei may also be found, whereas in subjects with rheumatoid arthritis the synovial membrane can obliterate the cystic lumen and thus mimic a solid lesion. In the even of rupture of the bursa the fluid diffuses in the soft tissue of the calf and the cysts appear as poorly defined hypoechoic areas [56,80] (Fig. 2.100). The **alternative causes** of a palpable popliteal mass include aneurysm of the popliteal artery or more rarely

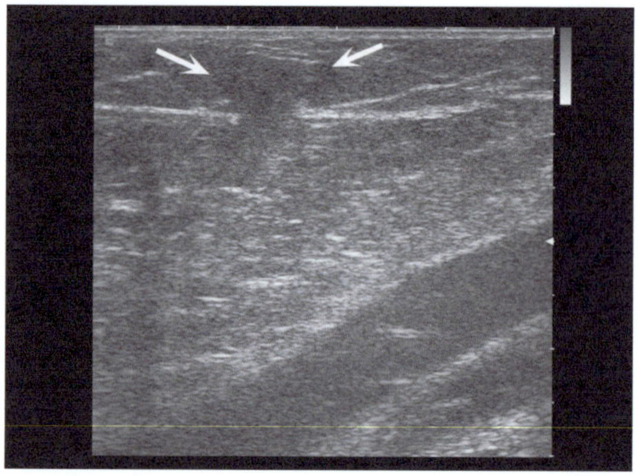

Fig. 2.101 Subcutaneous hernia of the popliteal fossa. Small adipose outpouching at the level of an interruption in the superficial fascia (*arrows*)

the popliteal vein, adventitial cysts of the popliteal artery, pseudoaneurysms of the popliteal artery or its branches, abscess, hematoma, muscular rupture, lipoma and sarcoma [80–82] (Figs. 2.101–2.105). In particular, the most typical location of synovial sarcoma is in fact the knee, especially when located posteriorly. The malignancy appears as a heterogeneous hypoechoic mass with possible internal calcification. A tumor should be suspected above all when the structure is mixed – cystic and solid – or when confronted with a solid heterogeneous mass. CD should also be used for a thorough search for relations with the relatively superficial popliteal vein and the deeper popliteal artery. In addition to a complicated Baker's cyst, the differential diagnosis of tumors should also include disease of vascular origin when the

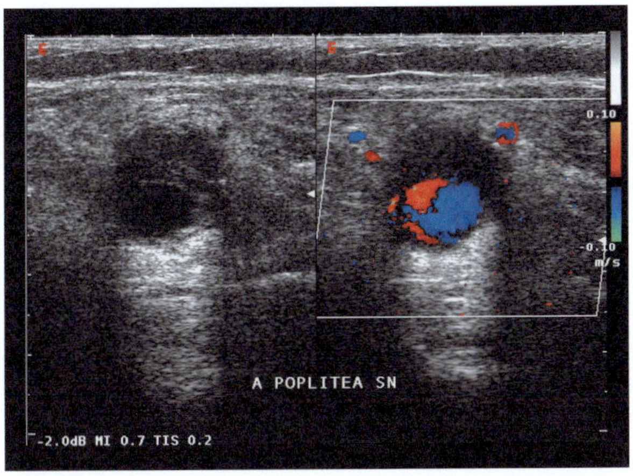

Fig. 2.102 Aneurysm of the popliteal artery. Spindle-shaped focal dilatation of the artery with eccentric luminal thrombosis

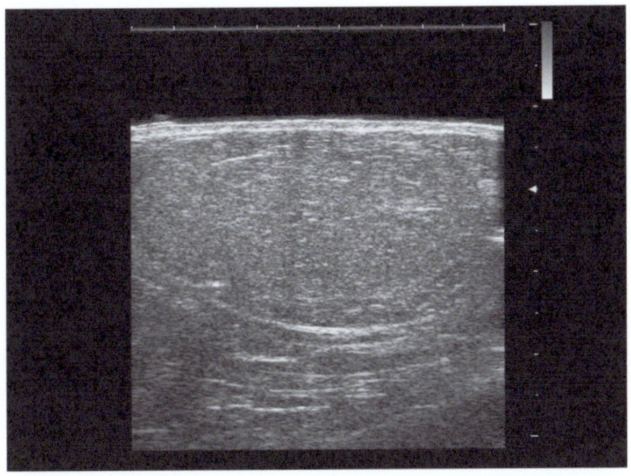

Fig. 2.103 Fibrolipoma of the popliteal fossa. Large oval mass with relatively homogeneous echogenic appearance

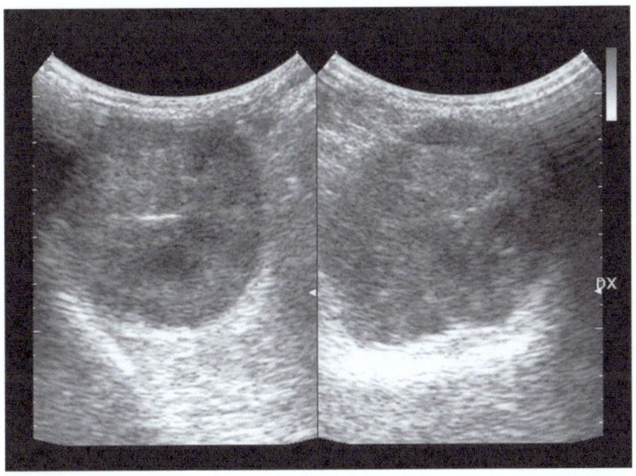

Fig. 2.104 Synovial sarcoma of the knee. Large and heterogeneous hypoechoic mass visualized with abdominal transducer

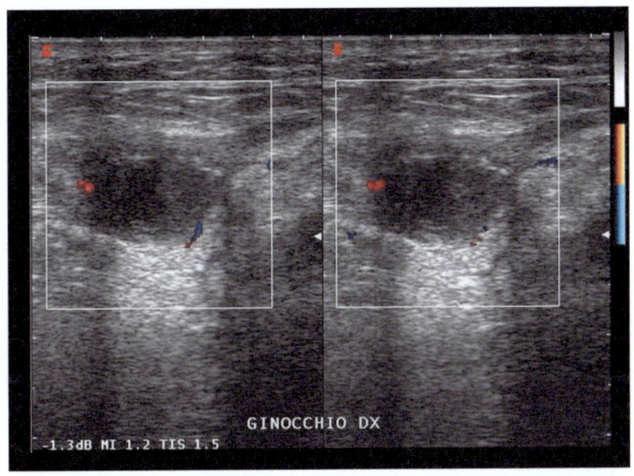

Fig. 2.105 Recurrence of popliteal sarcoma. Heterogeneous hypoechoic nodulation with some marginal signals at directional PD at the level of the surgical bed

lumen of the vessel itself is compressed or obliterated and therefore no longer identifiable.

Expansive lesions in the **hand** and **wrist** are for the most part dystrophic or hamartomatous rather than neoplastic. They are found in all age groups and without a particular prevalence in either sex. They include accessory muscles, circumscribed myositis ossificans, ganglia, giant cell tumors of the tendinous sheaths (63% of cases in the wrist and hand), hemangiomas, lipomas, Dupuytren's palmar fibromatosis, fibrolipoma of the median nerve, leiomyomas, neurofibromas, schwannomas, synovial sarcomas and epithelioid sarcomas (40% of cases in the hand and wrist) [53,83]. **Ganglia** (ganglia cysts) account for 59% of soft tissue focal lesions in the hand and wrist and are more common in young women. They are structures with mucinous content adjacent to the sheaths of the tendons (whereas synovial cysts are outpouchings of the synovial membrane through the capsule and are therefore communicating). Ganglia appear as rounded or oval, simple or complex, well-defined masses with anechoic or markedly hypoechoic structure and enhanced through-transmission (Fig. 2.106) [84]. More peculiar forms can be found in the **foot**, including Morton's neuroma and plantar fibromatosis, which appears in the form of oval hypoechoic nodulations of the plantar aponeurosis. Masses of the **fingers** and **toes** include ganglia and synovial cysts, epidermal inclusion cysts (ungueal bed), giant cell tumors of the tendinous sheath, fibromas of the tendinous sheath, extraskeletal chondromas, neurofibromas, lipomas, hemangiomas and glomus tumors

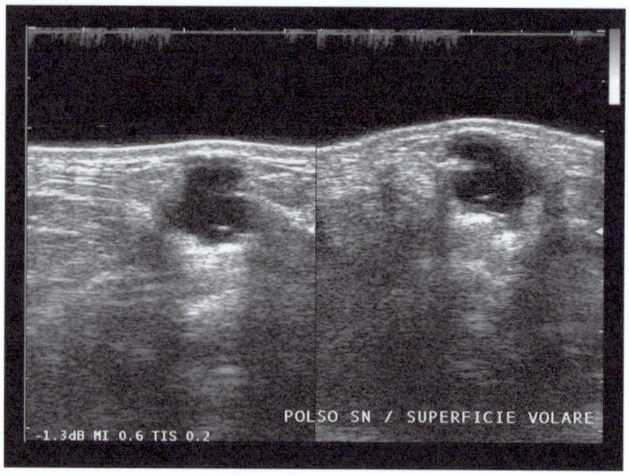

Fig. 2.106 Gamglion of the wrist. Lobulated anechoic mass at the level of the flexor compartment

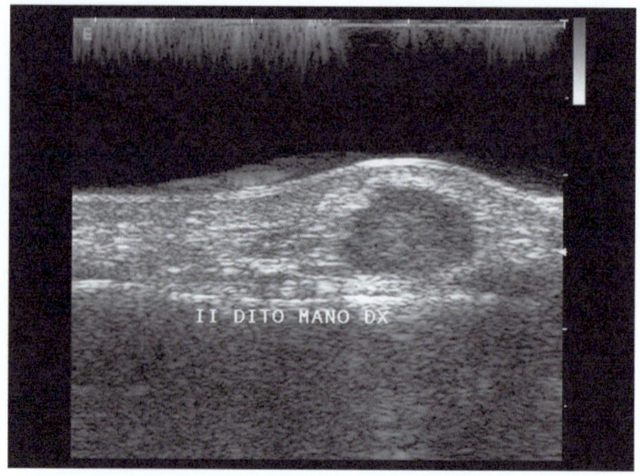

Fig. 2.107 Tumor of the tendinous sheath of the hand. Scan with spacer of the second finger shows a well-defined homogeneous hypoechoic nodule in a child with a painless palpable mass

(ungueal bed) [85]. Giant-cell tumors situated in the tendinous sheaths appear as more-or-less homogeneous hypoechoic masses of variable size and with moderate vascularity. These nodules are found adjacent to tendons, may erode or deform the bone cortex and can displace the digital arteries [86] (Fig. 2.107).

Soft tissue palpable lesions of the **scapular region** include subacromial-deltoid, scapular-thoracic and subscapular bursitis, acromioclavicular cysts, fluid collections (hematomas, abscesses, postoperative collections, etc.), synovial osteochondromatosis, myositis ossificans, lipomas, histiocytoma fibrosis, nodular fasciitis, fibromatosis, nerve sheath tumors, elastofibroma dorsi, sarcomas and masses arising from bone and cartilage [87] (Fig. 2.108). **Elastofibroma dorsi** is a not uncommon connective tissue proliferation, in part underestimated, which may be found unilaterally or occasionally bilaterally between the inferior scapular angle and the thoracic wall, and is produced by the friction from scapular movements. This pseudotumor is found in middle-aged and elderly subjects with a prevalence among females. Below the muscle plane a striated structure can be identified with an echogenic background (adipose) and hypoechoic linear or circular bands (fibroelastic) or a hypoechoic background with interposed echogenic strips. The margins may be sharp or poorly defined with respect to the adjacent soft tissue. No signs of infiltration or bone erosion are found. Abduction of the upper limb may facilitate the study; the moderate soreness and muscular-like US appearance make the finding typical, if known to the examiner, and help to avoid further examinations or biopsy [88,89] (Fig. 2.109).

Masses in the **gluteal region**, especially if deep, may reach a significant size before being identified, with symptoms associated with sciatic nerve compres-

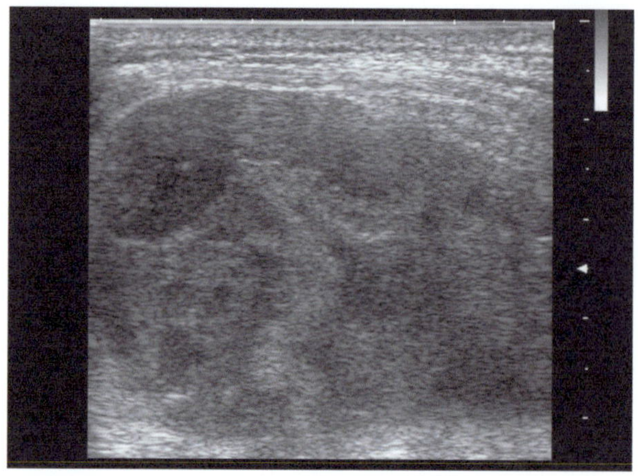

Fig. 2.108 Spontaneous shoulder hematoma in an elderly man. Large tumor-like lesion is identifiable within the posterior soft tissues of the shoulder

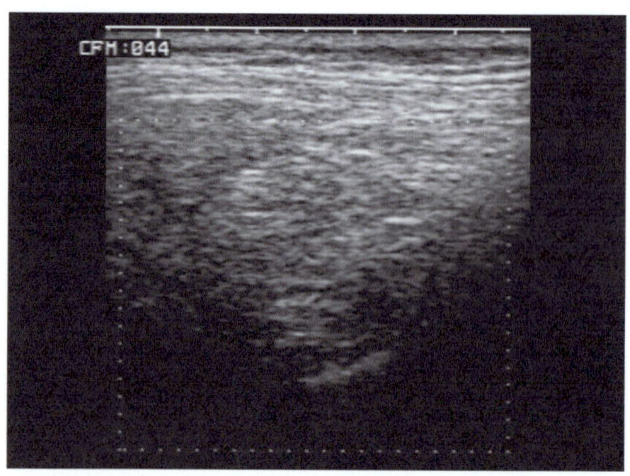

Fig. 2.109 Elastofibroma dorsi. Ill-defined and heterogeneous lesion is identifiable adjacent to the apex of the scapula

sion or swelling of the gluteal region. The pathologic processes which may be found unilaterally or occasionally bilaterally include sciatic bursitis (superficial to the tuberosity), masses arising from the posterior bony or cartilaginous structures of the pelvis, neurogenic tumors (sciatic nerve), muscle metastases, epidermoid inclusion cysts, rectal duplication cysts, aneurysm of the sciatic artery, lateral sacral meningocele, amyloidomas (chronic hemodialysis) and post-infection sequelae (tissue necrosis, abscesses, granulomas) (Fig. 2.110).

Masses of the thoracic wall, and even more so of the abdominal wall, are a frequent occurrence. They may give rise to symptoms of pain or not, they can be longstanding or of recent onset and they may be constant or intermittent. Not always, however, do they constitute an effective alteration when identified at palpation by the physician or patient themselves, because the finding may also be related to asymmetric conformations, such as of the underlying muscles or a bony protuberance (e.g. inversion of the xiphoid appendix or rib dysmorphisms). On the other hand, some lesions cannot be palpated, particularly in obese patients or at any rate patients with a thick panniculus: in this case the finding can be incidentally identified during an abdominal US study when a "bump" is felt when running the transducer over the skin or as an alteration in extreme close-up in the FOV of an abdominal transducer. In these cases reassessing the region with a high-frequency transducer is advisable.

The normal **thoracic wall** is formed by the ribs and their cartilaginous extensions alternated by the intercostal spaces. At the intercostal level the skin, subcutaneous fat, muscles, the thoracic fascia, extrapleural fat and the parietal pleural can be identified. The "pleural line" can be identified as a linear hyperechoic interface between the parietal tissue and the lung and is characterized during breathing by a movement of the ribs in the opposite direction [90]. The **abdominal wall** displays a number of layers: (1) skin – echogenic; (2) subcutaneous – generally reticular hypoechoic and of variable thickness; (3) muscle – fibrillar structure with intermediate echogenicity. The lateral muscles display three layers – oblique external, transverse abdominal and oblique internal. The echogenic aponeurotic membrane of these muscles widens to receive the rectus muscle of each side at the paramedian level, which has a lenticular appearance in the transverse plane, thus forming the anterior and posterior surface of the sheath of the rectus. Then the aponeurotic membranes from the two sides fuse on the median line, thus giving rise to the linea alba. Deep to the muscle plane are the echogenic transverse fascia, the hypoechoic extraperitoneal fat and the echogenic anterior parietal peritoneum [77,91].

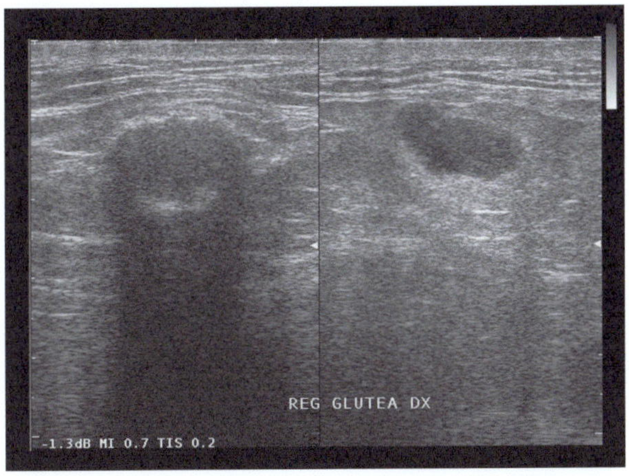

Fig. 2.110 Granuloma of the gluteus. In the gluteal region two granulomas can be identified in the gluteal region, one more recent with hypoechoic appearance and enhanced through-transmission (*right*) and the other less recent with broad calcified shell and posterior acoustic shadowing (*left*)

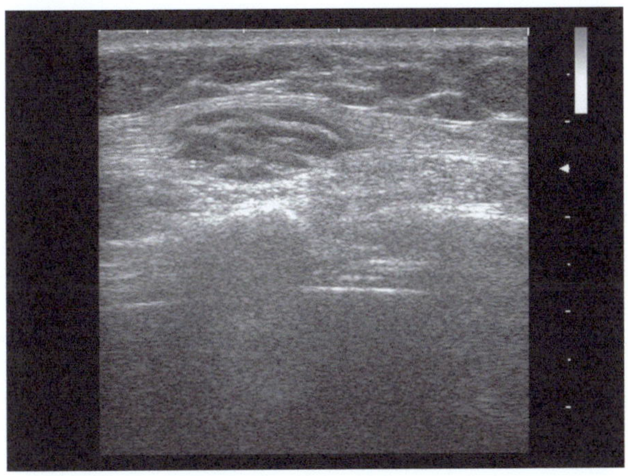

Fig. 2.111 Submammary leiomyoma. Hypoechoic nodule with echogenic bands located in the muscular layer of the thoracic wall

Masses of the thoracic wall include fluid collections, primary benign (lipomas, lymphangiomas, etc.) and malignant tumors (liposarcomas, histiocytomas, malignant fibrosis, fibrosarcomas, dermatofibrosarcomas, etc.) of the superficial soft tissues, bone tumors of the rib cage (especially chondromas and chondrosarcomas) and lymphomas (especially Hodgkin's lymphoma as an extension from the mediastinum) [58] (Figs. 2.111–2.113). A distinction needs to be made between these masses and pulmonary carcinomas that have invaded the thoracic wall (T3), which might not always be easy to do beyond a certain size. Unlike these, however, benign and malignant thoracic wall lesions usually appear as hypoechoic masses with smooth margins with a curved and smooth interface

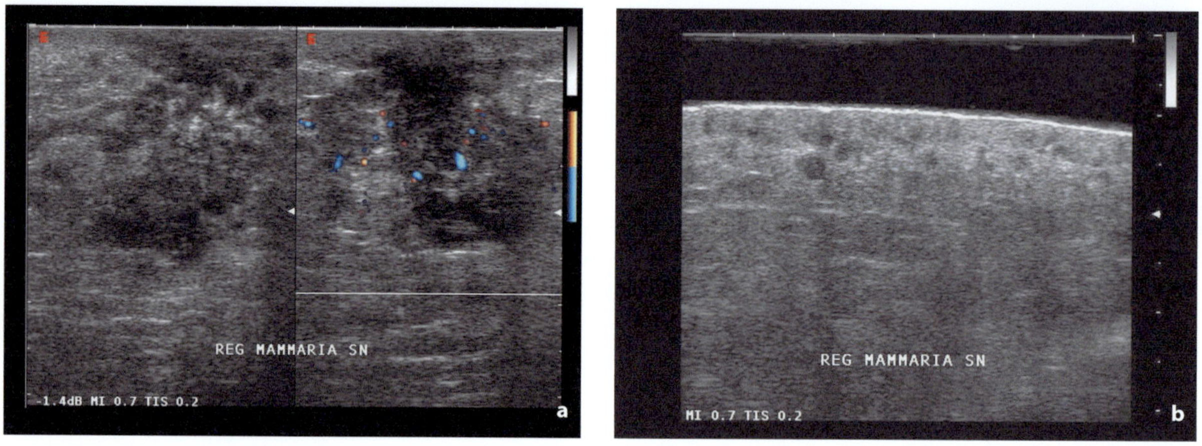

Fig. 2.112a,b Pectoral metastases from melanoma in male patient. Heterogeneous hypoechoic and poorly defined infiltrate with some flow signals at directional PD located in the retroareolar area (**a**). Superior to the metastatic lesion diffuse hypoechoic areas can be seen in the pectoral muscle (**b**)

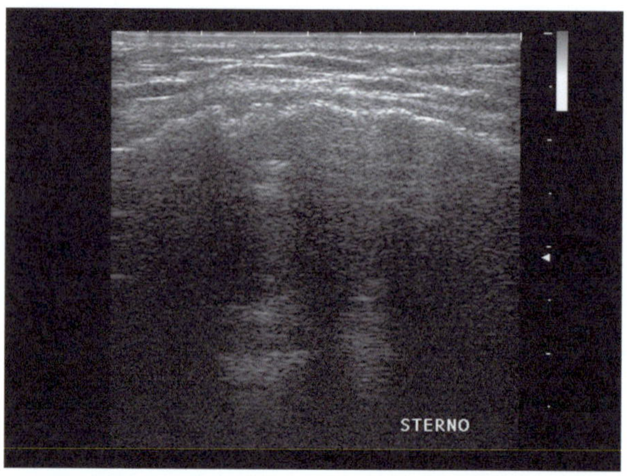

Fig. 2.113 Sternal metastases from breast cancer. Diffuse irregularity of the anterior sternal cortex view in the longitudinal plane

with the underlying lung. Moreover, the lesion appears firmly attached to the thoracic wall during respiratory motion [92]. Invasive pulmonary carcinoma interrupts the echogenic pleural line, crosses into soft parietal tissues and appears fixed during respiratory motion.

Primary malignant tumors of the **thoracic wall** account for around 2% of solid pediatric tumors and 3–8% of thoracic tumors in adults [93]. Since local recurrence occurs in 7–52% of cases, an accurate assessment of the tumor margins is crucial prior to resection. This applies to both the deep extension, which can be excellently defined with CT and MR particularly in terms of the cervicomediastinal vessels, and the superficial extension, for which US is superior to the other modalities in obtaining a wide lateral resection margin. CT and MR, in fact, are less able to define the relations with the various superficial layers of the thoracic wall and can therefore overstage, or, more frequently, understage the extension of the lesion leading to an insufficiently wide resection margin (bearing in mind that in this anatomic region the surgeon must preserve respiratory mechanics and therefore try not to excise beyond the tumor margins more than is necessary). US is also more accurate in identifying small satellite nodules, which characterize sarcomatous recurrence and the preoperative identification of which is crucial for en bloc excision [93] (Figs. 2.114, 2.115).

Costal metastases are identified with good accuracy by US, which, based on the site of referred pain, is able to explore the entire rib in question and detect irregular destruction of the bone cortex and the presence of a hypoechoic fleshy component. This is especially important because cancer patients are often elderly and/or cachectic, and can therefore suffer from rib fractures relatively easily after mild trauma, or even after a fit of coughing or exertion, such that fractures of this kind may not be present in the patient history. These fractures, which occur most frequently at the costochondral joint, may produce radiotracer uptake at bone scintigraphy. In this case a patent discontinuity can be seen ("step" image at the level of the echogenic cortical line), with possible hematoma of the pericostal tissue and callus formation (echoic nodulation with posterior acoustic shadowing) [90,94]. Three patterns of tumor involvement of the ribs have been identified: Pattern I, eccentric hyperechoic plate-like shadow inside a hypoechoic tumor (pattern characteristic of Pancoast tumor); Pattern II, rounded hyperechoic shadow or ring in the center of a hypoechoic tumor (metastasis); Pattern III, isolated hypoechoic tumor (metastasis or benign tumor). Unlike the patterns described, other elements such as the shape and

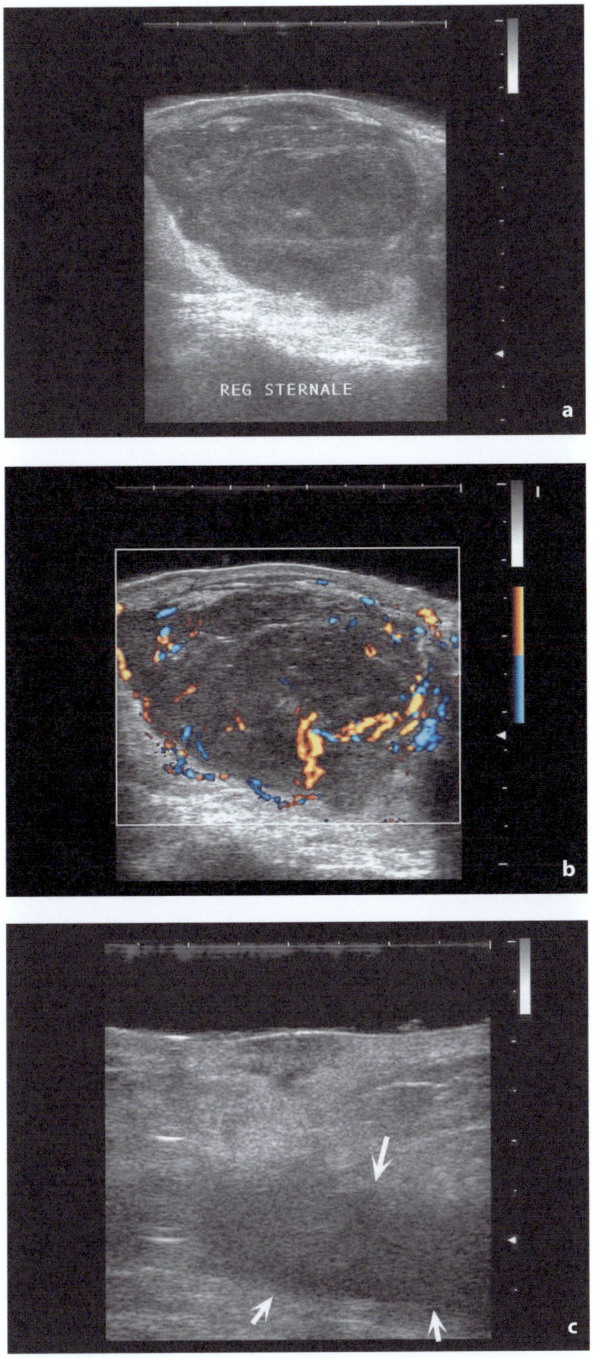

Fig. 2.114a-c Fibrosarcoma of the thoracic wall. Anterior to the sternal bone plane a large heterogeneous hypoechoic mass can be identified (**a**), which displays an irregular vascular network at PD, especially in the periphery (**b**). Normal postoperative appearance of the excision site, with deep fluid collection (**c**, *arrows*)

margins of the lesion and the characteristics of the costal acoustic shadow and the pleural line do not seem to help in the distinction between benign and malignant disease [95].

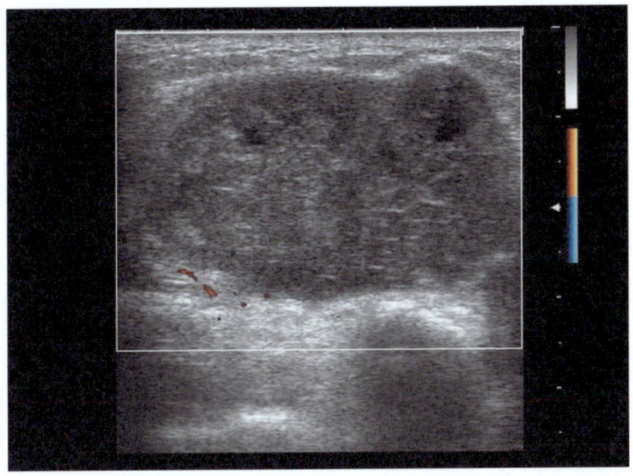

Fig. 2.115 Postoperative recurrence of chondrosarcoma of the thoracic wall. Large well-defined oval mass with hypoechoic appearance and practically no vascular signals at directional PD

Parietal **fluid collections** consist of postoperative seromas, which are generally anechoic and homogeneous when sterile, and abscesses and fluid hematomas, with the possible presence of internal debris, fluid-fluid levels and septations. Abscesses related to tubercular rib lesions are possible, in which case the rib appears remodeled and a heterogeneous fluid collection can be identified at the pericostal level [77]. **Hematomas of the rectus sheath** develop mainly in subjects treated with anticoagulants, or at any rate with a predisposition to hemorrhage, and can have marked extension, especially in the longitudinal direction. Generally oval-shaped, they tend to broaden the muscle and can cross over the median line at the hypogastric level and take on an oblong conformation. The hematoma is rather echogenic in the early phase, becoming increasing hypoechoic and heterogeneous [91] (Figs. 2.116, 2.117).

Tumors of the abdominal wall include subcutaneous or, more rarely, deep lipomas, desmoids, lymphomatous lesions (rare) and metastases (Figs. 2.118–2.124). Lipomas appear oval in shape and iso- or mildly hyperechoic to the muscles, and may be enclosed by a thin echogenic capsule. Identifying the lesions with respect to the normal subcutaneous fat can be challenging due to the frequent isoechogenicity. Desmoids arise from the fasciae or from the aponeurotic membrane, particularly in women and often in the vicinity of scar tissue. They appear as more-or-less well-defined heterogeneous hypoechoic masses with variable vascularity at CD. Differential diagnosis includes endometriomas and tumor implants [77]. Although rare, umbilical metastases (Sister Mary Joseph nodule) can be the first sign of the presentation

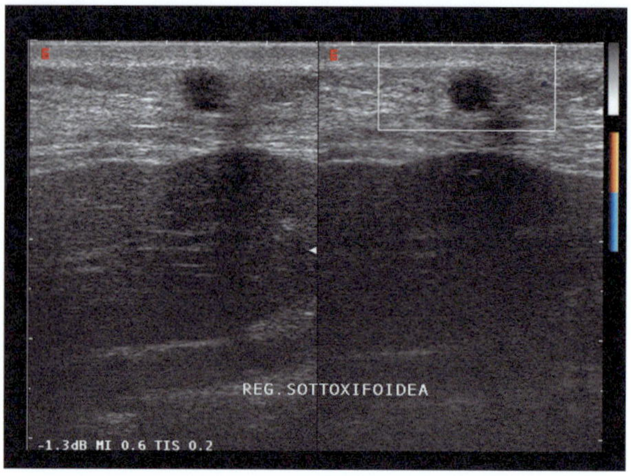

Fig. 2.116 Postoperative seroma of the abdominal wall. A small hypo-anechoic mass with no flow signals at PD can be identified at the level of a median laparotomic incision in the epigastric region

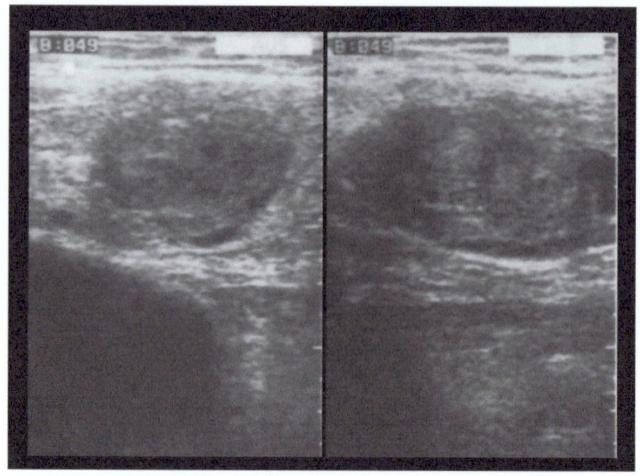

Fig. 2.117 Hematoma of the rectus sheath. Oval hypoechoic mass in the rectus muscle viewed in transverse and longitudinal scans

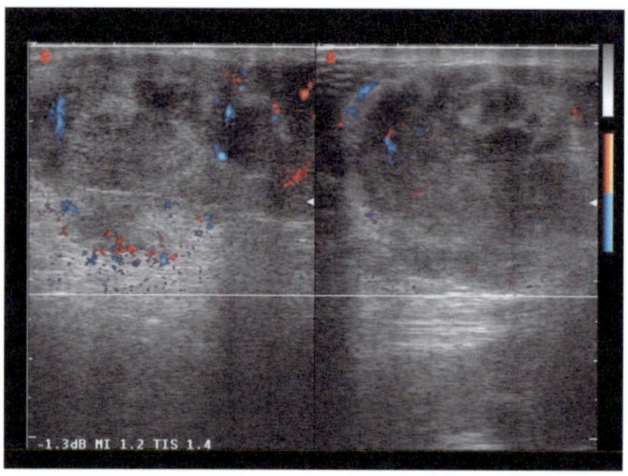

Fig. 2.118 Metastases of the abdominal wall from breast cancer. Large subcutaneous lesion with heterogeneous hypoechoic appearance and some flow signals at directional PD

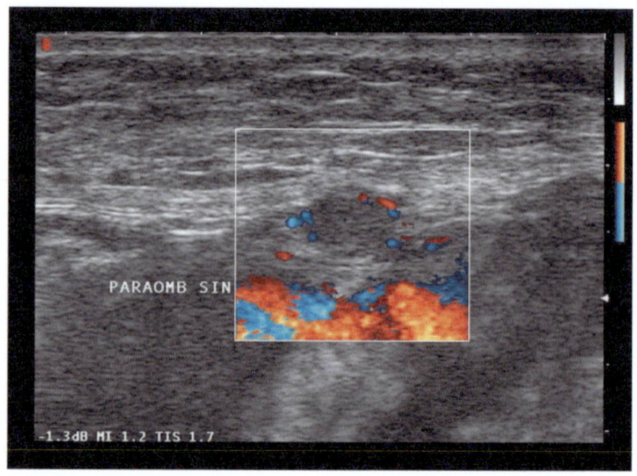

Fig. 2.119 Metastatic nodule of the abdominal wall from ovarian cancer. A small hypoechoic lesion with some peripheral vascular signals at directional PD can be seen at the level of the fascia

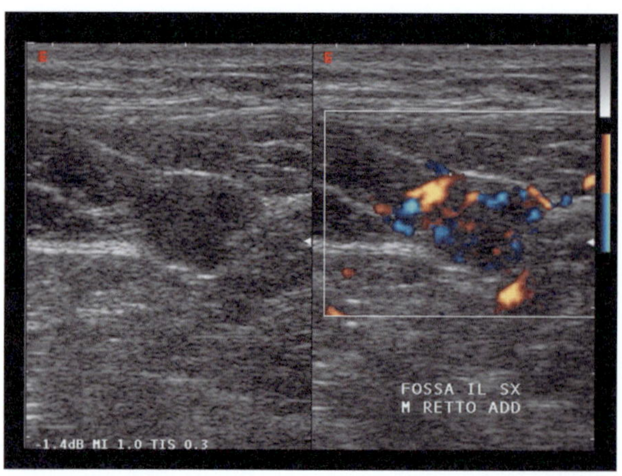

Fig. 2.120 Metastasis of the abdominal wall from melanoma. Hypoechoic nodule within the rectus muscle with moderate vascular signals especially in the periphery at directional PD

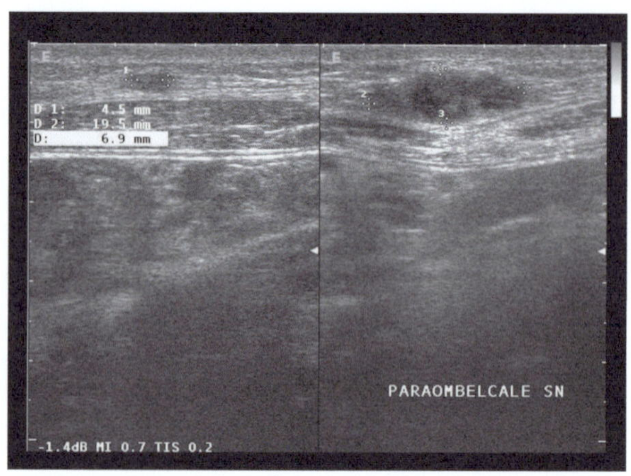

Fig. 2.121 Metastasis of the abdominal wall from melanoma. Two subcutaneous hypoechoic structures can be identified

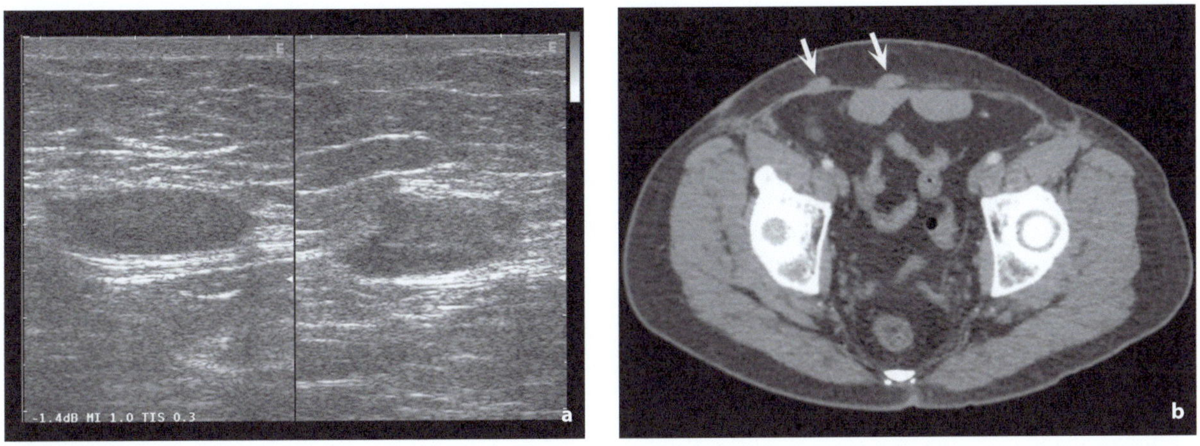

Fig. 2.122a,b Metastasis of the abdominal wall from melanoma in a patient operated on in that site. Two deep subcutaneous hypoechoic nodules can be discerned immediately superficial to the muscle plane which appears atrophic (**a**). Three other nodules were present but only the larger two could be identified by CT (**b**, *arrows*)

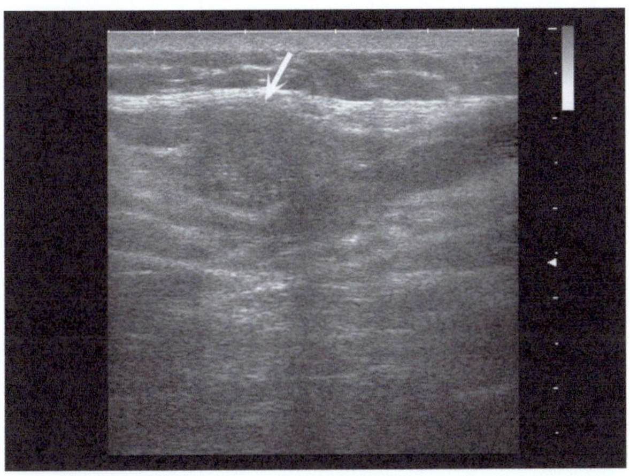

Fig. 2.123 Metastasis of the abdominal wall from Ewing's sarcoma. Rounded, ill-defined, hypoechoic nodule within the muscle plane (*arrow*)

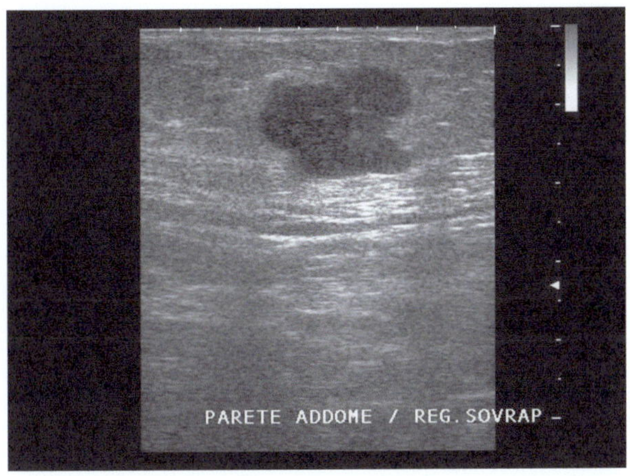

Fig. 2.124 Metastasis of the abdominal wall from melanoma. Markedly hypoechoic subcutaneous nodule at the suprapubic level

of an intra-abdominal tumor (pancreas, colon, etc.) and is characterized by erythematous skin nodules which may be painful or not. These lesions develop as a result of the embryonal development of this anatomic region and the ligamentous structures which connect it to various abdominal organs. US is able to identify the solid nodule and distinguish it from umbilical hernia and can be used to guide the biopsy [96,97].

A characteristic lesion is **endometriosis** of the abdominal wall, which should be suspected in all women who present a tender palpable mass in the vicinity of suprapubic scarring, especially if the pain is cyclic, if the mass is accentuated during menstruation, if the scar is due to a Caesarean section (0.03–1% of caesarean sections) and if the procedure was performed at least a year ago (mean 4 years). US can identify individual subcutaneous (deep and often lying on the muscular fascia) nodulations of varying size (generally 2–3 cm) which appear heterogeneous and hypoechoic with irregular and infiltrating margins and a possible peripheral echogenic halo of variable thickness and continuity. The vascular supply is variable but often intense (despite originating from a single arterial pole and being evenly distributed) with a variable RI (0.52–0.83). Larger lesions may show anechoic areas due to recent hemorrhagic phenomena [98] (Figs. 2.125, 2.126). The association of clinical data with the US findings is often enough to make the correct diagnosis. The US appearance alone requires differentiation from conditions such as abscesses, abdominal hernias, suture granulomas, desmoid tumors (which are also relatively hypervascular), metastases (melanomas), sarcomas, lymphomas, hemangiomas and sebaceous cysts [98].

External **hernias** are most commonly found at the abdominal-pelvic level (umbilical, linea alba, incisional, inguinal, femoral, etc.) and are identifiable as a fascial defect through which the protrusion occurs. The content may be at least in part reduced with delicate compression from the transducer and tends to increase during coughing or the Valsalva maneuver, thus constituting an element for differential diagnosis with solid lesions. The internal appearance is variable, with only the vaguely striated hypoechogenicity of the fat being visible or with the presence of collapsed, normally distended or dilated bowel loops with liquid and/or gas content. Occasionally, especially in cases of strangulation of the intestinal contents or abundant ascites, fluid may be detected around the bowel loops [77]. In oncology incisional hernias are particularly important, because these alterations, which generally arise in the first year after the surgical procedure, although they have been identified even later, can mimic a seeding both clinically and at US.

Seeding is the deposition of tumor cells with the subsequent growth of a macroscopic lesion as a consequence of "spillage" caused by surgical procedures, trocar placement for laparoscopic or thoracoscopic procedures, cytohistologic biopsies, percutaneous drainage of tumor collections or effusion or percutaneous ablation [99,100]. This occurs especially at the level of the soft tissue overlying the tumor, such as the tissue of the chest or abdominal wall, but it can obviously also occur within a cavity such as the peritoneum or the retroperitoneum, or within the organ itself which is the site of the tumor. In general, superficial lesions are more likely to provoke seeding, since spillage of cells is more probable from these. Moreover, in the case of therapeutic procedures such as PEI, "sterilizing" the needle track is much more difficult with superficial lesions. The risk of tumor cell dissemination is greater with biopsy needles than with fine needles for cytology, probably in part because only in the former is it possible to aspirate significant stromal fragments and therefore there is a greater probability of survival and growth of the "dragged" cells. Even a particularly low grade of tumor differentiation increases the probability of seeding [101]. The identification of seeding is important because this lesion does not necessarily indicate a negative prognosis, and if isolated it can be adequately treated [102]. In addition, in most cases the risk of seeding influences patient management: typically, in subjects who are candidates for liver transplant, percutaneous diagnostic or therapeutic procedures are avoided due to the risk of seeding, although the former could be important for having a certain diagnosis of the imaging findings and the latter could help the patient as bridging for the transplant [103]. In subjects with HCC the reported incidence of seeding after FNAC is 0.6–5.1%, whereas the incidence after histologic biopsy is 0.8–3.4% [103]. In patients with lung cancer parietal seeding is reported in 0.2% of FNAC [102]. After treatment procedures (drainage, ablation, etc.) seeding is described in 0.2–1.4% of cases, especially after RF thermoablation procedures, and it can be avoided by heating the electrode at the time of its withdrawal from the organ or by injecting ethanol along the needle track [99,104]. In the case of seeding from HCC the appear-

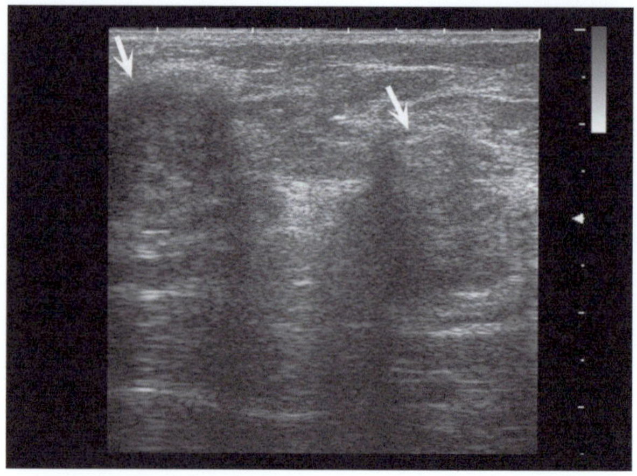

Fig. 2.125 Endometriosis of the abdominal wall. Double nodulation (*arrows*) with heterogeneous hypoechoic appearance and irregular shape located in correspondence to a prior Caesarean section

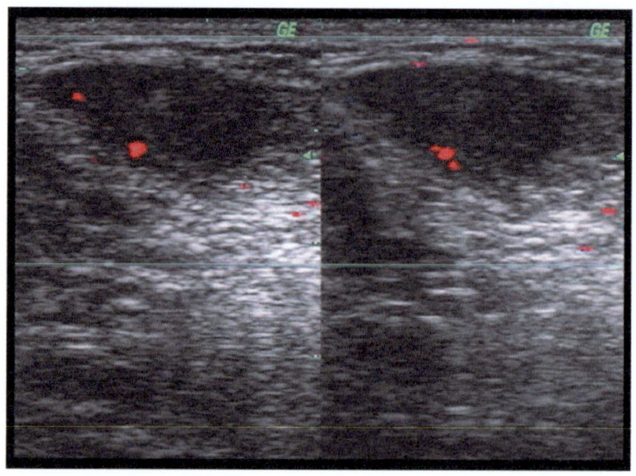

Fig. 2.126 Endometriosis of the abdominal wall. Heterogeneous hypoechoic nodulation with irregular shape and some peripheral vascular signals at PD, located in a site corresponding to a prior Caesarean section

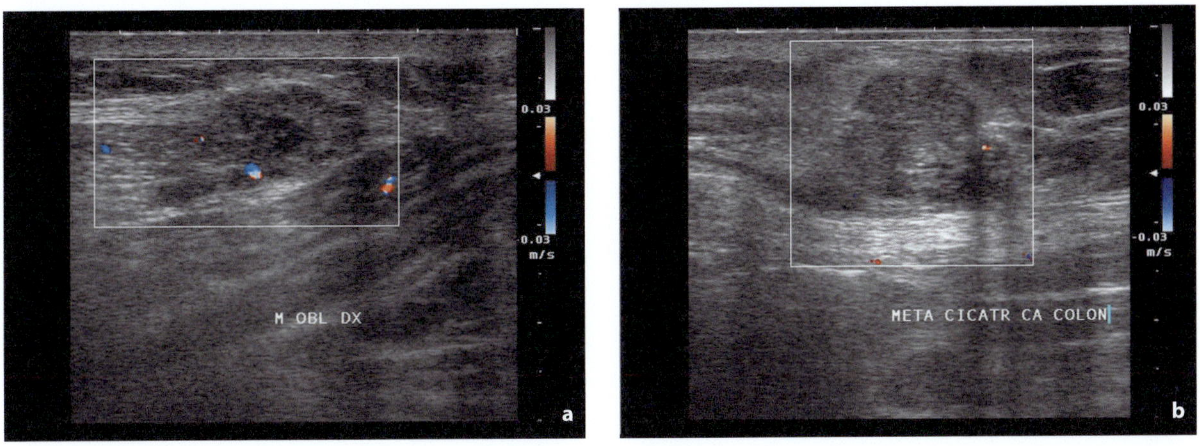

Fig. 2.127a,b Incisional tumor seeding in patient operated on for carcinoma of the right colic angle. A heterogeneous hypoechoic nodule with sporadic color signals at CD can be visualized in the muscle plane

ance is of nodulations with variable size, sharp and regular margins and hypoechoic echostructure with multiple intralesional signals [100]. In general, however, it appears that the incidence of this event is too low to justify routine surveillance with a surface transducer at the site of access in the abdominal wall. A study of this type is required, however, when the patient reports changes in the scar tissue or the access site of a percutaneous procedure, or if, when running an abdominal transducer across the skin to explore the internal organ, a superficial irregularity is perceived (Figs. 2.127, 2.128).

With regard to the **male breast**, masses at the level of this anatomic area and especially of the areolar region, whether uni- or bilateral, are anything but rare. US is the modality of choice for their study, in part also because of the technical difficulty of performing an adequate mammographic study [105]. The large majority of cases (>93%), however, regard lipomastia, retroareolar abscess, epidermal inclusion cyst, angiomatous stromal hyperplasia or, above all, gynecomastia (liver disease patients, patients undergoing treatment for prostate cancer, etc.). Only a minority of cases are due to tumors, including lipomas, hemangiomas, sarcomas, metastases from melanoma (subcutaneous or even exceptionally on retroareolar lymph nodes), lymphomas, intraductal papillomas and carcinomas [106,107] (Figs. 2.129–2.134). Carcinomas account for 0.2–1.5% of all male malignancies and 1% of all breast tumors, with a peak incidence between 60 and 75 years. Risk factors include cryptorchidism, Klinefelter syndrome (35% risk), testicular tumors, liver disease and thoracic radiation therapy treatment at pediatric age. The lesion usually presents as a slightly tender mass having appeared several months earlier and possibly associated with a dark or

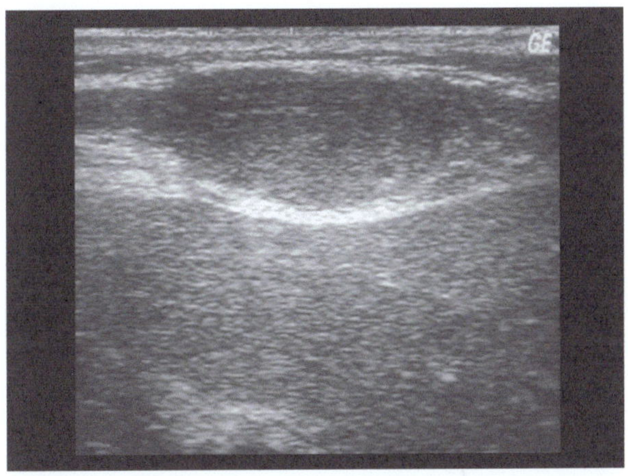

Fig. 2.128 Seeding of HCC after PEI. Parietal hypoechoic lesion protruding towards the underlying hepatic capsule

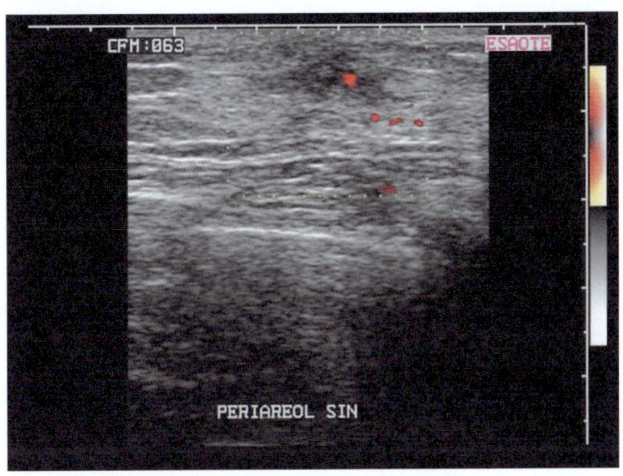

Fig. 2.129 Unilateral areolar thickening in cirrhotic patient. Non-nodular hypoechoic areola with some vascular signals at PD

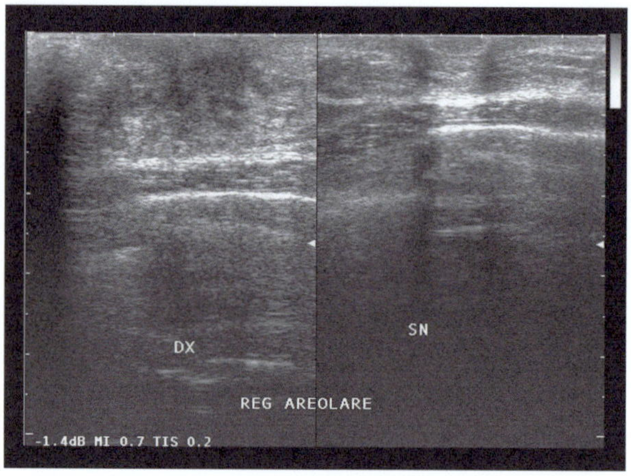

Fig. 2.130 Unilateral gynecomastia in patient undergoing hormone therapy for prostate cancer. Non-nodular heterogeneous hypoechoic thickening of the right retroareolar region (*left*) in comparison with the contralateral side

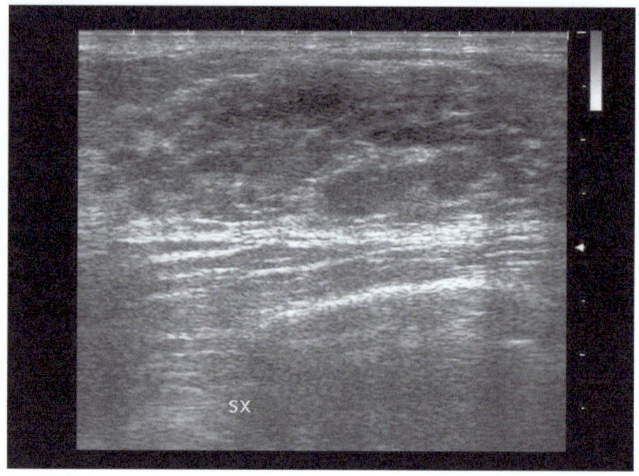

Fig. 2.131 Fibrocystic thickening of the male breast. Poorly defined hypoechoic area in the retroareolar region

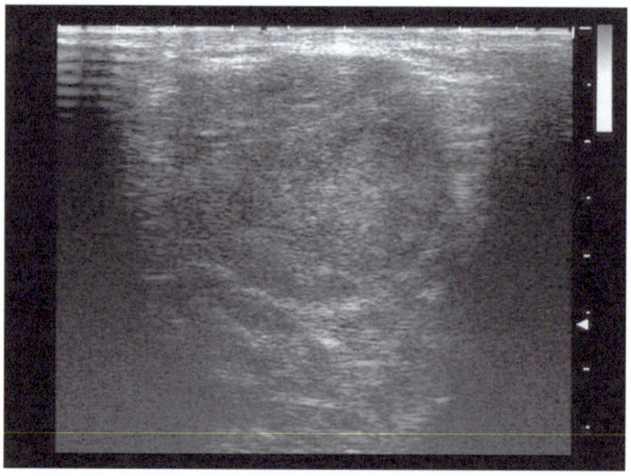

Fig. 2.132 Metastasis from melanoma of the male breast. Heterogeneous hypoechoic mass of the pectoral region

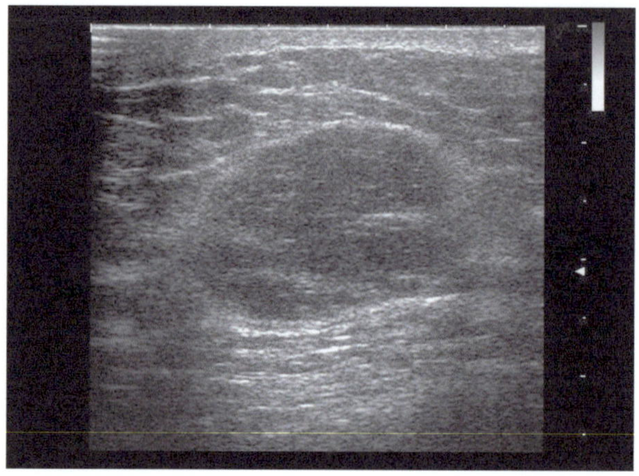

Fig. 2.133 Lymphoma of the male breast. Well-defined relatively heterogeneous hypoechoic nodule

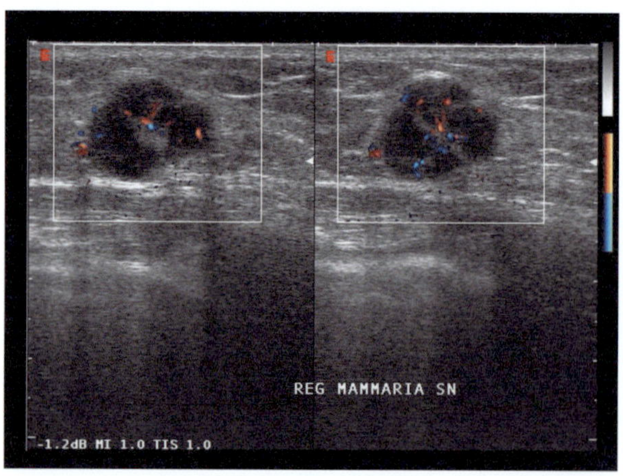

Fig. 2.134 Lymphoma of the male breast. Well-defined heterogeneous hypoechoic nodule with moderate and especially central vascular signals at directional PD

patently blood-stained nipple discharge. The lesions are in 85% of cases ductal infiltrating and can arise from the small amount of breast tissue present in the retroareolar area in the male or even develop from portions of ectopic breast tissue present at other sites in the pectoral region. Multifocality is also possible. At any rate, given the limited size of the male breast area, the tumor becomes invasive early on and relatively easily invades the adjacent structures. The appearance is generally of small hypoechoic nodules with irregular or ill-defined margins, possible acoustic shadowing and anarchic intralesional vascularity. Relatively common secondary signs include cutaneous thickening or ulceration and axillary adenopathies [106,107] (Figs. 2.135, 2.136).

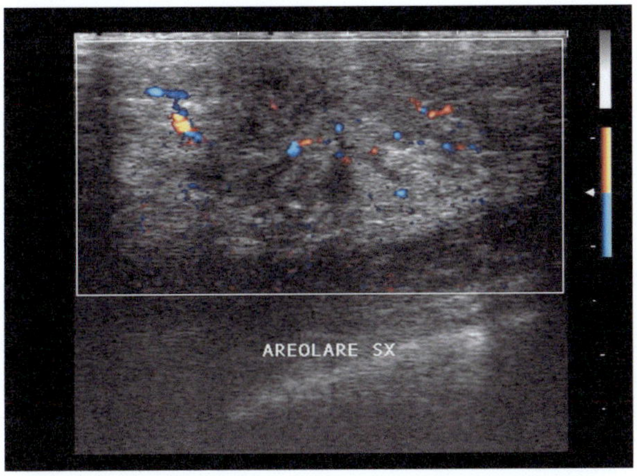

Fig. 2.135 Carcinoma of the male breast. Diffuse remodeling of the retroareolar tissue with moderate and irregular internal vasculature at directional PD

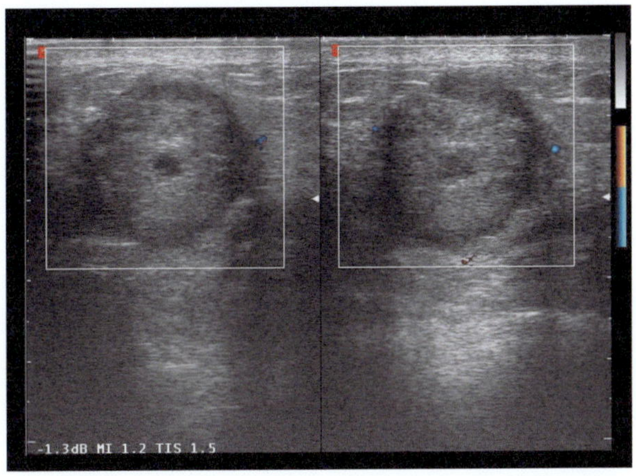

Fig. 2.136 Carcinoma of the male breast. Nodule with echogenic center and hypoechoic periphery located in the superior pectoral region and patently on ectopic breast tissue. Poor vascular supply at directional PD

2.4 Soft-Tissue Sarcomas

Superficial soft-tissue malignancies account for 1% of all adult tumors and 6% in pediatric patients, making them four times more frequent than the respective bone lesions [108]. They are predominantly found in the extremities (20% of cases of sarcoma in the upper extremities and 40% in the lower) and can arise from any structure: tendons, cartilage, adipose tissue, fibrous tissue, nerve tissue and vascular tissue. They mainly consist of liposarcomas (14% of cases), leiomyosarcomas (8%) and malignant fibrous histiocytomas (24%). Their growth pattern is centrifugal beginning from a single point, with the development of a kind of peripheral pseudocapsule due to compressed healthy tissue on the internal surface and neovascularized reactive and granulation tissue on the outer surface. In high-grade sarcomas the pseudocapsule is rapidly overtaken, with invasion of the surrounding tissue, both through direct extension and in the form of small satellite lesions. The staging of these lesions follows the TNM system (Fig. 2.137). The tumor is intracompartmental as long as it remains within a single muscle group, whereas it becomes extracompartmental when it extends from one muscle group to invade the adjacent vascular, nerve and bone structures.

All symptomatic lesions with rapid growth and/or size >5 cm should be investigated. Moreover, it should be borne in mind that the various imaging modalities are very often unable to definitively characterize these lesions and therefore, in many cases, FNAC and, above all, core biopsy (e.g. with 14G needles) or incisional biopsy are required. However, a biopsy incision in an inappropriate site can compromise the subsequent surgical approach. The consequences of an inaccurate preoperative evaluation are that even the surgery cases are operated on in a less than suitable manner, with the need for further surgery at a later date. Accurate pretreatment staging is instead fundamental. The principal prognostic factors are in fact histologic type and grade and resectability [108,109].

Modern imaging of sarcomas is largely based on the use of CT and especially MR, which are able to provide all the necessary information for the characterization (although possibly with the need for biopsy) and evaluation of extension (extracompartmental spread, involvement of the neurovascular bundle, bone involvement, etc.) for the purposes of treatment planning (radical operability or otherwise, conservation vs. amputation, possible neoadjuvant and/or adjuvant chemotherapy or radiation therapy, etc.). The grade of malignancy, however, cannot be defined with imaging modalities, although the less differentiated forms tend to have a more heterogeneous structure than well-differentiated masses [110].

US has a limited possibility of characterizing these lesions and should not be used for the definitive diagnosis [111,112]. Both benign and malignant mesenchymal tumors tend to be hypoechoic. However, the echostructure – hyperechoic or hypoechoic to the adjacent muscles – does not appear to be a major discriminating factor between benign and malignant musculoskeletal tumors, with sensitivity of 82% and specificity of 38%. Much the same can be said for the echotexture, with sensitivity of 85% and specificity of 40% for the diagnosis of malignancy [113]. It is in fact not uncommon for a soft tissue sarcoma to have a

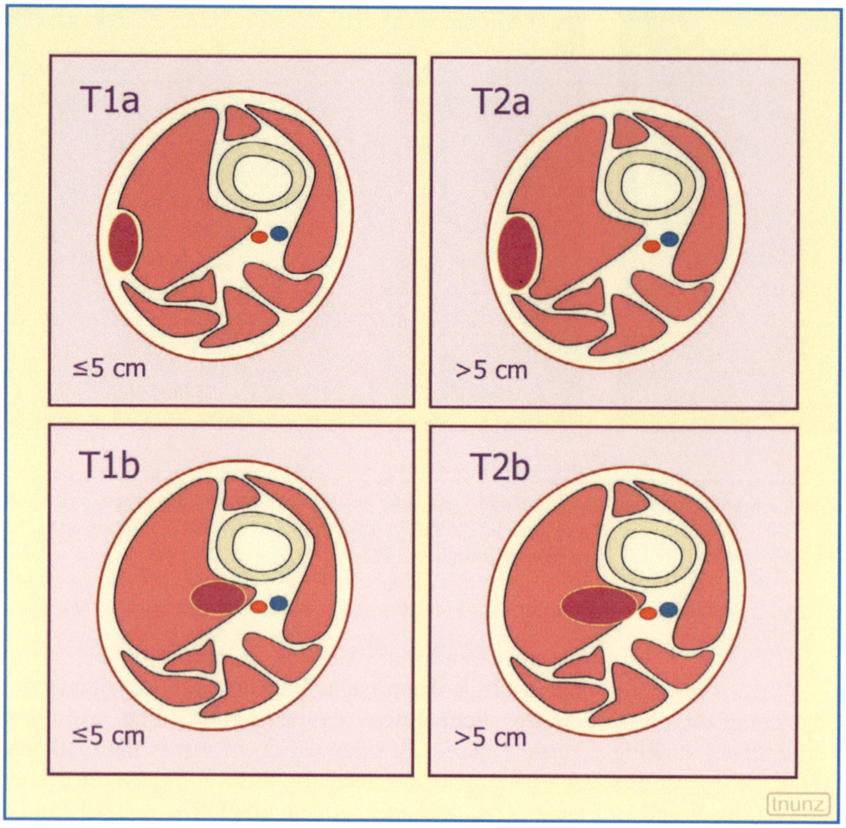

Fig. 2.137 Staging of soft-tissue sarcomas. *T1a*, superficial tumor (overlying the superficial fascia with no invasion) ≤5 cm; *T1b*, deep tumor (overlying the superficial fascia with invasion of this or the underlying fascia) ≤5 cm; *T2*a, superficial tumor >5 cm; *T2b*, deep tumor >5 cm

homogeneous echotexture and well-defined margins [112].

Spectral and color Doppler can provide additional information. In two studies of soft-tissue tumors of the limbs, US alone had sensitivity of 60–75% and specificity of 50–55%, which rose to 85–90% and 90–91%, respectively, when combined with the CD findings [114,115]. Benign lesions (except of course for hemangiomas) have a poor or absent vascular supply, with vessels that appear regular, displaced but not infiltrating, without particular changes to the perilesional vascular supply. The most indicative signs of malignancy are the presence of multiple vascular poles (>2) and the visibility of tortuous and irregular intralesional vessels [115]. Another study [113], which included both bone and soft-tissue lesions, identified the main Doppler criteria for the diagnosis of malignancy: stenosis (aliasing at CD and increase in V_{max} >100% of the distal value), obstruction (monophasic flow in a vessel, indicative of absent distal flow), trifurcation (subdivision of a vessel into three branches) and an anarchic vascular pattern. Three minor criteria were also defined: arteriovenous shunt (identified by RI <0.5), auto loop (vessel which connects with itself in a circle) and ratio between minimum and maximum RI on five vessels <0.67. In particular, the mean RI of all musculoskeletal tumors was 0.5 and the RI of the corresponding benign lesions was 0.79. The combination of any two of the main criteria improved results, with sensitivity 94% and specificity 93%. In other studies, however, spectral analysis did not prove useful for the purposes of differential diagnosis, especially due to wide variability and overlap of findings. The RI of a benign lesion is on average 0.72 (SD 0.42) and the RI of malignant lesions is 0.62 (SD 0.36) [116]. In particular, venous flow velocity and diastolic flow velocity do not appear to be useful, whereas discrimination can be helped by the systolic velocity, on average 27 cm/s in benign lesions and 55 cm/s in malignancies [114]. Compression of the transducer can be used to evaluate the deformability or otherwise of the superficial lesion, with malignancy being suggested in the latter case. In the same way, during a CD study the afferent arterial flow and internal color signals can be suppressed in benign lesions, but much less so in malignancies. Preliminary information has been obtained from analysis of the intensity/time curves obtained with CEUS, including in the variability of the curves themselves. This analysis has shown a rapid and regular peak during the wash-in phase of malignant lesions, and especially a characteristic trend in the wash-out phase, with a slow descent in values

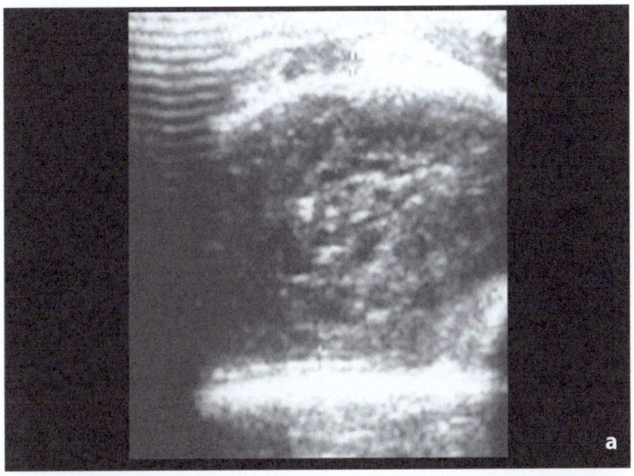

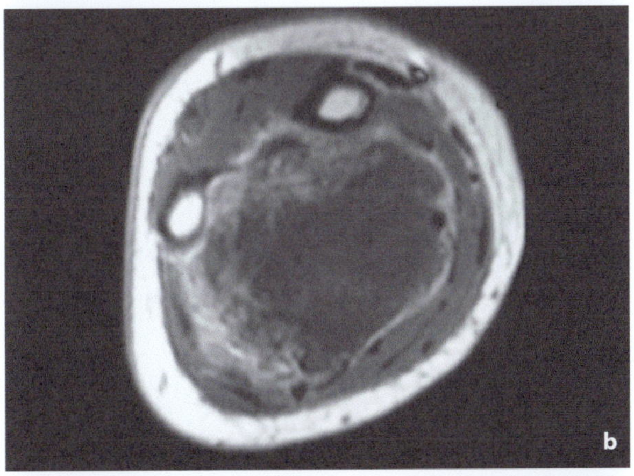

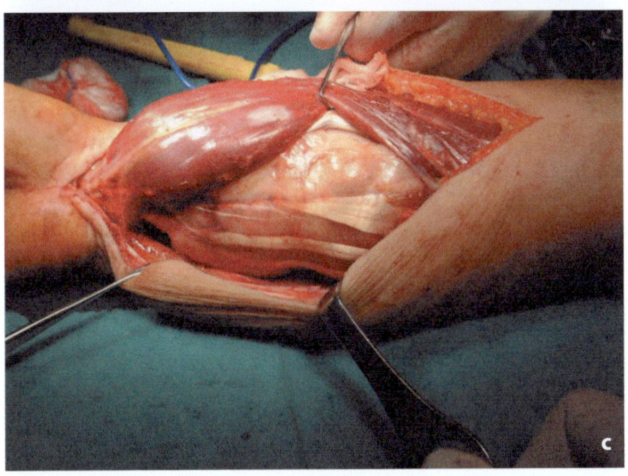

Fig. 2.138a-c Sarcoma of the forearm. Heterogeneous hypoechoic mass with anechoic areas at US (**a**). Axial MR appearance with irregular peripheral enhancement (**b**). Intraoperative view (**c**)

with smaller peaks closer together, or with a more rapid descent followed by smaller and less frequent peaks or lastly with a plateau of irregular peaks followed by a descent also with irregular peaks [117].

The site, size, extension and relations with adjacent structures (bone, vessels, nerves) of **soft-tissue**

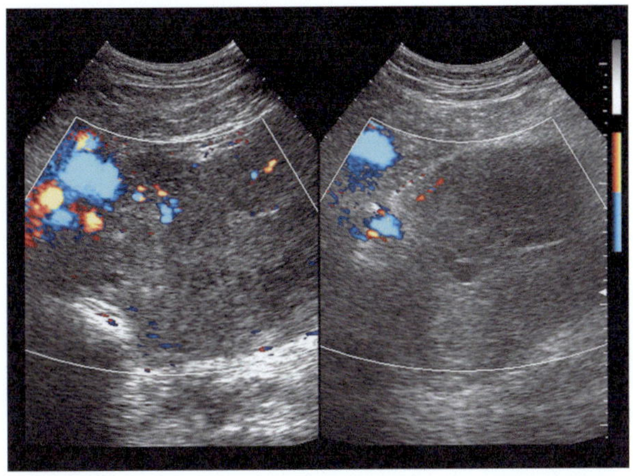

Fig. 2.139 Sarcoma of the thigh. A large heterogeneous hypoechoic mass can be identified at the level of the crural region, with some peripheral vascular signals at directional PD

sarcomas should be defined, even if this is performed more effectively with CT and MR [110]. The appearance is usually relatively well defined, lobulated and hypoechoic, even though some liposarcomas can appear hyperechoic. Calcifications may be present, especially in synovial sarcomas, as well as necrotic areas. Most of the lesions are hypervascular, with vessels distributed chaotically and heterogeneously in density and morphology, although there are also markedly hypovascular forms [56]. Lymph node metastases are more rare than hematogenous spread, although possible, and as such an exploration of the reference lymph node stations is required [108,109] (Figs. 2.138–2.140]. Up to 60% of liposarcomas present no macroscopic adipose components and therefore these lesions are more difficult to identify with US than with CT or MR [111]. In myxoid liposarcomas and synovial sarcomas the fluid component may prevail, with a cystic and hypovascular appearance. Well-differentiated liposarcomas may have an appearance that is very similar to that of the highly common simple superficial lipoma (lipoma-like liposarcoma), being characterized by slow growth, adipose appearance, homogeneous echotexture and well-defined margins (Fig. 2.141, 2.142). In these cases, especially if the mass is not subcutaneous, a thorough search for possible areas of heterogeneous echotexture or areas with vascular signals at CD should be made and biopsy guidance performed. Alternatively, an accurate definition of the dimensions of the lesion and monitoring over time are required.

Synovial sarcomas account for 8–10% of soft-tissue sarcomas and are characterized by a tendency to early extracompartmental spread with a typical para-articular, or in 5–10% of cases intraarticular, location.

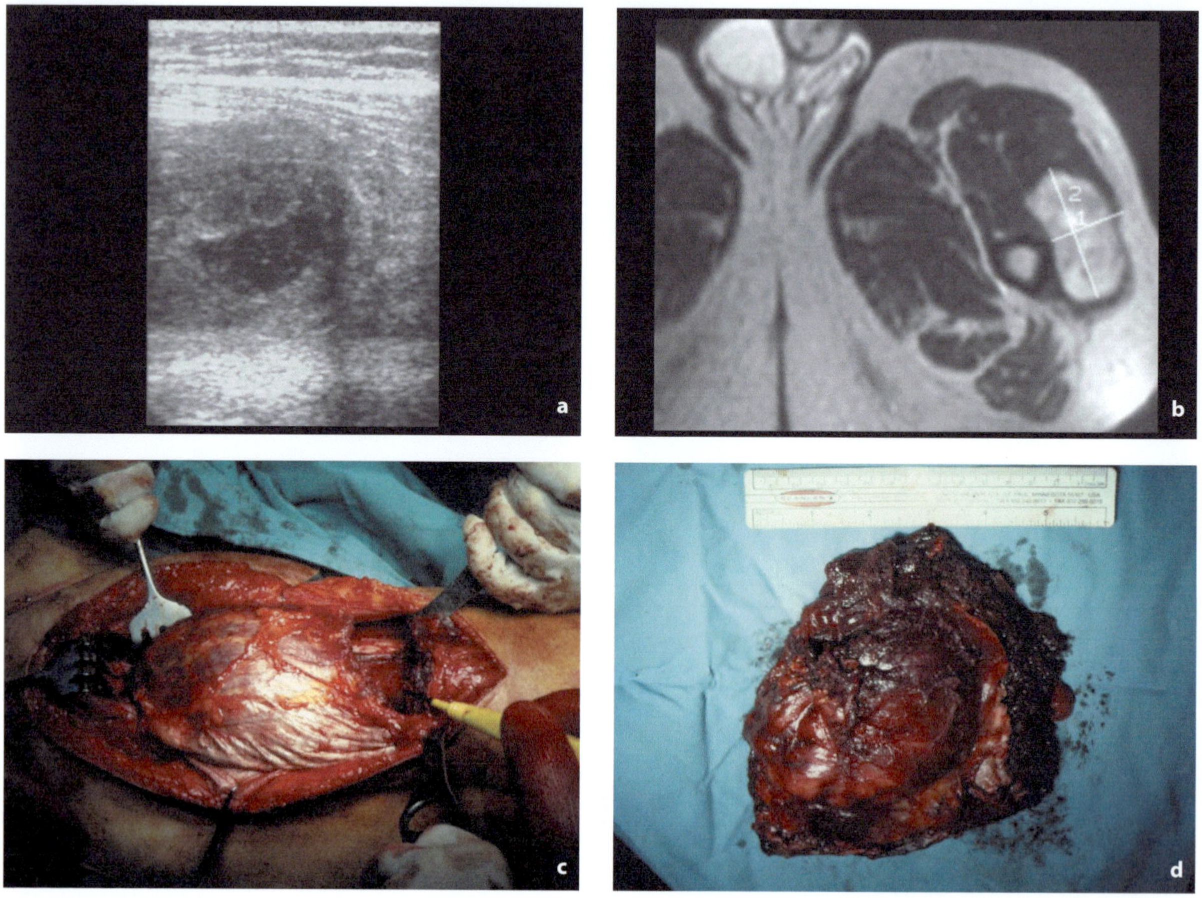

Fig. 2.140a-d Liposarcoma of the thigh. Heterogeneous hypoechoic mass with eccentric necrotic portion at US (**a**). Axial MR image (**b**). Intraoperative view (**c**). Surgical specimen (**d**)

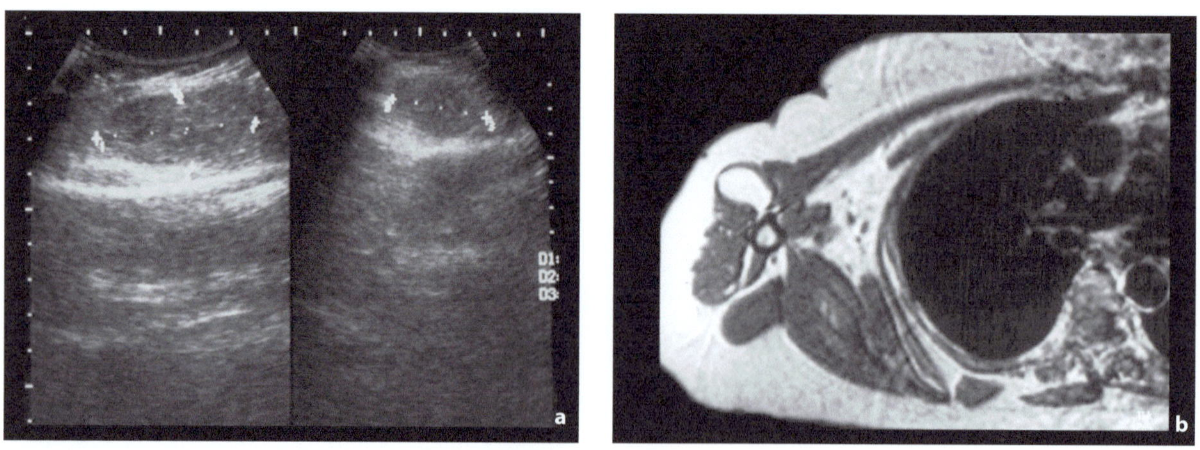

Fig. 2.141a,b Lipoma-like liposarcoma of the arm. Relatively well-defined and homogeneous hypoechoic mass at US (**a**), with a homogeneously hyperintense appearance on the axial MR image (**b**)

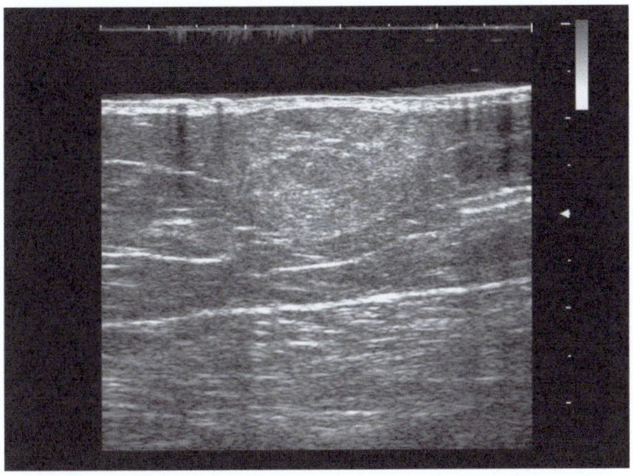

Fig. 2.142 Lipoma-like liposarcoma of the thigh. Heterogeneous echogenic subcutaneous mass

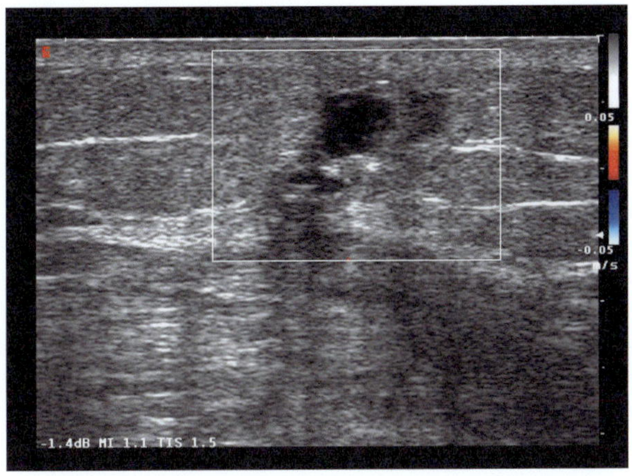

Fig. 2.143 Excision site of sarcoma. Several small fluid collections can be appreciated along the surgical scar, but no solid nodulations or areas of hypervascularity at CD can be seen

They are most frequently found in the lower limbs, especially at the level of the knee. US reveals nonspecific hypoechoic masses. In 20–30% of cases intralesional calcifications are present, which may suggest the correct diagnosis, along with signs of invasion of the adjacent bone structures [81,111].

Surgery, generally performed with adjuvant chemotherapy (especially effective in pediatric patients) is the treatment of choice for these tumors and should always aim at excision of the entire muscle compartment involved. **Local recurrence** is relatively frequent, even when analysis of the surgical specimen reveals adequate resection margins. It occurs in >50% of cases (16–51% in malignant fibrous histiocytoma and 66% in liposarcoma), generally in the first two years after resection [Manaster 2002]. The probability of recurrence depends on the size and grade of the resected tumor. Even the site of the original lesion is important because in the extremities, where the maximum radicality is easier to obtain, recurrence is 10–20%, but in the head and neck, where optimal resection is more difficult, the recurrence rate is 50% [108].

The early **diagnosis** of local recurrence is challenging, particularly in patients who have undergone surgery and radiation therapy [118]. Although important, the clinical evaluation can be obstructed by the depth of the recurrence or by the presence of changes associated with surgery and radiation therapy. In fact, up to one-third of recurrences identified at US are nonpalpable [119]. **US** has proven to be effective (sensitivity 92%, specificity 94%) in the follow-up and early identification of recurrence [118] (Fig. 2.143). It is comparable to MR (sensitivity 100% and 83%, respectively, and specificity 93% and 79%, respectively) in the detection of recurrences of soft-tissue sarcomas, since it loses on the panoramic view but gains on the high-resolution analysis of findings [120]. Recurrences are usually located in the vicinity of the surgical scar and appear as small rounded or oval nodulations, often multiple, with heterogeneous hypoechoic appearance and more-or-less well-defined margins. CD displays intralesional vascular signals and makes distinction from small cystic postoperative collections possible. However, it should be borne in mind that the scar tissue of the limbs is often highly vascular, particularly peripherally, so therefore the vascularity alone cannot be considered a discriminating factor [56] (Figs. 2.144–2.146, Video 2.6). US can encounter difficulty, particularly in the first 3–4 months postoperatively, due to limitations in differentiating between recent postoperative changes and disease recurrence [120]. A distinction also needs to be made between postoperative collections and recurrence, which may not always be easy especially in tumors with a significant liquid component such as myxoid liposarcoma and synovial sarcoma [108] (Fig. 2.147). Unlike the primary diagnosis of the sarcoma, diagnostic confirmation can generally be given by FNAC alone, with an accuracy of 88% [118,119].

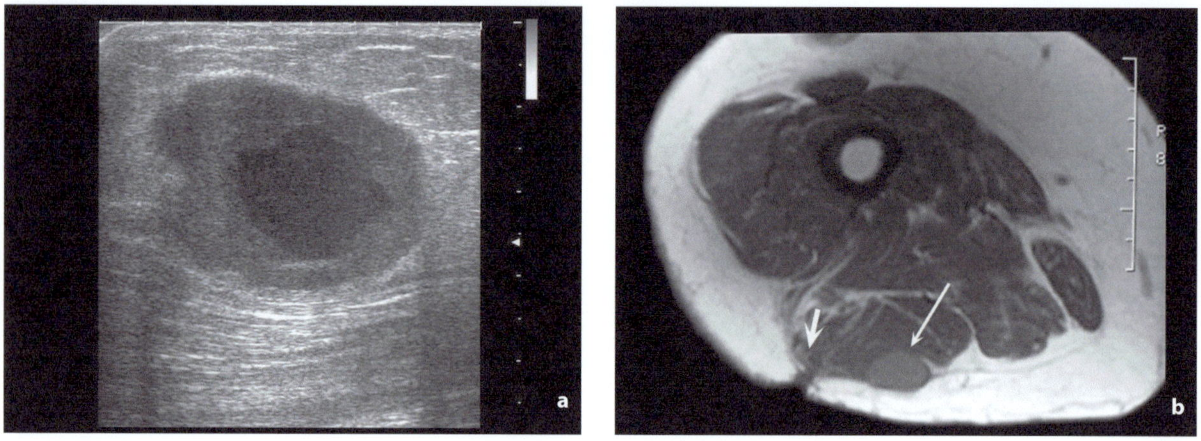

Fig. 2.144a,b Recurrence of malignant histiocytoma of the thigh. A hypoechoic mass with liquefactive center and well-defined margins can be appreciated at the level of the surgical scar between the subcutaneous layer and the muscle compartment (**a**) Axial MR correlation (**b**) which shows both the nodule (*long arrow*) and the scar (*short arrow*)

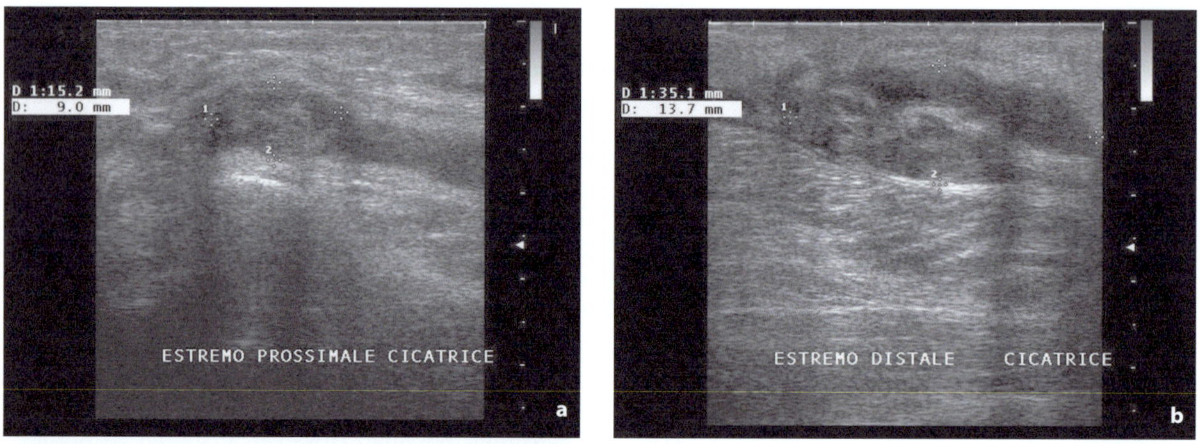

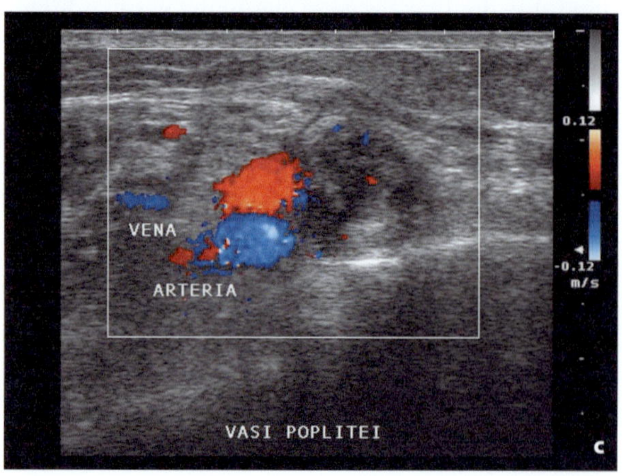

Fig. 2.145a-c Multicentric recurrence of aggressive fibromatosis. Heterogeneous hypoechoic nodule at the level of the proximal end of the scar (**a**), the distal end (**b**) and the intermediate portion (**c**). At the latter site CD demonstrates adherence to the popliteal vessels and the presence of some intralesional vascular signals

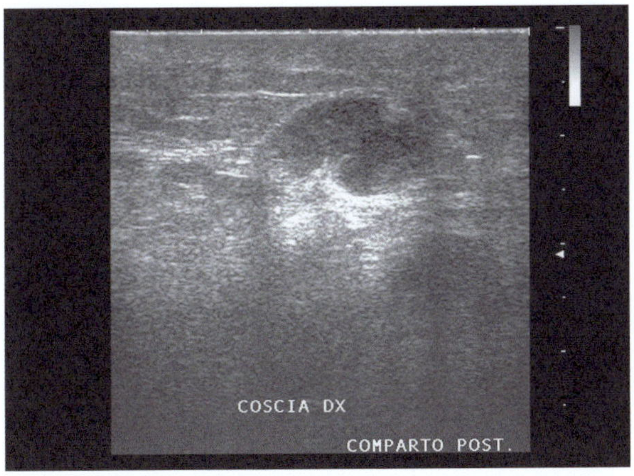

Fig. 2.146 Recurrence of liposarcoma of the thigh. A lobulated nodulation with relatively well-defined margins and homogeneous hypoechoic appearance can be identified between the subcutaneous layer and the deep compartment

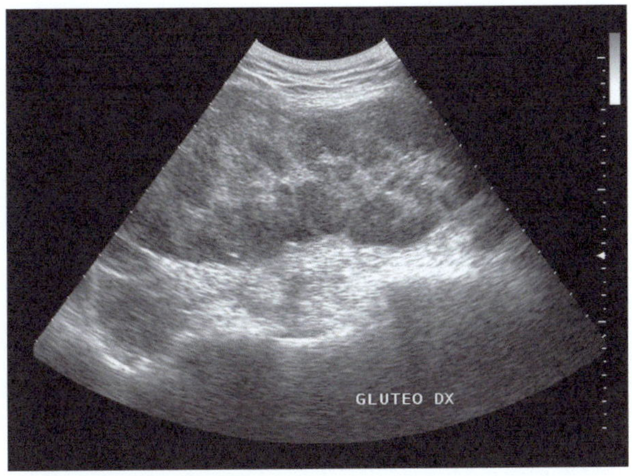

Fig. 2.147 Hematoma after excision of the gluteal compartment due to sarcoma. Large heterogeneous echogenic "mass" with significant hypo-anechoic areas five days after surgery

References

1. Bossi MC et al (2001) The skin. In: Meire H et al (eds) Abdominal and general ultrasound, II Edition. Churchill Livingstone, London, 955-982
2. Bessoud B et al (2003) High-frequency sonography and color Doppler in the management of pigmented skin lesions. Ultrasound Med Biol 29:875-879
3. Schmid-Wendtner M-H et al (2005) Ultrasound scanning in dermatology. Arch Dermatol 141:217-224
4. Karaman GC et al (2001) Power Doppler ultrasonography for the evaluation of skin tumors other than malignant melanoma. Eur Radiol 11:1111-1116
5. Wittekind Ch et al (2005) TNM atlas. Springer-Verlag Berlin
6. Lassau N et al (2006b) Prognostic value of angiogenesis evaluated with high-frequency and colour Doppler sonography for preoperative assessment of primary cutaneous melanomas: correlation with recurrence after a 5 year follow-up period. Cancer Imaging 6:24-29
7. Fanelli GP et al (2004) Skin metastases: clinical and sonographic characteristics. Giorn It Ecogr 7:257-262
8. Solivetti FM et al (2006) Sonographic evaluation of clinically occult in-transit and satellite metastases from cutaneous malignant melanoma. Radiol Med 111:702-708
9. Meier F et al (2002) Metastatic pathways and time courses in the orderly progression of cutaneous melanoma. Br J Dermatol 147:62-70
10. Blum A et al (2000) Ultrasound examination of regional lymph nodes significantly improves early detection of locoregional metastases during follow-up of patients with cutaneous melanoma: results of a prospective study of 1288 patients. Cancer 88:2534-2539
11. Burkill GJC et al (2004) Malignant tumours of the skin. In: Husband JE et al (eds) Imaging in oncology, II edition. Taylor & Francis, London, 1149-1168
12. Schäfer-Hesterberg G et al (2007) Use of ultrasound to early identify, diagnose and localize metastases in melanoma patients. Expert Rev Anticancer Ther 7:1707-1716
13. Voit C et al (2006) Ultrasound-guided fine needle aspiration cytology prior to sentinel lymph node biopsy in melanoma patients. Ann Surg Oncol 13:1682-1689
14. Nazarian LN et al (1998) Superficial melanoma metastases: appearances on grey scale and color Doppler sonography. AJR Am J Roentgenol 170:459-463
15. Fornage B et al (1989) Sonographic detection and fine-needle aspiration biopsy of nonpalpable recurrent or metastatic melanoma in subcutaneous tissues. J Ultrasound Med 8:421-424
16. Voit C et al (2001) Efficacy of ultrasound B-scan compared with physical examination in follow-up of melanoma patients. Cancer 91:2409-2416
17. Blum A et al (2006) Ultrasound mapping of lymph node and subcutaneous metastases in patients with cutaneous melanoma: results of a prospective multicenter study. Dermatology 212:47-52
18. Schmid-Wendtner M-H et al (2002) Improved differentiation of benign and malignant lymphadenopathy in patients with cutaneous melanoma by contrast-enhanced color Doppler sonography. Arch Dermatol 138:491-497
19. Kamel IR et al (1998) Imaging of abdominal manifestations of melanoma. Crit Rev Diagn Imaging 39:447-486
20. Holloway BJ et al (1997) Ultrasound diagnosis of metastatic melanoma of the gallbladder. Brit J Radiol 70:1122-1125
21. McDermott VG et al (1996) Malignant melanoma metastatic to the gastrointestinal tract. AJR Am J Roentgenol 166:809-813
22. Kawashima A et al (1991) CT of malignant melanoma: patterns of small bowel and mesenteric involvement. J Comput Assist Tomogr 15:570-574
23. Ying M et al (2003) Sonography of neck lymph nodes. Part I: normal lymph nodes. Clin Radiol 58:351-358
24. Rubaltelli L et al (2004a) Ultrasonography of superficial lymph nodes: results acquired and new trials. Radiol Med 107:388-400
25. Sakai F et al (1988) Ultrasonic evaluation of cervical metastatic lymphadenopathy. J Ultrasound Med 7:305-310
26. Ahuja A et al (2001) Lymph node hilus. Gray scale and

power Doppler sonography of cervical nodes. J Ultrasound Med 20:987-992
27. Ahuja A et al (2003) Sonography of neck lymph nodes. Part II: abnormal lymph nodes. Clin Radiol 58:359-366
28. Chong V (2004) Cervical lymphadenopathy: what radiologists need to know. Cancer Imaging 4:116-120
29. Shirakawa T et al (2001) Color-power Doppler sonographic differential diagnosis of superficial lymphadenopathy. Metastasis, malignant lymphoma, and benign process. J Ultrasound Med 20:525-532
30. Steinkamp HJ et al (1998) Differential diagnosis of lymph node lesions: a semiquantitative approach with colour Doppler ultrasound. Br J Radiol 71:828-833
31. Tschammler A et al (2002) Differential diagnosis of lymphadenopathy: power Doppler vs color Doppler sonography. Eur Radiol 12:1794-1799
32. Giovagnorio F et al (2002) Color Doppler sonography in the evaluation of superficial lymphomatous lymph nodes. J Ultrasound Med 21:403-408
33. Rubaltelli L et al (2004) Ultrasonography of superficial lymph nodes: results acquired and new trials. Radiol Med 107:388-400
34. Rickert D et al (2000) Color-coded duplex sonography of the cervical lymph nodes: improved differential diagnostic assessment after administration of the signal enhancer SH U 508A (Levovist). Eur Arch Otorhinolaryngol 257:453-458
35. Tschammler A et al (1998) Lymphadenopathy: differentiation of benign from malignant disease–Color Doppler US assessment of intranodal angioarchitecture. Radiology 208:117-123
36. Brniç Z et al (2003) Usefulness of Doppler waveform analysis in differential diagnosis of cervical lymphadenopathy. Eur Radiol 13:175-180
37. Steinkamp HJ et al (2002) Current status of power Doppler and color Doppler sonography in the differential diagnosis of lymph node lesions. Eur Radiol 12:1785-1783
38. Alam F et al (2008) Accuracy of sonographic elastography in the differential diagnosis of enlarged cervical lymph nodes: comparison with conventional B-mode sonography. AJR Am J Roentgenol 191:604-610
39. Asai S et al (2001) Ultrasonographic differentiation between tuberculous lymphadenitis and malignant lymph nodes. J Ultrasound Med 20:533-538
40. Reznek RH et al (2004b) Lymphoma. In: Husband JE et al (eds) Imaging in oncology, II Edition. Taylor & Francis, London, 817-874
41. Morton DL et al (1992) Technical details of intraoperative lymphatic mapping for early stage melanoma. Arch Surg 127:392-399
42. Mehta TS (2003) Current uses of ultrasound in the evaluation of the breast. Radiol Clin North Am 41:841-856
43. Nori J et al (2005) Role of axillary lymph node ultrasound and large core biopsy in the preoperative assessment of patients selected for sentinel node biopsy. Radiol Med 109:330-344
44. Roozendaal GK et al (2001) Sentinel nodes outside lymph node basins in patients with melanoma. Br J Surg 88:305-308
45. Alvarez S et al (2006) Role of sonography in the diagnosis of axillary lymph node metastases in breast cancer: a systematic review. AJR Am J Roentgenol 186:1342-1348
46. Thompson JF et al (2005) Lymphatic mapping in management of patients with primary cutaneous melanoma. Lancet Oncol 6:877-885
47. Carrington BM (2004) Lymph node metastases. In: Husband JE et al (eds) Imaging in oncology, II Edition. Taylor & Francis, London, 999-1022
48. Goldberg BB et al (2004) Sentinel lymph nodes in a swine model with melanoma: contrast-enhanced lymphatic US. Radiology 230:727-734
49. Goldberg BB (2005) Contrast-enhanced sonographic imaging of lymphatic channels and sentinel lymph nodes. J Ultrasound Med 24:953-965
50. Omoto K et al (2006) Sentinel node detection in breast cancer using contrast-enhanced sonography with 25% albumin – Initial clinical experience. J Clin Ultrasound 34:317-326
51. Starritt EC et al (2005) Ultrasound examination of sentinel nodes in the initial assessment of patients with primary cutaneous melanoma. Ann Surg Oncol 12:18-23
52. Sibon C et al (2007) The contribution of high-resolution ultrasonography in preoperatively detecting sentinel-node metastases in melanoma patients. Melanoma Research 17:233-237
53. Beaman FD et al (2007) Superficial soft-tissue masses: analysis, diagnosis, and differential considerations. Radiographics 27:509-523
54. Cappabianca S et al (2008) Lipomatous lesions of the head and neck region: imaging findings in comparison with histological type. Radiol Med 113:758-770
55. Bacaro D et al (2004) Ultrasonographic characterization of soft tissue lipomas: 127 cases. Giorn It Ecogr 7:263-265
56. Fornage BD (2000a) Soft-tissue masses: the case for increased utilization of sonography. Appl Radiol 10:8-22
57. An J-K et al (2005) Soft-tissue axillary masses (excluding metastases from breast cancer): sonographic appearances and correlative imaging. J Clin Ultrasound 33:288-297
58. Bergami G et al (1995) Ultrasonic diagnosis of "hematoma" of the sternocleidomastoid muscle. Radiol Med 89:766-768
59. Huang C-C et al (2005) Scapulothoracic bursitis of the chest wall. Sonographic features with pathologic correlation. J Ultrasound Med 24:1437-1440
60. Girish G et al (2006) Sonography of intramuscular myxomas. The bright rim and bright caps signs. J Ultrasound Med 25:865-869
61. Nikolaidis P et al (2006) Sonographic appearance of nodular fascitis. J Ultrasound Med 25:281-285
62. Thain LMF et al (2002) Sonography of peripheral nerves: technique, anatomy, and pathology. Ultrasound Q 18:225-245
63. Beggs I (1999) Sonographic appearances of nerve tumors. J Clin Ultrasound 27:363-368
64. Beggs I (1998) The ring sign: a new ultrasound sign of peripheral nerve tumours. Clin Radiol 53:849-850
65. Vignal P (2005) Sonographic appearance of a carcinoma developed in ectopic axillary breast tissue. J Ultrasound Med 33:468-470
66. Lernevall A (2000) Imaging of axillary lymph nodes. Acta Oncol 39:277-281
67. Shetty MK et al (2004) Sonographic evaluation of isolated abnormal axillary lymph nodes identified on mammograms. J Ultrasound Med 23:63-71
68. Bergvist L et al (1996) Management of accidentally found pathological lymph nodes on routine screening mammography. Eur J Surg Oncol 22:250-253

69. Given-Wilson RM et al (1997) The clinical importance of axillary lymphadenopathy detected on screening mammography. Clin Radiol 52:458-461
70. Fornage BD (2000b) Breast sonography. In: Shirkhoda A (ed) Variants and pitfalls in body imaging. Lippincott Williams & Wilkins, Philadelphia, 153-169
71. Oh SN et al (2007) Sonography of various cystic masses of the female groin. J Ultrasound Med 26:1735-1742
72. Sarna A et al (2005) Computed tomographic and ultrasonographic findings of endometrial carcinoma appearing as a fungating inguinal mass. J Ultrasound Med 24:1579-1582
73. Shadbolt CL et al (2001) Imaging of groin masses: inguinal anatomy and pathologic conditions revisited. RadioGraphics 21:S261-S271
74. Yang DM et al (2007) Sonographic findings of groin masses. J Ultrasound Med 26:605-614
75. van den Berg JC et al (1998) Masses and pain in the groin: a review of imaging findings. Eur Radiol 8:911-921
76. Hall TB et al (2003) The role of ultrasound-guided cytology of groin lymph nodes in the management of squamous cell carcinoma of the vulva: 5-year experience in 44 patients. Clin Radiol 58:367-371
77. Gokdale S et al (2006) Sonography in identification of abdominal wall lesions presenting as palpable masses. J Ultrasound Med 25:1199-1209
78. Gitschlag KF et al (1982) Diseases in the femoral triangle: sonographic appearance. AJR Am J Roentgenol 139:515-519
79. van den Berg JC et al (2000) Radiological anatomy of the groin region. Eur Radiol 10:661-670
80. Pathria MN et al (1988) Ultrasonography of the popliteal fossa and lower extremities. Radiol Clin North Am 26:77-85
81. Marzano L et al (2004) The role of diagnostic imaging in synovial sarcoma. Our experience. Radiol Med 107:533-540
82. Toolanen G et al (1988) Sonography of popliteal masses. Acta Orthop Scand 59:294-296
83. Garcia J et al (2001) Diagnostic imaging of tumors of the hand and wrist. Eur Radiol 11:1470-1842
84. Teefey SA et al (2008) Ganglia of the hand and wrist: a sonographic analysis. AJR Am J Roentgenol 191:716-720
85. Horcajadas AB et al (2003) Ultrasound and MR findings in tumor and tumor-like lesions of the fingers. Eur Radiol 13:672-685
86. Wang Y et al (2007) The value of sonography in diagnosing giant cell tumors of the tendon sheath. J Ultrasound Med 26:1333-1340
87. Harish S et al (2007) Soft-tissue masses in the shoulder girdle: an imaging perspective. Eur Radiol 17:768-783
88. Bianchi S et al (1997) Elastofibroma dorsi: sonographic findings. AJR Am J Roentgenol 169:1113-1115
89. Dalal A et al (2003) Sonographic detection of elastofibroma dorsi. J Clin Ultrsound 31:375-378
90. Mathis G (1997) Thorax sonography – Part I: Chest wall and pleura. Ultrasound Med Biol 1131-1139
91. Meire HB et al (2001) The anterior abdominal wall. In: Meire H et al (eds) Abdominal and general ultrasound, II Edition. Churchill Livingstone, London, 887-896
92. Saito T et al (1988) Ultrasonographic approach to diagnosing chest wall tumors. Chest 94:1271-1275
93. Briccoli A et al (2007) Ultrasonography is superior to computed tomography and magnetic resonance imaging in determining superficial resection margins of malignant chest wall tumors. J Ultrasound Med 26:157-162
94. Paik SH et al (2005) High-resolution sonography of the rib: can fracture and metastasis be differentiated? AJR Am J Roentgenol 184:969-974
95. Yang GG et al (1991) Sonographic patterns of ribs with tumor involvement. J Formos Med Asoc 90:141-145
96. Ching AS et al (2002) Sonography of umbilical metastasis (Sister Mary Joseph's nodule): from embryology to imaging. Abdom Imaging 27:746-749
97. Dodiuk-Gad R et al (2006) Sister Mary Joseph's nodule as a presenting sign of internal malignancy. Skinmed 5:256-258
98. Francica G et al (2003) Abdominal wall endometriomas near Cesarean delivery scars. Sonographic and color Doppler findings in a series of 12 patients. J Ultrasound Med 22:1041-1047
99. Shimizu Y et al (2004) Implantation metastasis along the percutaneous transhepatic biliary drainage sinus tract. Hepatogastroenterology 51:365-367
100. Tarantino L et al (2006) Seeding from hepatocellular carcinoma after percutaneous ablation: color Doppler ultrasound findings. Abdom Imaging 31:69-77
101. Bruix J et al (2005) Management of hepatocellular carcinoma. Hepatology 42:1208-1236
102. Kim JH et al (2003) Management for chest wall implantation of non-small cell lung cancer after fine-needle aspiration biopsy. Eur J Cardiothorac Surg 23:828-832
103. Maturen KE et al (2006) Lack of tumor seeding of hepatocellular carcinoma after percutaneous needle biopsy using coaxial cutting needle technique. AJR Am J Roentgenol 187:1184-1187
104. Ishii H et al (1998) Needle tract implantation of HCC after percutaneous ethanol injection. Cancer 82:1638-1642
105. Jellici E et al (2005) Imaging of the male breast. Radiol Med 110:574-588
106. Caruso G et al (2004) High-frequency ultrasound in the study of male breast palpable masses. Radiol Med 108:185-193
107. Chen L et al (2006) Imaging characteristics of malignant lesions of the male breast. RadioGraphics 26:993-1006
108. Tzeng CW et al (2007) Soft tissue sarcoma: preoperative and postoperative imaging for staging. Surg Oncol Clin N Am 16:389-402
109. Vanel DV et al (2002) New developments in imaging soft tissue sarcomas. Cancer Imaging 3:51-55
110. Hughes TMD et al (2000) Imaging of soft tissue tumours. Br J Surg 87:259-260
111. Manaster BJ (2002) Soft tissue tumors of the musculoskeletal system. In: Bragg DG et al (eds) Oncologic imaging. WB Saunders Company, Philadelphia, 668-694
112. Sintzoff SA et al (1992) Ultrasound evaluation of soft tissue tumors. J Belge Radiol 75:276-280
113. Bodner G et al (2002) Differentiation of malignant and benign musculoskeletal tumors: combined color and power Doppler US and spectral wave analysis. Radiology 223:410-416
114. Belli P et al (2000) Role of color Doppler sonography in the assessment of musculoskeletal soft tissue masses. J Ultrasound Med 19:823-930
115. Lagalla R et al (1998a) Color Doppler ultrasonography of soft-tissue masses. Acta Radiol 39:421-426
116. Kaushik S et al (2003) Spectral Doppler sonography of musculoskeletal soft tissue masses. J Ultrasound Med 22:1333-1336

117. De Marchi A et al (2002) A preliminary experience in the study of soft tissue superficial masses: color Doppler US and wash-in and wash-out curves with contrast media compared to histological results. Radiol Med 104:451-458
118. Arya S et al (2000) Soft tissue sarcomas: ultrasonographic evaluation of local recurrences. Clin Radiol 55:193-197
119. Alexander AA et al (1997) Superficial soft-tissue masses suggestive of recurrent malignancy: sonographic localization and biopsy. AJR Am J Roentgenol 169:1449-1451
120. Choi H et al (1991) Soft tissue sarcoma: MR imaging vs sonography for detection of local recurrence after surgery. AJR Am J Roentgenol 157:353-358

The Neck

3

3.1 Neck Masses

A number of **anatomic triangles** can be identified in the neck, the knowledge of which is vital for defining the site, and therefore the possible origin, of expansive lesions. The sternocleidomastoid muscle, which runs obliquely upwards and posteriorly, divides the neck into anterior and posterior triangles. The anterior triangle of each side is bounded by the anterior border of the sternocleidomastoid muscle, the inferior border of the mandible and the median line of the neck (from the manubrium of the sternum to the symphysis menti), and in turn is subdivided into four smaller triangles: submental, submandibular, carotid and muscular triangles. The posterior triangle is bounded, in addition to the sternocleidomastoid muscle anteriorly, by the trapezius and the middle third of the clavicle, and in turn is subdivided into two smaller triangles: supraclavicular and occipital triangles [1].

The **regional lymph nodes** corresponding to head and neck tumors (with the exception of primary tumors of the rhinopharynx and the thyroid) are classified as submental, submandibular, jugular or deep cervical (superior, middle and inferior), inferior deep cervical along the accessory nerve, supraclavicular, prelaryngeal, pretracheal, paratracheal, retropharyngeal, parathyroid, buccal, retroauricular and occipital nodes [2] (Fig. 3.1). However, for surgical purposes the lymph nodes are generally classified in the following groups [3]: IA – submental, between the anterior bellies of the digastric muscles), IB – submandibular, surrounding the submandibular gland, II – internal jugular, from the cranial base to the hyoid bone, III – internal jugular, from the hyoid bone to the cricoid cartilage, IV – internal jugular, from the cricoid cartilage to the supraclavicular fossa, V – accessory spinal or of the posterior triangle, posterior to the border of the sternocleidomastoid muscle, VI – central, from the hyoid bone to the sternal border, anterior to the carotid arteries, VII – from the sternal border to the superior mediastinum. The facial, parathyroid, mastoid and retropharyngeal lymph nodes are generally not removed during lymph node dissection of the neck and are therefore not included in this classification. In addition, not all of the sites listed are accessible to US. In general terms, pathologic lymph nodes are defined as cervical lymph nodes with longest diameter >10 mm (although at least 20% of lymph nodes >10 mm are in reality hyperplastic). It should also be borne in mind that up to 50% of metastatic cervical lymph nodes are <5 mm [4,5].

US is the diagnostic imaging modality of choice in the study of **palpable neck masses**. Sarcomas are rarely found in the neck, with <5% of liposarcomas found in this site [6]. Masses of the salivary glands, thyroid, parathyroid and lymph nodes are adequately identified with US and CD, although cytology is often required for the definitive diagnosis. Even many isolated neck masses, such as lateral cysts, thyroglossal duct cysts, dermoid cysts, glomus tumor of the carotid body, lipomas (0.1–5% of benign neck tumors, found predominantly in the posterior triangle), neurogenic tumors, angiomas (generally neonatal), lymphangiomas (pediatric, one of the preferential sites), hematomas and abscesses are relatively characteristic in site and appearance and can therefore be definitively characterized with US [1,7] (Figs. 3.2–3.15). In general US can also provide a valid definition of the relations between the expansive lesion and the adjacent anatomic structures, such as vessels, provided that the lesion itself is not excessively large and/or deep (Figs. 3.16–3.17).

Glomus tumors of the carotid body or **chemodectomas** are slow-growing painless masses found between the 3rd and 6th decade of life, with possible family history. They are typically found in the carotid triangle in close relation with the arterial bifurcation from which they cannot be separated. They may be

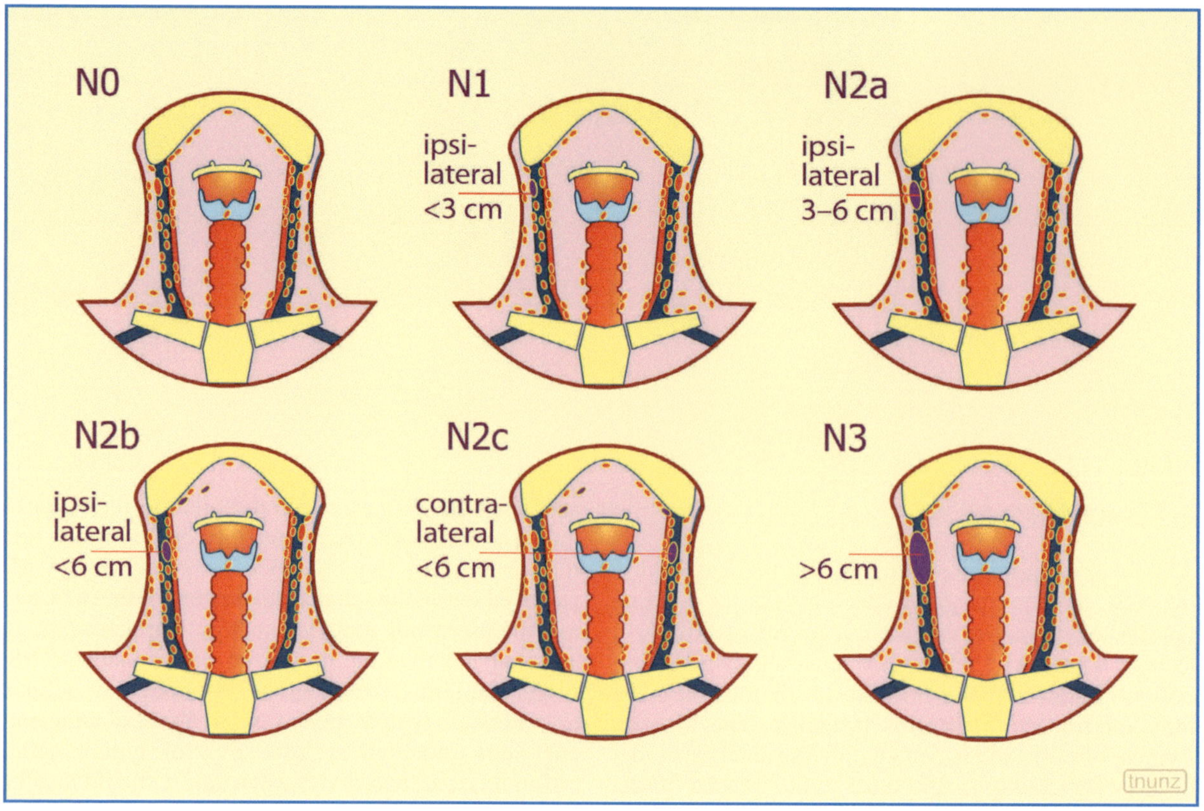

Fig. 3.1 N parameter for primary head and neck tumors (except rhinopharyngeal and thyroid tumors). Regional lymph nodes are considered *N1* if solitary, ipsilateral to the tumor and ≤3 cm in maximum diameter, *N2a* if solitary, ipsilateral and 3–6 cm, *N2b* if multiple, all ipsilateral and ≤6 cm, *N2c* if multiple, bilateral or contralateral, all ≤6 cm, *N3* if at least one lymph node, either ipsi- or contralateral, >6 cm. Lymph nodes of the median line are considered ipsilateral. Mediastinal lymph nodes are already M1. Modified from [2]

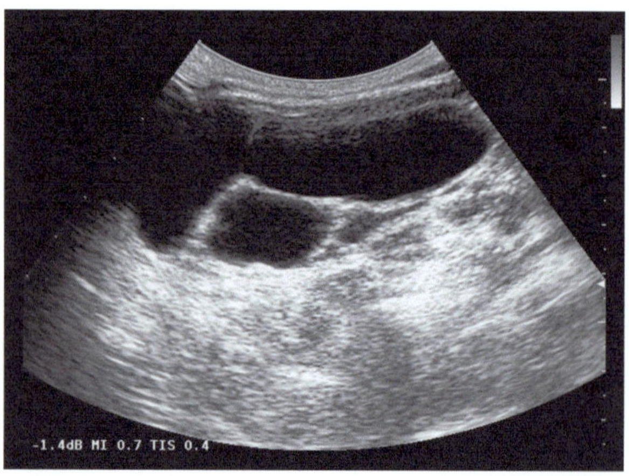

Fig. 3.2 Macrocystic lymphangioma of the neck. Anechoic, septated cystic mass

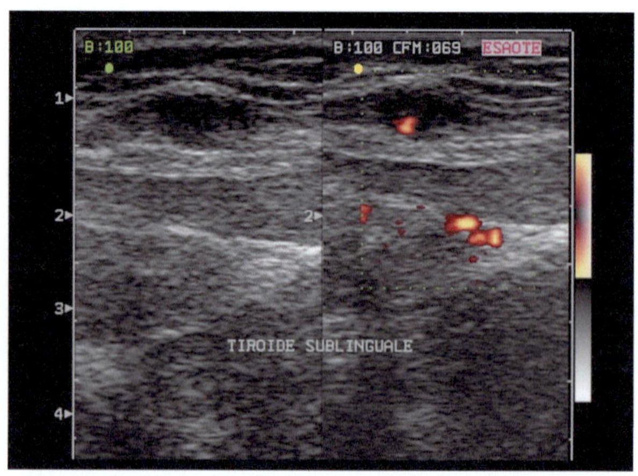

Fig. 3.3 Sublingual thyroid. Heterogeneous hypoechoic nodulation with ill-defined margins and some vascular signals at PD

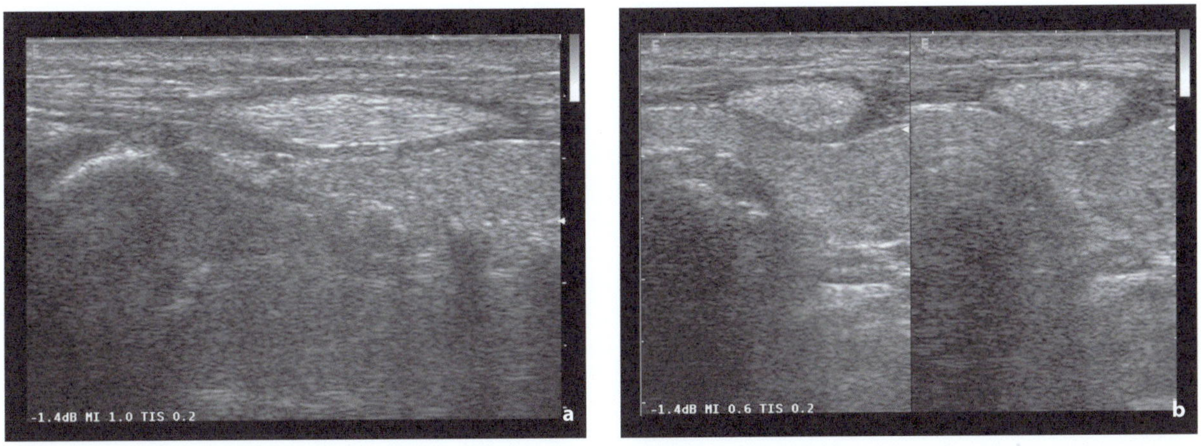

Fig. 3.4a,b Muscular fibroma. Spindle-shaped echogenic mass within the prethyroid muscles

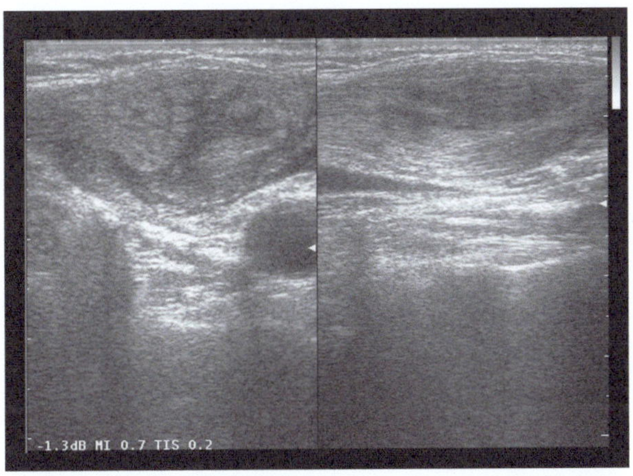

Fig. 3.5 Myositis of the neck. Heterogeneous alteration of the intermediate tract of the sternocleidomastoid muscle, which regressed after medical treatment, seen here in two orthogonal scans

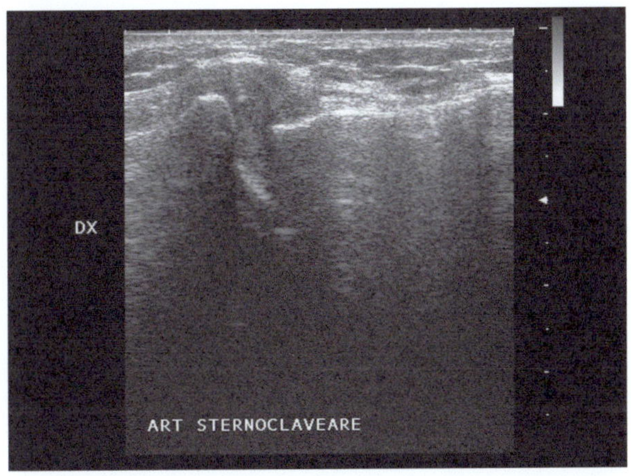

Fig. 3.6 Sternoclavicular arthritis. Abundant hypoechoic joint pannus, which protrudes at the jugular level

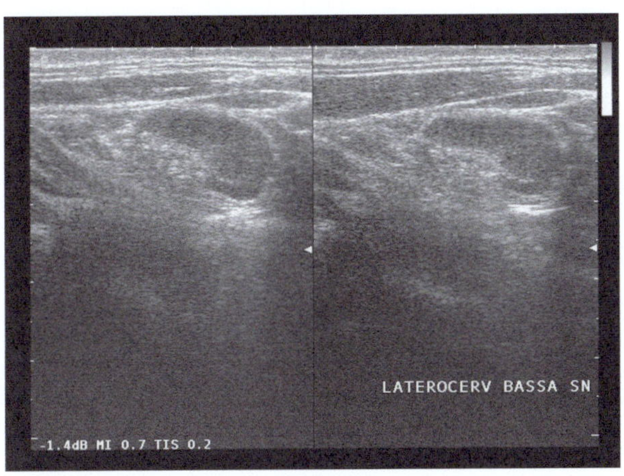

Fig. 3.7 Bilateral cervical lymphadenopathies from sarcoidosis. Several hypoechoic lymph nodes can be identified at the left supraclavicular level, with partial conservation of the central echogenic hilum

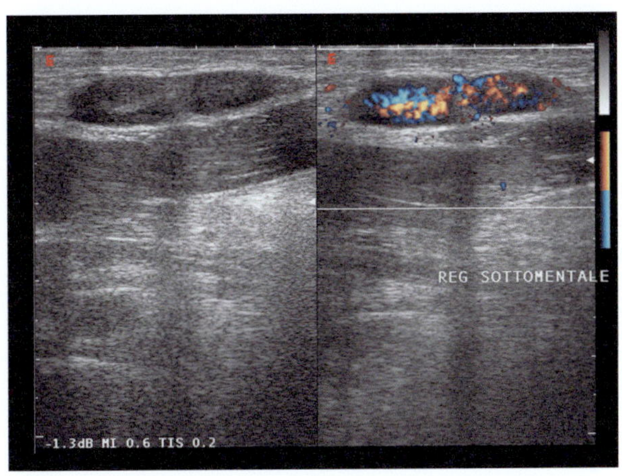

Fig. 3.8 Submental lymphadenitis. Hypoechoic, elongated lymph node with reduced central hilum still identifiable, characterized by intense but hilar and regularly distributed vascularity at directional PD

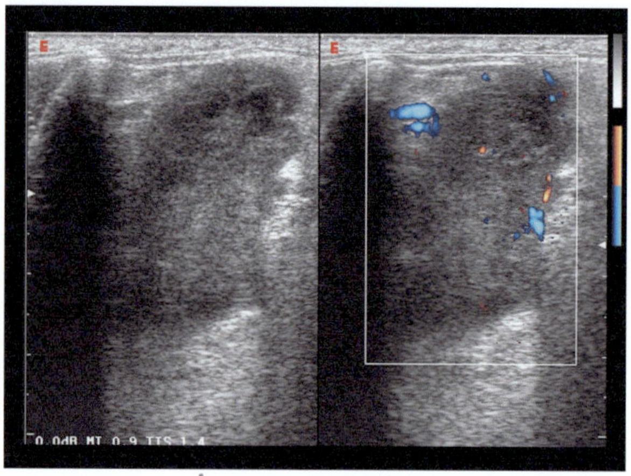

Fig. 3.9 Lymphomatous cervical lymphadenopathy. Elongated mass with heterogeneous hypoechoic appearance and some peripheral vascular signals at directional PD

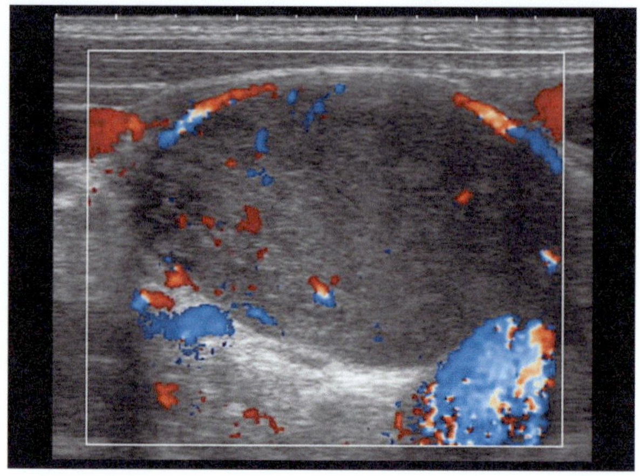

Fig. 3.10 Neurinoma of the vagus nerve. Large oval nodulation with relatively homogeneous hypoechoic appearance and some peripheral vascular signals at CD

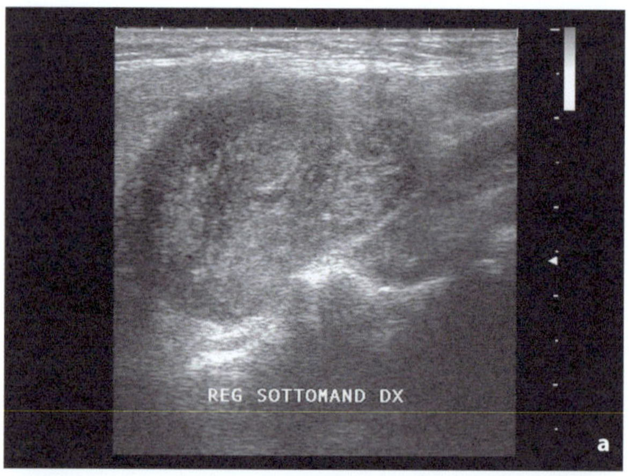

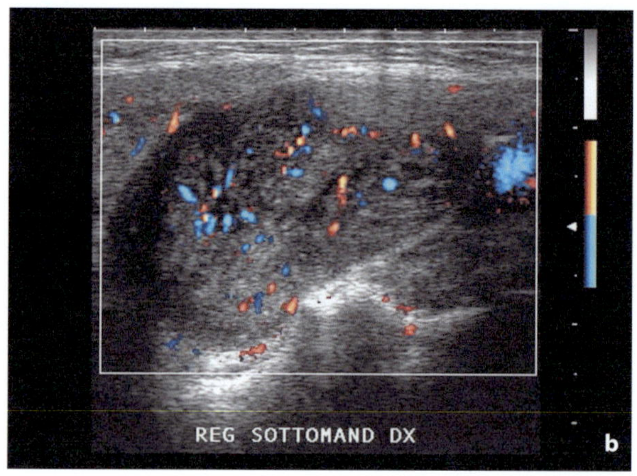

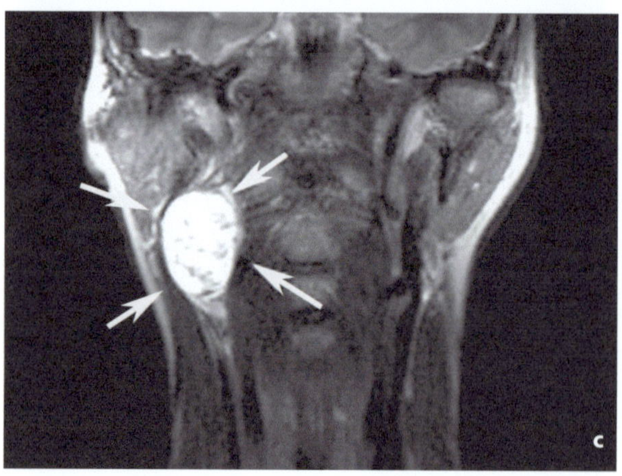

Fig. 3.11a-c Neurinoma of the vagus nerve. Spindle-shaped, well-defined, heterogeneous hypoechoic nodulation (**a**). Multiple color signals, particularly centrally at directional PD (**b**). Coronal T2-weighted MR image visualizes heterogeneous hyperintense mass (**c**, *arrows*)

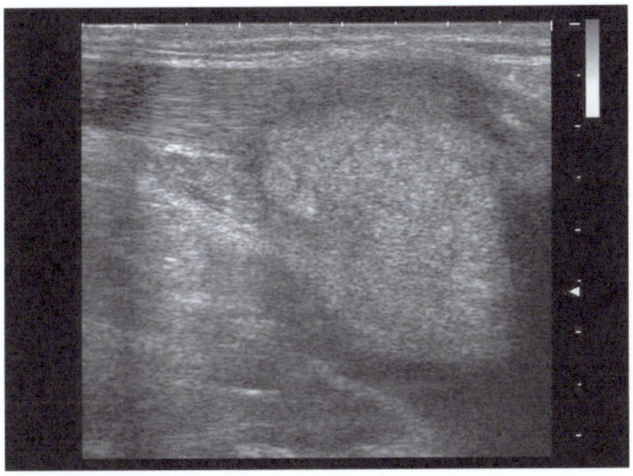

Fig. 3.12 Solitary postoperative contralateral recurrence of oropharyngeal carcinoma at the base of the neck. Heterogeneous echogenic nodulation below the sternocleidomastoid muscle

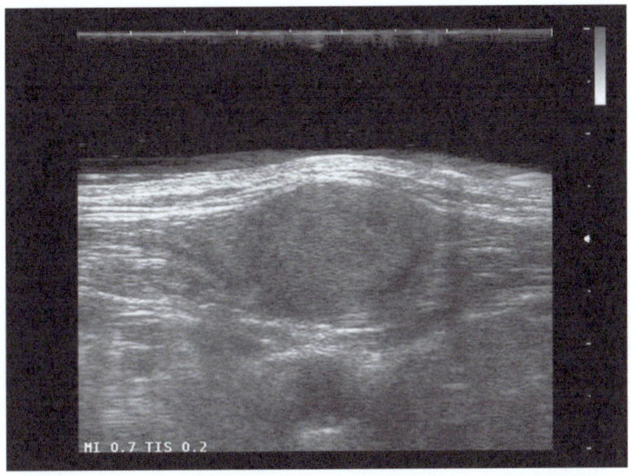

Fig. 3.13 Muscular metastases from lung cancer. Hypoechoic mass which locally widens the sternocleidomastoid muscle

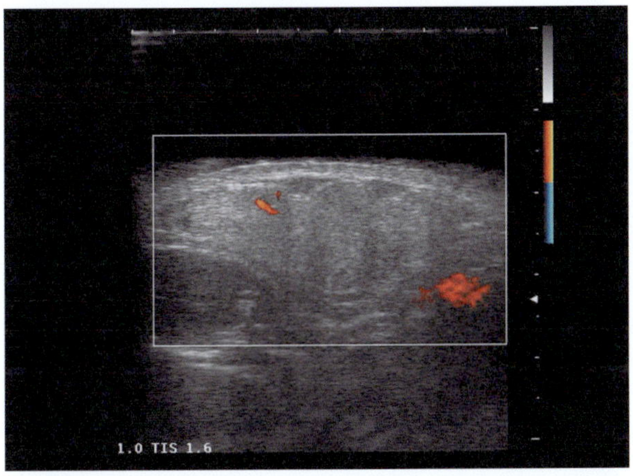

Fig. 3.14 Lipoma-like liposarcoma of the submandibular region. Relatively homogeneous echogenic mass with some vascular signs at directional PD

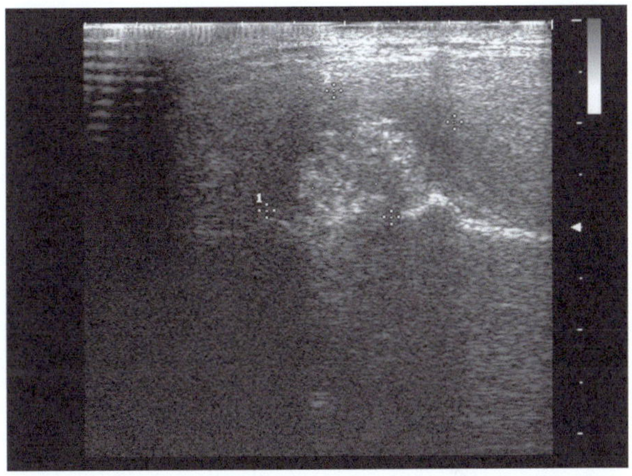

Fig. 3.15 Mandibular chondroma. Heterogeneous echogenic mass with peripheral hypoechoic halo and development towards the parotid gland. US study was performed for presumed parotid nodule

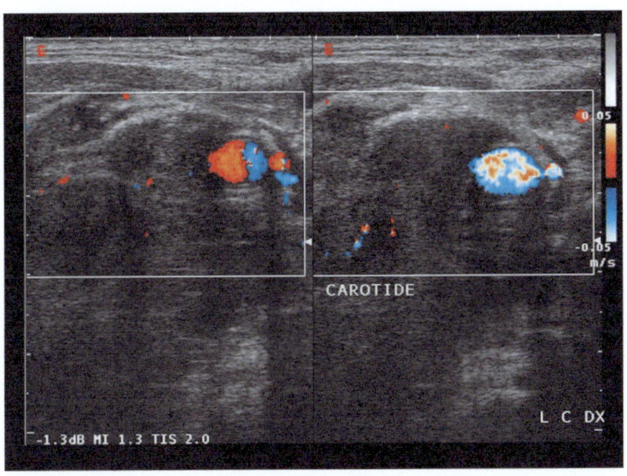

Fig. 3.16 Invasion of the vessels of the neck. Metastatic nodal tissue from occult primary neuroendocrine tumor totally invading the internal jugular vein, which is unrecognizable, and surrounding half of the carotid circumference

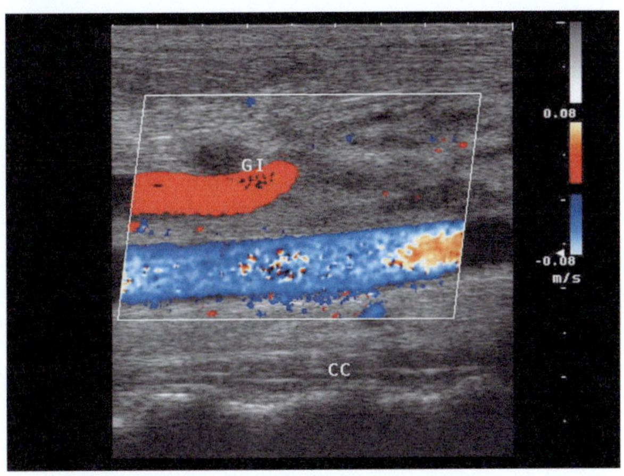

Fig. 3.17 Invasion of the internal jugular vein. Metastatic nodal tissue is seen encircling the jugular vein, which is unrecognizable distally

multiple and have a heterogeneous hypoechoic appearance, relatively well-defined margins and intense vascularity and high flow, even >100 cm/s. An unusually high diastolic component can be seen in the external carotid artery in these patients [1] (Fig. 3.18).

Thyroglossal duct cysts account for 70% of congenital neck cysts and are typically found in the superior portion of the muscular triangle of the neck, at the height of the inferior margin of the hyoid bone, although the site is variable on the median line from the base of the tongue to the pyramidal lobe of the thyroid. It appears as a cystic mass with possible internal echoes, solid components and thick walls, all of which are elements that do not directly correlate with a possible overlying infection of the cyst (Fig. 3.19). Malignant degeneration is rare but possible [1].

Lateral neck cysts arise in 95% of cases from the second branchial cleft and are usually located in the anterior triangle of the neck, in front of the sternocleidomastoid muscle or along its border, generally adjacent to the mandibular angle. These masses are usually found between the 2nd and 5th decade of life and present as rounded or oval cystic masses with heterogeneous hypo-anechoic appearance, which displace the sternocleidomastoid muscle dorsally or dorsolaterally, the neck vessels medially or posteromedially and the submandibular gland anteriorly [1] (Fig. 3.20).

The search for cervical **lymph node metastases** in head and neck tumors is crucial for staging, treatment planning and formulating the prognosis. In squamous cell tumors of the head and neck nodal metastases constitute the single most important prognostic parameter, with a five-year survival rate of 50% in the presence of a metastatic lymph node and 25% in the event of metastasis to a contralateral lymph node [4,8]. Often the primary tumor is occult, at least until the moment of the appearance of palpable cervical lymphadenopathies (41% of buccal cavity tumors, 36% of oropharyngeal tumors, 36% of hypopharyngeal tumors, 29% of supraglottic tumors) [4] (Fig. 3.21). In addition, neck metastases arise not only from head and neck cancers, but also from malignancies of other structures, such as the breast, lung or esophagus, as well as from skin melanomas. In patients with esophageal cancer, systematic study of the neck with US has identified nonpalpable lymph node metastases in 28% of examined cases, even when the tumor was situated in the thoracic esophagus. Palpation is inferior to imaging modalities, and the most accurate preoperative modality in the identification of metastases from head and neck cancers is US-guided FNAC, although it cannot be performed as a routine procedure and is usually reserved for suspicious lymph nodes. In most cases then the diagnosis is based on palpation, US and, in selected cases, CT or MR [9].

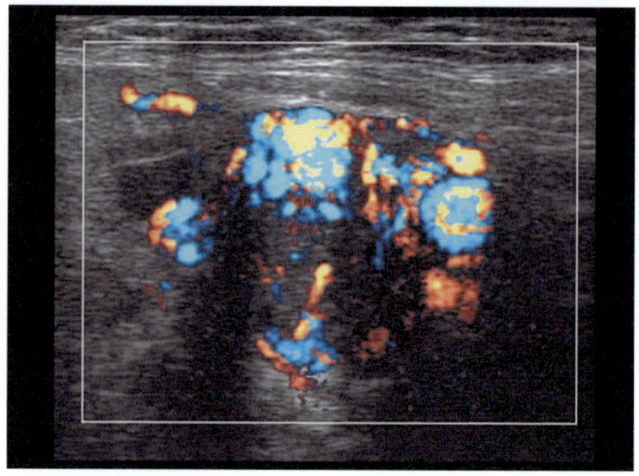

Fig. 3.18 Chemodectoma. Hypervascular nodule encircling the carotid bifurcation

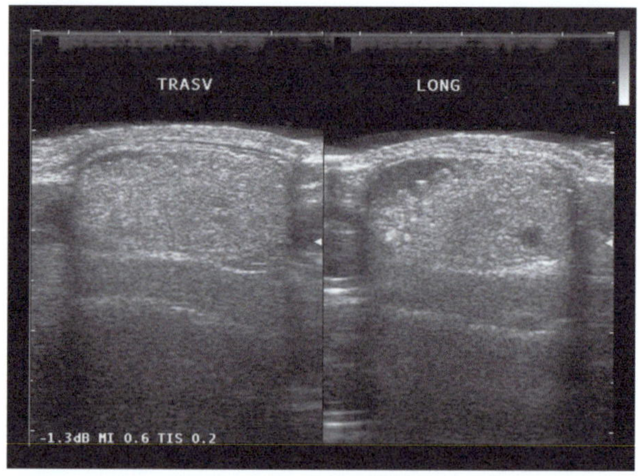

Fig. 3.19 Thyroglossal duct cyst. Median cystic mass of the neck, with internal echoes, scanned in the two orthogonal planes

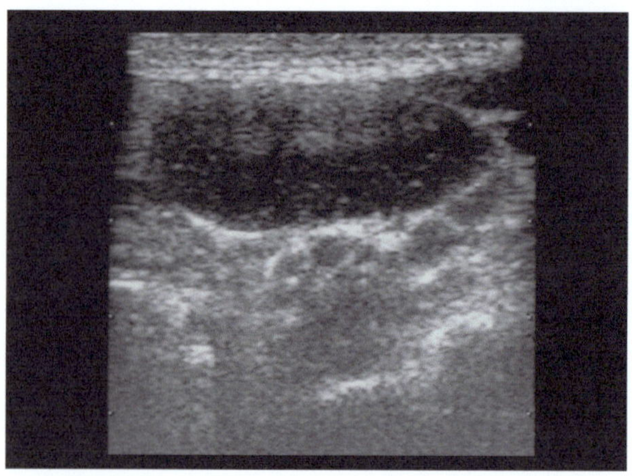

Fig. 3.20 Branchial cyst of the neck. Oval-shaped, unilocular cystic mass with some internal corpuscular heterogeneity

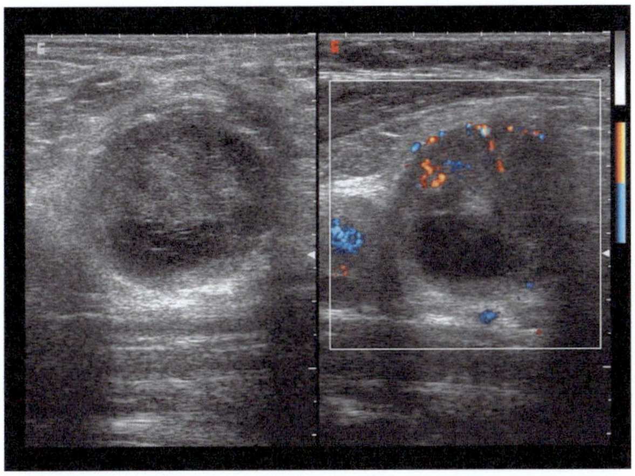

Fig. 3.21 Metastatic lymphadenopathy of the neck from unknown primary. Heterogeneous nodulation with patently necrotic component

Useful criteria for recognizing metastatic lymph nodes are described elsewhere in this book. Nonetheless, nodal morphology is of particular importance in the neck and is highly suspicious when rounded, regardless of its size. This is probably due to the fact that these lymph nodes, unlike axillary nodes for example, are immersed in dense tissue and therefore normally do not have a rounded appearance [1]. Lymph node metastases from squamous cell carcinoma, at least in larger metastases, have a predominantly necrotic structure which tends to be better visualized with CT than US (Figs. 3.22–3.26).

Tubercular lymphadenitis is not a rare condition, being found increasingly often in Western countries, especially in patients with AIDS, and consists of the most common extrapulmonary site of tuberculosis.

Parathyroid masses are caused by hyperplasia (generally involving all of the glands and present in

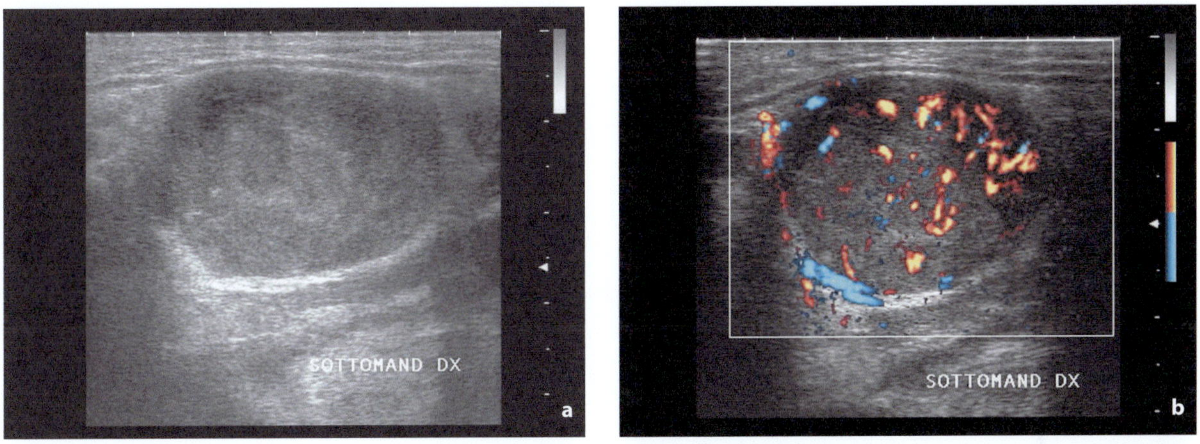

Fig. 3.22a,b Metastatic lymphadenopathy of the neck from melanoma. Enlarged heterogeneous hypoechoic lymph node (**a**), showing moderate and irregular vascularity with peripheral and central distribution at directional PD (**b**)

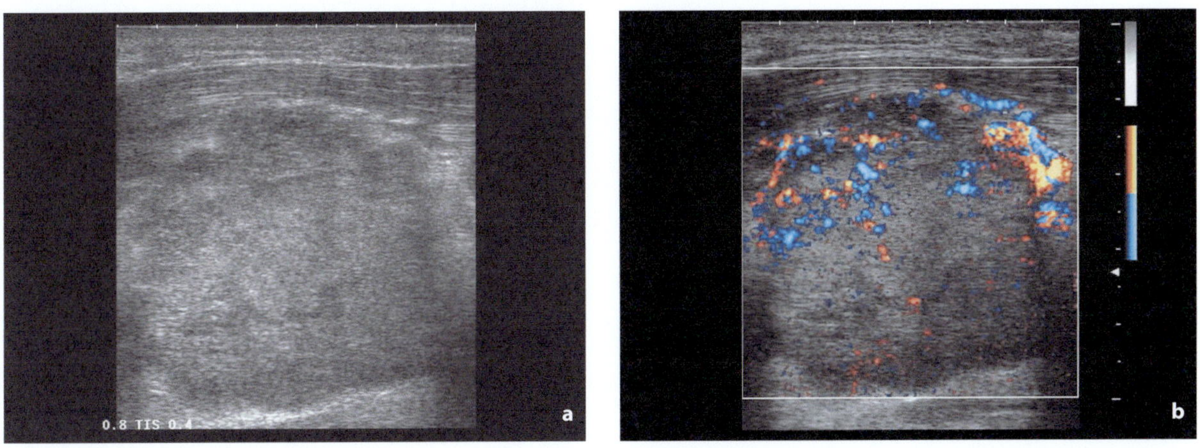

Fig. 3.23a,b Metastatic lymphadenopathy of the neck from oropharyngeal carcinoma. Large nodal mass anteriorly displacing the sternocleidomastoid muscle (**a**). Moderate capsular and irregularly distributed vascularity at directional PD (**b**). The poor vascular signal in the deep portion of the lesion is due to limited sampling ability of the Doppler signal with the transmit frequency used by the superficial transducer

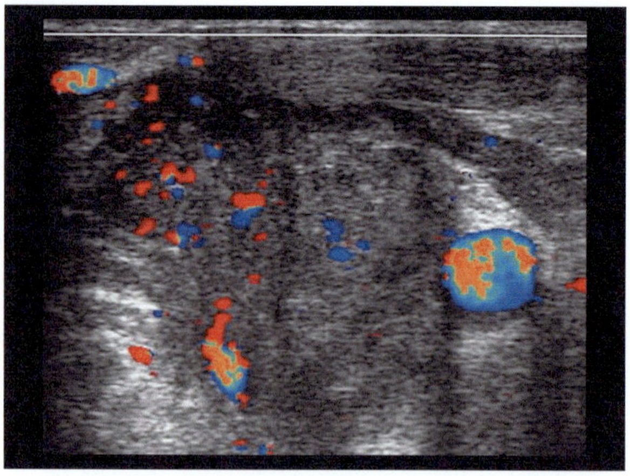

Fig. 3.24 Lymph node metastasis from anaplastic carcinoma of the thyroid. CD helps to define the relations of the common carotid artery with the adjacent structures and the absence of the internal jugular vein, which has been invaded and is no longer identifiable

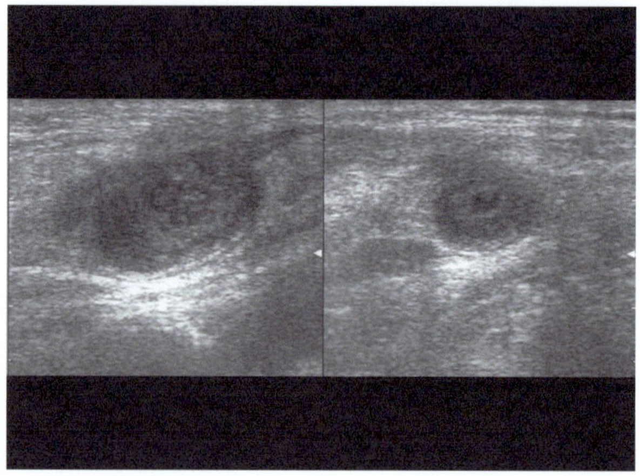

Fig. 3.25 Lymph node metastasis from carcinoma of the ear lobe. Heterogeneous hypoechoic lymphadenopathy at the high laterocervical level

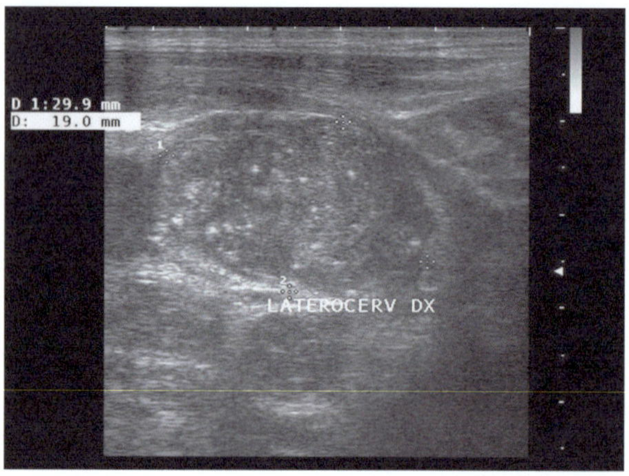

Fig. 3.26 Metastatic lymphadenopathy of the neck from medullary carcinoma of the thyroid. Hypoechoic lymph node with scattered microcalcifications

10–20% of subjects with primary hyperparathyroidism), adenoma (usually solitary, present in 80–90% of subjects with primary hyperparathyroidism) and carcinoma (solitary, present in 0.5–4% of subjects with primary hyperparathyroidism) [10,11]. They may be an incidental finding, e.g. during a US study of the thyroid, identified as a palpable lesion, or the result of a systematic search in subjects with hyperparathyroidism (primary, or secondary to events such as hypercalcemia from chronic renal failure). Primary hyperparathyroidism is a condition that is not as rare as thought in the past, and is more prevalent among women than men (F/M 2–3:1) and among postmenopausal than premenopausal women [1]. In subjects with endocrine alterations (elevated blood parathyroid hormone and calcium levels) the first challenge of imaging is to identify the site of a possible parathyroid lesion, which can be unusual (Fig. 3.27). Precisely defining the location offers the possibility of performing a minimally invasive approach, with a surgical incision <2 cm in place of conventional exploration of the neck. US easily identifies parathyroid lesions in the usual site – superior lesions are generally found dorsal to the middle third of the lateral thyroid lobe along the course of the inferior thyroid artery, whereas inferior lesions, the site of which tends to be more variable, are found inferoposterior to the base of the thyroid. The identification of patently ectopic lesions (1–3%) is more challenging, for which a CT or MR study is indicated, or better still a scintigraphy (Tc^{99m} sestamibi) [1]. US has shown a sensitivity for the identification of parathyroid adenoma of 24–92% [10,11]. The parathyroid nodules appear as small (<15–20 mm), rounded or more often oval or elongated masses with relatively homogeneous hypoechoic appearance and well-defined margins and often with a thin pseudocapsular echogenic rim [10,11]. The echogenicity can be similar or more often lower than the adjacent normal thyroid tissue, occasionally with marked hypoechogenicity. Heterogeneous internal signals can be due to hemorrhagic phenomena, degenerative cystic areas (2–4% of cases, whereas patently cystic lesions are rare) or internal or capsular calcifications (2–5%, especially in old secondary hyperplasias and carcinomas) [11] (Figs. 3.28–3.31).These lesions usually appear as loosely attached to the thyroid during swallowing and show no typical central hilum of the lymph nodes. There can

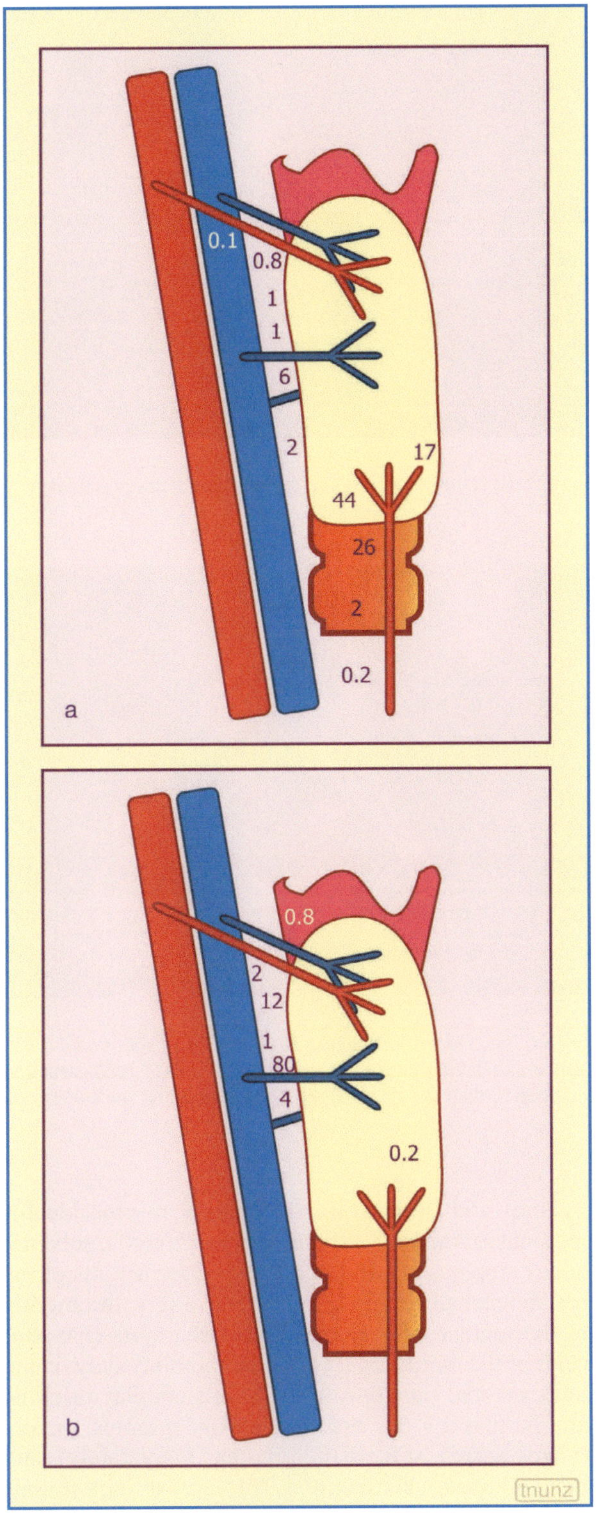

Fig. 3.27a,b Statistical location of the parathyroid glands, inferior (**a**) and superior (**b**). The percentage of locations of the parathyroid glands is indicated with respect to the surrounding structures and in particular to the thyroid

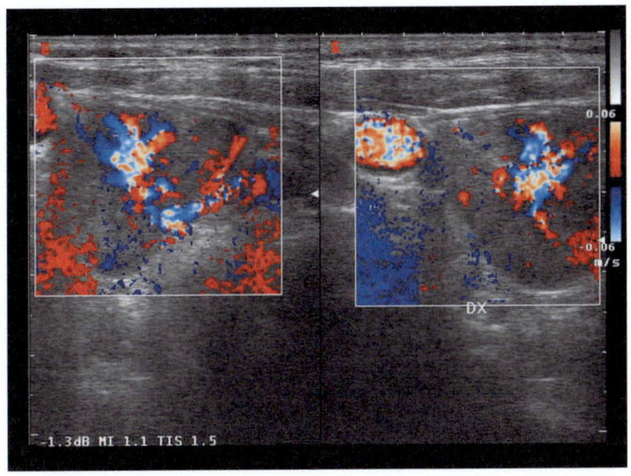

Fig. 3.28 Parathyroid adenoma. Hypervascular hypoechoic nodulation at the base of the neck

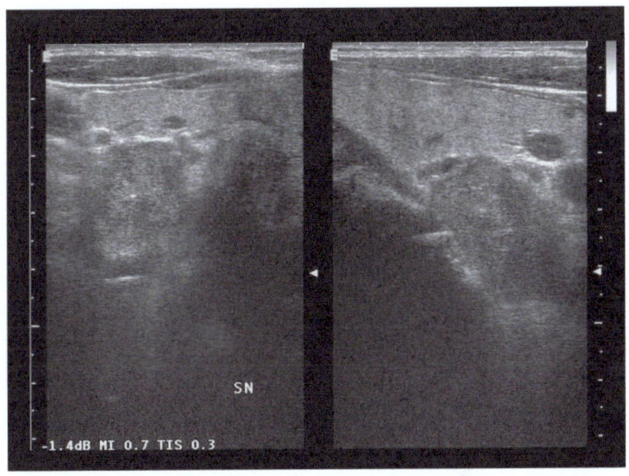

Fig. 3.29 Parathyroid adenoma. Relatively well-defined and homogeneous hypoechoic mass located dorsal to the base of the thyroid

also be difficulty in distinguishing between parathyroid lesions and thyroid nodules, especially when the former are particularly adherent to the thyroid or the latter are exophytic. CD usually reveals moderate central or diffuse hypervascularity with uniform or irregular distribution, but generally not marginal (as in many thyroid nodules). Avascularity is highly uncommon. A branch of the inferior thyroid artery can often be seen supplying the nodulation. The internal velocities are 20–30 cm/s and therefore similar to intrathyroid velocities and they have significant diastolic components with low RI values [11]. A carcinoma may be suspected when the lesion is of prominent size (>15 mm), displays fixity with swallowing and shows a heterogeneous echotexture with internal calcifications and signs of invasion of the adjacent muscular or vascular structures.

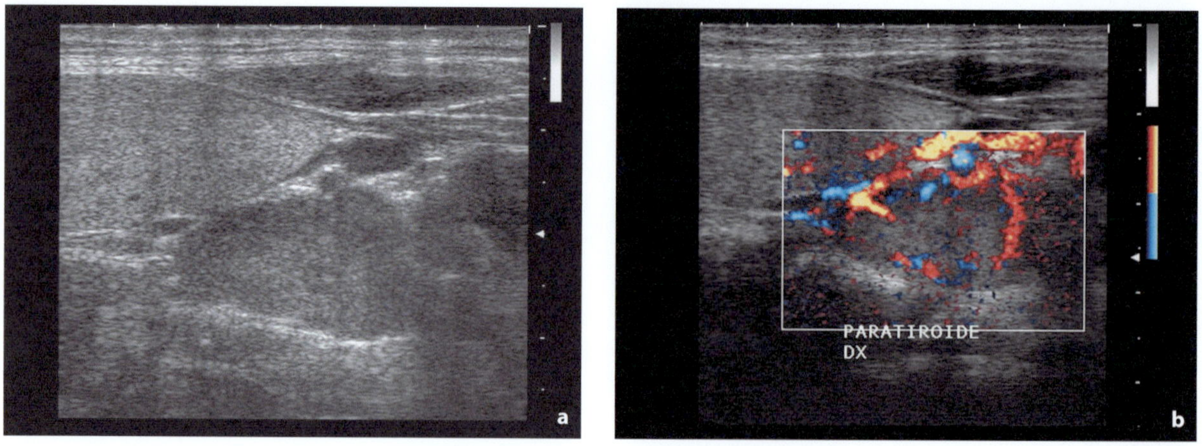

Fig. 3.30a,b Parathyroid adenoma. Well-defined, homogeneous, hypoechoic retrothyroid nodule (**a**) with moderate vascularity at directional PD (**b**)

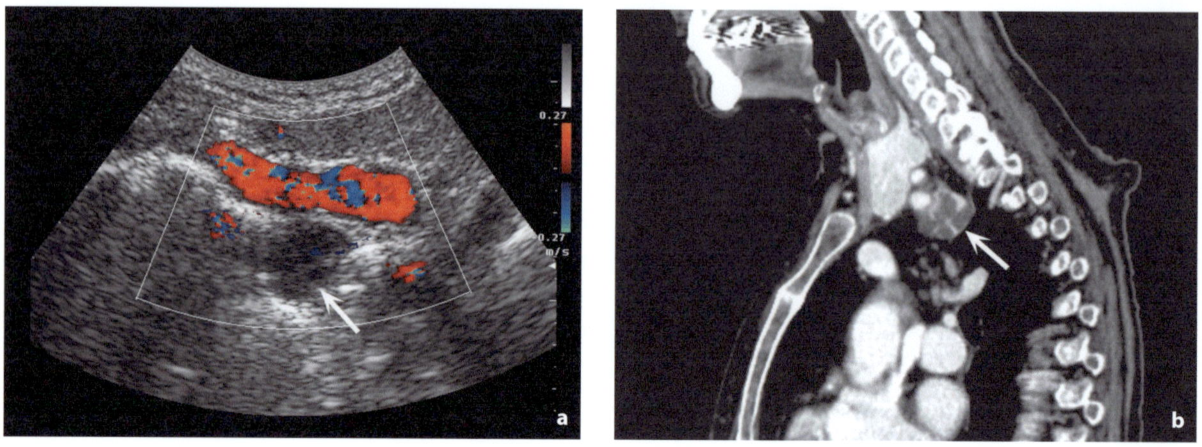

Fig. 3.31a,b Parathyroid adenoma. Heterogeneous hypoechoic nodulation can be identified (thanks to the use of an abdominal transducer) at the right superior thoracic aperture, immediately dorsal to the subclavian artery (**a**, *arrow*). Sagittal CT reconstruction confirms the heterogeneous hypoattenuating mass (**b**, *arrow*) located deep to the base of the right thyroid lobe and the subclavian artery

The distinction between hyperplasia and adenoma is not possible with US [11]. In addition to thyroid nodules (especially in cases of multinodular goiter), parathyroid lesions (and normal parathyroid glands) should be distinguished from normal vascular formations (in particular from a branch of the inferior thyroid vein which is often placed deep to the thyroid base), other neck tumors such as glomus tumors of the carotid body (which however have a characteristic location and higher flow velocities) and nodal masses (not so much normal or hyperplastic lymph nodes as metastatic, but in this case the vascularity is different, being capsular, and there is no fixity with the thyroid during swallowing) [10].

Palpable **supraclavicular masses** can be nodal or extranodal in origin. The non-nodal causes consist of lipomas and lipomatosis (commonly responsible for regional asymmetry and the reported "mass"), subcutaneous emphysema, fluid collections, aneurysms of the brachiocephalic artery or subclavian artery, thrombosis of the jugular vein, lymphangiectasis, cysts (lymphocele) of the thoracic duct (rare and possibly only on the left), ectopic parathyroid expanses, nodular fasciitis, neurinomas of the brachial plexus, glomus tumors (vagus nerve), soft tissue sarcomas (very rarely), and bone (clavicle), cartilaginous (first rib) or joint lesions (sternoclavicular joint) [6,12]. Lymphadenopathies should be sought with a thorough exploration, with an evaluation of the area immediately deep to the medial end of the clavicle and also possibly with the patient seated. These lymphadenopathies can have a wide range of origins, especially from the left side where the

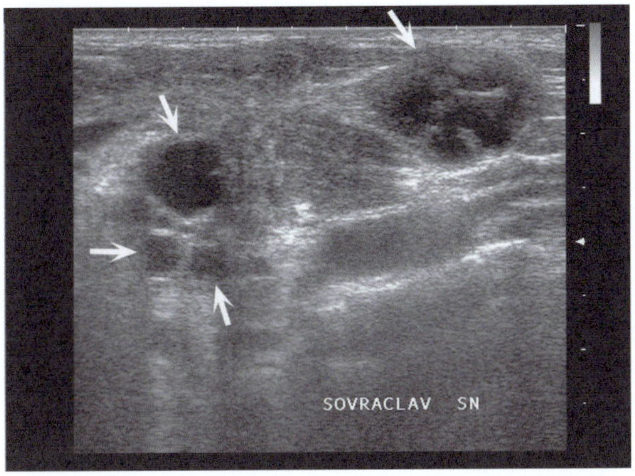

Fig. 3.32 Metastasis with cystic appearance, as the clinical presentation of a cystadenocarcinoma of the pancreas. Multiple hypo-anechoic lymph nodes at the left supraclavicular level (*arrows*)

venous confluence of the thoracic duct conveys the lymph of the lower part of the body. The origin may be descending from tumors of the head and neck, thyroid, ipsilateral but occasionally also contralateral breast, ipsilateral but occasionally also contralateral lung, or ascending from thoracoabdominal malignancies (thymus, lung, esophagus, stomach, kidney, colon, ovary, testicle, etc. – Troisier's sign) (Fig. 3.32). Generally in this site normal lymph nodes cannot be seen and therefore this is one of the few lymph node stations where the visualization of a lymph node is in itself suspicious. Very small supraclavicular lymph nodes (3–4 mm) but rounded and hypoechoic are highly suspicious of metastasis. In pulmonary carcinomas, where the incidence of supraclavicular lymphadenopathies is anything but negligible, palpation has been shown to have a low sensitivity (33%), so only the larger lymphadenopathies can be identified. US instead has a high sensitivity (100%), even higher than CT (83%), and the positive US finding can, if necessary, be confirmed with US-guided FNAC [13,14].

3.2 Salivary Tumors

US is the first-choice and in many cases conclusive imaging modality in patients with a suspected **mass of the major salivary glands** (Figs. 3.33–3.35). Limitations to the use of the technique include the inability to explore some deep regions (portions of the submandibular gland below the mandible and deep portions of the parotid gland), problems of differential diagnosis (partial overlap between solid benign and malignant lesions) and the difficulty in evaluating the

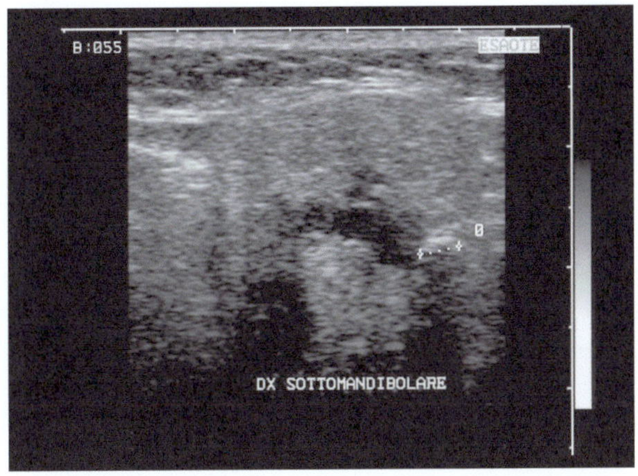

Fig. 3.33 Submandibular salivary calculus. Mass of the submandibular gland as the consequence of a large obstructive ductal calculus

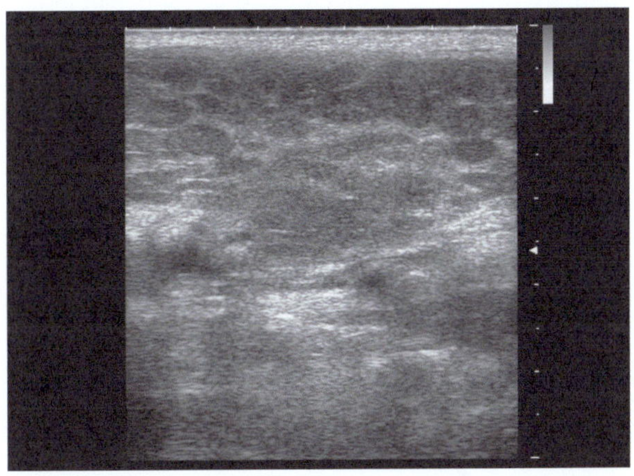

Fig. 3.34 Granulomatous parotitis. Hypoechoic glandular mass, with interposed echogenic bands

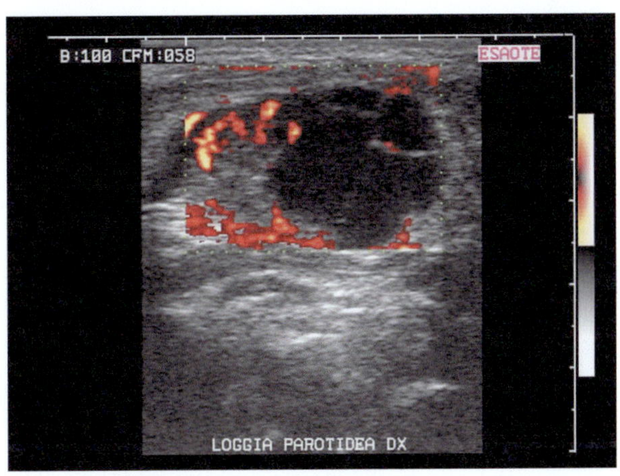

Fig. 3.35 Parotid cyst. Fluid-filled mass with some internal septations and some intraseptal and marginal color signals at PD

extent of expansive lesions. In the latter case a panoramic CT or better still MR study is indicated. For lesion characterization biopsy is used, possibly US-guided, whereas sialography and CT sialography are no longer indicated in the study of tumors.

Salivary gland tumors account for 5% of head and neck tumors. They are found at the level of the parotid in 80% of cases, the submandibular gland in 15% and sublingual gland or minor salivary glands in 5%. Malignant tumors account for around 30–40% of cases. In particular, at the level of the parotid gland 80% of lesions are benign, whereas this figure falls to 50% for the submandibular gland and 50–20% for the sublingual and minor glands [15,16].

US is able to identify the effective presence of a lesion, its exact site and topography, the number of lesions (nodules are often multiple or bilateral) and as much as possible the nature of the lesion. Malignancy can occasionally be suspected on the basis of clinical findings (up to 30% of cases of parotid carcinoma at presentation) in the presence of palpable lymphadenopathies (14–29% of cases of parotid carcinoma), peripheral paralysis of the facial nerve (14% of cases of parotid carcinoma), rapid growth and deep fixity, especially if combined [16,17]. Benign lesions tend to have the following characteristics: patently fluid-filled appearance, rounded shape, regular margins, homogeneous echotexture, separable from the adjacent structures and absence of adenopathies. Malignant tumors instead have a nodular appearance, with irregular or patently infiltrating margins ("stellate") and hypoechoic heterogeneous echotexture due in part to the presence of calcifications (especially suspicious if punctate) and hypo-anechoic necrotic-hemorrhagic areas (with irregular and disorderly arranged margins). Signs of local invasion, vascular infiltration or lymph node metastasis definitively clarify the nature of the lesions. However, these are not absolute criteria, there are benign lesions with internal heterogeneity and ill-defined margins, and malignant lesions such as acinar cell carcinoma which have a nodular, homogeneous appearance with well-defined margins. The overall accuracy of these morphologic signs in the identification of malignancy is 80–82%. A thorough search for diseased lymph nodes is crucial, which notably increases the suspicion of malignancy of the salivary lesion, as well as signs of invasion of the adjacent structures [16]. Especially at the level of the parotid gland the tumor nodules often have an exophytic appearance, which makes defining their precise origin challenging with respect to the submandibular gland, and also its exact nature with respect above all to the periparotid lymph nodes. The absence of a cleavage plane with respect to the parotid gland and the presence of an afferent vessel in relation with the gland enable the origin to be correctly defined.

At **CD** most salivary tumors, regardless of their nature, appear more vascular than the surrounding parenchyma. In at least half of the malignant lesions the subjectively evaluated vascularity is particularly emphasized, with multiple venous and above all arterial vessels, afferent from numerous poles and intertwined within the nodule with an irregular arrangement and relatively high-velocity flow (the threshold of 25 cm/s has a sensitivity of 72% and a specificity of 88%). The other half of malignant tumors are not as vascular, and although several intralesional vessels can be found there is generally no peripheral vascular network of the capsular kind which is characteristic of benign lesions (where there is also a predominance of venous flows). Contrast media tend to increase the visualization of the nodular vasculature, especially in pleomorphic adenomas, even in cases of unsatisfying baseline findings, so they therefore increase the ability of the technique to characterize lesions [18]. A useful sign is given by compression with the transducer. In adenomatous nodules, which have a prevalently venous flow, the intranodular color signals disappear in 58% of cases and attenuate in 29% of cases, whereas in carcinomas the color signals of the vascularity, which is for the most part arterial, increase in 1% of cases, remain unaltered in 75% and are attenuated in 24%, so are never completely cancelled. Occasionally, vessels common to the lesion and the surrounding parenchyma may be identified, which is a sign of invasion [16,19]. On the basis of the CD pattern and the response to the compression test, the accuracy of the technique is 87–88%. CD can also be useful in recognizing the retromandibular vein, which is identifiable in 70% of cases (possible, Valsalva maneuver), the relations of which with the parotid tumor need to be clarified preoperatively [15].

Pleomorphic adenoma accounts for 24–71% of salivary tumors and 75–80% of benign tumors of the parotid. Some 80% of lesions are located in the superficial part of the gland and 10% in the deep portion, with possible protrusion into the parapharyngeal space [15]. The tumor is predominant in females, with a peak between 35 and 50 years of age, may be bilateral and multifocal, and in 4–5% of cases it can also degenerate or be locally invasive and recurrent. In general it is a slow-growing lobulated nodule 2–4 cm in size with relatively homogeneous hypoechoic appearance (98% of cases) and well defined by a capsule. Only larger masses may show some internal heterogeneity or less well-defined margins [15]. Calcifications are common, and at the level of the parotid they are relatively specific for pleomorphic adenoma. CD generally displays (80% of cases)

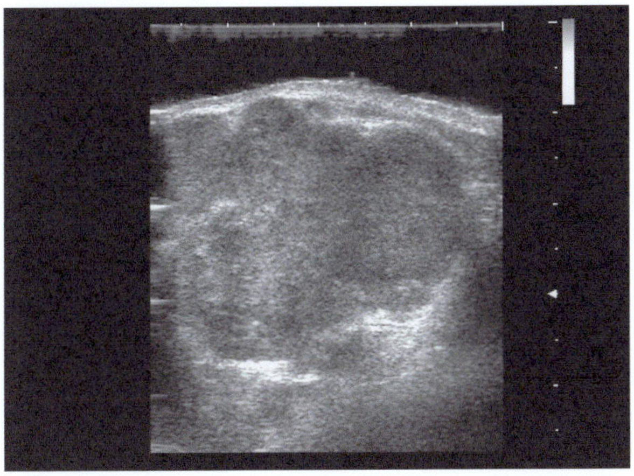

Fig. 3.36 Recurrence of pleomorphic parotid adenoma in a patient operated on seven years earlier. Large, relatively well-defined and heterogeneous hypoechoic nodule

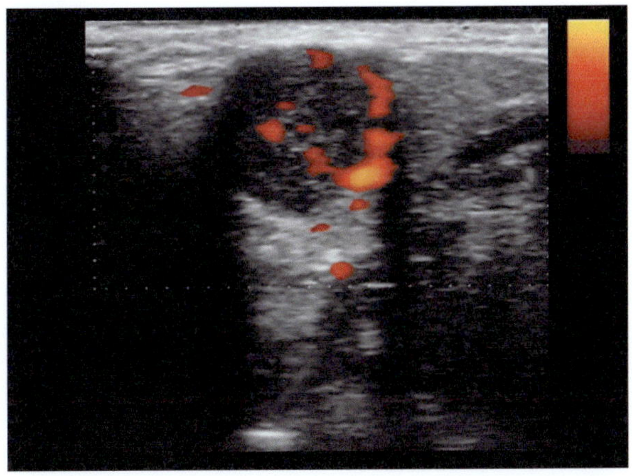

Fig. 3.37 Submandibular pleomorphic adenoma. Homogenous hypoechoic nodule with well-defined margins and some peripheral and central vascular signals at PD

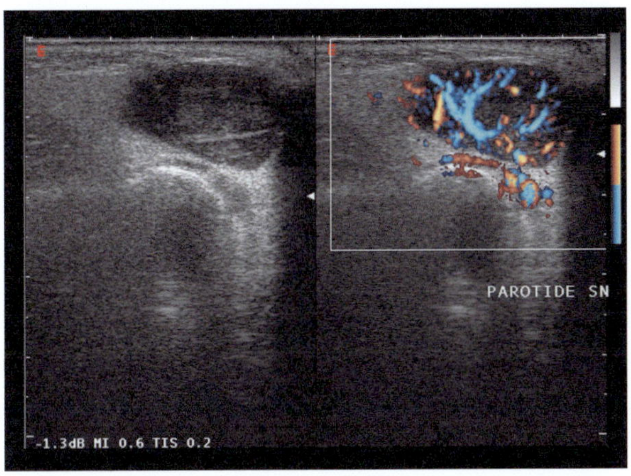

Fig. 3.38 Parotid pleomorphic adenoma. Homogeneous hypoechoic nodule with well-defined margins and a marked but central and homogeneously distributed vascular network

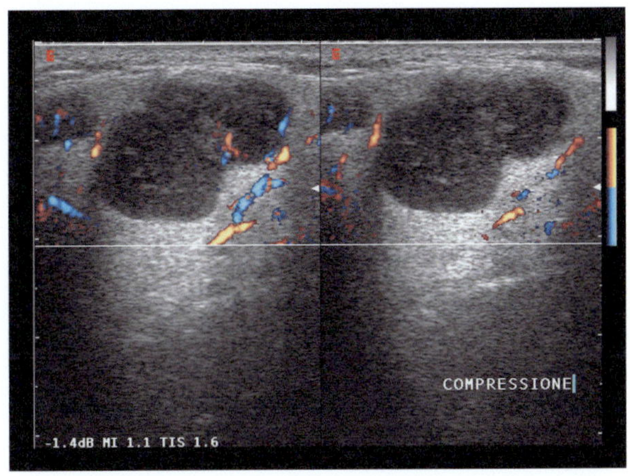

Fig. 3.39 Parotid pleomorphic adenomas, compression study. Two homogeneous hypoechoic nodules with well-defined margins and some peri- and intranodular vascular signals at directional PD. Transducer compression notably attenuates both flows

moderate vascularity, with complete or incomplete capsular branches and a single internal and generally venous vascular pole. The flow velocities recorded are <25 cm/s [15,16] (Figs 3.36–3.40).

Adenolymphoma (Warthin's tumor) accounts for 10–20% of parotid tumors, is prevalently found in the lower pole and is predominant among males, with a peak around 40 years of age. The tumor is multicentric in 30% of cases and bilateral in 7%, whereas they are rarely found in a submandibular location [15]. Adenolymphoma is a well-defined oval lesion with an internal structure rendered heterogeneous by hypo-anechoic areas of variable size, with a fan-shaped distribution. The finding of cystic components in a parotid lesion is practically diagnostic for adenolymphoma. CD reveals the moderate vascularity of the solid components, whereas a capsular-type vascular distribution is rare [16] (Fig. 3.41, Video 3.1, 3.2).

The major **malignant tumors** include mucoepidermoid carcinoma (the most frequent type in pediatric patients), adenoid cystic carcinoma (20% of submandibular tumors with a peak at 50–60 years), acinar cell carcinoma (2–4% of parotid tumors), adenocarcinoma (27% of malignant salivary lesions) and undifferentiated carcinoma (35% of malignant salivary tumors). These lesions have a variable growth rate and can reach significant dimensions. They generally appear as hypoechoic lesions which are homogeneous if <2 cm and heterogeneous if >2 cm, with necrotic or pseudocystic internal areas and microcalcifications. The vascular structure tends to be intense, anarchic with multiple vascular poles, and the margins

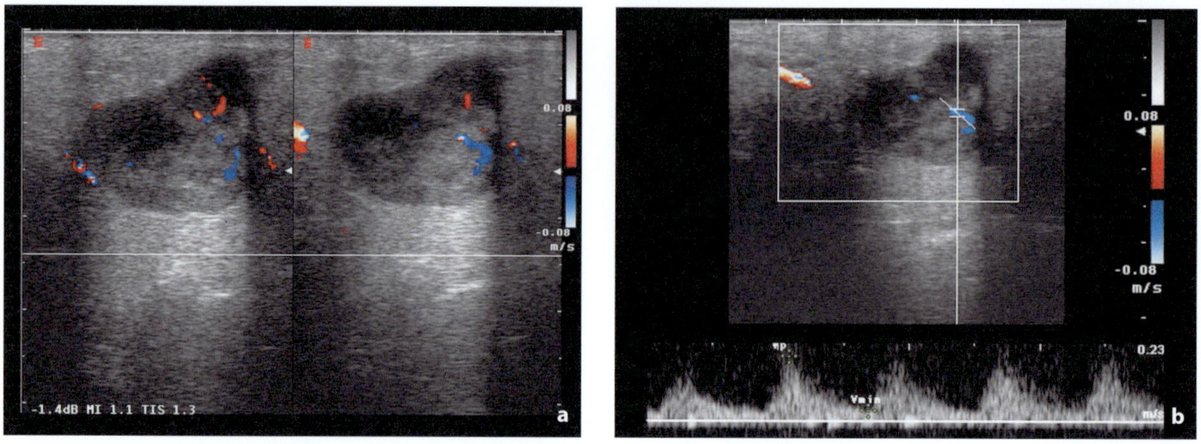

Fig. 3.40a,b Parotid pleomorphic adenoma. Lobulated hypoechoic nodule with relatively homogeneous echotexture and well-defined margins, with some vascular signals at CD (**a**). Spectral Doppler (**b**) shows low flow (V_{max} 18 cm/s) with a high RI (0.81)

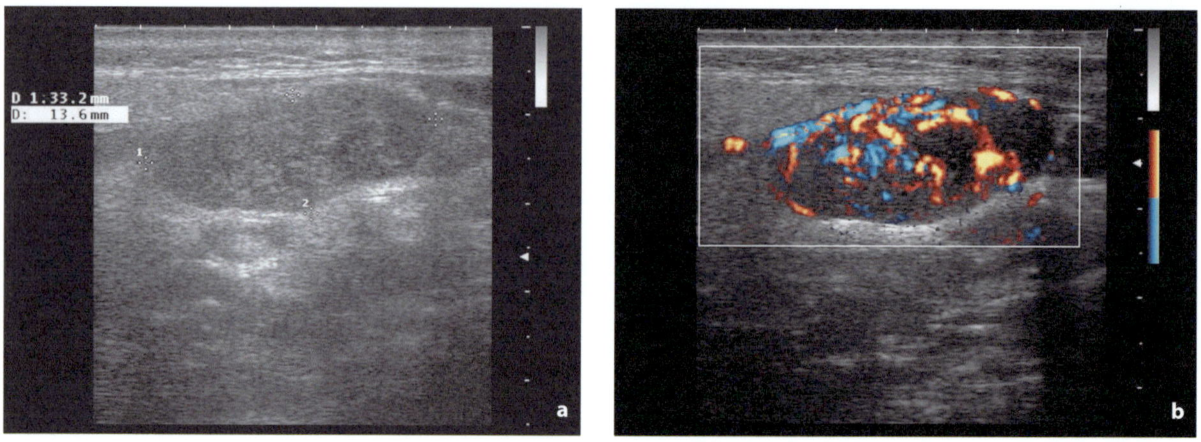

Fig. 3.41a,b Parotid cystadenolymphoma. Elongated hypoechoic mass with relatively homogeneous echotexture and well-defined margins (**a**), with mild central and peripheral vascularity at directional PD (**b**). Areas of abundant vessels alternate with hypovascular areas

appear poorly defined or patently infiltrating (occasionally clearly interrupted), especially in larger lesions. Smaller and especially low-malignancy lesions may appear homogeneous with well-defined margins, thus mimicking benign forms. The presence of hypervascularity or elevated flow velocity (>25 cm/s) should, however, prompt suspicion. Adenoid cystic carcinoma is characterized by a tendency to spread along the nerves more than via the lymphatic vessels, a characteristic which is difficult to identify with US. The lesion also presents internal pseudocystic formations [15,16] (Figs. 3.42, 3.43).

Lymphomas can be primary (2–5% of salivary gland tumors, especially including type-B lymphoma) or secondary (most of all non-Hodgkin's – 0.7% of all lymphomas) and Sjögren's syndrome is often associated. In these cases the glands appear enlarged, with

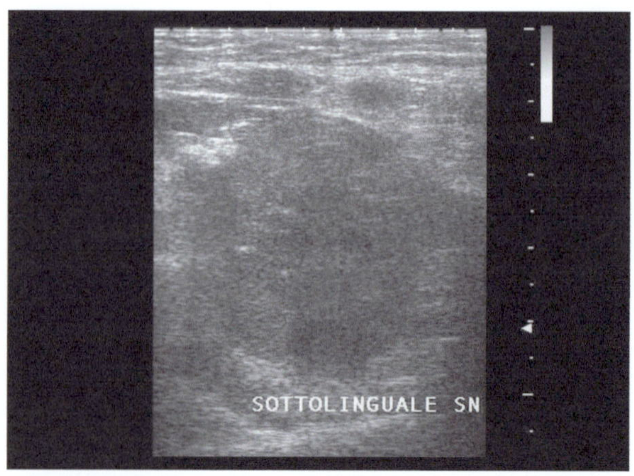

Fig. 3.42 Sublingual carcinoma. Heterogeneous, hypoechoic and ill-defined mass

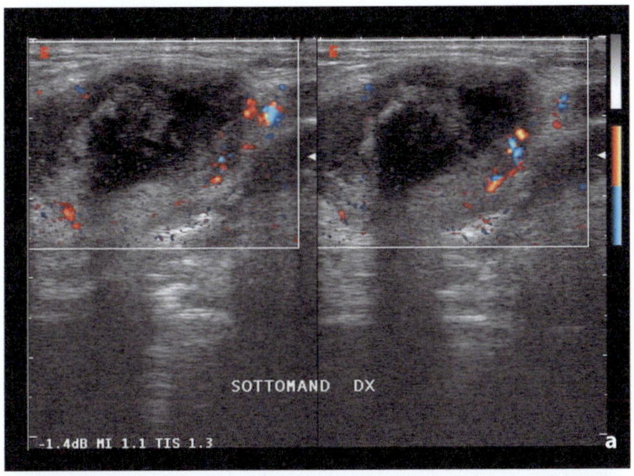

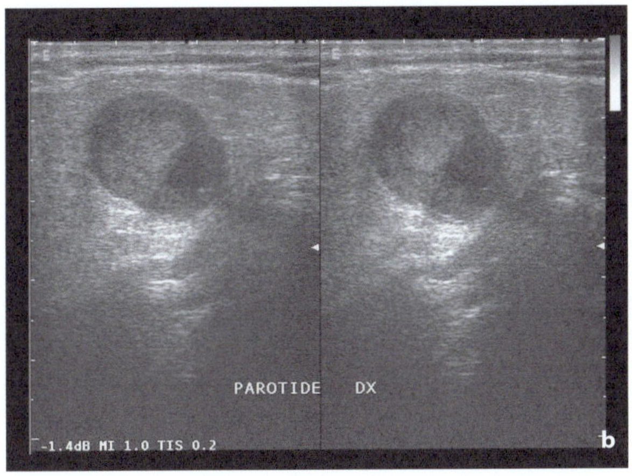

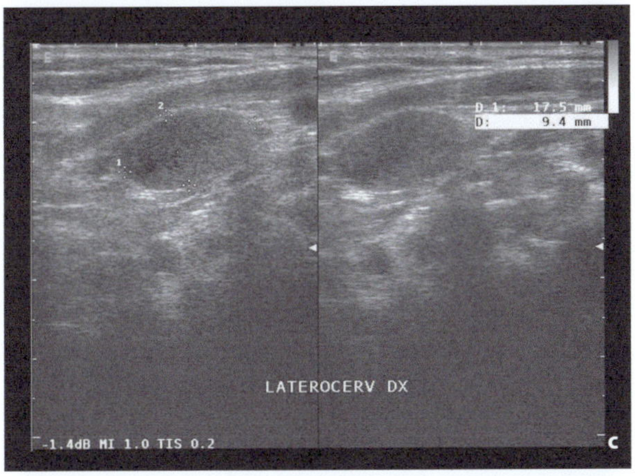

Fig. 3.43a-c Submandibular carcinoma with lymph node involvement associated with a parotid pleomorphic adenoma. Heterogeneous hypoechoic mass with central necrotic phenomena and capsular vascularity at directional PD in the submandibular site (**a**). Hypoechoic nodule with relatively homogeneous echotexture and well-defined margins of the homolateral parotid gland (**b**). Oval-shaped metastatic lymph node, but without central echogenic structure, situated in the upper neck (**c**)

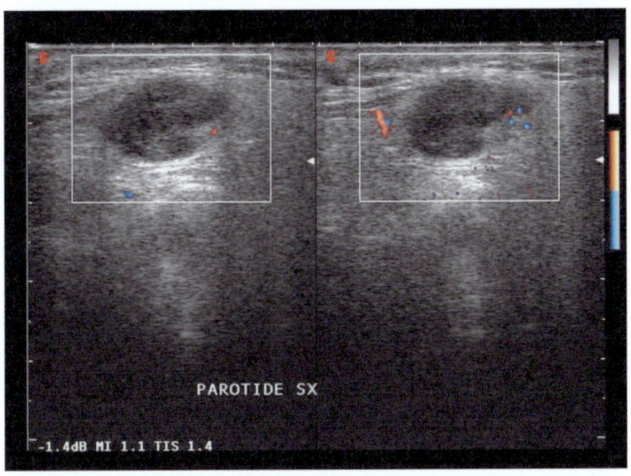

Fig. 3.44 Intraparotid metastatic lymph node from carcinoma of the face. Enlarged lymph node with echogenic residual eccentric hilum showing some vascular signals at directional PD

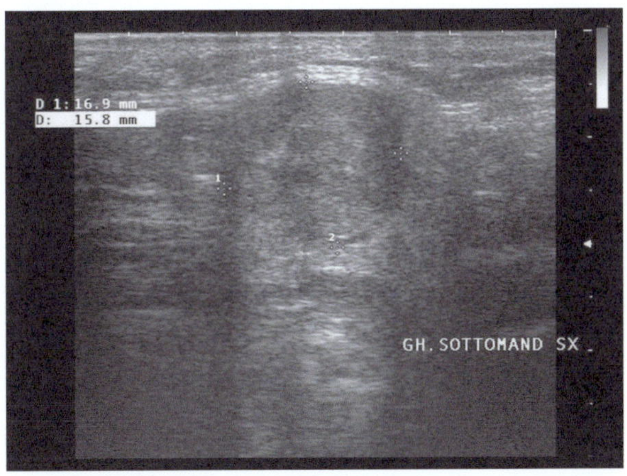

Fig. 3.45 Submandibular metastasis from lung cancer. US, performed subsequent to the finding of radiotracer uptake at PET, shows a heterogeneous hypoechoic lesion of the salivary gland

heterogeneous hypoechoic areas and more-or-less well-defined margins. Occasionally they may appear almost pseudocystic anechoic [16]. Other salivary gland tumors include lipomas, angiomas (typical in children), oncocytoma and metastases. The latter may be found in the intraglandular lymph nodes or directly in the salivary parenchyma (Figs. 3.44, 3.45).

In some cases, attributing an expansive lesion to a salivary gland may be challenging, both because the margins of these glands are often poorly defined, particularly in the elderly, and because salivary tumors are often exophytic. The problem of **differential diagnosis** therefore arises with adjacent lesions, such as those of nodal origin. Especially in the context of the parotid gland, small subcapsular or intraparenchymal lymph nodes are often present, which should not be confused with nodules and which can develop their own hyperplastic, inflammatory or neoplastic disease. The presence of multiple lesions within the salivary gland may be the expression of reactive or inflammatory lymph nodes, but also of tumors, especially adenolymphomas or, less frequently, acinar cell tumors or pleomorphic adenomas (particularly in the recurrent form).

3.3 Thyroid Nodules

Palpable **thyroid nodules** identified incidentally with imaging techniques, especially US, are a daily and almost "epidemic" problem. A palpable thyroid nodule is identified in 5% of individuals, particularly middle-aged and elderly women, and subcentimeter nodules are detected at US in up to 70% of normal thyroids, generally in a multinodular setting [10,20,21] (Figs. 3.46–3.52, Video 3.3). Developments in instrumentation, with the possibility of high-resolution and compound imaging, has increased the identification of small areas of structural heterogeneity in the thyroid, with the consequent problems of patient management (even though the term nodule should be reserved for focal lesions >6 mm) [22]. In a patient population with nonpalpable nodules between 8 mm and 15 mm in size, 9% of solitary nodules and 6% of nodules on multinodular goiter were malignant, with no particular correlation with the size of the lesion itself [23]. Nonetheless, thyroid carcinoma is rather infrequent, accounting for 0.5% of all cancer deaths. The probability that a solitary nodule in a euthyroid patient is malignant is 5–10%. Carcinomas account for <5% of thyroid nodules, whereas 15–20% consist of adenomas, and the remaining 75–85% are non-neoplastic nodules (hyperplastic or colloid-cystic) [21,24].

Thyroid tumors are predominant in women (F/M ratio 1.5–4:1) and include the more common forms with slow growth and the rarer highly aggressive forms. **Papillary carcinomas**, the incidence of which is increasing, account for around 60–80% of cases, with a peak in the 3rd and 4th decade of life. Although little aggressive and multicentric in 10–20% of cases, they do tend to spread early to the lymph nodes (this is the first sign of disease presentation in up to 15% of cases). Forms with a maximum diameter ≤10 mm are an increasing incidental finding and are defined as "microcarcinoma" [10]. **Follicular tumors** are included in this group because the distinction adenoma/carcinoma is generally only possible after surgery. However, follicular carcinoma accounts for only 10–25% of thyroid cancers and is found most of all in geographic areas of iodine deficiency, with age of onset >40 years (mean 50 years) and a greater tendency to distant hematogenous spread rather than lymph node involvement. **Medullary carcinoma** of the thyroid is relatively infrequent (5–10% of thyroid cancers, occasionally in the setting of type II MEN in which parathyroid nodules may also be evident adjacent to the thyroid nodules) and arises from parafollicular C cells. Peak incidence is in the 4th and 5th decade of life (even earlier in subjects with MEN) and there is no predominance in either sex. Lymph node metastases are found at the time of diagnosis in 50% of cases and distant metastases (lung, liver and bone)

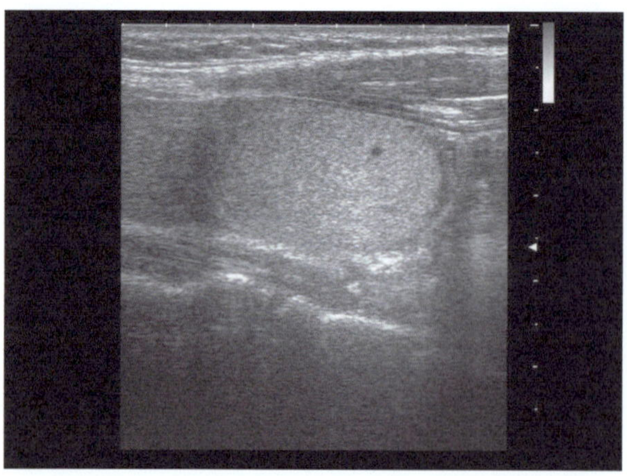

Fig. 3.46 Benign thyroid nodule. Large, oval, echogenic mass with relatively homogeneous echotexture

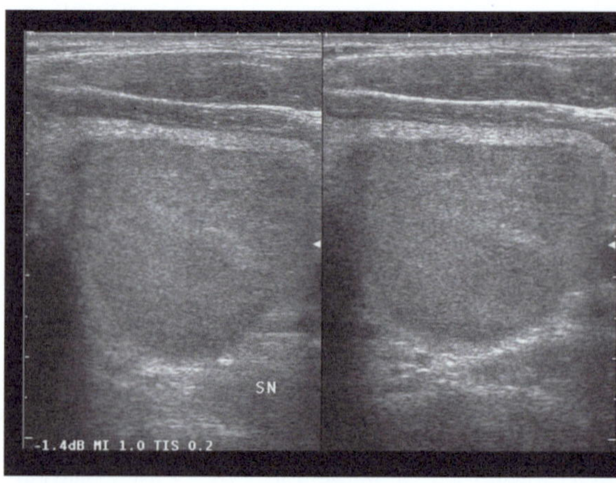

Fig. 3.47 Benign thyroid nodule. Large, oval, echogenic mass with relatively homogeneous echotexture

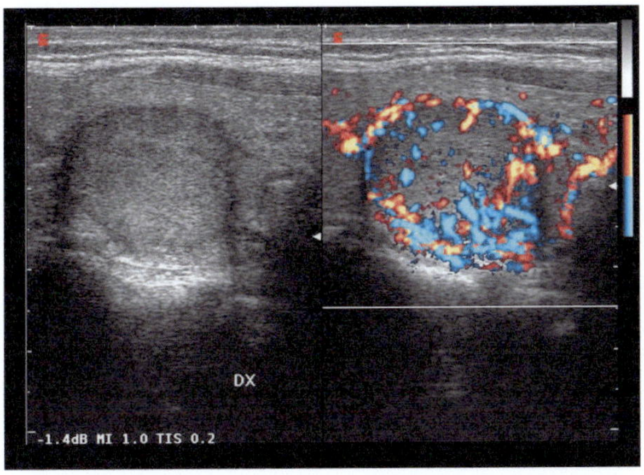

Fig. 3.48 Benign thyroid nodule. Large rounded hypoechoic mass with relatively homogeneous echotexture and moderate, prevalently peripheral and irregularly distributed vascular network at direction PD

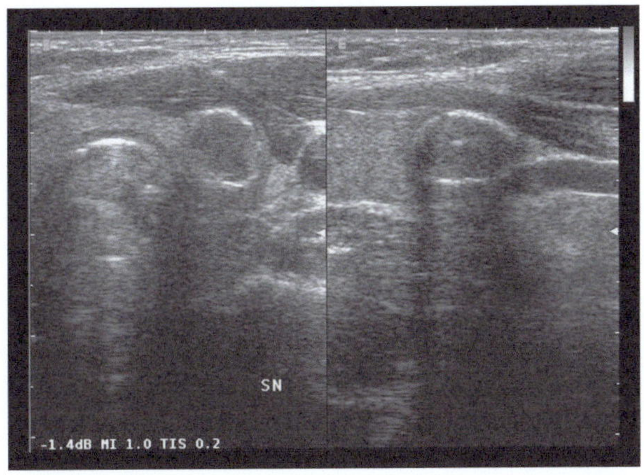

Fig. 3.49 Benign thyroid nodule. Mass with thick and regular calcified shell

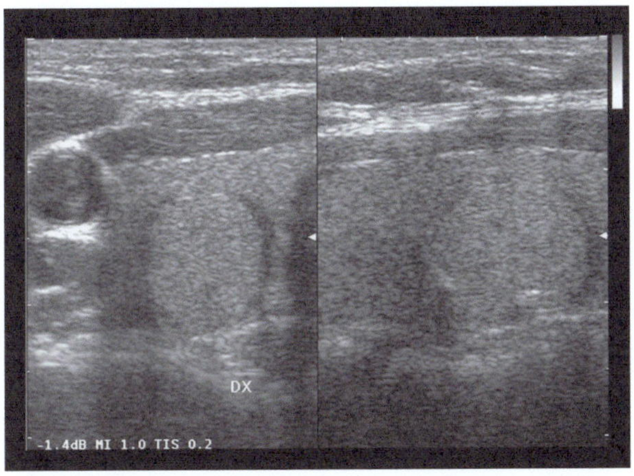

Fig. 3.50 Benign thyroid nodule. Large oval mass with heterogeneous hypoechoic appearance and a thin, uniform and hypoechoic peripheral halo "of safety"

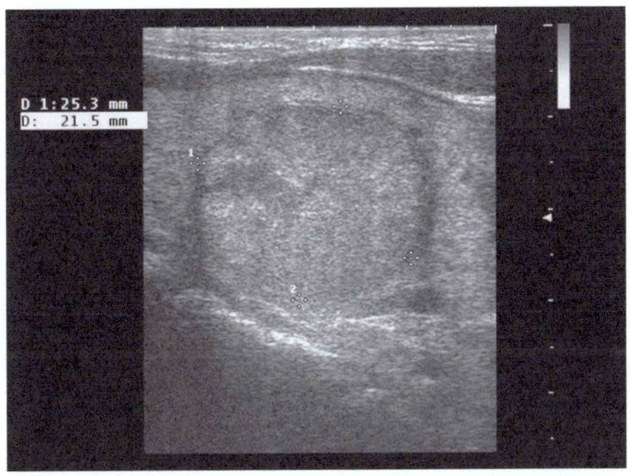

Fig. 3.51 Benign thyroid nodule. Large rounded mass with relatively homogeneous hypoechoic appearance and peripheral hypoechoic halo

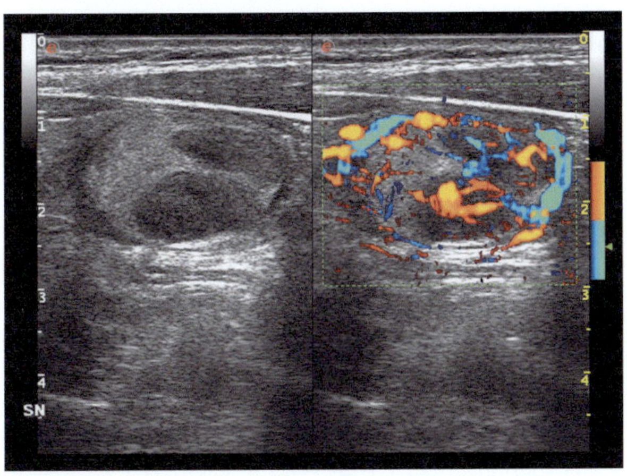

Fig. 3.52 Benign thyroid nodule, "nodule in a nodule" appearance. Hypovascular echogenic nodule can be seen with two internal hyperechoic hypervascular nodules

in 15–25%, and there is moderate tendency to neck or mediastinal recurrence. **Anaplastic carcinoma** is a particularly virulent lesion which accounts for 10–15% of thyroid tumors, with onset above 50 years of age.

The finding of a carcinoma can be incidental, during a US study for various reasons, or linked to the finding of a palpable mass or at any rate to symptoms of local growth or laterocervical lymph node spread, with compression/infiltration of adjacent structures such as the trachea, esophagus, lateral neck vessels or the recurrent laryngeal nerve. Occasionally there may be endocrine symptoms of a medullary carcinoma (diarrhea, electrolyte imbalance, flushing, etc.). Subjects with thyroid carcinoma are usually euthyroid, and therefore with normal laboratory findings. In fact a hyperfunctioning nodule with TSH suppression is rare, although there are carcinomas capable of producing sufficient hormones to cause hyperthyroidism. Antithyroglobulin antibodies may be increased. Medullary carcinoma may give rise to hypercalcemia and increased serum levels of calcitonin. At scintigraphy these nodules are generally "cold" to the scan with Tc^{99m}.

US is the first and fundamental imaging modality in the study of the patient with a thyroid nodule, especially with normal or increased TSH. In the subject with a palpable nodule and serum TSH levels below the norm, the initial approach is instead scintigraphy, in order to identify the hyperfunctioning, "hot" nodules [11]. In addition to detecting and characterizing lesions, US is also important in preoperative planning, being able to provide an early demonstration of local invasion and lymph node involvement. This is particularly important since not all subjects are treated with radical thyroidectomy, and in the event of a perfectly homogeneous contralateral lobe, a lobar resection may be feasible. Clearly, US also has a role to play in the identification of locoregional recurrence.

Characterization of the nodule is important. While it is true that **FNAC** plays a central role in this sense, in general being indicated in all new non-palpable nodules >10 mm, it is also true that unlike scintigraphy US can suggest a probable benignity or malignancy of the nodule and therefore influence patient management. In the presence of multiple nodules US can suggest which should be aspirated – this is not necessarily the largest nodule but can be the nodule with the most suspicious US structural and vascular characteristics – and may also be used to guide the biopsy needle to the most anomalous or vascular area of a nodule. FNAC has a sensitivity of 65–98% and a specificity of 72–100% in the diagnosis of malignancy [11]. The percentage of FNAC with insufficient or nondiagnostic material is around 20%, and in such cases the biopsy tends to be repeated. Masses with significant cystic components have a high probability of being negative at the first FNAC and therefore as a routine require a repeat procedure. Centrifugation of the aspirated liquid is also important [25]. Serial controls are also crucial, because in the event of a nodule with prior negative FNAC for malignant cells but with a suspicious appearance, such as a progressive increase in size, repetition of the FNAC may be indicated (even though many benign nodules display significant growth over time, even >15% in 5 years) [26].

The **suspicion of malignancy** increases in the presence of male sex, age <20 years or >70 years, family history, prior breast cancer, neck irradiation in infancy, monofocal lesion, rapid growth, presence of enlarged lymph nodes and a "cold" appearance at scintigraphy. The solitary nodule is often more suspicious for malignancy than the nodule encountered in a multinodular setting, especially among males. However, some 10–20% of papillary carcinomas can be multicentric, and therefore each nodule in the context of multinodular thyroid disease needs to be carefully evaluated. In fact there is the risk of underestimating the finding simply because it appears in a multinodular setting. The size of nodules is not a criterion of the differential diagnosis [10]. In terms of echostructure there are a number of elements suggestive of possible malignancy, although the individual weight of each is rather limited, particularly for subcentimeter lesions. At least one sign potentially indicative of malignancy is revealed in 69% of benign lesions and only the combined presence of multiple signs can indicate malignancy, although to the detriment of sensitivity [24,27–29]. Thyroid carcinomas are more often hypoechoic: the incidence of malignancy is 26% in cases of hypoechogenicity and 4% in cases of hyperechogenicity. In addition, the hypoechoic appearance has a low specificity (49–83%) and a low positive predictive value (40%). The arrangement of malignant thyroid nodules tends to be more longitudinal with respect to benign nodules, in practice following the long axis of the thyroid lobes ("taller than wide"). The nodular margins tend to be ill-defined. The perinodular hypoechoic halo, due to the capsule, the compressed parenchyma and/or perinodular vessels, is identified mostly in benign nodules. Its absence has a sensitivity of 56–67% and a specificity of 77–80% for malignancy, and especially in papillary carcinomas <10% show a partial or complete halo [20,24]. Nodules with a significant fluid component are generally benign (cystic or hemorrhagic degeneration) and the finding of punctate foci with posterior shadowing within the fluid (comet tail sign) indicates the colloidal nature and therefore benignity. Nonetheless there are some carcinomas, especially papillary carcinomas, which can have cystic components (other indicative signs will be present such as punctate calcifications in the solid parts) [21]. Whereas large calcifications with acoustic shadowing, especially if peripheral or with a "shell-like" appearance, are indicative of benignity, small punctate calcifications, especially if lacking an acoustic shadow, are found relatively frequently in malignant lesions (up to 29% of nonpalpable carcinomas <15 mm) and especially in papillary carcinomas (25–42% of cases). Microcalcifications (calcified psammomatous bodies) have a specificity of 93% and a positive predictive value of 70% for the diagnosis of malignancy (but with a sensitivity as low as 36–59%) [20,23,30]. In a multicenter retrospective study, statistically significant findings of malignancy were a taller-than-wide shape (sensitivity 48%, specificity 91%), a spiculated margin (sensitivity 48%, specificity 92%), marked hypoechogenicity (sensitivity 41%, specificity 92%), microcalcification (sensitivity 44%, specificity 91%), and macrocalcification (sensitivity 10%, specificity 96%). The US findings for benign nodules were isoechogenicity (sensitivity 57%, specificity 88%) and spongiform appearance (sensitivity 10%, specificity 100%) [31].

In the presence of a hypoechoic nodule with ill-defined margins, microcalcifications and a hypervascular appearance at CD, FNAC is indicated even in subcentimeter lesions [23,27]. In the absence of these indicators of risk, clinical monitoring alone may be a feasible proposition, while bearing in mind the risk of not recognizing follicular carcinomas, which occasionally can have a benign US appearance. The elements most suggestive of the benignity of a thyroid nodule are marked prevalence of a fluid content, hyperechoic appearance, the presence of "shell-like" calcifications, and avascularity, although some exceptions are possible [1]. At **CD**, malignant nodules often appear more hypervascular in relation to the adjacent parenchyma than benign lesions, which particularly produces good positive predictability. Hypovascularity, on the other hand, does not exclude malignancy. A classic division of lesion flow is as follows: type I, absence of demonstrable color signal; type II, marginal signals (peripheral intranodular and/or perinodular); type III, presence of patently intranodular flows, either isolated (IIIa) or associated with marginal flows (IIIb); type IV, multiple vascular poles with irregularly distributed diffuse intranodular flows. This classification has lost some of its validity, even though a type I pattern, which has become rather rare given the sensitivity of the current instrumentation, or even a type II pattern is suggestive of benignity [32,33]. Evaluating the distribution of these vessels can be important, whether perinodular (color halo sign), peripheral intranodular or also central intranodular. Some 22% of papillary carcinomas present a prevalently perinodular flow, whereas 69% of cases are hypervascular [20]. A classification of nodular distribution patterns includes three types: A (ring sign) with perinodular ring, identifiable especially in benign lesions; B (complex ring sign) characterized by peri- and intranodular vessels which may be very fine and regularly distributed in hyperplastic forms or numerous, large and irregular in adenomas and carcinomas; C (delta sign) with peri- and intranodular circulation supplied by a single arterial vessel, which is relatively infrequent but rather specific for carcinoma [34]. In small nodules a quantitative analysis of vascularity may have benefits over visual inspection of PD patterns and help differentiating malignant from benign lesions [35]. The wash-in and wash-out curves after contrast medium injection seem to be different in hyperplastic, adenomatous and carcinomatous lesions. The latter display a rapid time to peak intensity and a slow and gradual wash-out phase [36]. Preliminary data with CEUS show an overlap between the behavior of different types of lesions, with a diffuse, homogeneous or heterogeneous nodular enhancement in benign nodules and a diffuse, faint dotted or absent enhancement in malignant lesions [37].

With regard to the morphostructural characteristics of the different tumor histotypes, **papillary carcinoma** is generally solid (70% of cases), hypoechoic (77–90% of cases), with irregular margins, punctate calcifications (25–90% of cases), intense and chaotic internal vascularity (69% of cases) and cervical lymphadenopathies. In addition, the atypical forms are not rare, have a patently cystic appearance (6%, but still with vascular signals in the moderate solid components), large or peripheral calcifications, regular margins (47%) and hypovascularity (never avascularity) [20,21] (Figs. 3.53–3.60, Video 3.4). The **follicular form** displays a hypoechoic echostructure but also iso- or hyperechoic, often with a homogeneous echotexture (70% of cases) and a well-visualized peripheral halo (80%of cases). Follicular carcinomas tend to be more vascular than adenomas, with generally peripheral flows in the benign forms and diffuse flows in the malignant lesions, and a cut-off for malignancy of PI >1.35, RI >0.78 and V_{max}/V_{min} ratio >0.89 [38,39] (Fig. 3.61). Moreover, the CD appearance can be misleading in follicular carcinoma as well, displaying a limited and prevalently perilesional or peripheral intralesional vascular network. Due to the often "benign" US appearance of these lesions, the correct preoperative diagnosis is often difficult

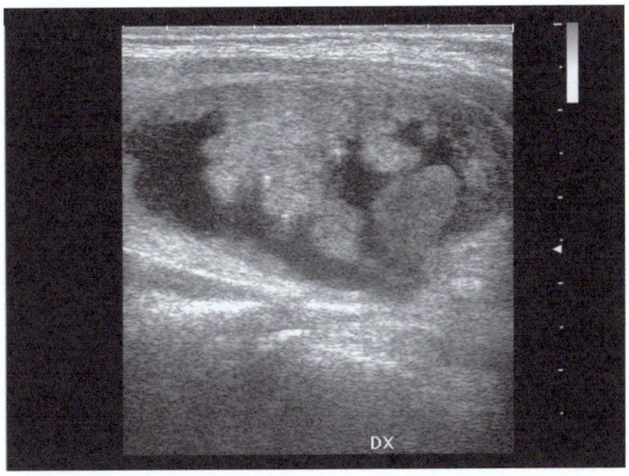

Fig. 3.53 Papillary carcinoma of the thyroid. Partially cystic mass with large internal solid projections and some small calcified nuclei

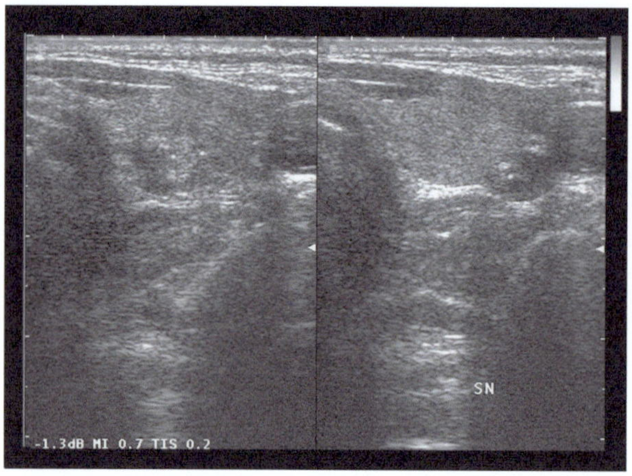

Fig. 3.54 Bifocal papillary carcinoma of the thyroid. Two small heterogeneous hypoechoic nodules with ill-defined margins and several microcalcifications

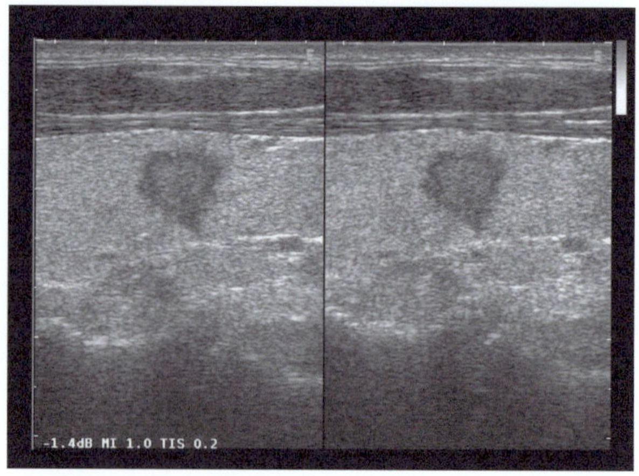

Fig. 3.55 Papillary carcinoma of the thyroid. Hypoechoic nodule, especially in the periphery, and relatively well defined

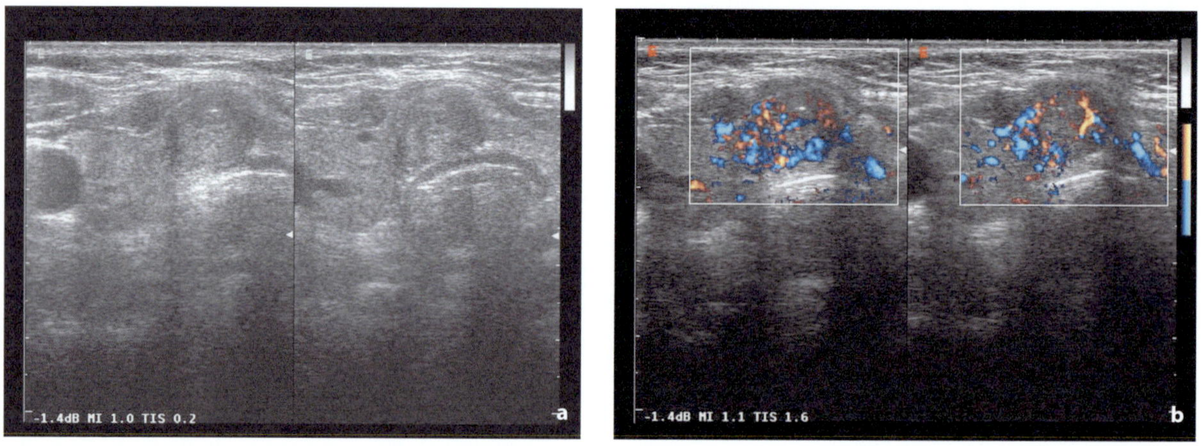

Fig. 3.56a,b Papillary carcinoma of the thyroid. Heterogeneous hypoechoic nodule with ill-defined margins and several microcalcifications (**a**). Moderate and irregular vascularity at directional PD (**b**)

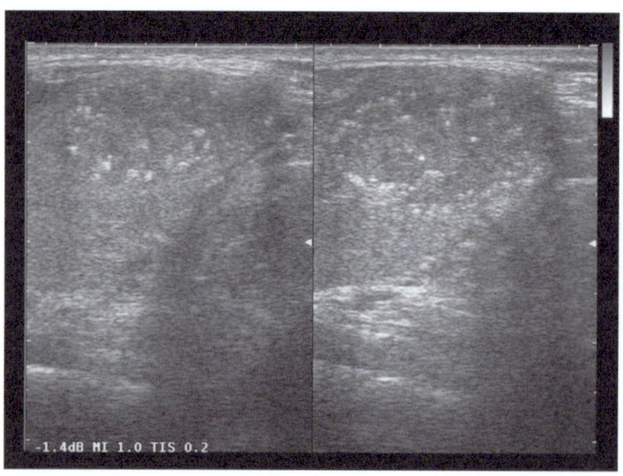

Fig. 3.57 Papillary carcinoma of the thyroid. Heterogeneous and mildly hypoechoic nodule with multiple microcalcifications

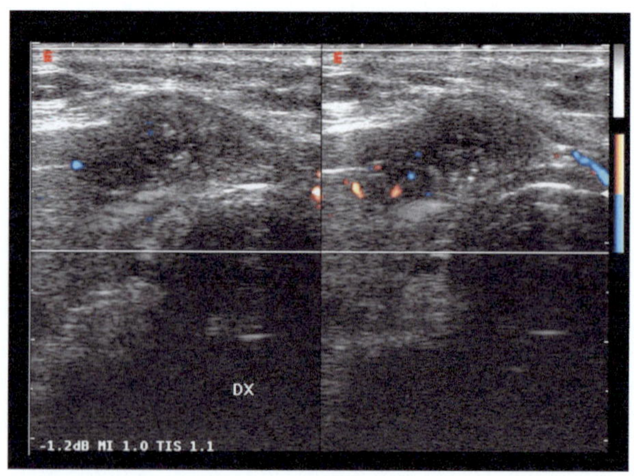

Fig. 3.58 Papillary carcinoma of the thyroid. Heterogeneous hypoechoic nodule with ill-defined margins and several microcalcifications. Poor vascularity at directional PD

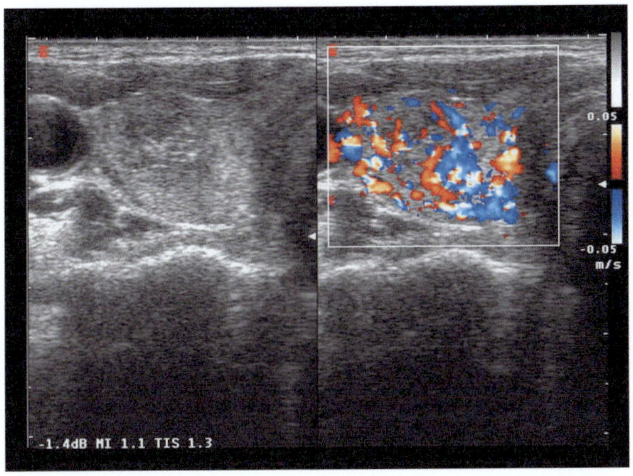

Fig. 3.59 Papillary carcinoma of the thyroid. Heterogeneous hypoechoic nodule with very poorly defined margins and moderate vascularity at CD although hypovascular in relation to the glandular tissue

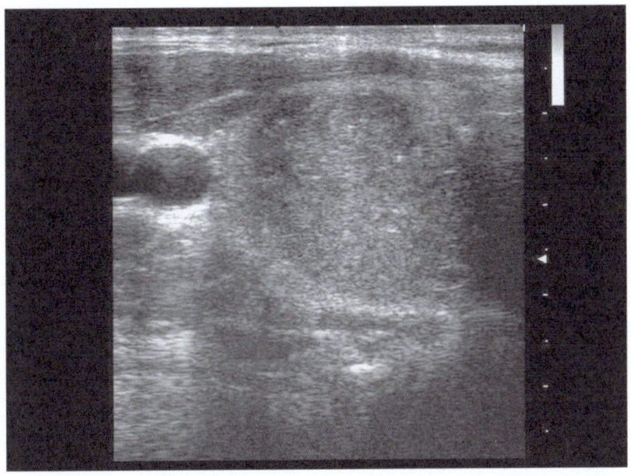

Fig. 3.60 Papillary carcinoma of the thyroid. Large heterogeneous hypoechoic nodule

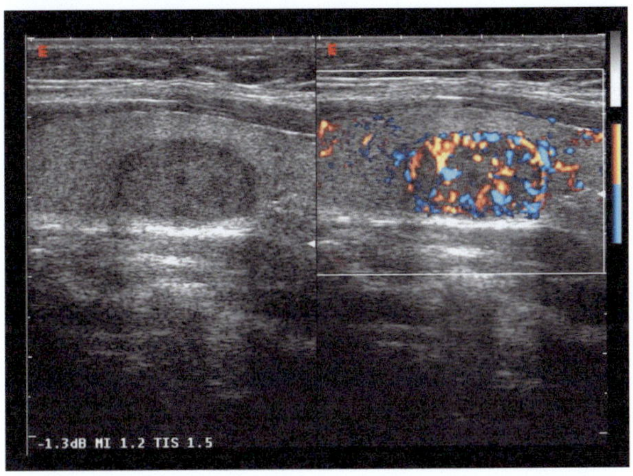

Fig. 3.61 Follicular carcinoma of the thyroid. Hypoechoic nodule with relatively homogeneous echotexture and well-defined margins as well as marked hypervascularity at directional PD with both peripheral and central vessels

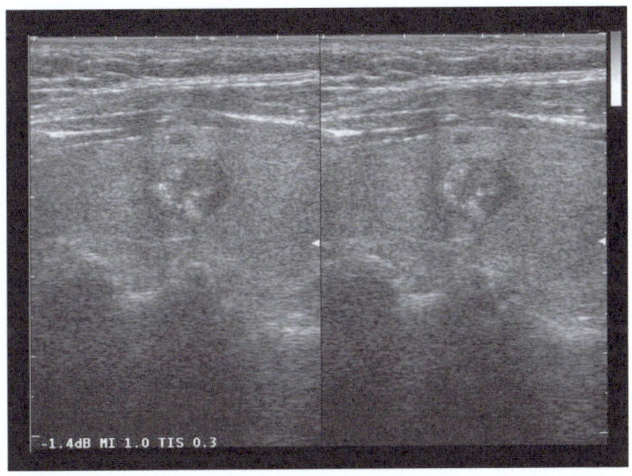

Fig. 3.62 Medullary carcinoma of the thyroid. Heterogeneous hypoechoic nodule with microcalcifications

(sensitivity of 18% against the 86.5% of nonfollicular forms, and specificity of 89% against the 92% of nonfollicular forms) [40]. The nodules of **medullary carcinoma** are generally solid, hypoechoic, with echogenic foci in 80–90% of cases (calcified amyloid deposits) and evident and irregularly distributed vessels [10] (Figs. 3.62–3.65). **Anaplastic carcinoma** often manifests as rapidly growing nodules which may develop to the point of occupying an entire lobe. Its appearance is poorly defined, hypoechoic with heterogeneous echotexture due to necrotic areas (78% of cases), hypervascular with numerous small internal vessels but also hypo-avascular areas. Signs of extrathyroid spread may be present with enlarged and

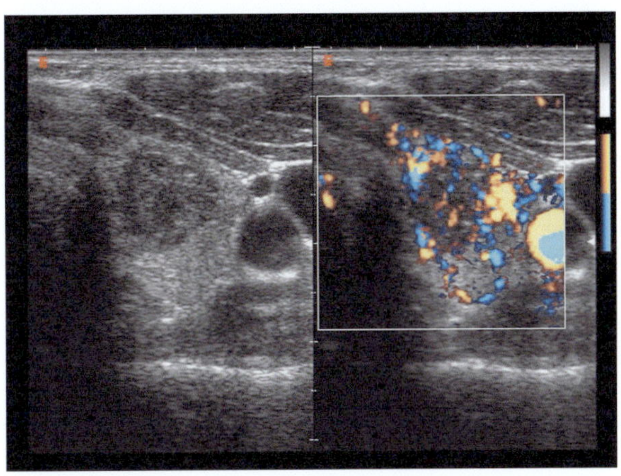

Fig. 3.63 Medullary carcinoma of the thyroid. Heterogeneous hypoechoic nodule with moderate vascularity at directional PD but still hypovascular in relation to the glandular tissue

often necrotic cervical lymph nodes (50% of cases) [10,21] (Figs. 3.66–3.68).

Primary **thyroid lymphomas** (1–10% of thyroid tumors) are generally non-Hodgkin's type (usually B-cell lymphomas), which often arise in the presence of an underlying chronic thyroiditis. The typical appearance is hypoechoic with echogenic bands. It should be noted that in Hashimoto thyroiditis the nodular areas, or more correctly the pseudonodular areas, are not rare, although they are mostly of the homogeneous hyperechoic type (Fig. 3.69). Thyroid lymphomas, on the other hand, manifest as hypoechoic heterogeneous or patently pseudocystic nodules with well-defined margins and associated with cervical lymphadenopathies [41]. There are also diffuse forms, with extraglandular spread and vascular invasion. FNAC or core biopsy usually make an adequate diagnosis possible [42].

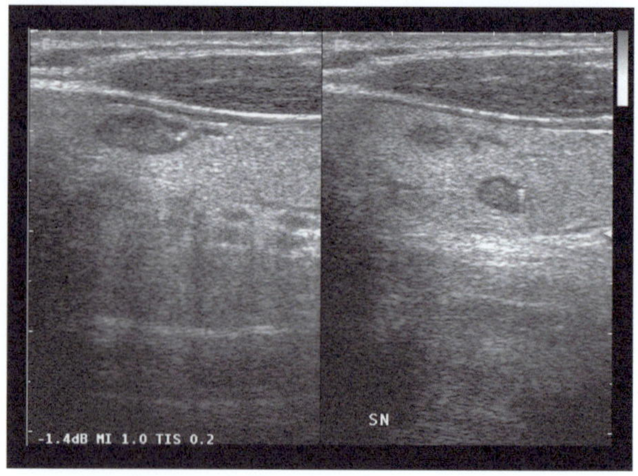

Fig. 3.64 Bifocal medullary carcinoma of the thyroid. Two small heterogeneous hypoechoic nodules with some microcalcifications

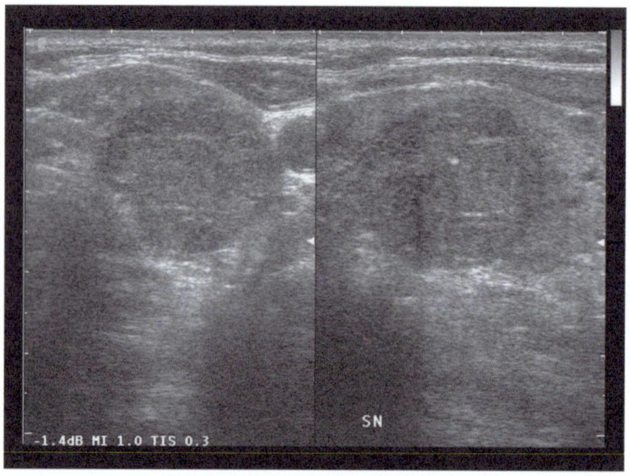

Fig. 3.65 Medullary carcinoma of the thyroid. Large heterogeneous hypoechoic nodule with some microcalcifications

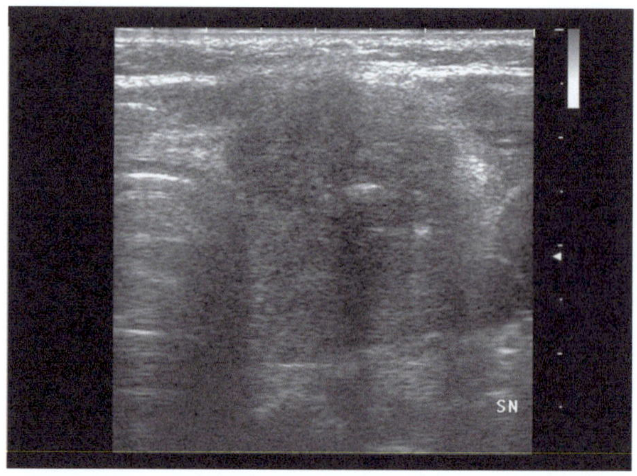

Fig. 3.66 Anaplastic carcinoma of the thyroid. Large, heterogeneous, hypoechoic and invasive nodule

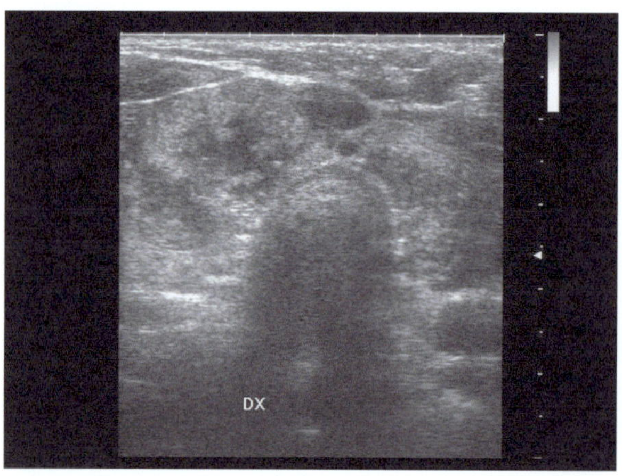

Fig. 3.67 Anaplastic carcinoma of the thyroid. Diffuse remodeling, almost thyroiditis-like, of the gland with scattered hypoechoic areas and some microcalcifications

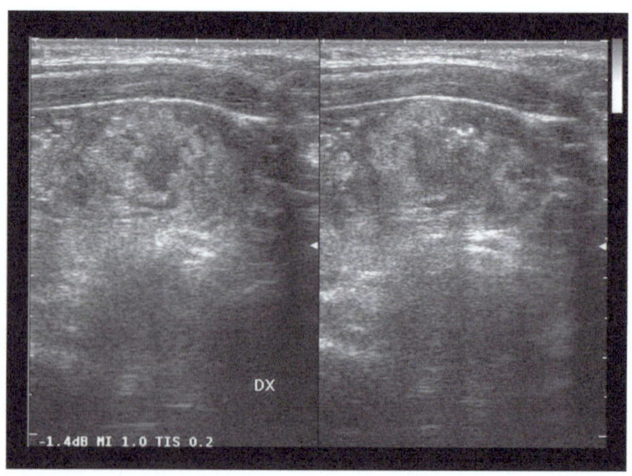

Fig. 3.68 Anaplastic carcinoma of the thyroid. Diffuse remodeling of the gland with ill-defined hypoechoic areas and multiple microcalcifications

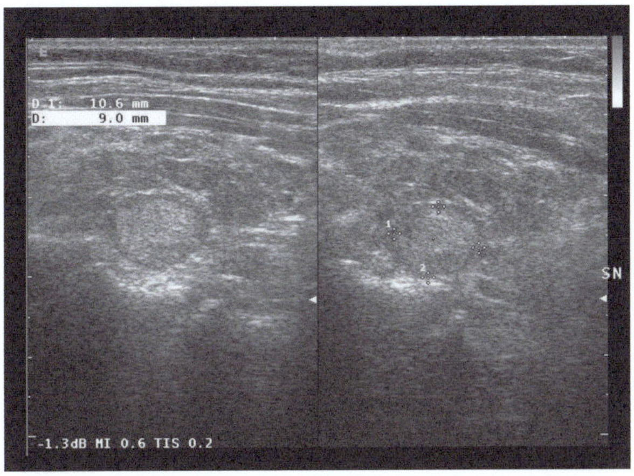

Fig. 3.69 Echogenic nodule with underlying chronic Hashimoto thyroiditis. Hyperechoic mass with relatively homogeneous echotexture and well-defined margins on a background of thyroiditis with hypoechoic areas of lymphocyte infiltration and hyperechoic bands

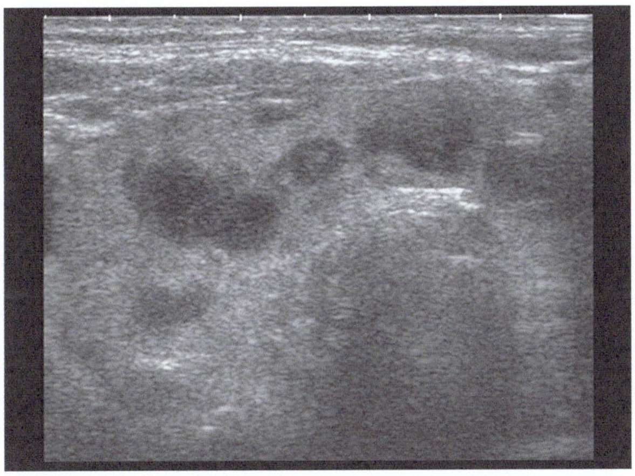

Fig. 3.70 Thyroid metastasis from melanoma. Multiple markedly hypoechoic heterogeneous nodules with ill-defined margins

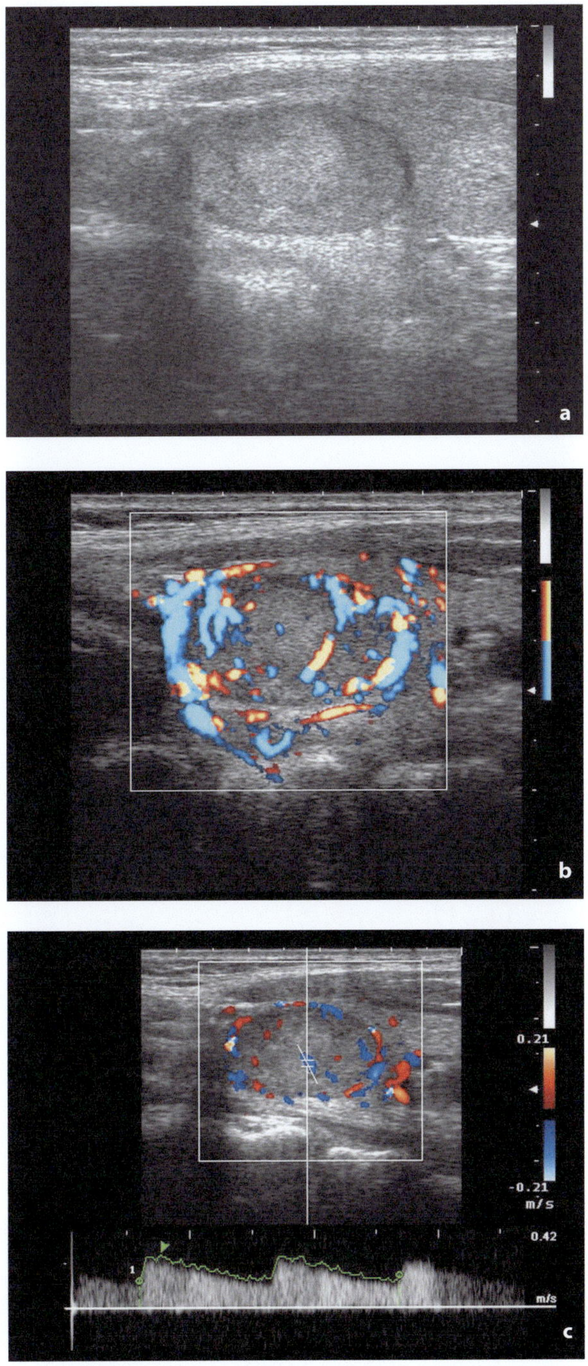

Fig. 3.71a–c Follicular adenoma of the thyroid. Mildly heterogeneous isoechoic nodule with a peripheral hypoechoic halo (**a**) and moderate vascularity especially in the periphery at directional PD (**b**). Spectral Doppler identifies low-velocity and low-resistance flow (**c**)

Thyroid metastases (2–17% of patients with a known primary tumor, 1–2 % of thyroid tumors) are generally hematogenous and associated with melanomas and breast, lung, kidney and colon cancers. Contiguity spread is rare [21]. They generally manifest as homogeneous hypoechoic lesions with well-defined margins, although they can be multiple and heterogeneous as well as profoundly altering the thyroid parenchyma [43] (Fig. 3.70).

Adenomas (follicular and nonfollicular) have US morphologic and vascular characteristics that cannot be individually separated from malignant lesions. In particular, toxic adenoma (Plummer's disease) may appear rather vascular at CD, with mean velocity around 70 cm/s and therefore higher than normal thyroid tissue or malignant tissue. Differentiation is performed with FNAC and, above all, scintigraphy ("hot" nodule) (Figs. 3.71, 3.72).

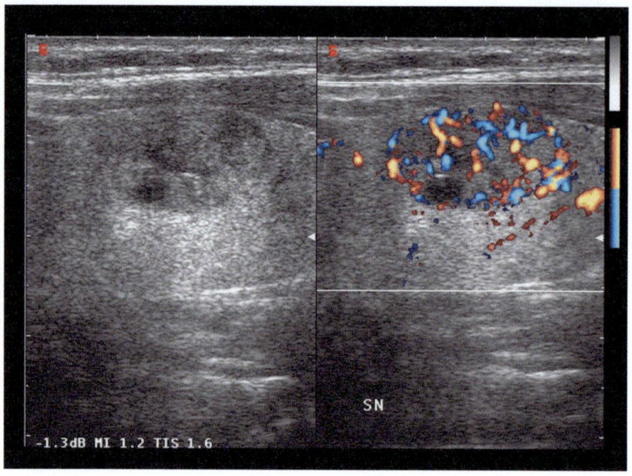

Fig. 3.72 Benign thyroid nodule appearing "hot" at scintigraphy. Oval slightly hypoechoic and relatively homogeneous (small colloidal area) lesion with moderate vascularity in the periphery but not centrally at directional PD

3.4 Staging and Follow-up of Thyroid Cancer

One of the tasks of US in the study of thyroid nodules is to provide information for tumor staging (Figs. 3.73, 3.74). This involves searching for irregularities in the thyroid profile at the level of the nodule in question and clear signs of extrathyroid spread. **Extracapsular growth** should be sought, bearing in mind that such growth not only involves the presence of lesions of a certain size, but also includes subcentimeter carcinomas [23]. Signs of invasion of the adjacent structures such as prethyroid muscles should be investigated. Involvement of the vascular bundle of the neck, and especially the venous structures, occurs in advanced forms, and a thorough search should be done for the purposes of treatment planning [44]. US is able to reveal adhesion to the vessel walls and thrombotic luminal obliteration, or in the case of a vein its nonvisualization for a certain tract associated with the

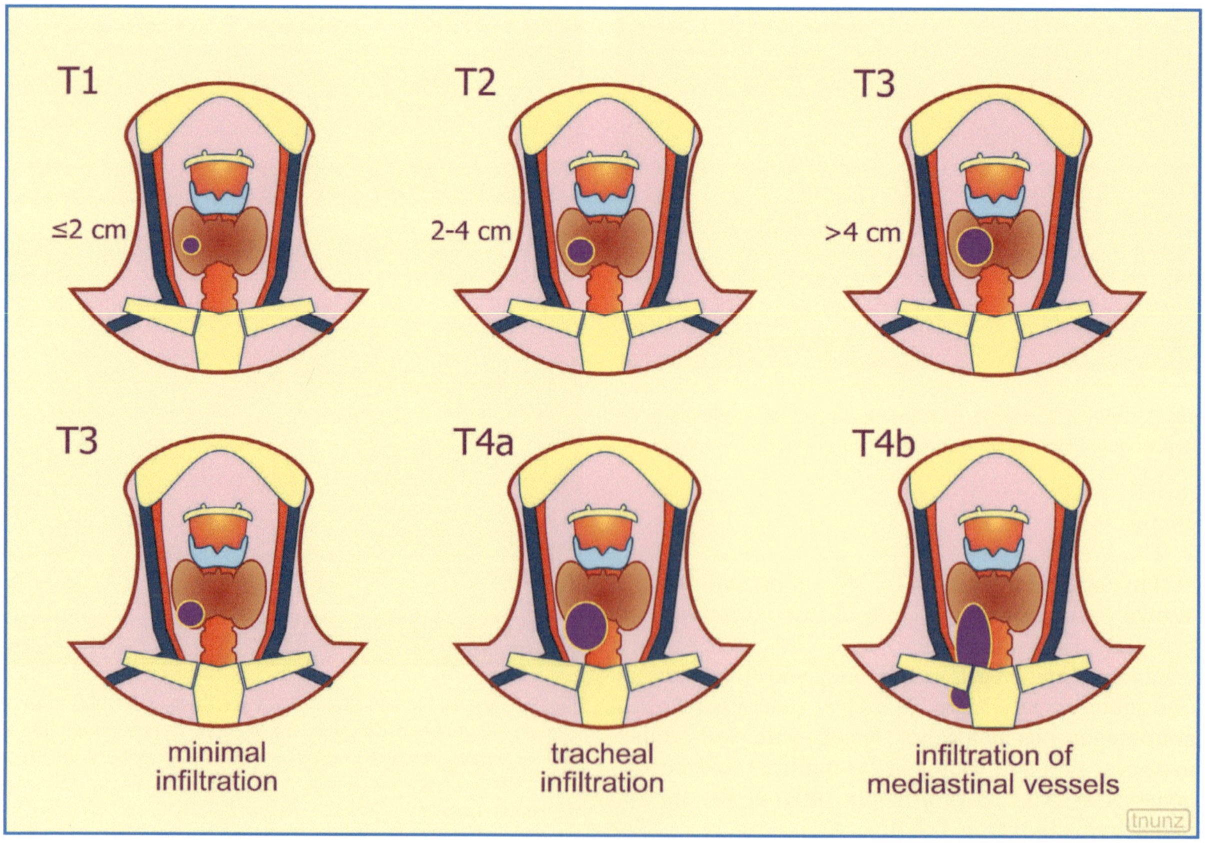

Fig. 3.73 Staging of differentiated thyroid cancers. *T1*, tumor ≤2 cm and confined to the gland; *T2*, tumor 2–4 cm confined to the gland; *T3*, tumor >4 cm confined to the gland, or tumor of any size with initial extraglandular spread (e.g. invasion of prethyroid soft tissues or sternocleidomastoid muscle); *T4a*, tumor of any size with invasion of the subcutaneous tissue, larynx, trachea, esophagus or inferior laryngeal nerve; *T4b*, tumor of any size with invasion of the prevertebral fascia, carotid or mediastinal vessels. Anaplastic carcinoma is classified separately and is by definition a *T4* tumor. Modified from [2]

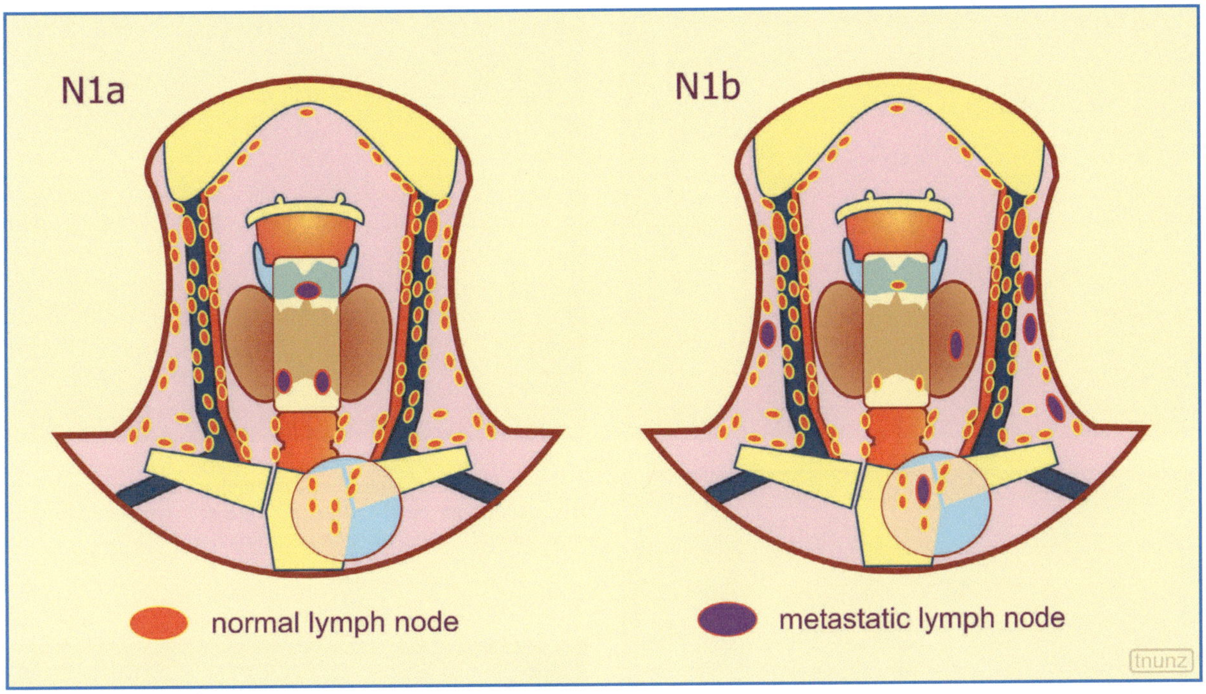

Fig. 3.74 N parameter for thyroid cancer. Regional lymph nodes include the cervical lymph nodes and the superior mediastinal lymph nodes. *N1a* includes metastases to the VI level lymph nodes (pretracheal and paratracheal, including the prelaryngeal), whereas *N1b* relates to metastases to the other cervical lymph nodes (whether ipsi- or contralateral) and upper mediastinal lymph nodes. Modified from [2]

presence of multiple collateral vessels. EUS is able to evaluate esophageal invasion. In a study on the staging of papillary carcinoma, US proved to be superior to MR in identifying the primary tumor, even in multifocal forms, and inferior in recognizing extracapsular diffusion and tracheal or esophageal invasion. The two techniques are comparable in identifying lymphadenopathies, with difficulty mainly in the central location. The study concluded by emphasizing the utility of US as a first-choice modality and the need for MR integration in cases where the carcinoma is not completely surrounded by normal thyroid tissue [45].

The study of the **lymph nodes** of the neck is an integral part of any thyroid examination, especially when suspicious nodules are identified. It is not uncommon for cervical lymphadenopathies, even significantly enlarged lymph nodes, to be revealed in subjects with mild thyroid alterations. In a patient population with nonpalpable lesions, there was no difference in the incidence of lymph node metastases between cases with a thyroid nodule <10 mm and those with a nodule 10–15 mm [23]. Occasionally it is in fact the identification of enlarged cervical lymph nodes, especially with the morphostructural characteristics described below, that prompts a more thorough investigation of the thyroid and a re-evaluation of an initially underestimated nodule or repetition of an initially negative thyroid FNAC.

Lymph node metastases from thyroid cancer are often difficult to identify with palpation, especially if small or situated deep to the sternocleidomastoid muscle, the jugular vein or the carotid artery [46]. During US study, the finding of lymph node metastases is a relatively common occurrence in subjects with thyroid cancer (15–20% of cases), especially in the event of papillary or medullary carcinomas. In general, the most important criteria for differentiation between benign and malignant lymph nodes are size of the lymph node (transverse diameter >7 mm for lymph nodes of the superior internal jugular chain – level II – and >6 mm for the others), rounded shape (in 80% of metastases from papillary carcinoma but also in 29.5% of normal lymph nodes), absence of an echogenic hilum, presence of cystic-like areas (infrequent but highly specific), overall nodal echogenicity greater than that of the regional muscles (at least in papillary carcinoma) and the presence of calcifications (infrequent but highly specific) [46,47]. Metastatic lymph nodes often appear hypervascular at **CD**, with multiple vascular branches and peripheral entry and the presence of heterogeneous spectra for peak velocity and RI. A bilateral manifestation should be cause for suspicion. Even the site of the lymph node is important, because most metastatic lymph nodes (67%) are found in the lower third of the neck, whereas 20% are found

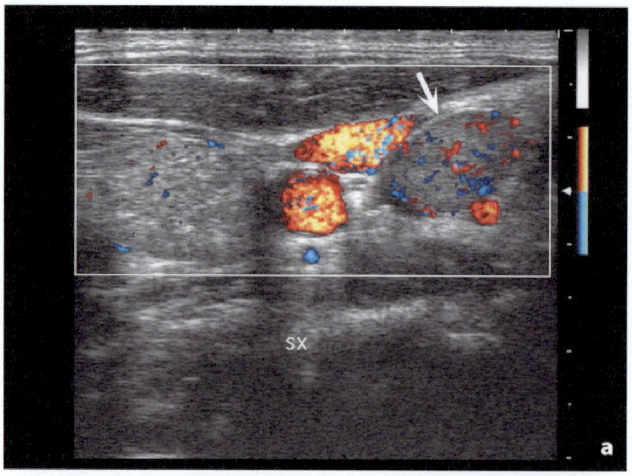

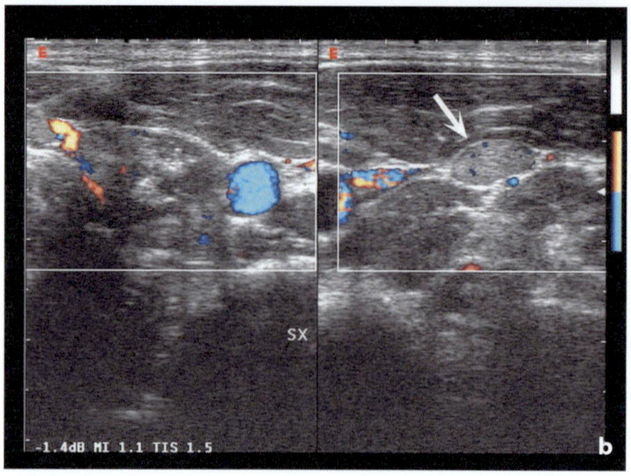

Fig. 3.75a,b Papillary carcinoma of the thyroid with lymph node metastases. Remodeling of the left lobe of the thyroid with amorphous calcifications, associated with two relatively homogeneous oval lymphadenopathies (*arrows*). Poor vascularity of both the tumor and the lymph nodes at directional PD

in the middle third and only 13% in the upper third, while reactive lymph nodes are distributed in the opposite manner [46]. There is in fact an overlap in the imaging characteristics between metastatic lymph nodes and reactive lymph nodes, but at least US has proven to be effective in selecting the suspicious lymph nodes to undergo FNAC, which has proven very useful for their definitive characterization [46]. In cases of papillary carcinoma, the diseased lymph nodes are mostly found in the pretracheal, paratracheal and laterocervical sites and display internal cystic-necrotic phenomena in 25% of cases and punctate calcifications in 50%. The appearance therefore becomes very similar to that of the primary tumor. Internal calcifications are also frequently found (50–60% of cases) in medullary carcinoma as well, whereas necrotic phenomena are common (50% of cases) in anaplastic carcinoma (Figs. 3.75–3.84).

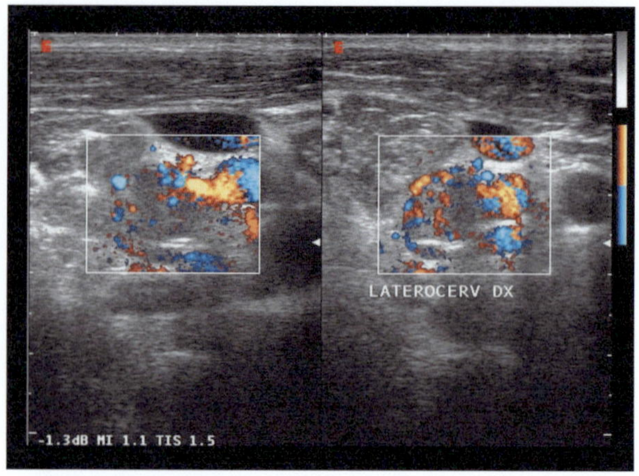

Fig. 3.76 Metastatic laterocervical lymphadenopathy from papillary carcinoma of the thyroid. Enlarged lymph node with capsular and central vascularity at directional PD

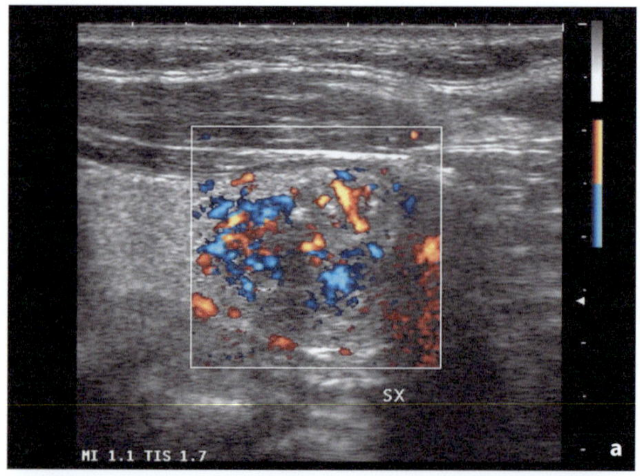

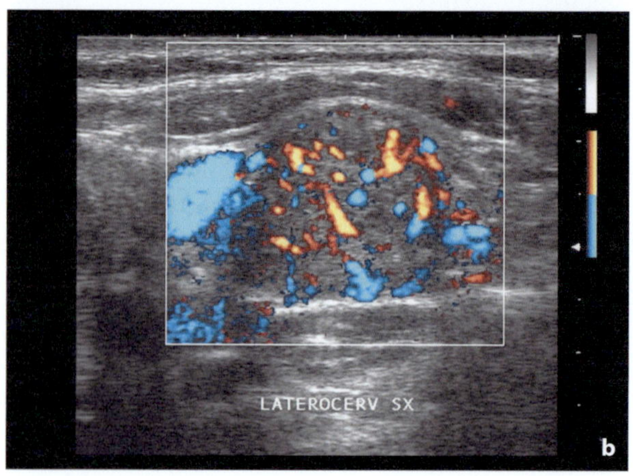

Fig. 3.77a,b Papillary carcinoma of the thyroid with lymph node metastasis. Heterogeneous hypoechoic mass, with amorphous calcifications and moderate, irregular vascularity at directional PD in the left thyroid lobe (**a**). Large adenopathy with US structure and vascularity very similar to the tumor (**b**)

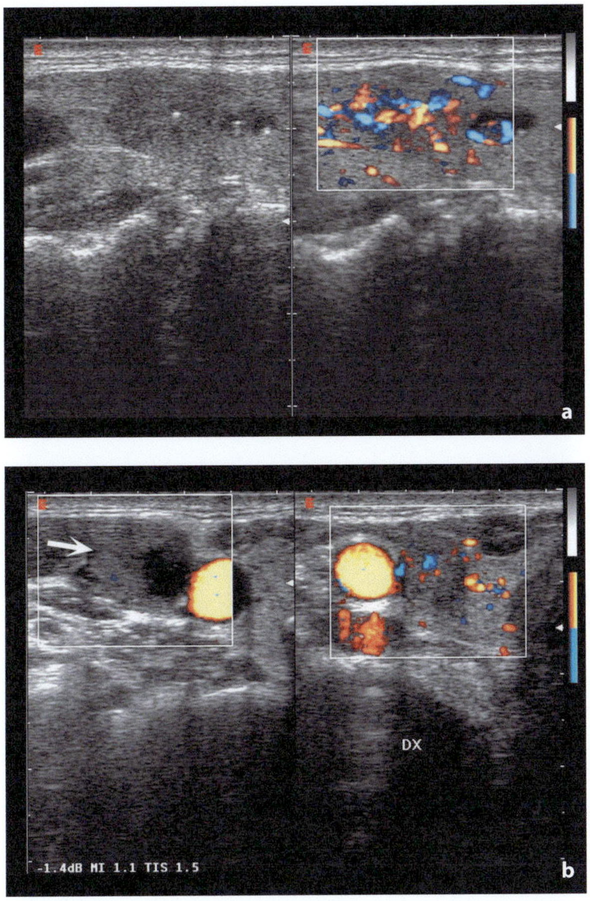

Fig. 3.78a,b Papillary carcinoma of the thyroid with lymph node metastasis. Heterogeneous, hypo-anechoic, multinodular mass with several amorphous calcifications and moderate vascularity (**a**). Relatively homogeneous, hypoechoic and hypovascular adenopathy (**b**, *arrow*)

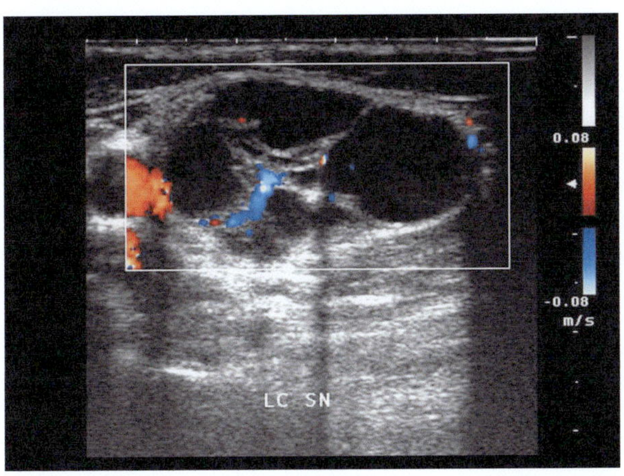

Fig. 3.79 Lymph node metastasis from papillary carcinoma of the thyroid. Large formation with cystic multilocular appearance and septal vascular signals at CD

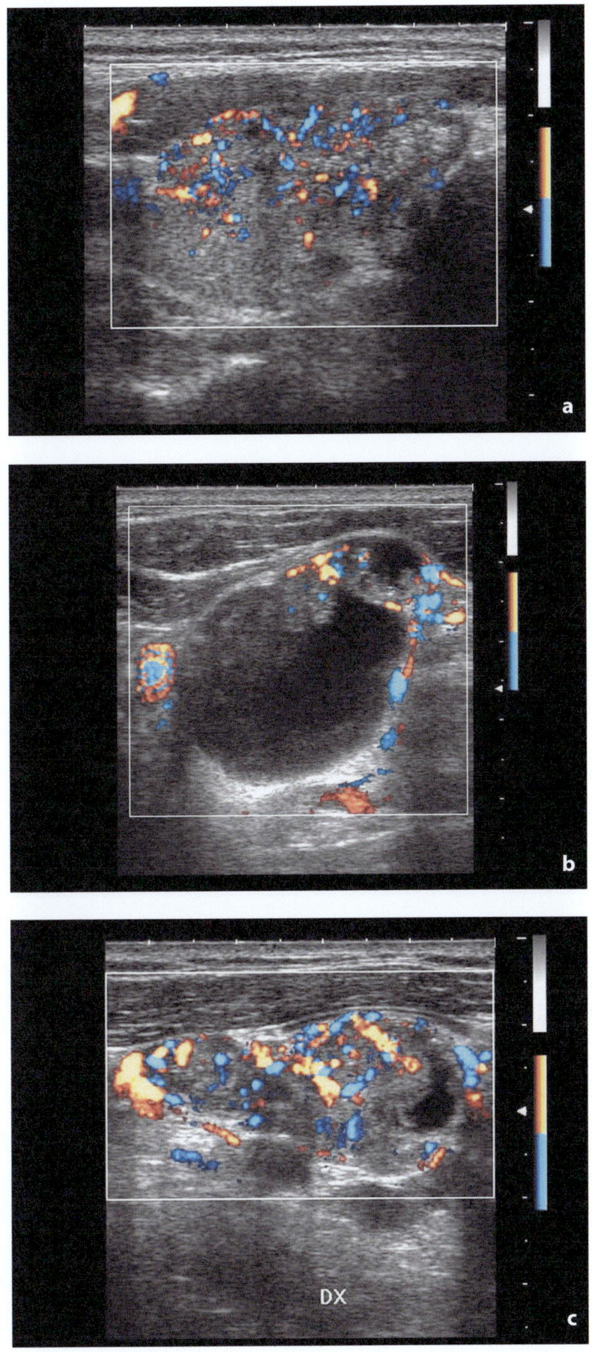

Fig. 3.80a-c Papillary carcinoma of the thyroid with lymph node metastasis. Ill-defined lesion with some microcalcifications and moderate anarchic vascularity at directional PD at the level of the right thyroid lobe (**a**). Large cystic adenopathy with several vascular papillary projections (**b**). Another two enlarged lymph nodes with a predominantly solid structure (**c**)

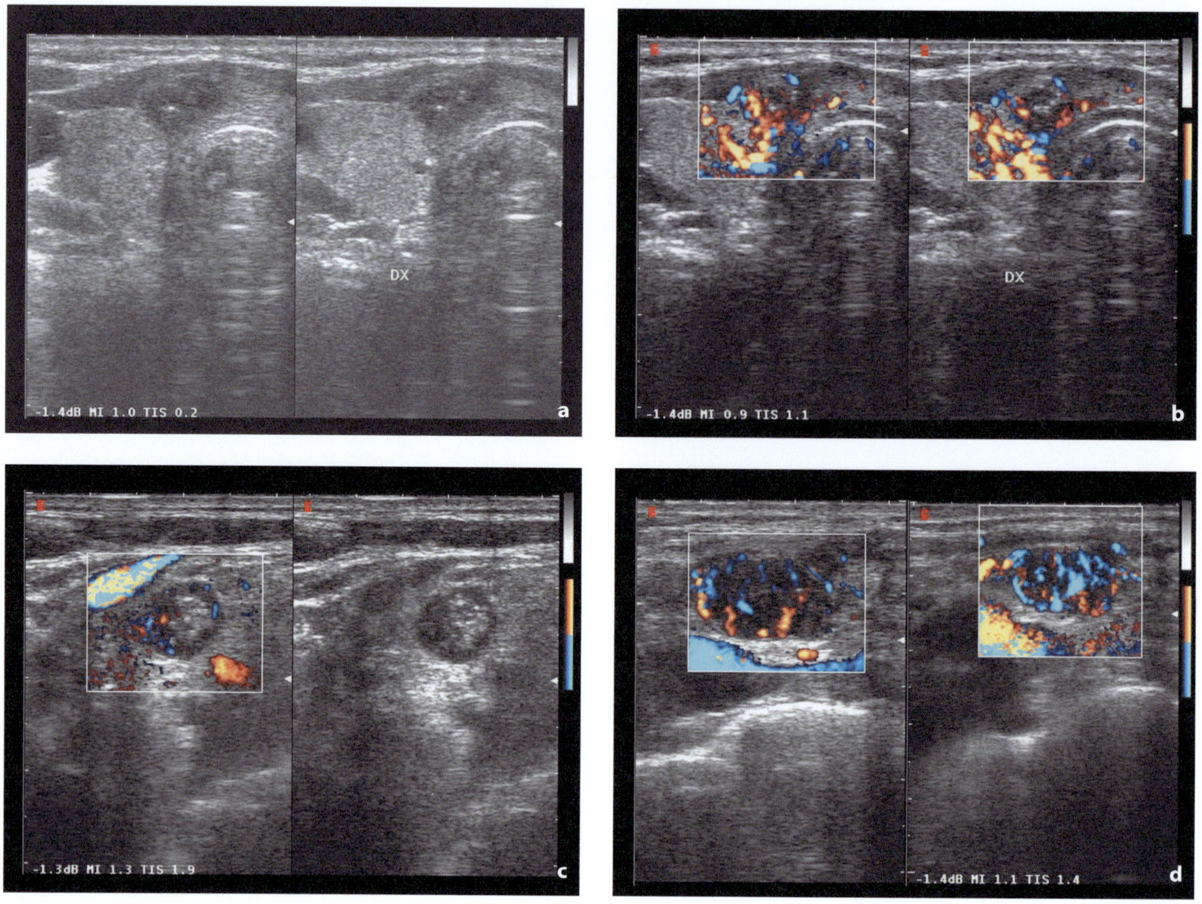

Fig. 3.81a-d Papillary carcinoma of the thyroid with lymph node metastasis. Heterogeneous and slightly hypoechoic lesion with ill-defined margins and some small calcifications (**a**). The nodule displays vascular signs at directional PD which are less evident with respect to the adjacent parenchyma (**b**). Metastatic lymphadenopathy with heterogeneity and internal microcalcifications but hypovascular (**c**). Another two adenopathies with more marked hypoechoic echostructure and more manifest and irregular vascular network (**d**)

The monitoring of subjects operated on for thyroid cancer is entrusted to thyroglobulin and calcitonin assay (medullary carcinoma). An important role in the identification of **residual disease** or **locoregional recurrence** is played by scintigraphy, especially with the use of total body scans with I-131 (bearing in mind also the role of metabolic therapy in their treatment), PET-FDG and octreotide PET (for medullary carcinoma). However, US can also perform some important tasks, such as evaluation of the surgical bed, fibrosis of any residual parenchyma and the cervical lymph node stations, given that around 2/3 of recurrences occur in the neck, particularly in the lymph nodes [47,48] (Figs. 3.85, 3.86). The contribution of CD is debatable, because it is very dependent on the size of the suspicious area. In the first six months after surgery the fibrous scar tissue is notably vascular. Surgical bed recurrence usually appears as an oval, well-defined, hypoechoic nodule, but these findings are not constant [49]. Microcalcifications are seen in 10% of cases. Care should be taken not to confuse **suture granulomas**, which have a hypoechoic appearance and amorphous calcifications, with nodules (especially in papillary carcinoma) [21]. Knowledge of this possibility and its avascular appearance at CD are generally enough for a correct differentiation. Other causes of surgical bed pseudolesions being considered in the differential diagnosis include residual thyroid tissue, fibrosis, strap muscle, reactive lymph nodes, cyst, tracheal cartilage and fat necrosis [49]. Availability of previous follow-up scans for comparison is mandatory. In patients with suspected local or regional recurrence, FNAC is usually the next step in the diagnostic algorithm (Figs. 3.87–3.89).

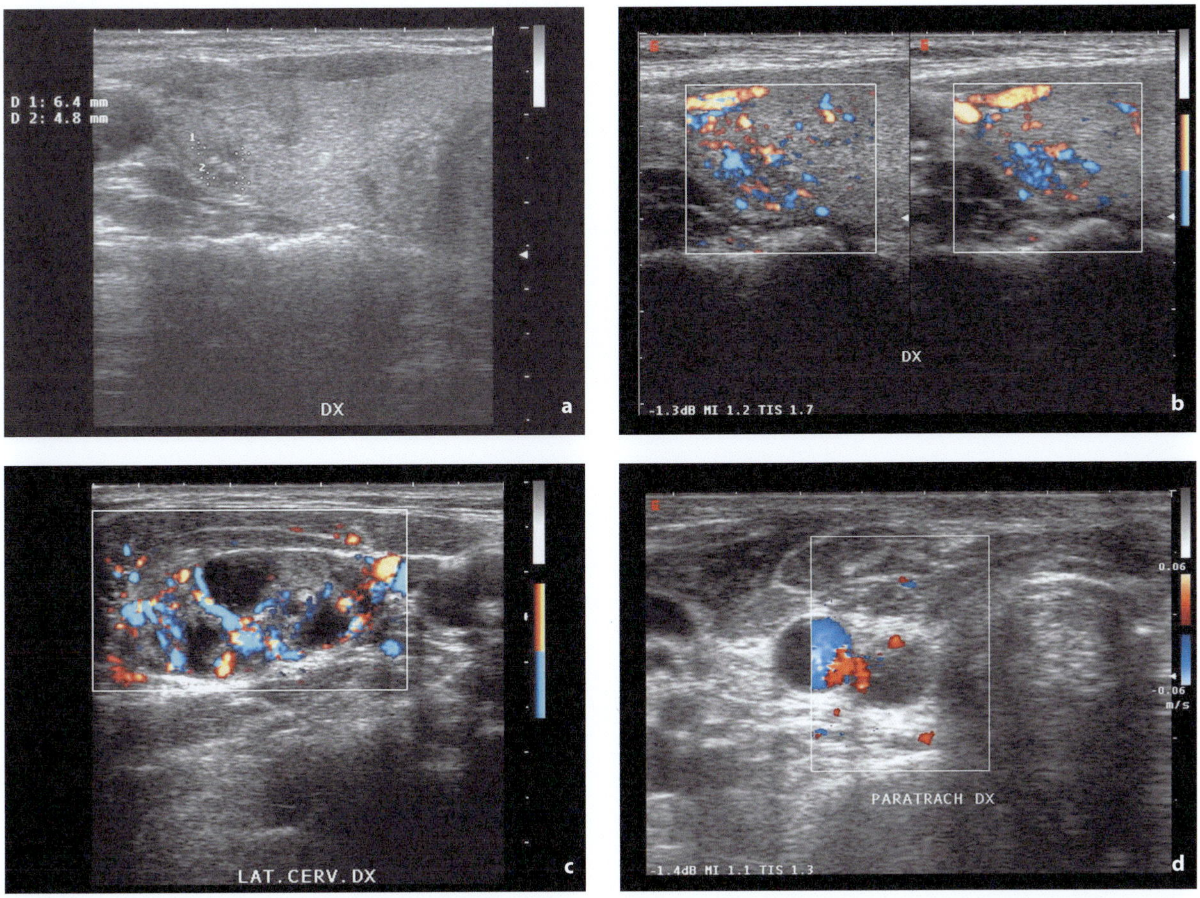

Fig. 3.82a-d Papillary microcarcinoma of the thyroid with lymph node metastasis. Small, heterogeneous, hypoechoic nodule with ill-defined margins and microcalcifications (**a**). Lesion displays heterogeneous hypervascularity at directional PD (**b**). Large homolateral laterocervical adenopathy with anechoic areas and moderate, irregular hypervascularity at directional PD (**c**). Paracarotid lymph node smaller and less vascular than the previous at CD located caudal to the base of the thyroid (**d**)

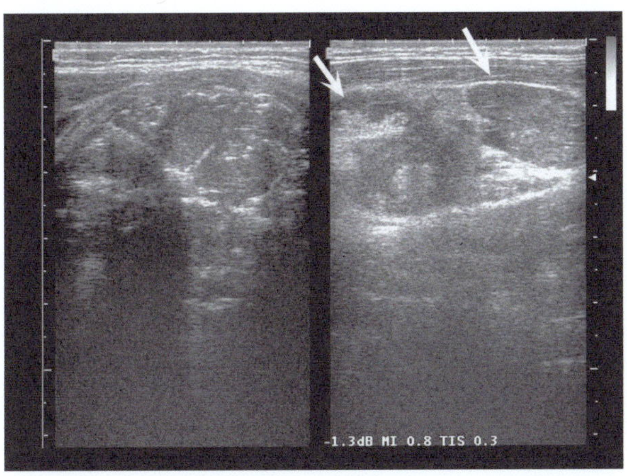

Fig. 3.83 Anaplastic carcinoma of the thyroid with lymph node metastasis. Profound structural hypoechoic change of the right thyroid lobe which appears widened, with enlarged ipsilateral laterocervical lymph nodes (*arrows*)

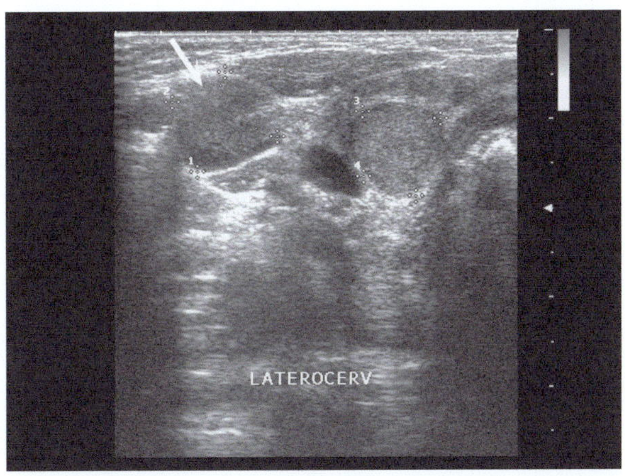

Fig. 3.84 Follicular carcinoma of the thyroid with lymph node metastasis. Hypoechoic nodule with relatively homogenous echotexture and well-defined margins at the level of the right thyroid lobe. Hypo-anechoic adenopathies are associated (*arrow*)

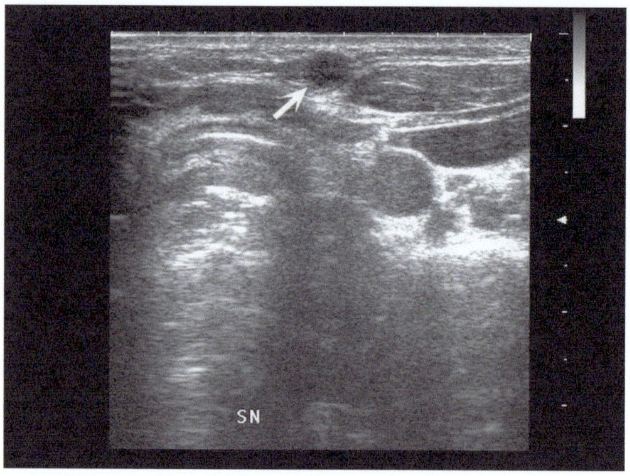

Fig. 3.85 Recurrence of medullary carcinoma after total thyroidectomy. Small superficial hypoechoic nodule (*arrow*)

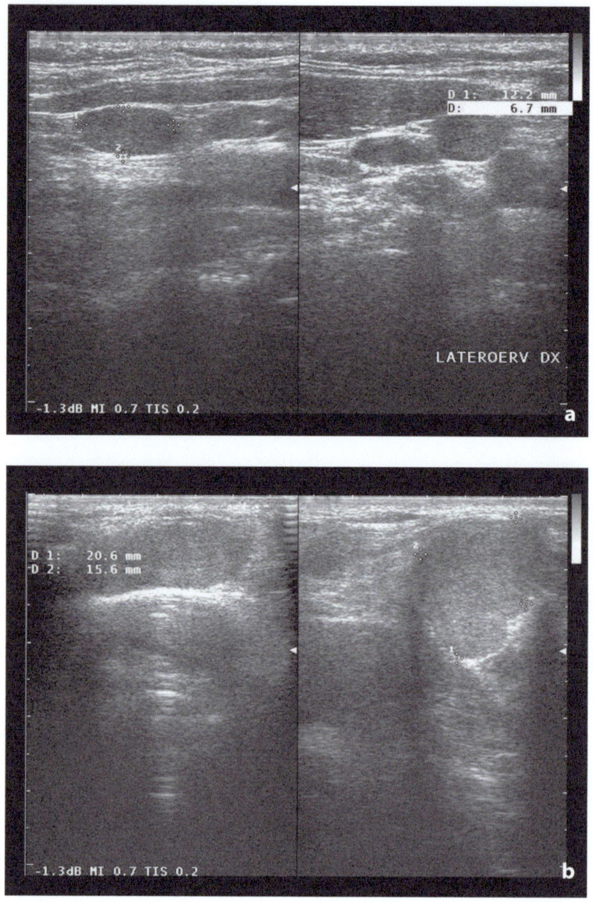

Fig. 3.86a,b Lymph node recurrence after thyroidectomy for follicular carcinoma. Multiple oval enlarged lymph nodes with hypoechoic and relatively homogeneous appearance, well-defined margins and no signs of confluence

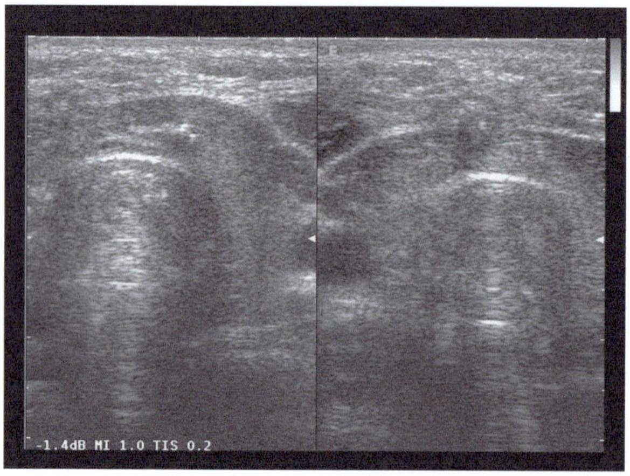

Fig. 3.87 Granuloma after right hemithyroidectomy and isthmectomy. A heterogeneous hypoechoic area with small calcifications can be appreciated at the level of the isthmus

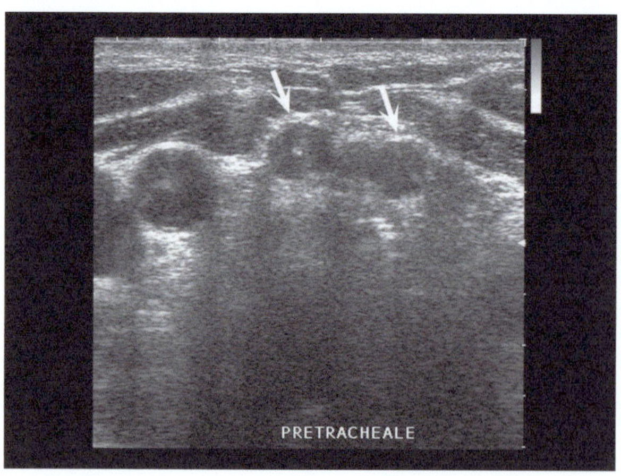

Fig. 3.88 Granuloma after thyroidectomy. In a patient with prior radical thyroidectomy for papillary carcinoma, two small hypoechoic nodules (*arrows*) can be visualized in the pretracheal region due to granulomas

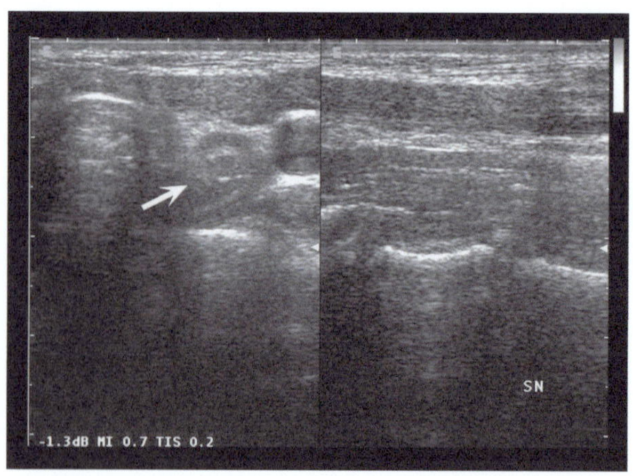

Fig. 3.89 False image of recurrence of thyroid carcinoma after total thyroidectomy. The cervical esophagus is located in the left paratracheal site (*arrow*), mimicking a local recurrence. Longitudinal scan displays the digestive structure (*right*)

References

1. Branstetter BF 4th et al (2000) Normal anatomy of the neck with CT and MR imaging correlation. Radiol Clin North Am 38:925-940
2. Wittekind Ch et al (2005) TNM atlas. Springer-Verlag Berlin
3. Som PM et al (1999) An imaging-based classification for the cervical nodes designed as an adjunct to recent clinically based nodal classification. Arch Otolaryngol Head Neck Surg 125:388-396
4. Chong V (2004) Cervical lymphadenopathy: what radiologists need to know. Cancer Imaging 4:116-120
5. Ying M et al (2003) Sonography of neck lymph nodes. Part I: normal lymph nodes. Clin Radiol 58:351-358
6. Morse MA et al (2000) Myxoid liposarcoma of the supraclavicular fossa. Chest 117:1518-1520
7. Gritzmann N et al (2002) Sonography of soft tissue masses of the neck. J Clin Ultrasound 30:356-373
8. Ahuja A et al (2003) Sonography of neck lymph nodes. Part II: abnormal lymph nodes. Clin Radiol 58:359-366
9. Nilssen ELK et al (1999) Radiological staging for squamous carcinoma of the head and neck: a standardised practice? J R Coll Surg Edinb 44:303-306
10. Khati N et al (2003) Ultrasound of the thyroid and parathyroid glands. Ultrasound Q 19:162-176
11. Solbiati L et al (2001) Ultrasound of thyroid, parathyroid glands and neck lymph nodes. Eur Radiol 11:2411-2424
12. Graif M et al (2004) Sonographic evaluation of brachial plexus pathology. Eur Radiol 14:193-200
13. Fultz PJ et al (2002) Detection and diagnosis of nonpalpable supraclavicular lymph nodes in lung cancer at CT and US. Radiology 222:245-251
14. van Overhagen H et al (2004) Metastases in supraclavicular lymph nodes in lung cancer: assessment with palpation, US, and CT. Radiology 232:75-80
15. Gritzmann N et al (2003b) Sonography of the salivary glands. Eur Radiol 13:964-975
16. Salaffi F et al (2006) Usefulness of ultrasonography and color Doppler sonography in the diagnosis of major salivary gland diseases. Reumatismo 58:138-156
17. Wong DSY (2001) Signs and symptoms of malignant parotid tumours: an objective assessment. J R Coll Surg Edinb 46:91-95
18. Gallipoli A et al (2005) Ultrasound contrast media in the study of salivary gland tumors. Anticancer Res 25:2477-2482
19. Schick S et al (1998) Differentiation of benign and malignant tumors of the parotid gland: value of pulsed Doppler and color Doppler sonography. Eur Radiol 8:1462-1467
20. Chan BK et al (2003) Common and uncommon sonographic features of papillary thyroid carcinoma. J Ultrasound Med 22:1083-1090
21. Wong KT et al (2005) Ultrasound of thyroid cancer. Cancer Imaging 5:157-166
22. Bartolotta TV et al (2006a) Incidentally discovered thyroid nodules: incidence, and greyscale and colour Doppler pattern in an adult population screened by real-time compound spatial sonography. Radiol Med 111:989-998
23. Papini E et al (2002) Risk of malignancy in nonpalpable thyroid nodules: predictive value of ultrasound and color-Doppler features. J Clin Endocrinol Metab 87:1941-1946
24. Rago T et al (1998) Role of conventional ultrasonography and color flow-Doppler sonography in predicting malignancy in "cold" thyroid nodules. Eur J Endocrinol 138:41-46
25. Alexander EK et al (2002) Assessment of nondiagnostic ultrasound-guided fine needle aspirations of thyroid nodules. J Clin Endocrinol Metab 87:4924-4927
26. Kane RA et al (2003) Ultrasound of the thyroid and parathyroid glands. Controversies in the diagnosis of thyroid cancer. Ultrasound Q 19:177-178
27. Iannuccilli JD et al (2004) Risk for malignancy of thyroid nodules as assessed by sonographic criteria: the need for biopsy. J Ultrasound Med 23:1455-1464
28. Lyschchik A et al (2005) Diagnosis of thyroid cancer in children: value of gray-scale and power Doppler US. Radiology 235:604-613
29. Wienke JR et al (2003) Sonographic features of benign thyroid nodules. Interobserver reliability and overlap with malignancy. J Ultrasound Med 22:1027-1031
30. Takashima S et al (1995) Thyroid nodules: re-evaluation with ultrasound. J Clin Ultrasound 23:179-184
31. Moon W-J et al (2008) Benign and malignant thyroid nodules: US differentiation. Multicenter retrospective study. Radiology 247:762-770
32. Chammas MC et al (2005) Thyroid nodules: evaluation with power Doppler and duplex Doppler ultrasound. Otolaryngol Head Neck Surg 132:874-882
33. Lagalla R et al (1992) Echo-Doppler couleru et pathologie thyroidienne. J Echograph Med Ultrasons 13:44-47
34. Spiezia S et al (1997) Usefulness of power Doppler in the diagnostic management of hypoechoic thyroid nodules. Eur J Ultrasound 6:165-170
35. Lyshchik A et al (2007) Quantitative analysis of tumor vascularity in benign and malignant solid thyroid nodules. J Ultrasound Med 26:837-846
36. Spiezia S et al (2001) Analysis of color Doppler signal intensity variation after Levovist injection: a new approach to the diagnosis of thyroid nodules. J Ultrasound Med 20:223-231
37. Bartolotta TV et al (2006b) Qualitative and quantitative evaluation of solitary thyroid nodules with contrast-enhanced ultrasound: initial results. Eur Radiol 16:2234-2241
38. De Nicola H et al (2005) Flow pattern and vascular resistive index as predictors of malignancy risk in thyroid follicular neoplasms. J Ultrasound Med 24:897-904
39. Miyakawa M et al (2005) Diagnosis of thyroid follicular carcinoma by vascular pattern and velocimetric parameters using high resolution pulsed and power Doppler ultrasonography. Endocr J 52:207-212
40. Hoike E et al (2001) Ultrasonographic characteristics of thyroid nodules: prediction of malignancy. Arch Surg 136:334-337
41. Takashima S et al (1988) Primary thyroid lymphoma: comparison of CT and US assessment. Radiology 171:439-443
42. Kwak JY et al (2007) Primary thyroid lymphoma: role of ultrasound-guided needle biopsy. J Ultrasound Med 26:1761-1765
43. Ahuja AT et al (1994) Role of ultrasonography in thyroid metastases. Clin Radiol 49:627-62
44. Gross M et al (2004) Internal jugular vein tumor thrombus associated with thyroid carcinoma. Ann Otol Rhinol Laryngol 113:738-74
45. King AD et al (2000) Staging papillary carcinoma of the thyroid: magnetic resonance imaging vs ultrasound of the neck. Clin Radiol 55:222-226

46. Kusasic Kuna S et al (2006) Ultrasonographic differentiation of benign from malignant neck lymphadenopathy in thyroid cancer. J Ultrasound Med 25:1531-1537
47. Weslley Souza Rosário P et al (2005) Ultrasonographic differentiation between metastatic and benign lymph nodes in patients with papillary thyroid carcinoma. J Ultrasound Med 24:1385-1389
48. Gorges R et al (2003) Diagnostic value of high-resolution B-mode and power-mode sonography in the follow-up of thyroid cancer. Eur J Ultrasound 16:191-206
49. Shin JH et al (2007) Sonographic findings in the surgical bed after thyroidectomy: comparison of recurrent tumors and nonrecurrent lesions. J Ultrasound Med 26:1359-1366

The Breast

4

4.1 Breast Nodules

Breast cancer is the most common female neoplasm (31% of tumors in women) and the second-leading cause of death in women after lung cancer. Some 25% of cases involve subjects with increased risk: family history (first-degree relative), genetic predisposition (carriers of *BRCA1* and *BRCA2* mutations), personal history, previous biopsy of precancerous breast changes (atypical ductal hyperplasia and lobular carcinoma in situ), early onset of menstruation and/or late menopause, nulliparity, first pregnancy at older age and radiation exposure [1]. Around 90% of cases are epithelial tumors arising from the cells lining the ducts or lobules: ductal carcinomas (70–80% of total cases) include in situ and invasive forms; lobular carcinoma (5–10%) is invasive by definition (in situ cases are considered more as risk markers than as overt cancer precursors), and is often multifocal and bilateral [2]. The remaining 10% of cases include other histotypes: from most to least common – medullary (5% of cases), mucinous (colloid), papillary and tubular [1]. The main prognostic indicators are size and histologic grade of the lesion (low, medium and high), and the presence and number of axillary lymphadenopathies.

The **breast nodule** is a daily challenge in the setting of US, although in most cases the finding can be put down to cysts, fibroadenomas or nodular adenosis. In fact cancer is found in only 4% of symptomatic women, because in most women who report a palpable mass no effective focal lesion can be found (e.g. confirmed in only 34% of adolescents) or the mass is benign in nature [3]. The majority of palpable lesions which undergo cytologic analysis are benign [4]. The use of US modifies patient management in 64% of cases, and is able to avoid 22% of unnecessary biopsies [2]. Moreover at least 10–15% of breast cancer patients who undergo surgery do not have palpable lesions, in that even an expert breast specialist is unable to palpate the lesions, even after having viewed the mammography and US findings. A prospective study [5] showed that the negative predictive value of a combination mammography-US was 100%: none of the women with palpable masses evaluated as negative developed a carcinoma in that site after 29 months of follow-up.

The evaluation of breast nodules, whether palpable or not, is based on the central role of mammography, despite its known limitations in young women, and the additional roles of US, FNAC and contrast-enhanced MR. The latter has taken on an increasingly prominent role in recent years. In the surveillance of women at high risk due to hereditary disease, MR has in fact produced better results than mammography and US and is currently considered the modality of choice [6].

For the sonographer, clinical evaluation of the breast is fundamental, as is the combination of the US findings with the mammography, which should precede the US even when the two examinations are performed on the same day [4]. As a rule, the **US** study is intended as a panoramic bilateral examination extended to the axilla (whole breast US) and is particularly useful in the case of a dense breast, a problem which is growing due to the increasingly widespread use of hormone replacement therapy. The evidence tends to support an additional use of US in the screening of women with a dense or heterogeneous breast [7]. In one study the sensitivity of mammography and US for nonpalpable carcinoma was 80% and 88%, respectively, for the BI-RADS grades of breast density D1 and D2, but 56% and 88% for grades D3 and D4 (with the exclusion of women with totally adipose breasts and negative physical examination) [8]. In a study on women <36 years of age, US proved to be more sensitive than mammography, although with no statistical significance (79% vs. 74%) [9]. In young women both the clinical and mammographic diagnosis is more difficult – perhaps in part due to the

O. Catalano, A. Nunziata, A. Siani, *Fundamentals in Oncologic Ultrasound*.

greater tendency to underestimate minimal signs – prompting the need to integrate the different diagnostic options. In women >36 years of age, the sensitivity of the clinical examination was found to be 70%, mammography 76%, US 60% and FNAC 81% [9]. In a study of symptomatic women <55 years of age [10] the combined mammography-US assessment increased the sensitivity by 11.6% with respect to the use of US alone and 17.5% with respect to mammography alone. At least in general terms, however, the US study of the breast should not be performed in the absence of adequate mammographic support for studying middle-aged and elderly women. This is because the background of a predominantly or totally adipose breast can conceal carcinomas that are barely detectable if at all with US.

US has shown good accuracy in the characterization of nodules, with a negative predictive value for malignancy of 98–100% [11,12]. US follow-up has proven to be an effective alternative to biopsy for solid lesions with a benign appearance seen at initial US [12]. The mammography-US combination has significantly increased the percentage of detection of breast cancers, with a combined sensitivity in the different study populations of 83–91%. In four large retrospective studies, occult palpable cancers at both mammography and US were 0.2% overall [5]. The use of tissue harmonic imaging can in theory increase the lesion-parenchyma contrast, especially in adipose and adipose-glandular breasts (with some difficulty however in dense breast due to intense reflection), with greater spatial and contrast resolution and with sharper lesion margins, internal content and possible shadowing [8,13,14]. However, tissue harmonic imaging does not seem to show a significantly greater accuracy than fundamental imaging in the benign vs. malignant distinction and its greater utility may be in the identification of poorly visualized lesions, such as isoechoic lesions [15]. Compound imaging also increases the contrast and definition between lesion and parenchyma, although it does reduce posterior shadowing, which is an important finding [16].

The additional use of **Doppler** techniques increases accuracy (in particular, it reduces false positives). In one study the sensitivity of mammography and US with color and spectral Doppler was 99% and the specificity was 76%. The use of the Doppler techniques increases specificity both for nodules ≤10 mm (from 89% to 100%) and those >10 mm (from 70% to 97 %) [17].

PD with vocal fremitus, i.e. with the evaluation of vibration artifacts induced by the oscillation of the thoracic wall of the patient during phonation, does not seem helpful in the benign vs. malignant distinction, as initially hypothesized. However, it does appear to help in the differentiation between normal tissue (presence of artifacts) and pathologic tissue (absence of artifacts in the abnormal area). This technique can be used for identifying isoechoic nodules (distinction from glandular lumps or from adipose lobules) and for demonstrating adhesion to the cystic wall of possible luminal echoes [18].

The description and classification of breast lesions can be enhanced with the terminology and classification of the **US BI-RADS**, drawn up by the ACR. The system takes into consideration shape, margins, borders, echostructure, posterior shadowing or enhancement and alteration of the surrounding tissue. Five categories can be identified: (1) negative finding; (2) benign finding (benign cyst or nodule unmodified since previous study); (3) probably benign finding – indication for 6-month follow-up or biopsy; (4) suspicious abnormality, indication for biopsy; (5) highly suspicious of malignancy, appropriate action should be taken [19]. The use of the BI-RADS terminology has shown a sensitivity of 98%, a specificity of 33% and an accuracy of 71% in the differentiation between benign and malignant breast lesions [20].

Malignant lesions usually present an irregular shape which tends to be rounded or slightly oval but not patently elongated, with spiculated margins and lobulated contours (especially if microlobulated). The echo pattern tends to be hypoechoic with heterogeneous echotexture and growth predominantly in height (perpendicular orientation of the nodule with respect to the skin profile or nonparallel arrangement) [20,21] (Figs. 4.1–4.6, Videos 4.1–4.4). These predictors of malignancy are dependent on the size of the lesion. Apart from irregular margins and marked hypoe-

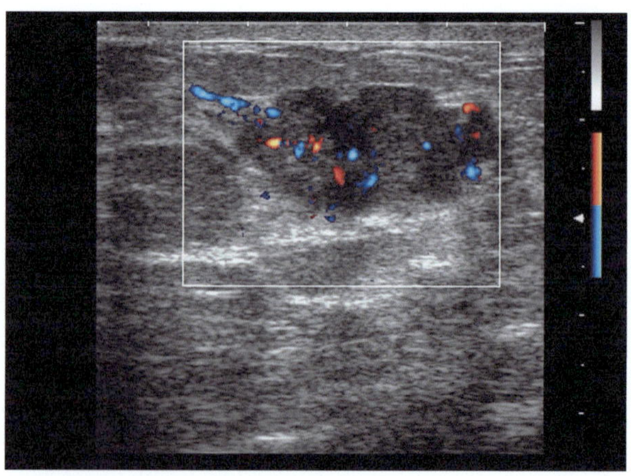

Fig. 4.1 Breast cancer. Lobulated hypoechoic nodule with parallel orientation and overall homogeneous echotexture, mild posterior acoustic shadowing and moderate vascular signals at directional PD. In particular an afferent artery is identifiable

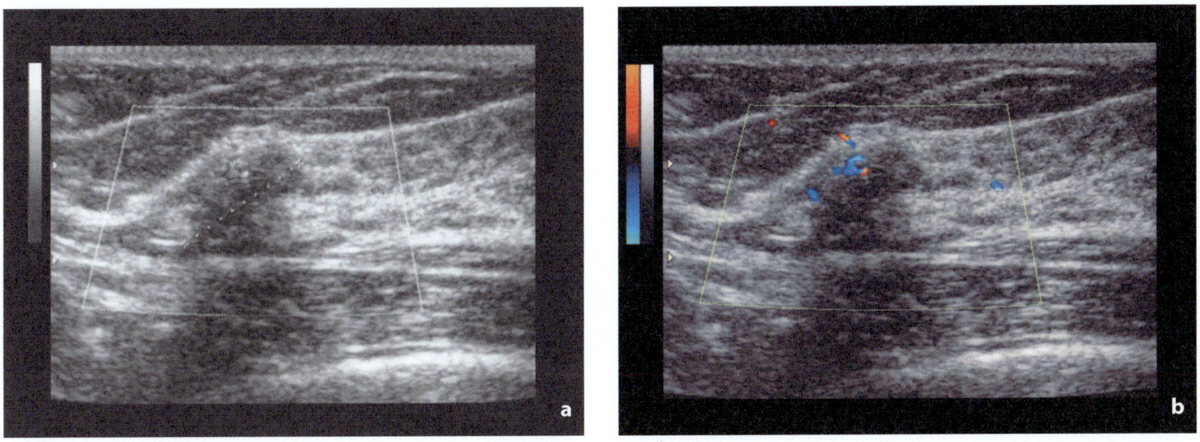

Fig. 4.2a,b Breast cancer. Heterogeneous hypoechoic nodule with nonparallel orientation, irregular margins, microcalcifications and acoustic shadowing (**a**). CD shows some peripheral vascular signal (**b**). The nodule is rather deep and adheres to the fascial plane

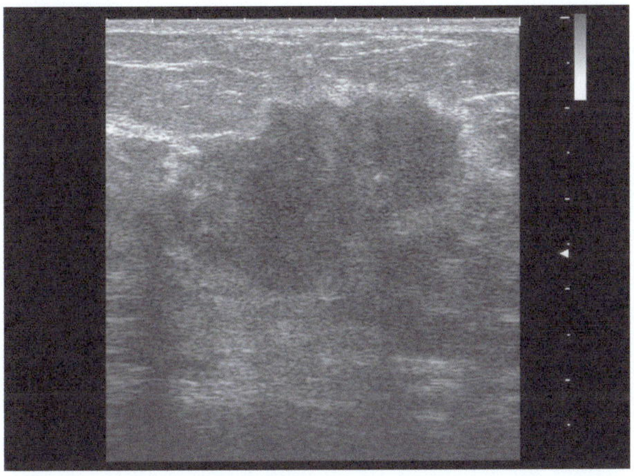

Fig. 4.3 Breast cancer. Hypoechoic lesion with microlobulated margins, superficial echogenic rim and deep acoustic shadowing

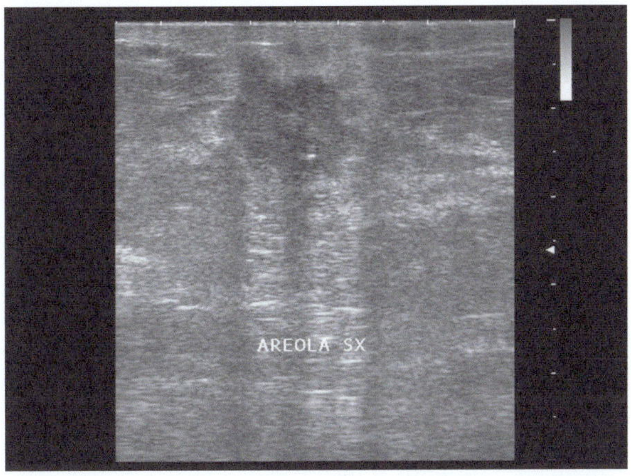

Fig. 4.4 Breast cancer. Heterogeneous hypoechoic lesion with microcalcifications, irregular margins and an evident echogenic border. Both acoustic shadowing and enhanced through-transmission can be identified deep

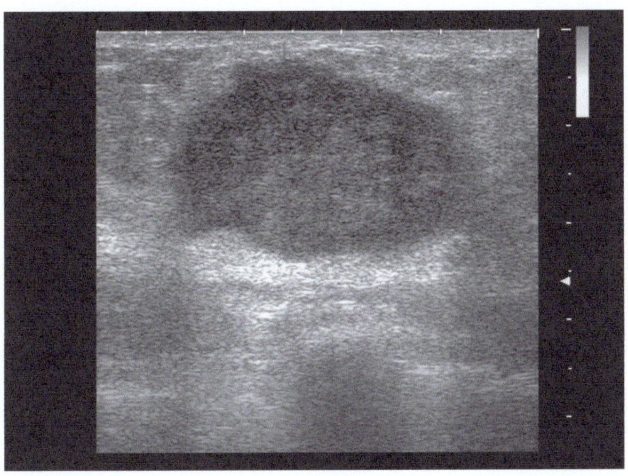

Fig. 4.5 Breast cancer. Large hypoechoic mass with parallel orientation and moderately enhanced through-transmission

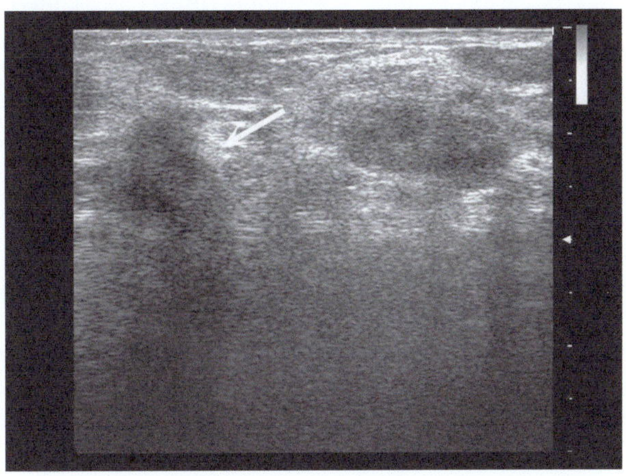

Fig. 4.6 Adjacent carcinoma and fibroadenoma. Hypoechoic neoplastic nodule with irregular margins and patent posterior acoustic shadowing (*arrow*). Adjacent to this a more homogeneous and circumscribed nodule with moderately enhanced through-transmission and parallel orientation can be identified, attributable to fibroadenoma

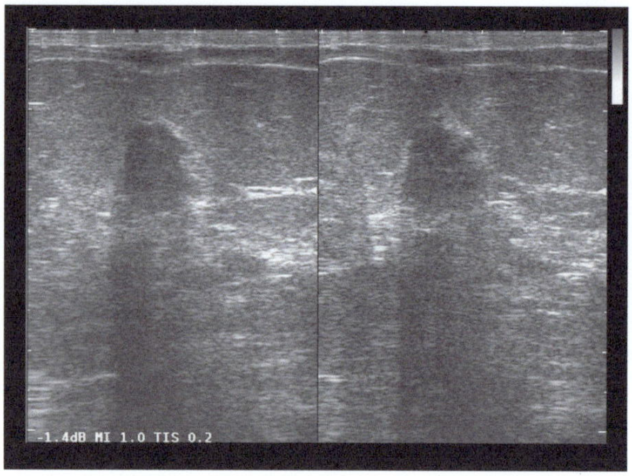

Fig. 4.7 Breast cancer. Irregularly shaped, vaguely rounded lesion with evident posterior acoustic shadowing

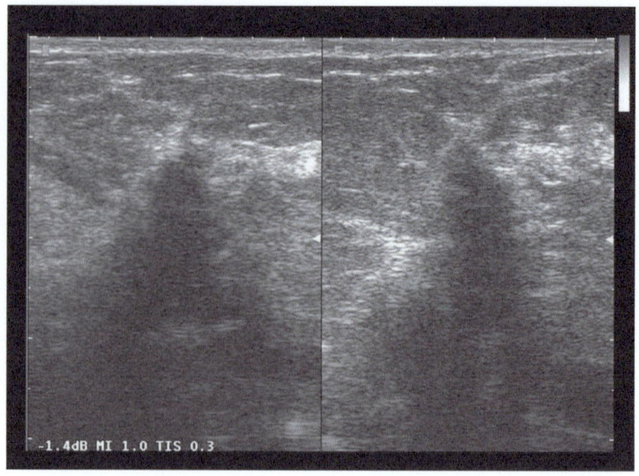

Fig. 4.8 Breast cancer. Heterogeneous hypoechoic lesion with infiltrating margins and intense posterior acoustic shadowing

chogenicity, in fact, the other signs are particularly noticeable in lesions >7 mm [22]. There is also a more-or-less intense posterior **shadowing**, with difficulty visualizing the deeper part of the lesion and the parenchyma immediately deep to it. The degree of shadowing is correlated with the intensity and extension of the desmoplastic phenomena connected to the neoplasm, which can be irregularly distributed [20,21] (Figs. 4.7, 4.8). Beam attenuation is inconstant, being present fully or in part in only 35% of carcinomas (especially if tubular, tubulo-lobular or invasive lobular). In around 28% of cases there is even enhanced through-transmission (particularly for medullary or mucinous carcinomas) [23]. Posterior acoustic shadowing can also be found in benign lesions (regardless of the presence of calcifications). It can be found in noncalcified fibroadenomas (up to 30% of cases), granular cell tumors (most cases), phyllodes tumors (16% of cases), radial scars (most cases), postoperative scarring, focal fibrosis and sclerosing adenosis, diabetic mastopathy and fat necrosis [24]. However, there are differential diagnostic elements. For example, in hyalinizing fibroadenoma the shadowing is revealed deep to the nodule, whereas in carcinoma the shadowing completely conceals the posterior portion of the lesion, rendering it unrecognizable. In addition, many of the lesions described above – such as sclerosing adenosis, focal fibrosis and diabetic mastopathy – have the appearance more of an area of heterogeneous and poorly defined hypoechogenicity than a nodule proper. The vascularity of these pseudonodular images also is not abnormal.

The carcinoma does not display images indicating a pseudocapsule, whereas hypo-anechoic bands at the margin of a lesion with possible ramifications can be suggestive of intraductal extension (differentiate from dilated ducts) [25]. In many cases an echogenic halo may be seen at the periphery of a nodule, caused by infiltration and/or desmoplastic reaction of the surrounding tissues. 3D US may better display the effects on the adjacent parenchyma: a "converging" pattern, with echogenic bands converging radially towards the perifocal echogenic halo, suggests malignancy, whereas a "compressive" pattern, with echogenic bands displaced by the central image, is suggestive of benignity [26]. The neoplasm tends to be bounded by the anterior mammary fascia, which separates it from the subcutaneous layer, and tends to extend above all at the points where Cooper's ligaments are inserted into the fascia itself [23]. The ill-defined margins, non-compressibility and distortion of the adjacent structures (in particular the interruption of Cooper's ligaments) are highly indicative imaging characteristics of malignancy [27]. Occasionally the overlying skin may be locally thickened and hypoechoic due to invasion.

Microcalcifications (calcifications <5 mm) are identifiable at US only in some cases, having the appearance of small echogenic foci without posterior shadowing. They are especially identifiable if within a nodular hypoechoic area or anechoic ductal structures [28,29]. Differential diagnosis is made with the echogenic parenchymal bands, which nonetheless take on a linear appearance if the transducer is rotated, and with speckle artifacts, which however are not confirmed if the same areas is insonated from different angles. US has proven to be sensitive to the identification of microcalcifications, especially in ductal carcinoma in situ, and their finding in a nodule increases the suspicion of malignancy [30]. If the mammography images are used as a guide, US with a high-frequency transducer (10–13 MHz) can identify up to

23% of cases of microcalcification clusters not associated with nodules defined at mammography, and be used to guide biopsy [23,30] (Figs. 4.9, 4.10).

Invasive ductal carcinomas appear as typical hypoechoic nodules with irregular shape, distortion of the surrounding parenchyma and acoustic shadowing. This appearance tends to be found most of all in lower-grade lesions, whereas, paradoxically, higher-grade lesions tend to have a more "benign" appearance, occasionally with well-defined margins or enhanced through-transmission [31]. In some cases the lesion appears in the form of a ductal dilatation involving a single segment, and in this case the ducts involved display thick and irregular walls and papillary or fine luminal echoes [32]. **Invasive lobular carcinoma** instead causes a limited desmoplastic reaction and slight distortion of the adjacent tissues, characteristics which make it more difficult to detect. Occasionally only a hazy area of attenuation of the beam may be seen, without the clear appearance of a mass, or in contrast a nodulation without acoustic absorption [16]. **Ductal carcinomas in situ**, which are identified at mammography most of all because of the elevated frequency of microcalcification clusters, may be identified at US as nodular lesions or focal dilatations of the ducts (especially in higher-grade lesions) or as echogenic nuclei not associated with a mass or ductal dilatation but bordered by an edematous hypoechoic halo (particularly in low-grade lesions). The presentation as a cystic mass is instead rare [30]. **Medullary carcinomas**, which are more frequent in young women and have a better outcome, can have a misleading appearance, manifesting as homogenous, well-defined lesions occasionally with increased through-transmission, although in some cases there may be a partial irregularity in the margins or partial beam attenuation. The lymph node metastases can be isoechoic and therefore be missed [16]. The main sign found in **tubular carcinomas** is a nonspecific parenchymal distortion. Last of all, **mucinous carcinomas** have a nodular, lobulated and relatively echogenic appearance [13].

The possibility of identifying vascular signals with **Doppler techniques** depends on a number of factors. The ability to reveal flows with the first Doppler devices was very low, and as such they allowed a specificity of 100% for the diagnosis of malignancy. Today modern instrumentation has achieved the detection of flow in 14–86% of fibroadenomas and 65–98% of carcinomas [16,17] (Fig. 4.11). Regardless of the sensitivity of the various devices and their appropriate settings, the main factors that increase the possibility of identifying flow signals are the use of PD in place of CD, superficial location of the nodule and significant size of the nodule. The use of contrast media clearly increases the sensitivity of CD, even though the cost–benefit feasibility with respect to FNAC for example has not been demonstrated. Contrast media increase the number of identifiable vessels and also enable the visualization of an early and intense enhancement in carcinomas and a more slow and persistent enhancement in fibroadenomas. In addition, the number of vessels and the time to peak seem to be less significant parameters with respect to the morphology and course of the vessels (see below). The use of contrast media may be able to reduce the number of biopsies performed [33–34].

At **CD**, malignant lesions display intense vascularity with multiple vascular poles and a greater number of vessels identifiable than in benign lesions, which are distributed anarchically in both the center

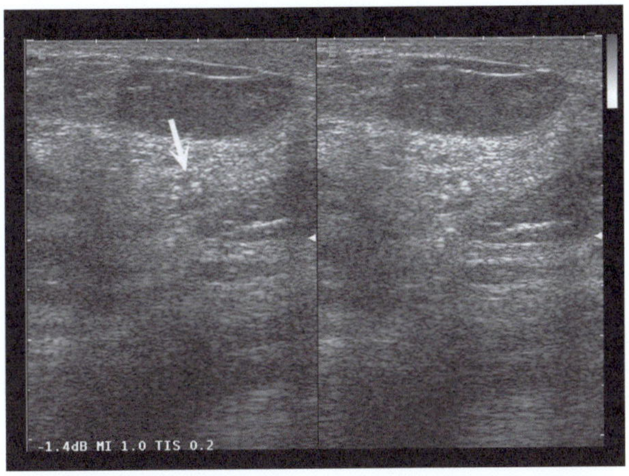

Fig. 4.9 Sclerosing lobular hyperplasia and cluster of microcalcifications. Superficial hypoechoic nodule with thin peripheral septation. Deep to this a hypoechoic area is identifiable with multiple punctate echogenic foci (*arrow*)

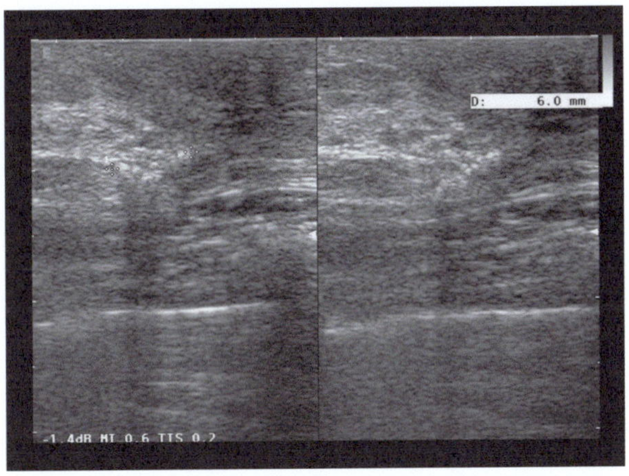

Fig. 4.10 Cluster of microcalcifications. Multiple small hyperechoic areas contiguous to each other

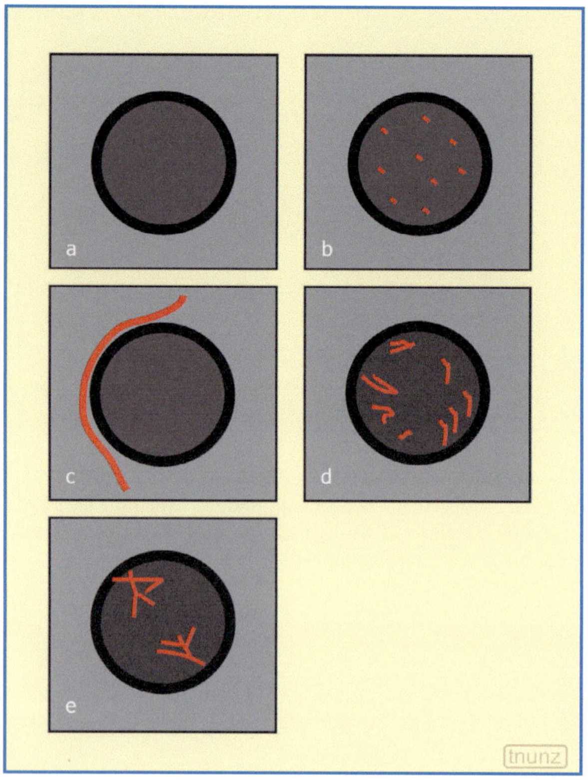

Fig. 4.11a-e Main CD patterns of focal breast lesions. **a** avascularity (pattern 1); **b** multiple spots of intranodular color (pattern 2a); **c** vessel detouring (pattern 2b); **d** multiple and prevalently peripheral intranodular vessels (pattern 3a); **e** multiple vascular poles with intranodular branching (pattern 3b)

and the periphery (Figs. 4.12–4.15). Particularly suspicious are vessels that are only identifiable at the center, or "penetrating" vessels, i.e. terminal arterioles which arrive from outside the lesion, penetrate in the periphery at or almost at right angles to it then reach the center and anastomose in an evident intranodular network. The fastest and most evident flows are peripheral, whereas in the center the signals are generally less marked and at any rate flow is slower. These vessels also have a variable diameter and direction and a tortuous course and may even present bidirectional flows due to fistulas or "mosaic" signals indicative of variable flow velocity. The overall vasculature is chaotic and heterogeneous (polychromatic) [17]. There is, however, a certain overlap of the CD findings between benign and malignant nodules and it has been seen that the semiquantitative parameters measured with CD, in addition to being subject to an intra- and interobserver variability related to the sampling, are also influenced by features such as menopausal status and hormone replacement therapy. It should also be borne in mind that some carcinomas, especially

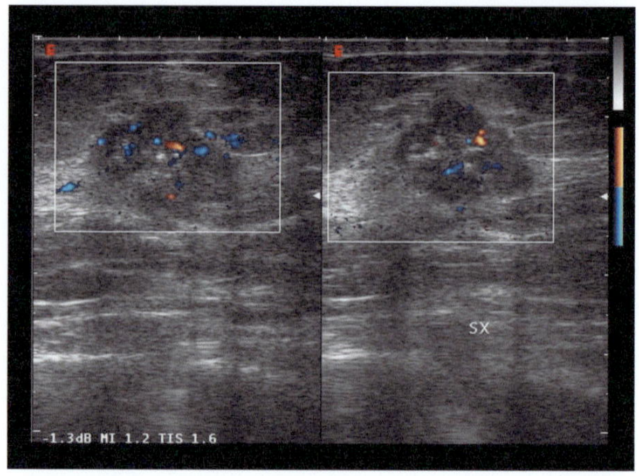

Fig. 4.12 Breast cancer. Lobulated, hypoechoic lesion with moderate internal microcalcifications and irregular vascularity at directional PD

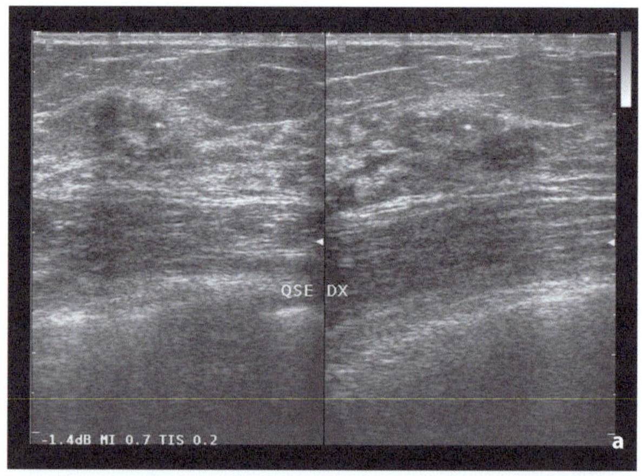

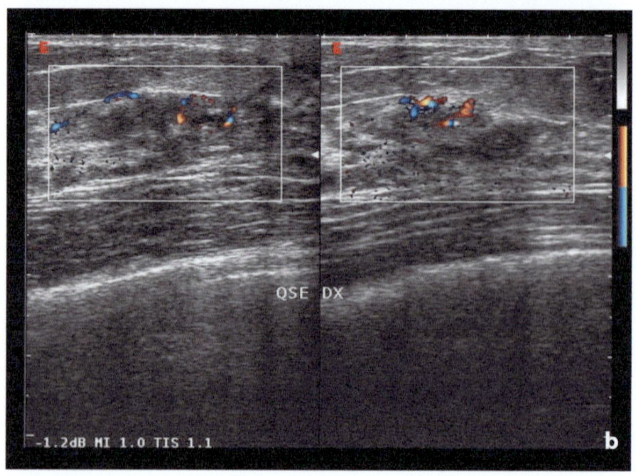

Fig. 4.13a,b Breast cancer. Heterogeneous hypoechoic nodule with some microcalcifications is poorly defined in terms of the adjacent parenchyma (**a**). Directional PD identifies moderate diffuse vascularity and therefore better visualizes the lesion (**b**)

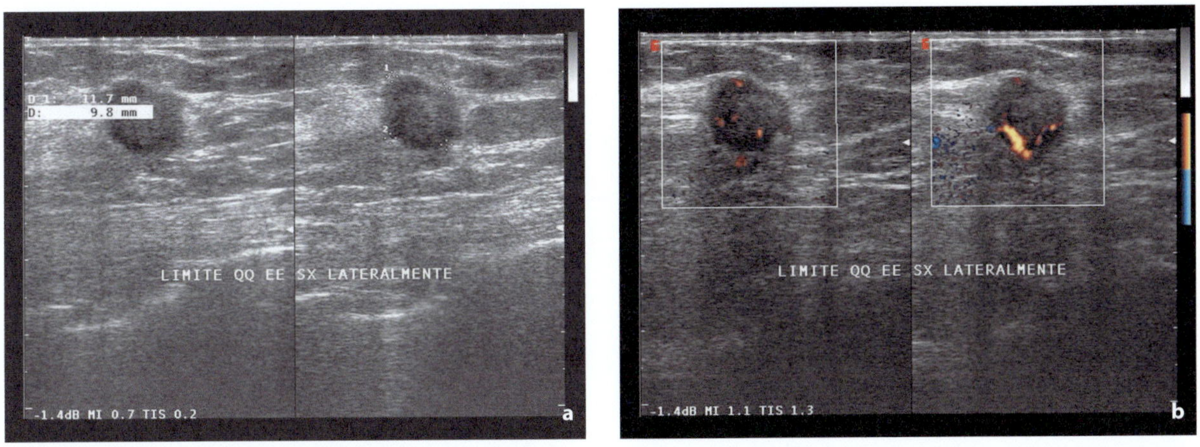

Fig. 4.14a,b Breast cancer. Oval, hypoechoic and relatively homogeneous and well-defined mass with oblique orientation and mild posterior acoustic shadowing (**a**). Multiple vascular poles are evident at directional PD (**b**)

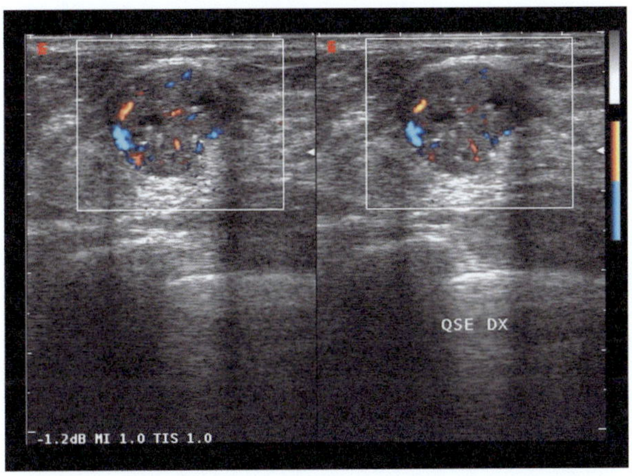

Fig. 4.15 Breast cancer. Oval lesion with well-defined margins, internal calcifications and some anechoic areas. Moderate vascularity also at the center of the lesion at directional PD

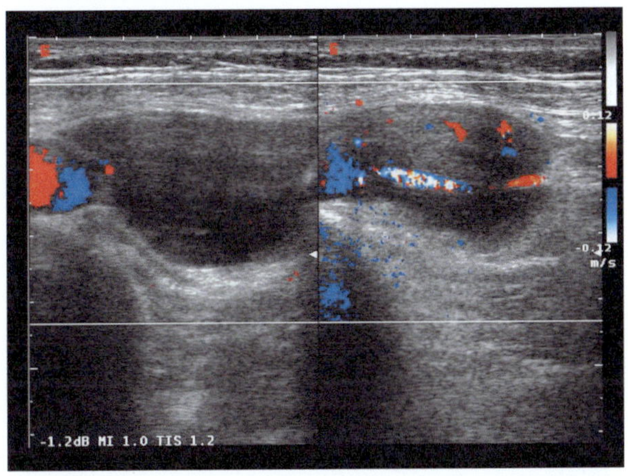

Fig. 4.16 Medullary carcinoma of the breast. Mass with a relatively "benign" appearance, with oval shape, relatively homogeneous hypoechoic structure, parallel orientation and hypovascularity at CD

lobular carcinomas, can be hypovascular, and that some benign lesions, such as inflammation and fibroadenomas, can be rather vascular [16,36] (Figs. 4.16, 4.17). The presence alone of vessels within the nodule has a sensitivity of 68% and a specificity of 64% [37].

With regard to semiquantitative **spectral analysis**, the literature has not provided a consensus, in part because the indices, and in particular the RI, are influenced by the pre- or postmenopausal status of the woman. In one study all nodules (except for one) with an RI>0.99 (i.e. with absent or inverted diastolic flow) or with a PI >4 were malignant [37]. Others consider an RI>0.7 or 0.8 suggestive of malignancy if associated with appropriate morphologic findings [37]. In another study [16], no significant differences were found between benign and malignant lesions: the RI

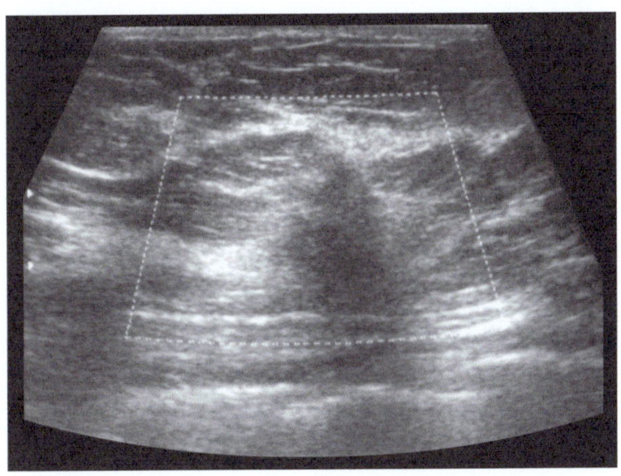

Fig. 4.17 Breast cancer. Heterogeneous hypoechoic nodule with irregular margins and acoustic shadowing. CD shows no vascular signals

was 0.64±0.12 in benign lesions and 0.66±0.09 in malignant lesions; the PI was 1.07±0.30 in benign lesions and 1.10±0.25 in malignant lesions; and the AI was 5.6±2.8 in benign lesions and 7.0±2.8 in malignant lesions. In general it can be stated that RI and PI tend to be higher in malignant lesions, even though they do not seem to be correlated with MVD. The systolic velocity is in itself hardly discriminating, but it does correlate better with MVD and prognosis. In one study, the 5-year survival rate was 82% for women with carcinoma with V_{max} <0.25 cm/s and 37% for women with V_{max} >0.25 cm/s [38].

With regard to **elastography**, carcinomas tend to be harder (less compressible) than benign nodules and even more so than cysts. In a comparative series, elastography proved more specific (96%) than US and mammography in differentiating benign and malignant lesions, while the three modalities showed a similar sensitivity: it was suggested that a combination of US and elastography had the best results and could reduce the number of biopsies [39].

The number of studies with **CEUS** is still rather limited. The possibility of highlighting nodular enhancement as an indicator of the microcirculation is interesting, particularly given the availability of effective systems for its quantification. In one study, CEUS patterns and parameters correlated more closely with MVD than VEGF expression [40]. CEUS has demonstrated good application in the study of suspicious lesions with a nondiagnostic FNAC, achieving a sensitivity of 100% and a specificity of 91% in defining biologic behavior (whereas PD reported a sensitivity of 45% and a specificity of 78%) [41]. Indubitably the presence or absence of contrast enhancement increases the confidence of the diagnosis in terms of malignancy and benignity, respectively, but the possible practical applications have not yet been adequately defined.

In addition to a thorough morphostructural analysis of the nodule, US study should evaluate and describe in the report the site (single quadrant or union of two adjacent quadrants), distance from the areola, depth and relations with adjacent structures (pectoral fascia, skin, etc.) (Fig. 4.18). The dimensions of the nodule are not always accurately defined by US, which tends to slightly underestimate the size (whereas mammography tends to overestimate) (Fig. 4.19). The grade of the lesion cannot be defined, even though the high-grade forms tend to be larger at diagnosis and are more likely to display posterior acoustic shadowing. It has been noted that nodules with Doppler hypervascularity are more likely to be associated with axillary lymphadenopathies than hypovascular lesions, although there is little agreement in the literature [16,37]. In all women with a new diagnosis of breast cancer, an accurate study of the other quadrants of the diseased side as well as the contralateral breast is required. US has in fact demonstrated its ability to identify one or more additional nodules in 14% of cases (although MR is the most effective modality in identifying multiple focal tumors) [16]. **Multifocal** breast cancer is defined as the presence of >2 synchronous tumors located at a distance from each other <4–5 cm and generally situated in the same quadrant or along the same ductal unit. In contrast, **multicentric** breast cancer is defined as >2 synchronous lesions distant >4–5 cm from each other and typically located in different quadrants (Figs. 4.20–4.22). Of course the lesions synchronous to carcinoma may also be benign: 11% of synchronous lesions with BI-RADS 3

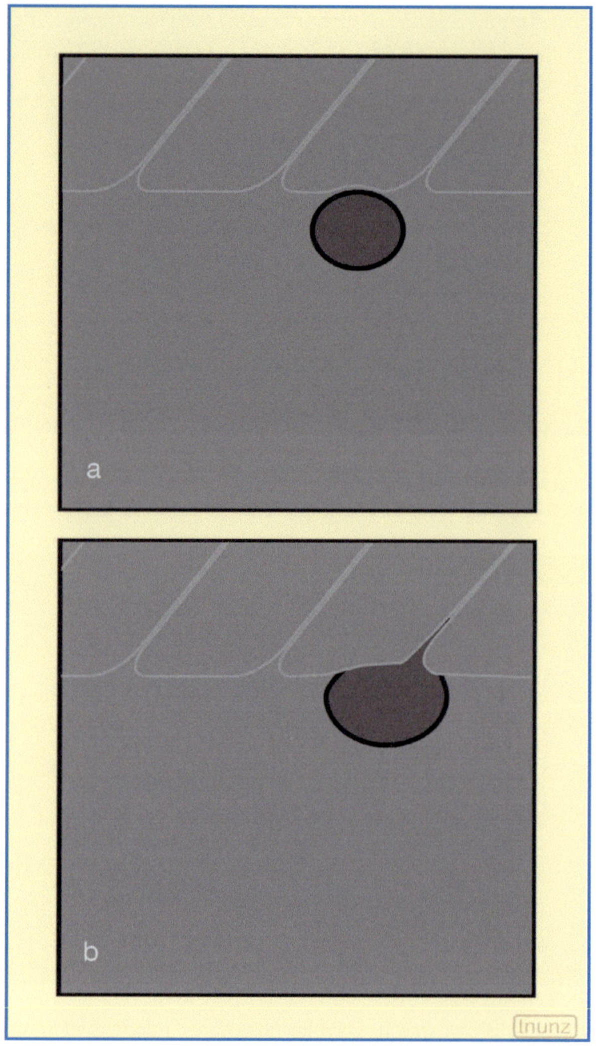

Fig. 4.18 Spread of breast cancer. Due to the relative resistance of the anterior breast fascia, the nodule initially tends to grow transversally. With further growth the nodule infiltrates along the insertions of Cooper's ligaments where resistance is minor, distorting the adjacent structures. Modified from [42]

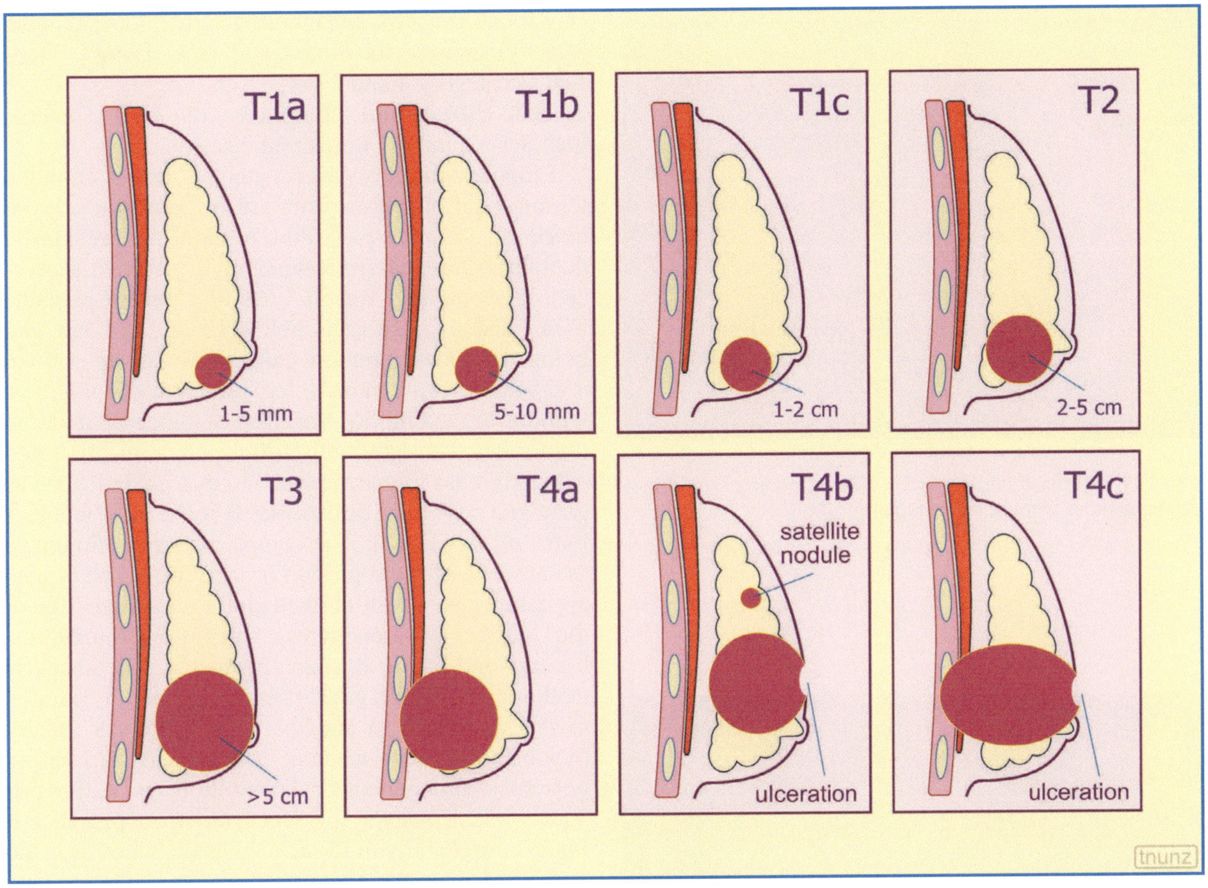

Fig. 4.19 Staging of breast cancer. *T1a*, nodule ≤5 mm; *T1b*, nodule 5–10 mm; *T1c* nodule 1–2 cm; *T2*, nodule 2–5 cm; *T3*, nodule >5 cm; *T4a,* tumor of any size invading the thoracic wall (ribs, intercostal muscles, serratus anterior muscle but not the pectoral muscle); *T4b*, edema with peau d'orange appearance, skin ulceration or satellite nodules in the same breast; *T4c*, combination of criteria of 4a and 4b. Inflammatory carcinoma is classified *T4d*. Skin alterations other than those mentioned, including retraction of the nipple and sinking of the skin, do not modify the stage. Modified from [43]

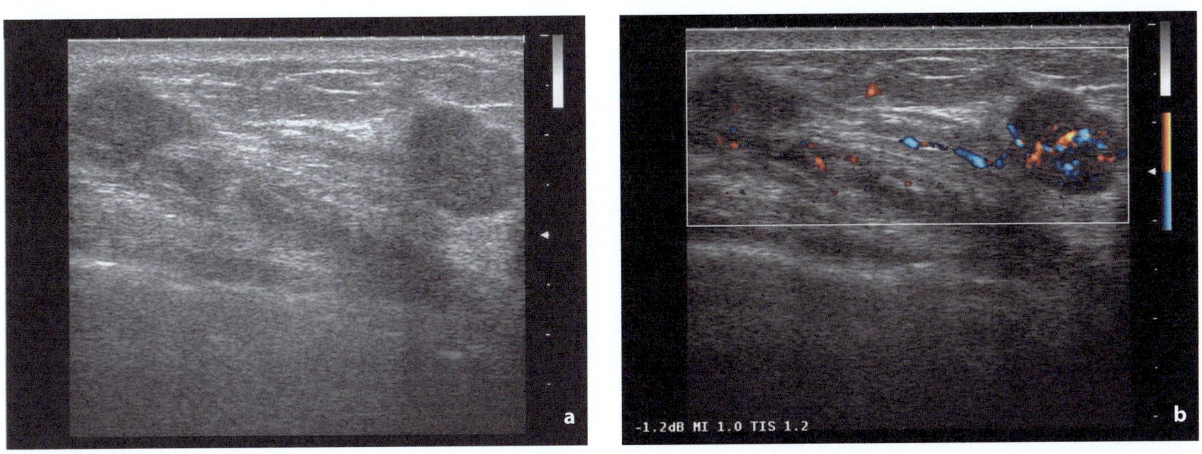

Fig. 4.20a,b Multifocal breast cancer. Two neoplastic nodules in the same quadrant, one of which appears more vascular at directional PD

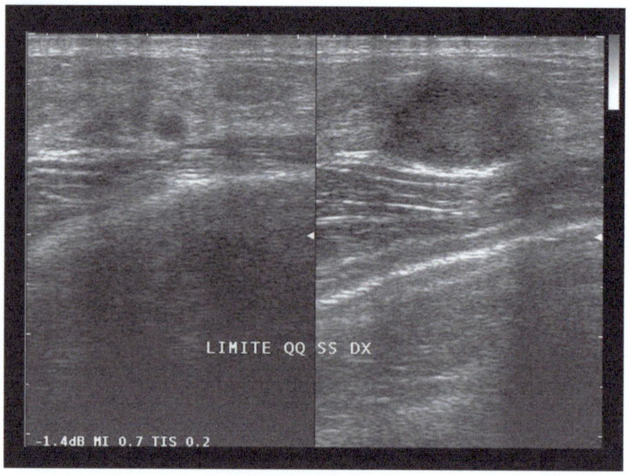

Fig. 4.21 Multifocal breast cancer. Two differently sized hypoechoic nodules in the same quadrant

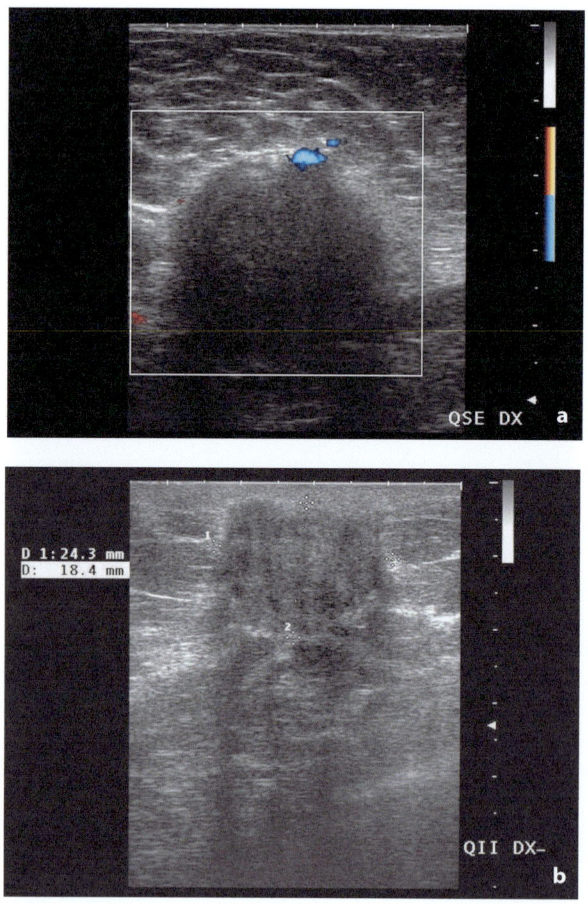

Fig. 4.22a,b Multicentric breast cancer. Two neoplastic lesions in different quadrants of the same breast

classification are malignant (especially if located in the same quadrant as the tumor) and 48% of those classified as category 4 and 5 [44].

The **differential diagnosis** of breast cancer includes a number of different diseases.

Fibroadenoma is very frequent. It derives from the terminal ductal lobular unit and is due to the coexistence of stromal proliferation and non-neoplastic ductules. Onset of fibroadenomas is often in adolescence (accounting for 50–75% of cases of palpable breast lesions in subjects below 19 years of age, and being the most common palpable lesion in women <35 years), with a more or less rapid growth and then, without exceeding 20 mm, they stabilize or undergo involution with age, with atrophy, hyalinization and calcification. Fibroadenomas >40 mm are indicated as giant and need to be differentiated above all from phyllodes tumors [3,13]. The symptoms are minimum in the absence of rapid growth or infarction. The typical appearance is of well-defined nodules (compression of the adjacent parenchyma), with macrolobulated borders and a thin echogenic capsule. The shape is oval or patently elongated (long axis generally parallel to the skin surface) and the echo pattern is usually hypoechoic (often isoechoic to the breast fat) with a generally homogeneous echotexture (Figs. 4.23–4.32, Video 4.5). However, this characteristic appearance is found entirely only in 15–55% of cases, whereas in the remaining cases there is some variation in the imaging characteristics. Internal pseudocystic areas and macrocalcifications may be present. In 30% of cases there is posterior acoustic shadowing, although it is generally weak in the absence of calcifications and does not completely conceal the deep profile of the nodule (Figs. 4.33, 4.34). At CD the vascularity appears more intense in the younger prevalently adenomatous forms

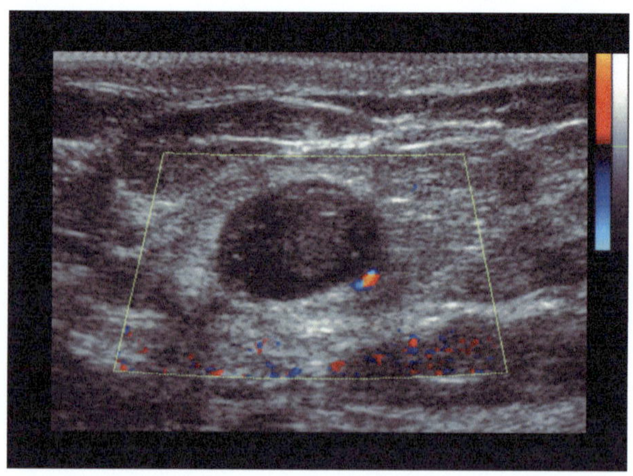

Fig. 4.23 Fibroadenoma. Oval hypoechoic nodule with parallel orientation and overall homogeneous echotexture and no internal color signals at CD

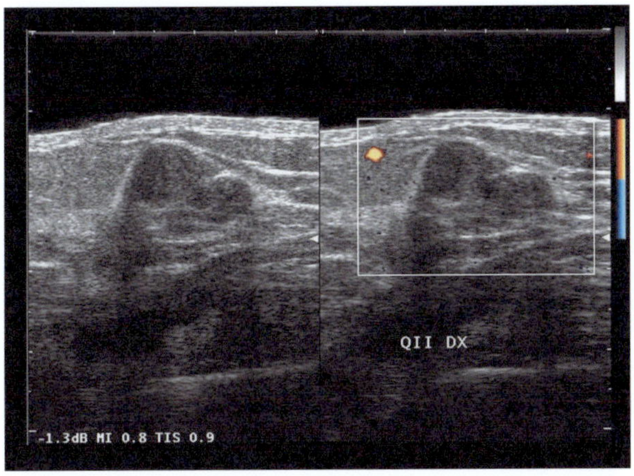

Fig. 4.24 Fibroadenoma. Macrolobulated hypoechoic nodule with no color signals at directional PD

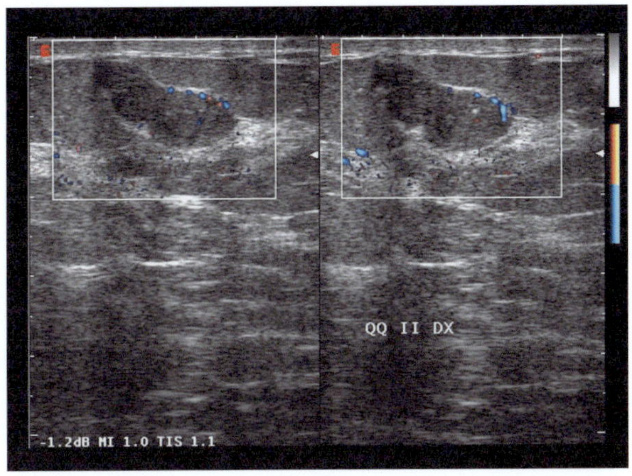

Fig. 4.25 Fibroadenoma. Superficial, macrolobulated, hypoechoic nodule with some small calcifications and prevalently marginal flow signals at directional PD

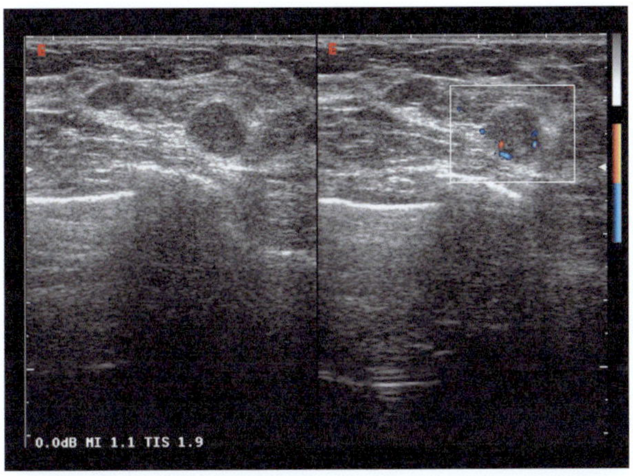

Fig. 4.26 Fibroadenoma. Small oval nodule with homogeneous hypoechoic structure, well-defined margins and some peripheral vascular signals at directional PD

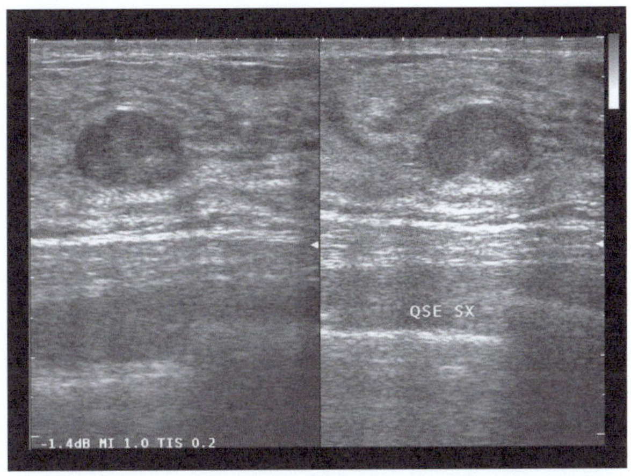

Fig. 4.27 Fibroadenoma. Oval hypoechoic mass with well-defined margins and parallel orientation

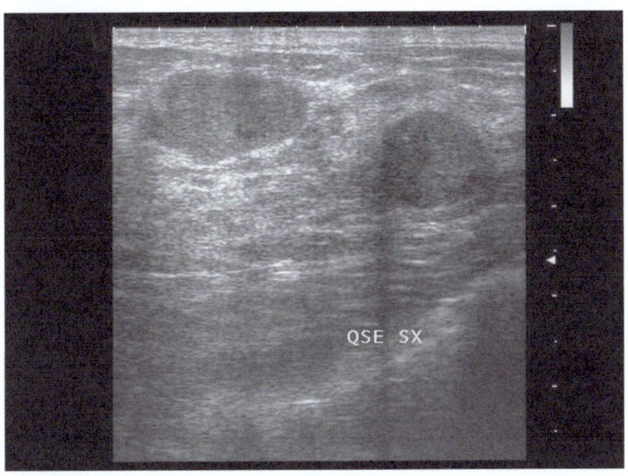

Fig. 4.28 Fibroadenomas. Two adjacent, relatively homogeneous and well-defined nodules with enhanced through-transmission

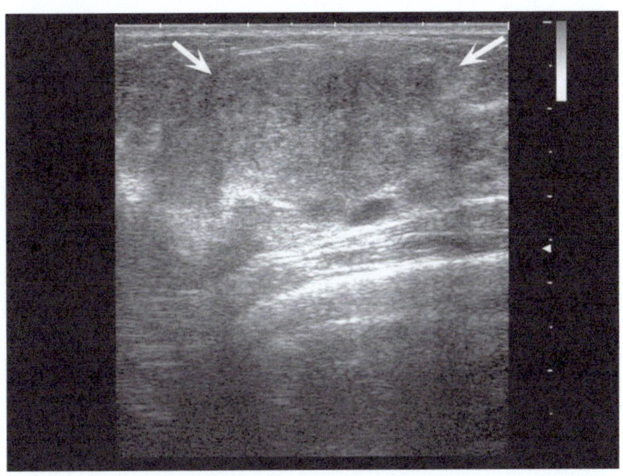

Fig. 4.29 Fibroadenoma. Large oval homogeneous nodule with parallel orientation (*arrows*). The echostructure is prevalently isoechoic to the surrounding parenchyma, making identification of the lesion difficult despite its size

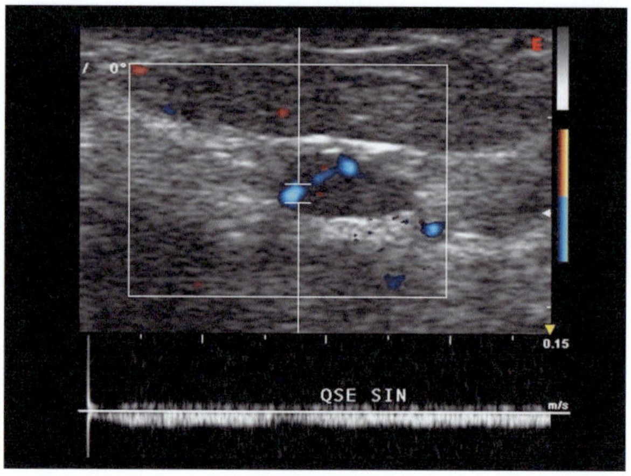

Fig. 4.30 Fibroadenoma. Directional PD and spectral Doppler identify continuous venous flow at the intranodular level

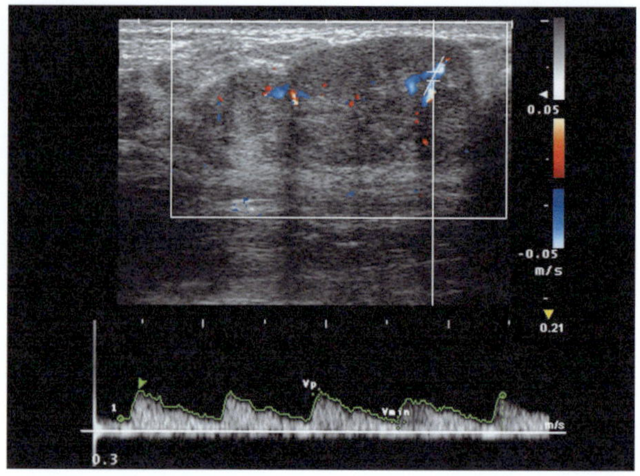

Fig. 4.31 Fibroadenoma. Bilobular nodule with some internal vascular signals at CD and low-resistance spectrum at spectral analysis

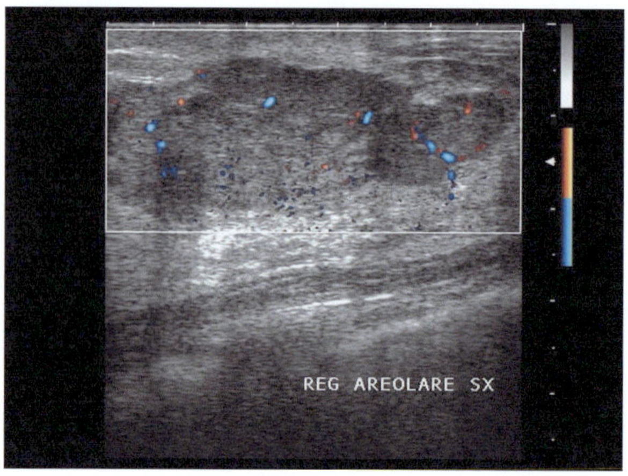

Fig. 4.32 Recurrence of fibroadenoma in 15-year-old patient. Large, macrolobulated, hypoechoic and relatively homogeneous mass with parallel orientation, well-defined margins and some vascular signals at directional PD can be identified in the retroareolar region, already operated on in the past

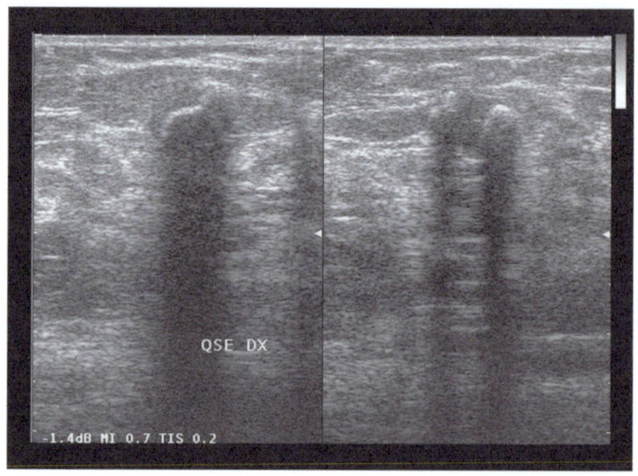

Fig. 4.33 Breast fibroadenoma with macrocalcifications. Oval hypoechoic nodule with large internal calcified nuclei characterized by patent posterior acoustic shadowing

than in the older and predominantly sclerotic lesions. Even the size of the lesion influences the possibility of recognizing flow signals, which are present most of all in medium-sized and large lesions (Figs. 4.35–4.37). When vascular signs are identifiable, the distribution is regular and prevalently peripheral, occasionally with an overall "basket" appearance, which is best appreciated with 3D PD. The vessels tend to be relatively uniform in terms of flow velocity and diameter, and therefore the overall appearance tends to be "monochromatic". Central vessels are only seen in young fibroadenomas or during hormone stimulation or pregnancy. When the vascularity is conspicuous the possibility of a phyllodes tumor should be considered, or of course a carcinoma, even when the B-mode appearance is benign. A correct diagnosis of fibroadenoma can avoid unnecessary surgery, which is usually reserved for symptomatic, rapidly growing lesions >20 mm, with or without hypervascularity at CD.

The **phyllodes tumor** (0.3–1% of all breast tumors) is a rare fibroepithelial neoplasm found prevalently in women aged between 35 and 55 years, although it may be found at any age. It can be distinguished in benign, borderline and malignant disease with a tendency for local recurrence but only with rare cases of metastasis. The tumor generally appears as lobulated nodulations of moderate size (median 46 mm) with well-defined margins, mildly hypoechoic heterogeneous echo pattern and possible posterior acoustic shadowing. Calcifications are rare and generally macroscopic

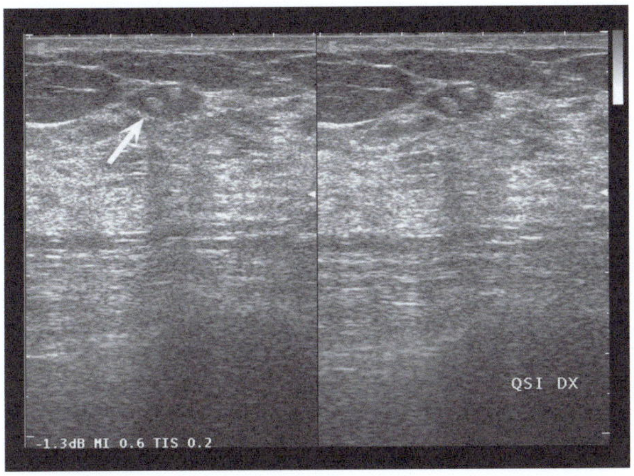

Fig. 4.34 Calcified fibroadenoma. Hypoechoic nodule with well-defined margins and internal macrocalcifications (*arrow*)

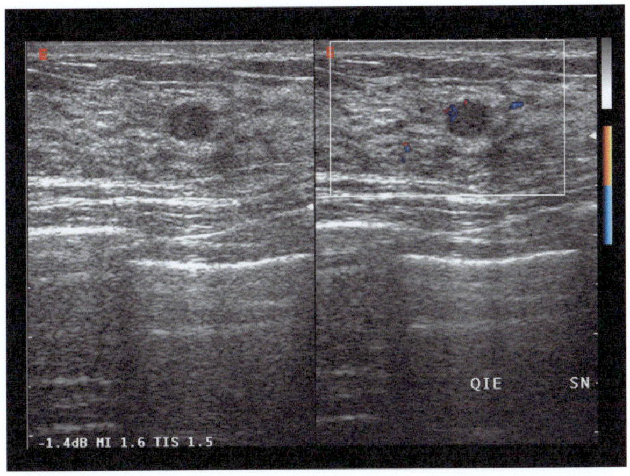

Fig. 4.35 Fibroadenoma mimicking a "dirty" cyst. Small rounded hypoechoic mass with well-defined margins and enhanced through-transmission. Nevertheless, directional PD shows some intralesional flow signals

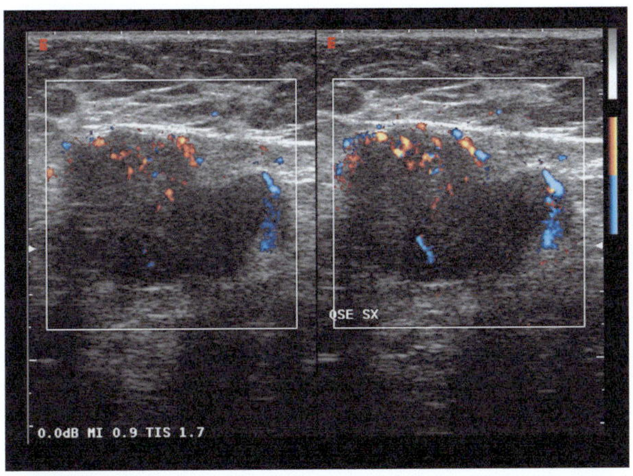

Fig. 4.36 "Young" fibroadenoma. Large macrolobulated nodule with parallel orientation, well-defined margins and moderate peripheral vascularity at directional PD

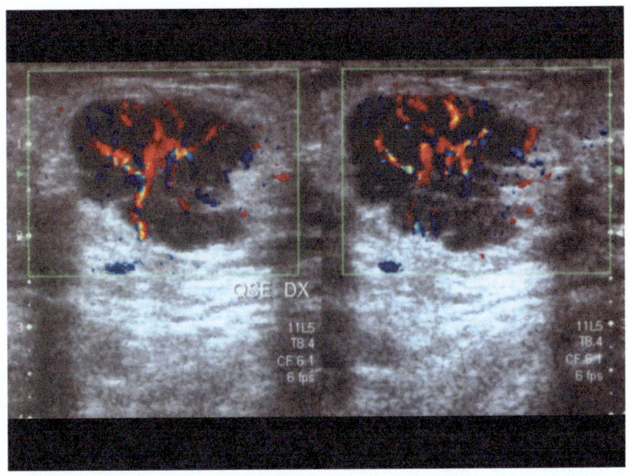

Fig. 4.37 "Young" fibroadenoma. Heterogeneous hypoechoic nodule with multiple vascular poles visible at CD

(Figs. 4.38–4.40, Video 4.6). Vascular signals are found in 97% of cases, with an RI >0.7 in most cases, PI often >1.3 and V_{max} often >15 cm/s. There is therefore a certain amount of overlap with fibroadenoma, although phyllodes tends to have onset in older women, is on average larger and generally without calcifications or posterior acoustic shadowing. Adequate preoperative definition, which may be difficult even at FNAC or core biopsy, can be important due to the risk of a positive resection margin and therefore greater likelihood of recurrence. There is also the risk that a phyllodes tumor with a particularly hypoechoic appearance, posterior acoustic shadowing and signs of intense vascularity at color and spectral Doppler mimics a carcinoma [24,45].

Sclerosing lobular hyperplasia is a relatively infrequent benign proliferative lesion (3–7% of benign biopsies) found especially in young women. It is characterized by hyperplasia of the lobules with interposed sclerosis of the stroma, and is therefore similar to fibroadenoma. Since it is not associated with malignant neoplasms and may spontaneously regress, the lesion does not require surgical resection and therefore a correct diagnosis prior to possible surgery is ideal. At US the lesion appears as well-defined oval or lobulated nodules with a parallel orientation. The only imaging sign that can enable a differential diagnosis with fibroadenoma is the finding of a thin echogenic intralesional septation, especially if it arises from the periphery (incidentally, the presence of echogenic

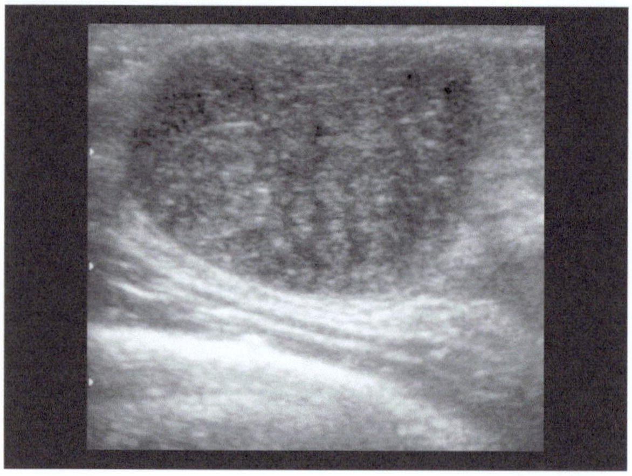

Fig. 4.38 Phyllodes tumor. Large oval nodule with parallel orientation, well-defined margins and heterogeneous echotexture

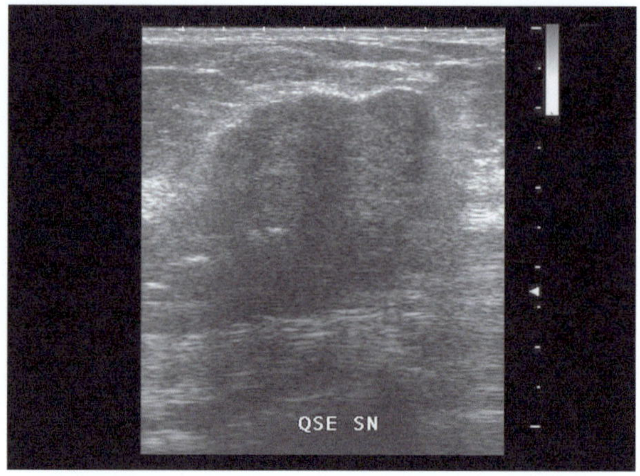

Fig. 4.39 Phyllodes tumor. Large macrolobulated nodule with parallel orientation, mildly heterogeneous echotexture and acoustic shadowing. The anterior margin shows a thin pseudocapsular echogenic image which cannot be identified at the deep margin

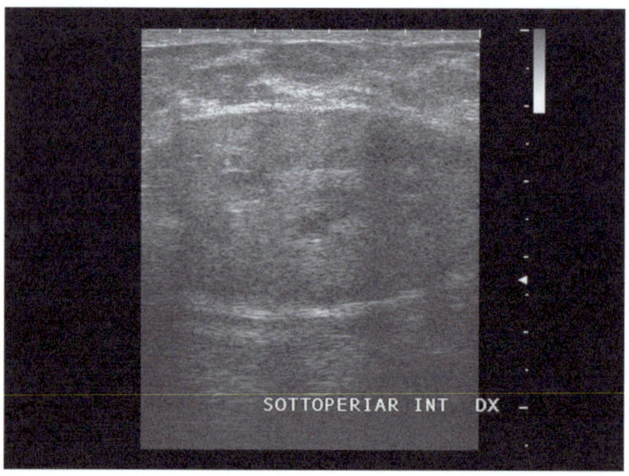

Fig. 4.40 Phyllodes tumor. Large, para-areolar, deep and hypoechoic mass with relatively homogeneous echotexture (central anechoic area) and parallel orientation

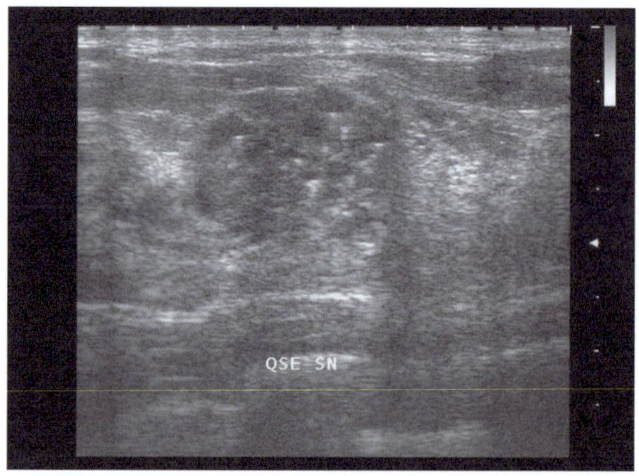

Fig. 4.41 Cystic dysplasia of the breast. Vaguely nodular and thickened area with multiple small cystic masses within

intranodular septations is a sign suggestive of benignity, being found occasionally in fibroadenomas, benign phyllodes tumors and hamartomas) [45].

Cystic lesions are very common, being found in 1 in 4 women between 35 and 50 years of age. They are, however, less frequent below and above this age range, unless the subject is undergoing hormone replacement therapy [13]. Apart from dysplastic and sebaceous cysts, numerous other lesions can have a cystic-like appearance, at least in part or during a phase of their development. These include galactocele, abscess, plasma cell mastitis, seroma, hematoma, lymphocele, fat necrosis, superficial thrombophlebitis of the breast, hemangioma, lymphangioma and arteriovenous malformation [23] (Figs. 4.41–4.43). "Simple" cysts are extremely variable in size and shape and appear homogeneous and anechoic with thin walls and enhanced through-transmission. The lesions may display linear echoes on the anterior side due to reverberation artifacts, or thin internal septations producing a complete or incomplete multilocular structure, often the result of clusters of confluent microcysts. "Complicated" or "dirty" cysts are characterized by multiple low-level internal echoes which may be mobile (this may be demonstrated with M-mode or CD) and in various patient populations have proven to be malignant in 0–0.3% of cases [46]. Internal echoes in a cyst can be due to numerous causes other than papilloma

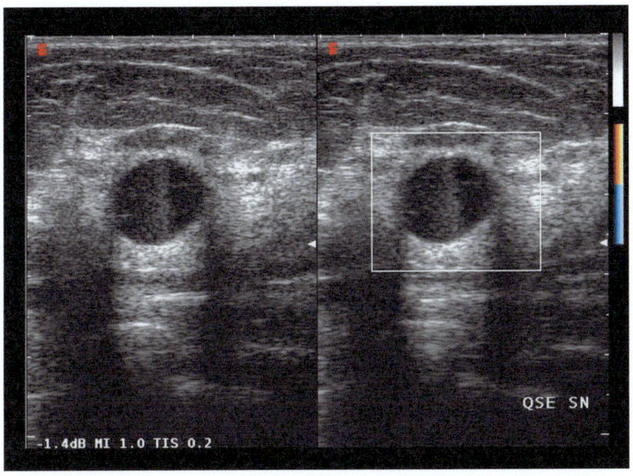

Fig. 4.42 "Dirty" cyst. Hypoechoic mass with well-defined margins, enhanced through-transmission and no vascular signs

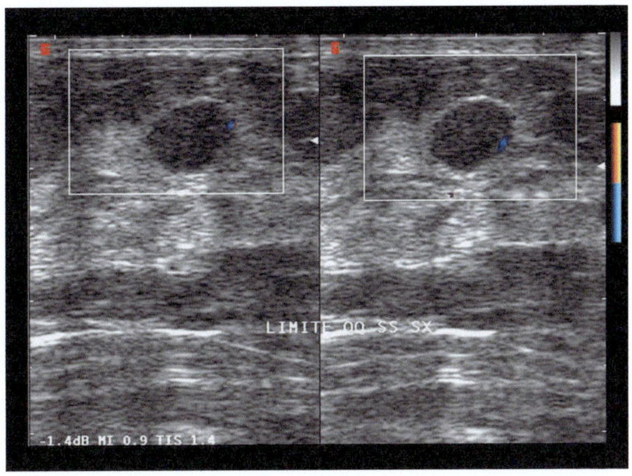

Fig. 4.43 "Dirty" cyst. Well-defined hypoechoic mass with some marginal color signals at directional PD but no internal flow

and carcinoma, such as cell debris, protein globules, cholesterol crystals, floating cells and blood clots [23] (Video 4.7). "Complex" cysts are those that show signs of atypia, such as mural nodules, thick septations or irregular walls, and that are classified as BI-RADS 4. The US appearance of cystic lesions can be subdivided into six patterns (Fig. 4.44): I (simple), anechoic circumscribed mass with imperceptible border and enhanced through-transmission; II (cluster), anechoic cluster mass with no solid components; III (septated), mass with thin septations (<0.5 mm thick); IV (complicated), mass with low-level homogeneous internal echoes or floating debris or fluid-debris levels; V mass with thick walls or septations (>0.5 mm) or with nodules but nonetheless with a fluid component >50%; VI (complex), essentially solid mass with fluid component <50% and eccentric cystic foci corresponding to dilated ductules, acini or necrosis. Types I to IV are always benign, with pattern IV often corresponding to abscesses. Types V and VI are malignant (usually ductal invasive) in 26% and 62% of cases, respectively, or are the expression of fibroadenomas, phyllodes tumors or abscesses [46] (Figs. 4.45–4.50). **Intracystic carcinomas** (0.3–2% of breast cancers) are generally papillary and should be distinguished from papillomas, solid necrotic tumors and blood clots adhering to the wall of the cyst [16,46]. Although the presence of vascular signals in an intracystic solid component increases the suspicion of malignancy (but also benign intracystic solid components may display internal vessels, generally with a low RI spectrum), in reality all complex cysts should be aspirated and subject to cytologic evaluation. In the event of incomplete emptying after aspiration, a core biopsy of the residue is indicated. It should be recalled how some carcinomas, especially large and/or with rapid growth,

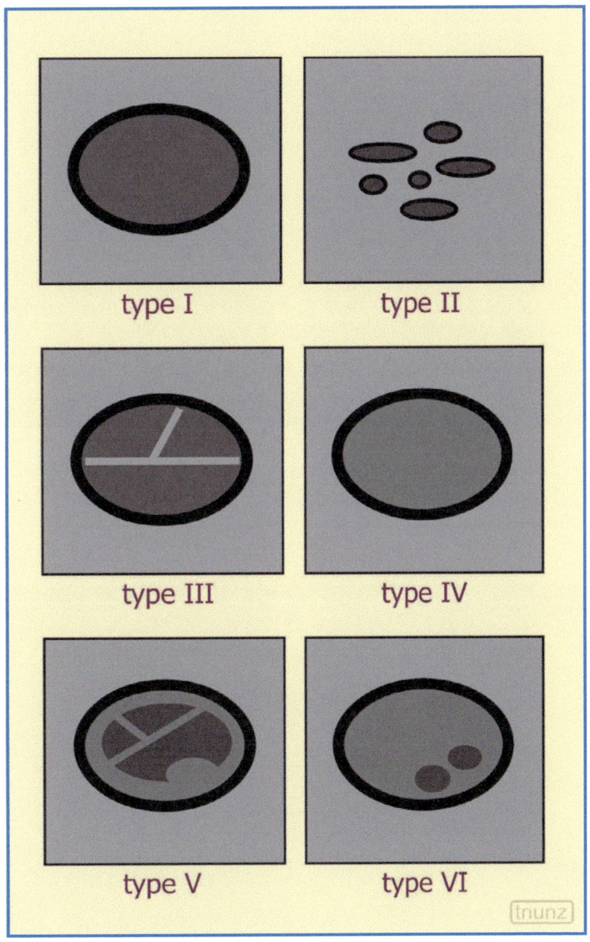

Fig. 4.44 Morphostructural pattern of breast cysts. *Type I*, simple; *Type II*, cluster; *Type III*, septated; *Type IV*, complicated; *Type V*, with thick walls or septations or with nodules, but with a prevalently fluid component; *Type VI*, prevalently solid with eccentric cystic foci. Modified from [46]

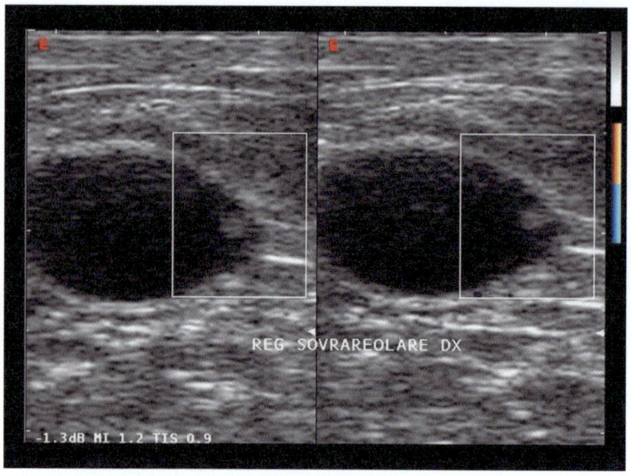

Fig. 4.45 Intracystic papilloma. Small parietal outgrowth with no vascular signals at directional PD

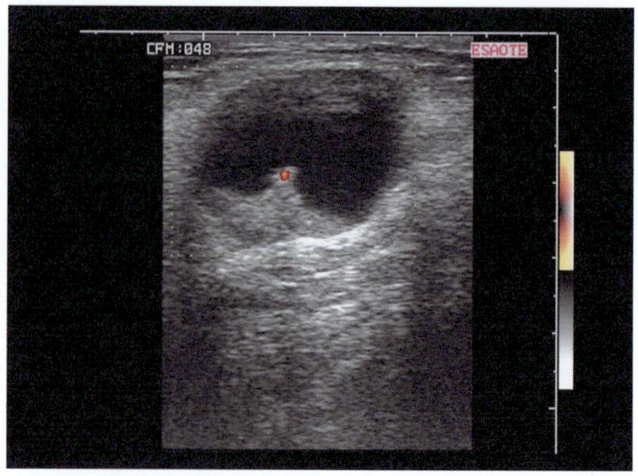

Fig. 4.46 Intracystic papillary carcinoma of the breast. Polypoid mass with vascular signals at directional PD

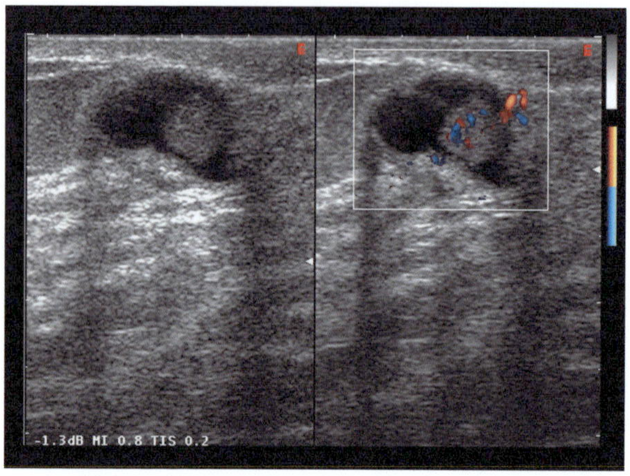

Fig. 4.47 Intracystic carcinoma of the breast. Hypo-anechoic polypoid lesion with a slender base appearing vascular at directional PD

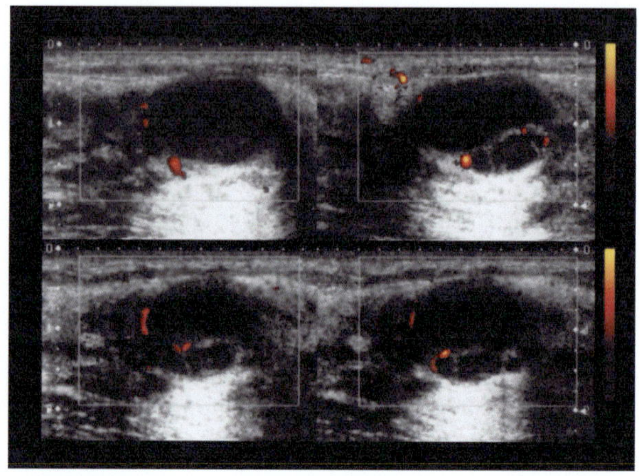

Fig. 4.48 Cystic carcinoma of the breast. Heterogeneous hypo-anechoic solid mass with internal septations and intraseptal color signals at PD

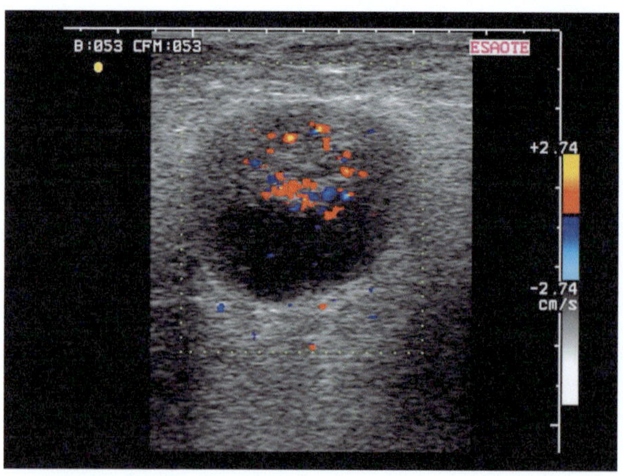

Fig. 4.49 Intracystic carcinoma of the breast. Large solid intracystic outgrowth with evident color signals at CD

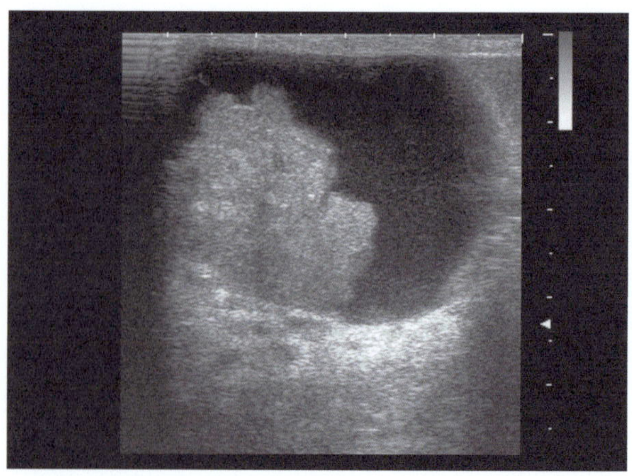

Fig. 4.50 Intracystic carcinoma of the breast. Large broad-based lesion

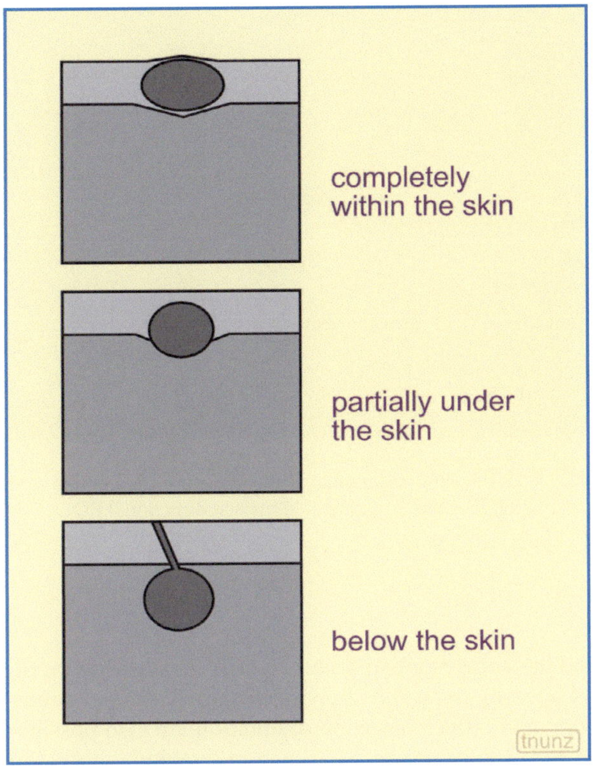

Fig. 4.51 Sebaceous cysts. The lesions may be located completely intradermally, partially subcutaneous or totally below the subcutaneous, but in communication with the surface. Modified from [42]

can be massively necrotic and therefore mimic a "dirty" cyst or an abscess. The demonstration of some flow signals at CD can be misleading [13,47].

Sebaceous cysts have a hypoechoic appearance and are found at the level of the skin or the subcutaneous layer, but generally with a visible hypoechoic duct which reaches the skin, or a deformity of the skin at the margins of the mass itself [23] (Fig. 4.51). The site itself is indicative of benignity and these lesions do not require further study. Suppuration may render the content of the cyst particularly heterogeneous and produce hyperemia of the surrounding tissue at CD.

Galactocele is generally found in pregnant women or women who are or have recently been breast-feeding. It consists of a cystic mass varying in size from a few millimeters to several centimeters which contains milk and is due to obstruction (inflammatory and occasionally neoplastic). The appearance is variable and may include generally well-defined uni- or multilocular cystic images with enhanced through-transmission, intraluminal findings of fat-fluid levels (lower hypoechoic fatty component and upper anechoic fluid component) and pseudosolid echogenic components (occasionally throughout the entire mass). The appearance can at times mimic a solid nodule, with pronounced posterior acoustic shadowing and ill-defined or microlobulated margins. However, galactocele is characteristically a small rounded lesion with a partial anterior or posterior thin echogenic rim (due to the residual of the original ductal walls) and no vascular signals at CD. FNAC, which is indicated in the suspicion of an intracystic neoformation, shows the milk content of the lesion with negative content of malignant cells [48,49] (Figs. 4.52, 4.53).

Lactating adenoma is a slightly tender adenomatous-hyperplastic mass which develops as a response to physiologic hormone stimuli in advanced pregnancy or during breast-feeding. The US appearance is an oval mass with parallel orientation and generally well-defined margins, relatively homogenous hypoechoic structure and enhanced through-transmission. Nonetheless there are atypical forms with irregular margins and acoustic shadowing. The definitive

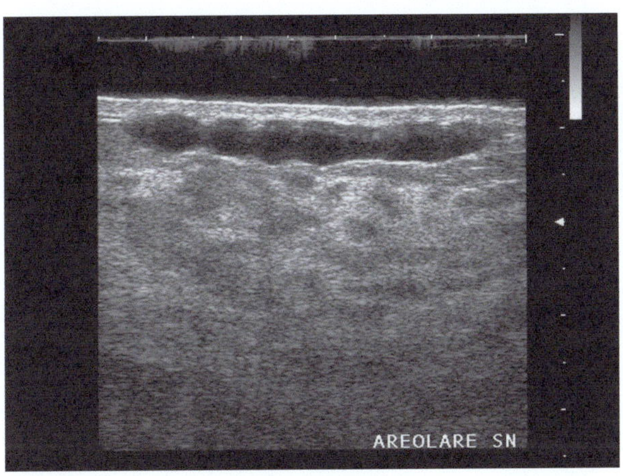

Fig. 4.52 Galactocele. Superficial anechoic mass with extremely elongated shape. Venous thrombosis may have a similar appearance

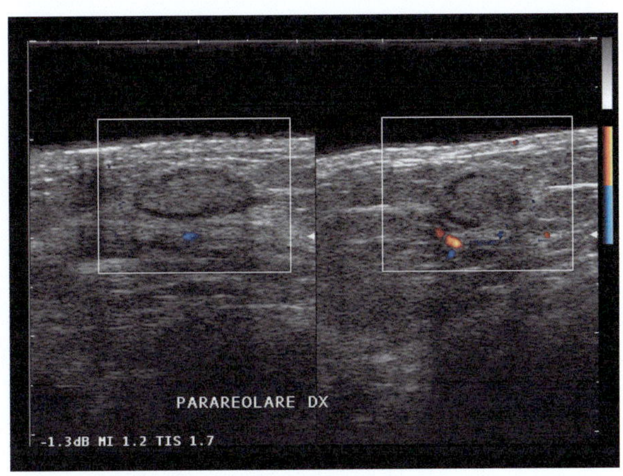

Fig. 4.53 Galactocele. Oval echogenic mass with hypoechoic rim and no vascular signals at directional PD

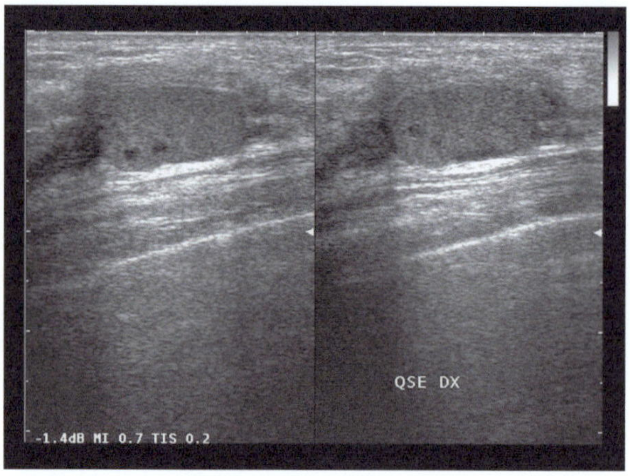

Fig. 4.54 Lactating adenoma of the breast. Oval nodulation with well-defined margins, relatively homogeneous echotexture except for some anechoic areas, and enhanced through-transmission. The lesion is found in a typical location immediately superficial to the fascia

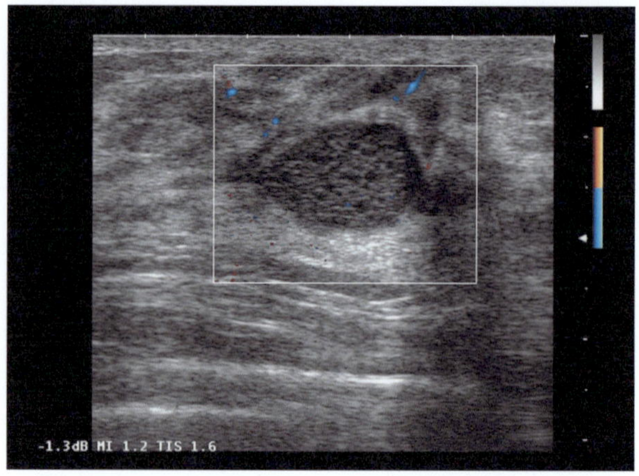

Fig. 4.55 Lactating adenoma of the breast. Cystic lesion with fine septations and no vascular signals at directional PD

diagnosis, which may be hypothesized on the basis of patient history, is the domain of FNAC or, better still, core biopsy, which does however risk creating a "milk fistula" [50] (Figs. 4.54, 4.55).

Intraductal papillomas are relatively common, particularly in women aged between 35 and 55 years, and may be multiple. Intraductal papillary carcinomas on the other hand are rather rare and generally found in middle-aged or elderly women. The lesion clinically presents with a serous or blood secretion from the nipple. US has proven to be a useful complement or alternative to galactography in the study of patients with breast secretion, palpable retroareolar lesions or retroareolar thickening at mammography [51]. US study, especially if performed with the transducer parallel to the long axis of the duct and prior to breast expression, which would otherwise empty the duct itself, is able to identify hypoechoic tissue partially or totally occupying the anechoic ductal lumen [13] (Figs. 4.56–4.59).

Abscesses are not uncommon either in adolescents or in adult subjects, regardless of milk production. The lesion is characterized as a complex mass with areas of differing echogenicity due to the coexistence of edematous and inflamed echogenic portions and other liquefactive hypo-anechoic areas. CD can demonstrate perifocal hyperemia but with a low-resistance "benign" spectrum (Fig. 4.60).

Granular cell tumor is a relatively infrequent lesion with a mean peak incidence at 52 years. The lesion may occasionally be locally aggressive and has an appearance of hypoechoic or rarely hyperechoic nodules with heterogeneous echotexture and occasionally irregular margins. An echogenic halo may be seen on the superficial wall and acoustic shadowing on the deep wall, as well as hypervascularity. Beam attenuation and taller-than-wide orientation are also possible. The US appearance, as at mammography, is therefore nonspecific and may mimic malignancy [52,53].

Lipomas appear as generally superficial lesions which are often completely contained in a lobule of fat. They have a generally pronounced hyperechoic appearance occasionally with mild internal heterogeneity. The hyperechogenicity of a breast nodule is a reliable indicator of presumed benignity [13] (Figs. 4.61, 4.62, Video 4.8).

Hemangiomas are rather rare and appear as oval superficial lesions varying in size and usually with well-defined margins. They present a hypoechoic, isoechoic or complex echo pattern and are only rarely hyperechoic [54].

Fat necrosis refers to an area of necrosis of the adipose tissue which is progressively circumscribed by an encapsulating fibrocalcific reaction. The condition may appear after trauma or surgery (distinct from recurrence after breast-sparing surgery) [13,55]. The cystic forms ("oil cysts") appear complex, heterogeneous and hyperechoic, with a generally thick and continuous external echogenic layer and possible internal echogenic areas or bands and evident posterior acoustic shadowing. In the fibrotic forms the appearance is more solid, heterogeneous and hypoechoic (occasionally even homogeneous hyperechoic), with irregular margins, calcifications and possible posterior acoustic shadowing. The identification of internal oil microcysts can nonetheless correctly characterize the lesion, and the combined mammographic and US findings may be sufficient, in typical cases, for a definitive

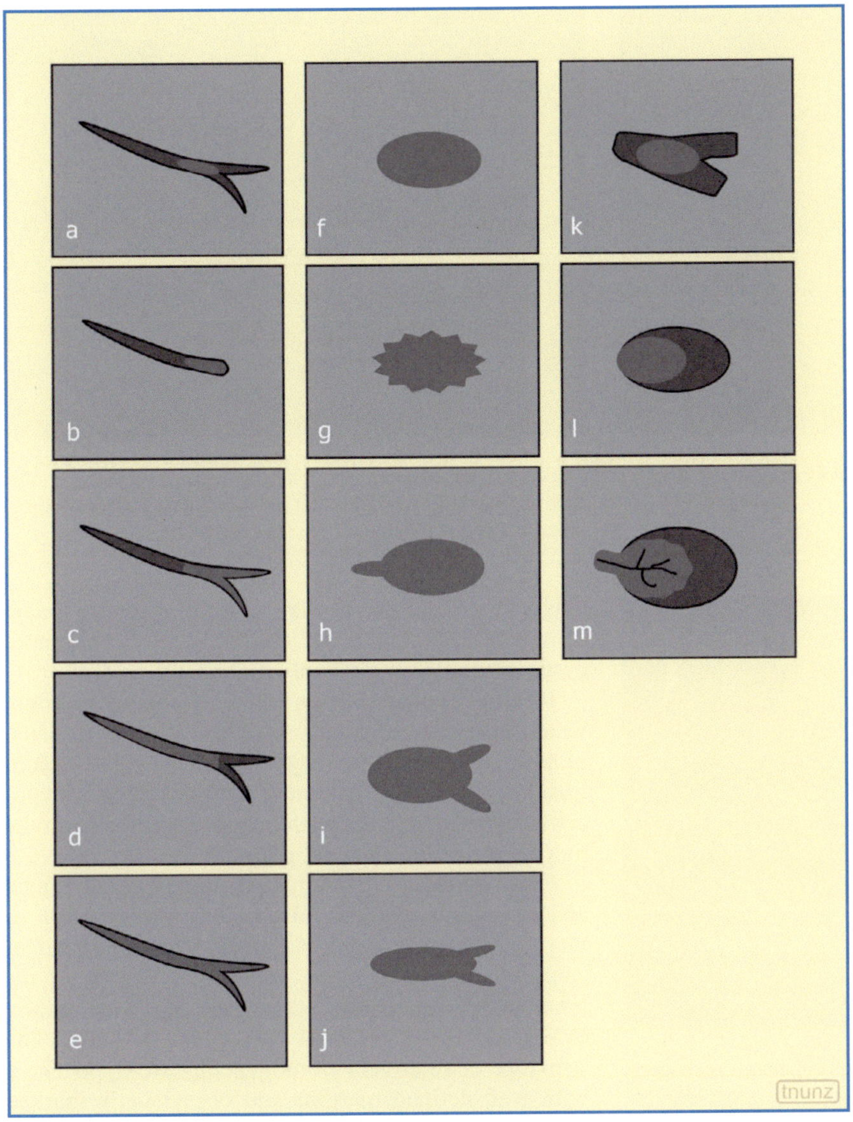

Fig. 4.56 Morphostructural pattern of intraductal tumors. The three columns show the different appearances of these lesions in the presence of ductal dilatation, absent dilatation and ductal extension and branching. Modified from [42]

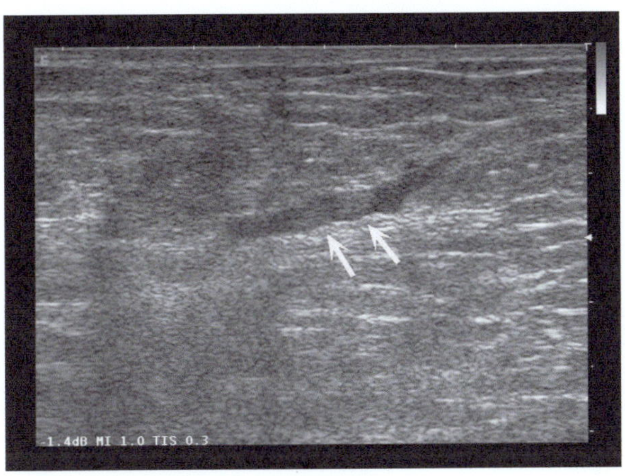

Fig. 4.57 Intraductal papillomas. Two small hypoechoic lesions (*arrows*) within a dilated duct

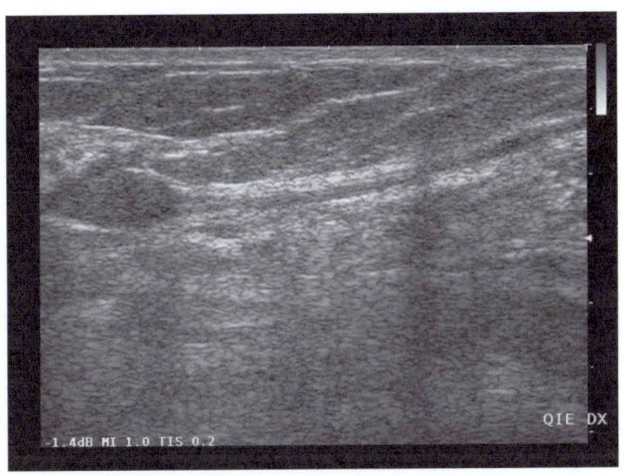

Fig. 4.58 Intraductal papilloma. Moderately-sized lesion located at the end of a dilated lactiferous duct

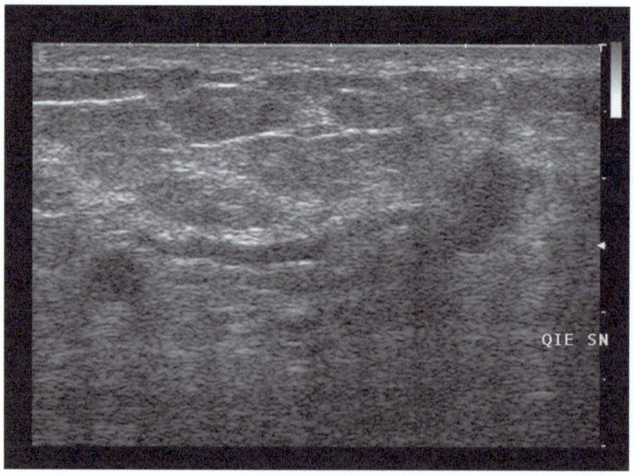

Fig. 4.59 Intraductal papilloma. Moderately-sized lesion located at the end of a dilated duct

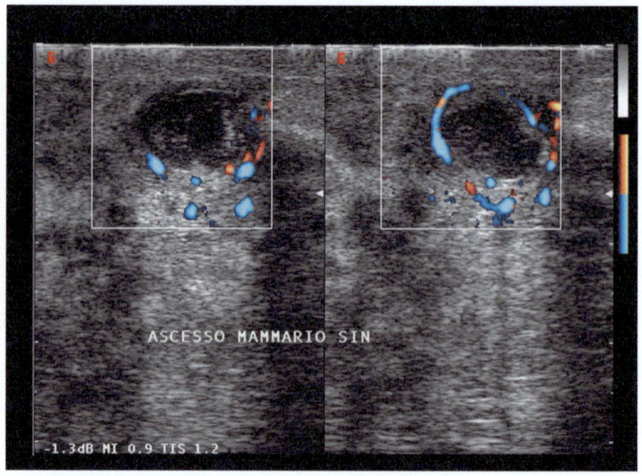

Fig. 4.60 Breast abscess. Small heterogeneous hypoechoic mass with a hyperemic appearance of the surrounding tissue at directional PD and thickening of the skin surface

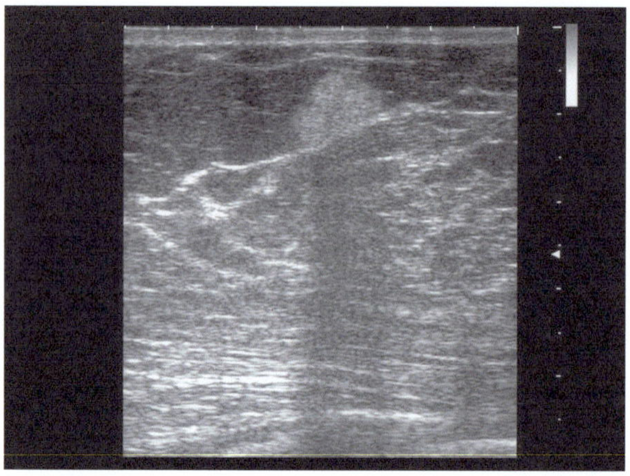

Fig. 4.61 Intramammary lipoma. Subcutaneous echogenic nodule with posterior acoustic shadowing

diagnosis. At follow-up the lesions may appear stable or undergo involution while tending to become more cystic internally or generally more solid.

Radial scars are benign lesions of unknown origin which develop particularly after resection or excision biopsy. When >1 cm they may be palpable and at imaging mimic a neoplasm. The appearance is hypoechoic with intense deep attenuation and as such invite biopsy, possibly excision biopsy.

Focal fibrosis is a stromal proliferation with ductal and lobular obliteration. It is rather common (4–8% of biopsied breast lesions) and arises from a number of causative factors, such as regional involution of the breast tissue. Its appearance is variable, with usually oval nodulations oriented parallel to the skin. The structure is relatively homogeneous iso-hypoechoic with well-defined margins and occasionally marked

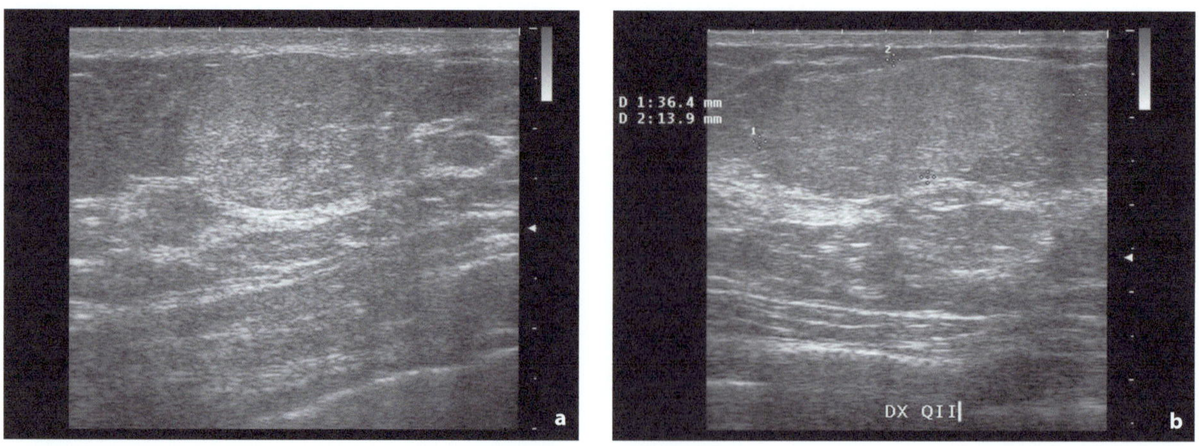

Fig. 4.62a,b Multiple lipomas of the breast. Two superficial, oval, echogenic nodulations, one more homogeneous than the other and both with parallel orientation

posterior acoustic shadowing. Given its nonspecific nature, FNAC or, better still, core biopsy is generally indicated [56].

Diabetic mastopathy arises in patients with long-term diabetes mellitus and in postmenopause. The pseudonodular lesion varies in size from a few millimeters to several centimeters and is usually poorly defined at mammography although better visualized at US. The appearance is nonetheless nonspecific: hypoechoic ill-defined nodule with posterior acoustic shadowing such that FNAC is generally indicated (provided that the patient history is indicative) [23].

Lymphomatous breast lesions are uncommon but possible, in both women (1% of all breast tumors) and men. They appear as generally well-defined, hypervascular, hypoechoic nodules with or without enhanced through-transmission. On rare occasions diffuse architectural undermining may be found. Axillary lymphadenopathies may be associated [57,58] (Fig. 4.63).

Metastases to the breast are rare, with possible development via lymphatic or hematogenous spread, especially from lymphomas and melanomas, and may even manifest as "mastitis". The lesions are often multiple and bilateral with a variable appearance, often as masses similar to fibroadenomas (well-defined, homogeneous and without particular acoustic shadowing), but often with intense and chaotic vascular signals (Fig. 4.64).

Nonepithelial primary tumors of the breast are rare (Fig. 4.65).

Lastly, **false nodular images** need to be considered [47]. Several physiologic findings can mimic a focal lesion, particularly in a predominantly adipose breast. Cooper's ligaments, suspended between the parenchyma and the subcutaneous layer, and various connective structures can create posterior acoustic shadowing, particularly when oblique to the ultrasound beam, and therefore mimic a hypoechoic focal lesion. However, the finding is attenuated if not completely resolved by varying the scan plane and/or compressing the image with the transducer. It is therefore possible to differentiate these images from real focal lesions: the posterior shadow is not associated with any lesion so that with a little experience its cause can be found in more superficial echogenic structures. The nipple-areola complex can mimic beam attenuation secondary to a focal lesion, although awareness of the event and the possibility of scanning at different insonation angles or with the use of a spacer can generally identify the false images. Posterior acoustic shadowing can be created by an artery with a calcified wall, especially when the vessel is scanned in a transverse section. The rotation of the transducer, however,

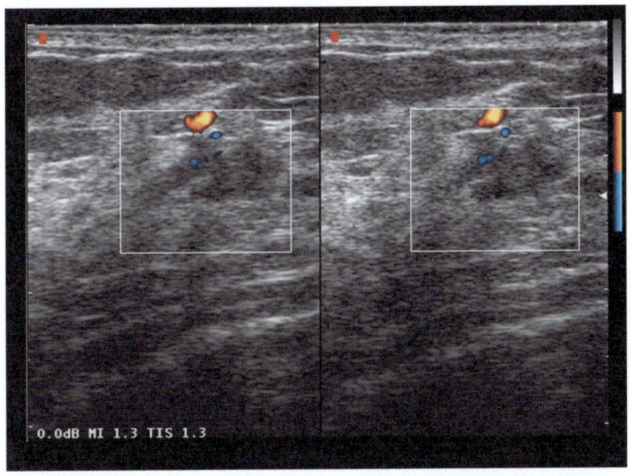

Fig. 4.63 Breast MALToma. Ill-defined, hypoechoic nodule

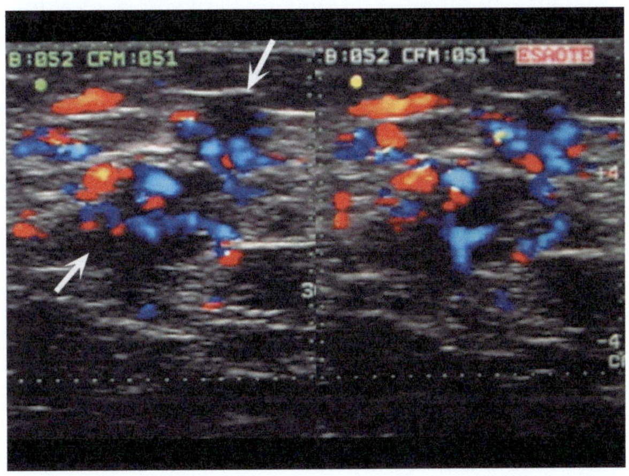

Fig. 4.64 Intramammary metastasis from melanoma. Two hypoechoic nodules with hypervascular appearance at CD (*arrows*)

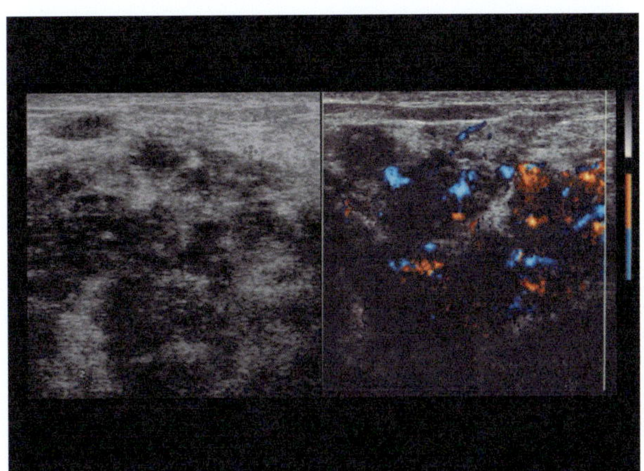

Fig. 4.65 Primary angiosarcoma of the breast. Large, irregular and infiltrating breast tumor tissue with heterogeneous hypoechoic echostructure and irregular vascular appearance at directional PD (where several avascular areas can also be identified)

reveals the characteristic binary vessel image. The adipose lobules of the normal glandular structure can mimic a nodular lesion, especially a fibroadenoma. Careful rotation of the transducer, however, is able to demonstrate the continuity between the nodular-like lobule and the surrounding adipose tissue. The intramammary lymph nodes, which may occasionally be identified in the axillary tail or the upper outer quadrant, or more rarely in the lower external quadrant, can mimic a tumor, especially when the shape is rounded and the echogenic center is poorly identifiable or absent. In general, however, the characteristic US signs of the nodal structure can be identified and CD usually shows a single vessel penetrating the echogenic hilum (Fig. 4.66). The port chambers of port-catheter systems in women undergoing chemotherapy and the valves of expandable breast implants can mimic a lesion with acoustic shadowing, but these cases can generally be resolved with an appropriate analysis of the patient history. Silicon granulomas, which particularly arise in the event of extracapsular rupture of a prosthesis, appear as echogenic areas with posterior shadowing, reverberation and snowstorm pattern and may mimic hyperechoic nodules, whereas the collections of free silicon appear as cystic-like masses with a typical anteroposterior development. The costal cartilage, with its homogeneous hypoechoic appearance, or hypoechoic appearance with echogenic foci in the event of calcifications, can mimic a focal lesion (especially a cyst or a fibroadenoma) when transversely scanned. The rotation of the transducer however shows the entire length of the cartilage, which is also deeper than the breast tissue.

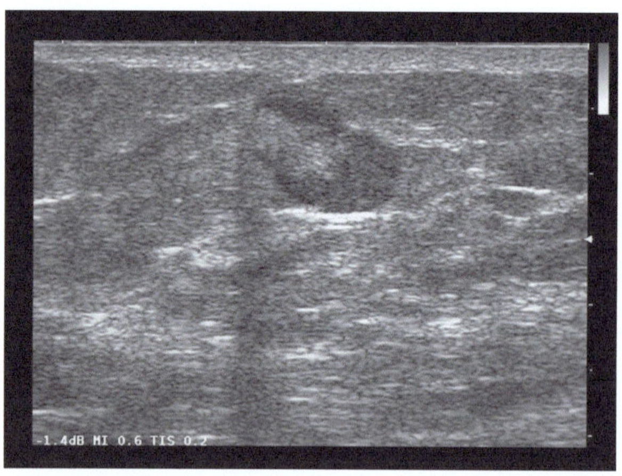

Fig. 4.66 Hyperplastic inflammatory lymph node. Enlarged lymph node with asymmetric cortical thickening

4.2 Locally Advanced Breast Cancer

Inflammatory carcinoma (carcinomatous mastitis) accounts for 1–6% of newly diagnosed breast cancers, with an incidence of 0.7 cases/100,000/year and a mean age at diagnosis of 55 years (although in recent years the number of cases in women <50 years has increased) [1,59,60]. It may consist of any histotype and is by definition a form of locally advanced carcinoma (T4d), with frequent axillary adenopathies and distant metastasis at presentation (five-year survival rate of 25–48%). It is associated with thickening and induration of the skin, edema and erythema and is due to infiltration of the dermal lymphatic vessels by tumor cells which can be shown histologically. A distinction needs to be made between the form which emerges secondary to the spread of an advanced carcinoma and the form which presents an inflammatory appearance right from the outset, a distinction which is not always possible in practice. The primary form of inflammatory carcinoma is characterized by its marked aggressiveness, its relatively sudden onset and its typical intense angiogenesis and angioinvasiveness [59]. It may in turn be subdivided into "common" (50% of cases), where clinical evidence of inflammatory carcinoma and histologic findings are associated, "clinical" (40% of cases), where histologic findings are absent, and "clinical occult", where dermal lymphatic invasion histologically is not associated with corresponding clinical findings [60]. Skin thickening is a nonspecific finding, since it may also be found in edematous forms of various origin (such as secondary to axillary dissection or even venous thrombosis), in mastitis from breast-feeding and infectious mastitis (where nonetheless liquefactive-abscess components may be found) [16]. In addition to skin thickening, US is able to identify the signs of diffuse subcutaneous edema, with transverse hypoechoic bands and strips, and neoplastic infiltration of the corpus mammae which presents heterogeneous, hypoechoic and ill-defined areas, which take on a nodular appearance only in part. The cytologic or microhistologic sampling of the areas with the greatest nodularity and vascular signals at CD usually confirms the diagnosis [59] (Figs. 4.67, 4.68).

Locally advanced breast cancer (LABC) is defined by a lesion with a diameter >3 cm and/or with positive axillary lymph nodes [61]. The state of the axillary region is especially important for the staging and therapeutic management of these patients and should be evaluated cytologically. In one study population, US-guided FNAC produced a sensitivity and specificity of 100% for the diagnosis of lymph node metastases [61] (Figs. 4.69, 4.70).

Women with inflammatory carcinoma or LABC are

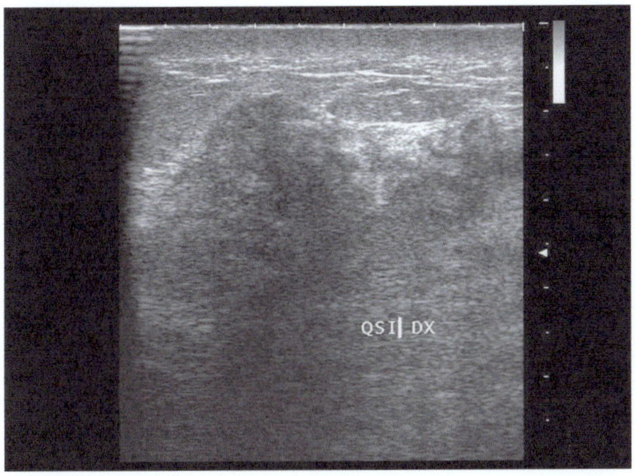

Fig. 4.67 Inflammatory carcinoma of the breast. Diffuse echostructural remodeling of the breast with thickening of the overlying skin

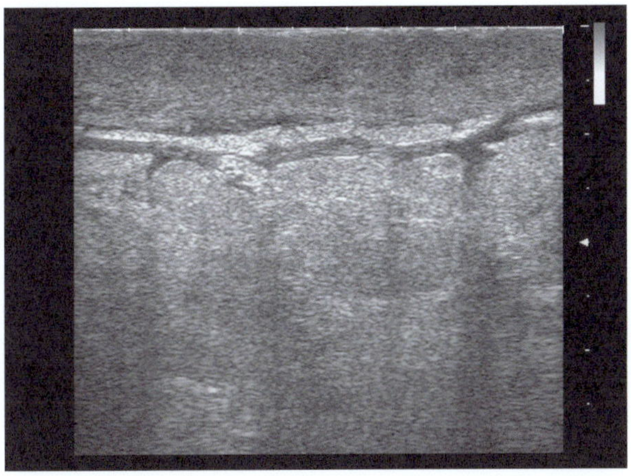

Fig. 4.68 Carcinomatous mastitis. Marked hypoechoic thickening of the skin associated with edematous hypoechoic strips and bands between the echogenic lobules of subcutaneous fat

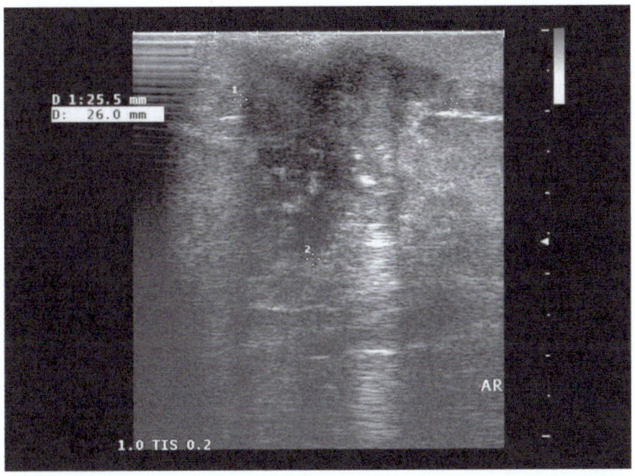

Fig. 4.69 Locally advanced breast cancer. Tumor with infiltrating margins and microcalcifications extended to the areolar skin

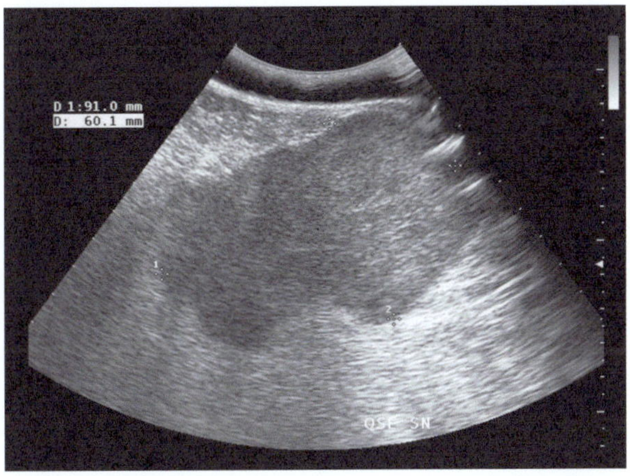

Fig. 4.70 Locally advanced breast cancer. Solid and very large breast mass (>9 cm) with hypoechoic echostructure, relatively homogeneous echotexture and well-defined margins, which can be visualized and measured only with the use of an abdominal probe

generally treated with neoadjuvant **chemotherapy** or **hormone therapy** with the aim of reducing the stage of the disease and rendering the lesion operable. A complete response is obtained in 10% of cases and a partial response in 75% [62]. However, no standard procedures have been developed with regard to the duration and intensity of the neoadjuvant treatment. Microscopic residual tumor, which is present in almost all cases, is not particularly significant, and the treatment result is considered excellent if no macroscopic residual disease is found at the subsequent surgical resection. An effective response is correlated with a better outlook than in cases with residual, since it is associated with an increased disease-free interval and better survival. Being able to preoperatively verify the disappearance of macroscopic tumor is nonetheless crucial, since this can enable breast-sparing surgery. Similarly, a negative finding for the axillary lymph nodes makes a sentinel lymph node procedure possible in place of surgical dissection of all the axillary lymph nodes [63,64]. Even the choice of postoperative medical therapy is influenced by the presence or otherwise of residual tumor [62].

Traditionally, **evaluation of the response** of LABC to neoadjuvant treatment is entrusted to the physical examination and mammography, with the more recent introduction of US. It should, however, be noted that in this setting contrast-enhanced MR is taking on an increasingly important role, thanks to the possibility of quantifying the treatment response on perfusion maps.

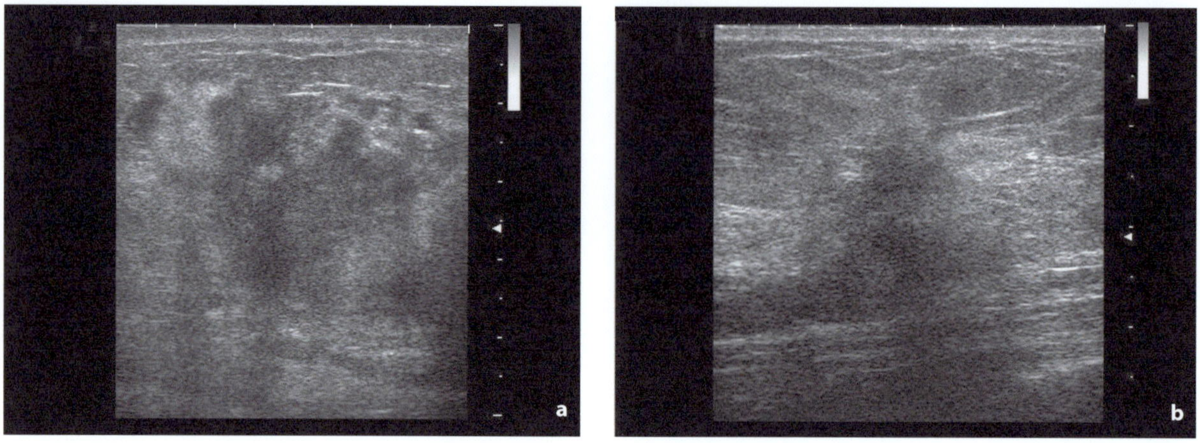

Fig. 4.71a,b Locally advanced breast cancer, before and after chemotherapy. Diffuse echostructural remodeling of the breast (**a**) which is notably reduced after neoadjuvant chemotherapy (**b**)

Other suggested options are scintimammography with Tc^{99m} MIBI, PET and CT [62,65]. It is not uncommon for there to be disagreement between clinical, mammographic, US and surgical findings in women with LABC who have undergone neoadjuvant treatment [63]. In nearly half of cases with a complete response according to clinical findings residual tumor is found at subsequent surgery, and around 20% of women with an apparently partial response are found to have had a complete response at surgery. Palpation can be undermined by a number of factors, with false positives in the case of residual fibrotic or necrotic tissue mimicking the persistence of disease and false negatives if the regression of post-biopsy edematous or hemorrhagic changes mimics a reduction in neoplastic tissue [62]. PET and MR have proven to be accurate in the early definition of response and the latter is today considered the morphologic and functional reference modality [64]. The physical examination and mammography are superior to US in defining the size of residual disease after neoadjuvant treatment, and the use of US has not influenced the predictive accuracy of the preoperative evaluation [63]. Nonetheless, US has proven superior to the physical examination and mammography in determining residual lymph node status. Therefore, a combined use of physical examination, mammography and US in all cases appears desirable [63].

The US measurement of **residual tumor** is often problematic since in addition to the known panoramic limitations and problems of objectivity with the technique is the fact that the lesions are often ill-defined and multifocal, with a mixture of zones of healthy tissue and zones of diseased tissue. There are also the problems of the fibrous phenomena induced by the treatment and the subsequent increase in echogenicity of the lesion and the greater difficulty identifying it against the parenchymal background [62,64,65]. Particularly extensive or deep lesions can be difficult to include in the US FOV, thus creating difficulties in evaluating the size of the lesion. Monofocal forms which are relatively circumscribed and hypoechoic can be well-defined and followed up with US [66]. In addition, the CD study may show a reduction or disappearance of vascular signals and therefore provide early indication of positive treatment response, just as an increase in vascularity may predict disease progression. CD appears to be reliable when there is no macroscopic residual tumor, but may produce false negatives in the event of persistence of such residual disease [62,66]. The use of contrast media can increase the detection of intralesional vascular signals both before and possibly after treatment, thus rendering the CD evaluation more reliable [67]. The skin thickness should also be measured, since it is an indicator of edema, and its progression should be monitored (Figs. 4.71–4.73).

4.3 Lymph Node Metastasis

Axillary lymphadenopathies are the single most important prognostic factor for operable breast cancer (Fig. 4.74). Lymphadenopathies are present in 20% of T1 and 35% of T2 tumors, and the likelihood of their presence is correlated with the size of the nodule. In some cases the evidently small-sized primary breast tumor is occult (CUP syndrome) and lymph node metastasis is the first manifestation of disease.

Three levels of surgical lymph nodes can be identified in the axilla: proximal (level I), caudal and lateral to the inferior margin of the pectoralis minor muscle;

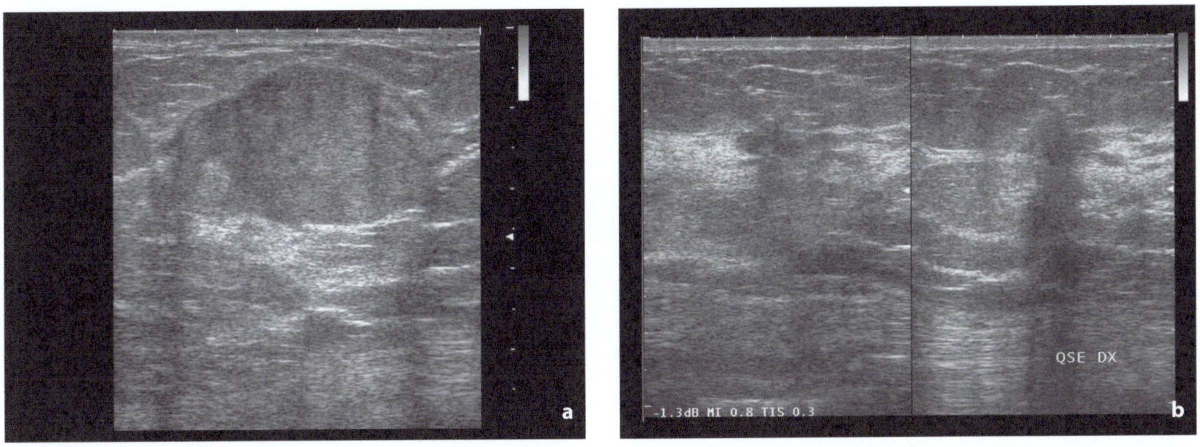

Fig. 4.72a,b Locally advanced breast cancer, before and after chemotherapy. Large breast tumor (**a**) is notably reduced in size after neoadjuvant chemotherapy (**b**)

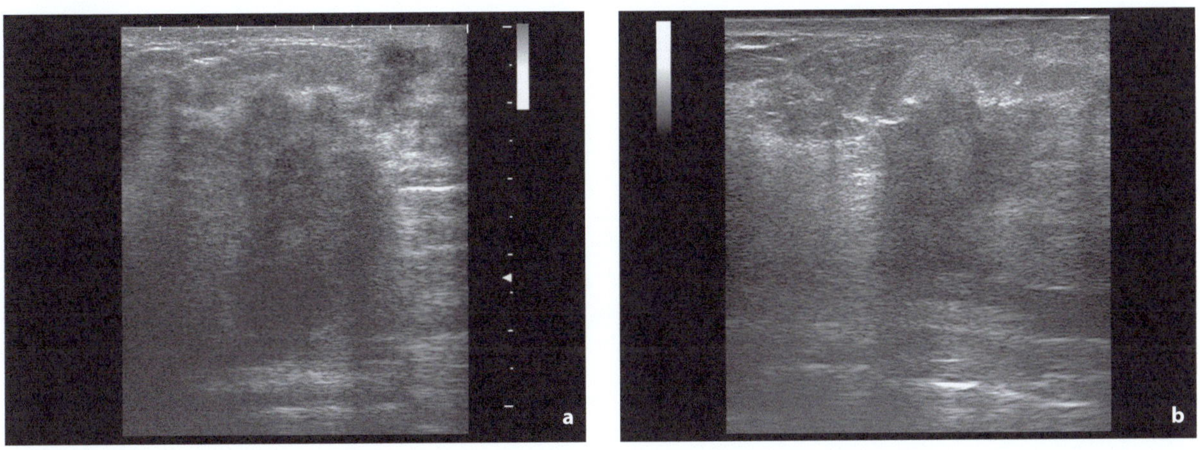

Fig. 4.73a,b Locally advanced breast cancer, before and after chemotherapy. Large breast lesion with satellite lesions towards the skin (**a**) appears markedly reduced after neoadjuvant therapy (**b**)

middle (level II), lying underneath the pectoralis minor muscle; distal (level III), between the superior margin of the pectoralis minor muscle and the thoracic inlet of the axillary vein (Fig. 4.75). These levels are usually involved in a progressive manner (although in 30% of cases levels II and III can be metastasized without involvement of level I nodes) and the extent of their involvement correlates with prognosis [68].

Palpable axillary lymph nodes are metastatic in around 75% of cases, whereas nonpalpable axillary lymph nodes are metastatic in around 30% of cases. Overall the physical examination has shown a sensitivity of 50–74% and a specificity of 48–91% in different patient populations. US is more accurate than both the physical examination and mammography in identifying metastatic axillary lymph nodes, although even its accuracy is not optimal, especially for lymph nodes at the axillary apex, such that a negative study cannot definitively rule out the presence of metastases [69]. Patently abnormal lymph nodes at US leave little diagnostic doubt, especially when the study reveals disappearance of the central echogenic hilum (whereas asymmetric thickening of the cortex is nonspecific and can lead to false positives), rounded shape, size >10 mm and fixity. If the size criterion alone is considered, US has a sensitivity of 49–87% and a specificity of 56–97% in the identification of nonpalpable lymph nodes, whereas when morphologic criteria are associated, the sensitivity is 26–76% and specificity 88–98% [69]. In a study on patients with BI-RADS 5 nodules, the most common lymph node patterns were diffuse hypoechoic (45% of cases, with metastasis in 87% of these), focal cortical thickening (20% of cases, with metastasis in 53% of these) and diffuse cortical thickening (35% of cases, with metastasis on 30% of these). These findings underline the need for further

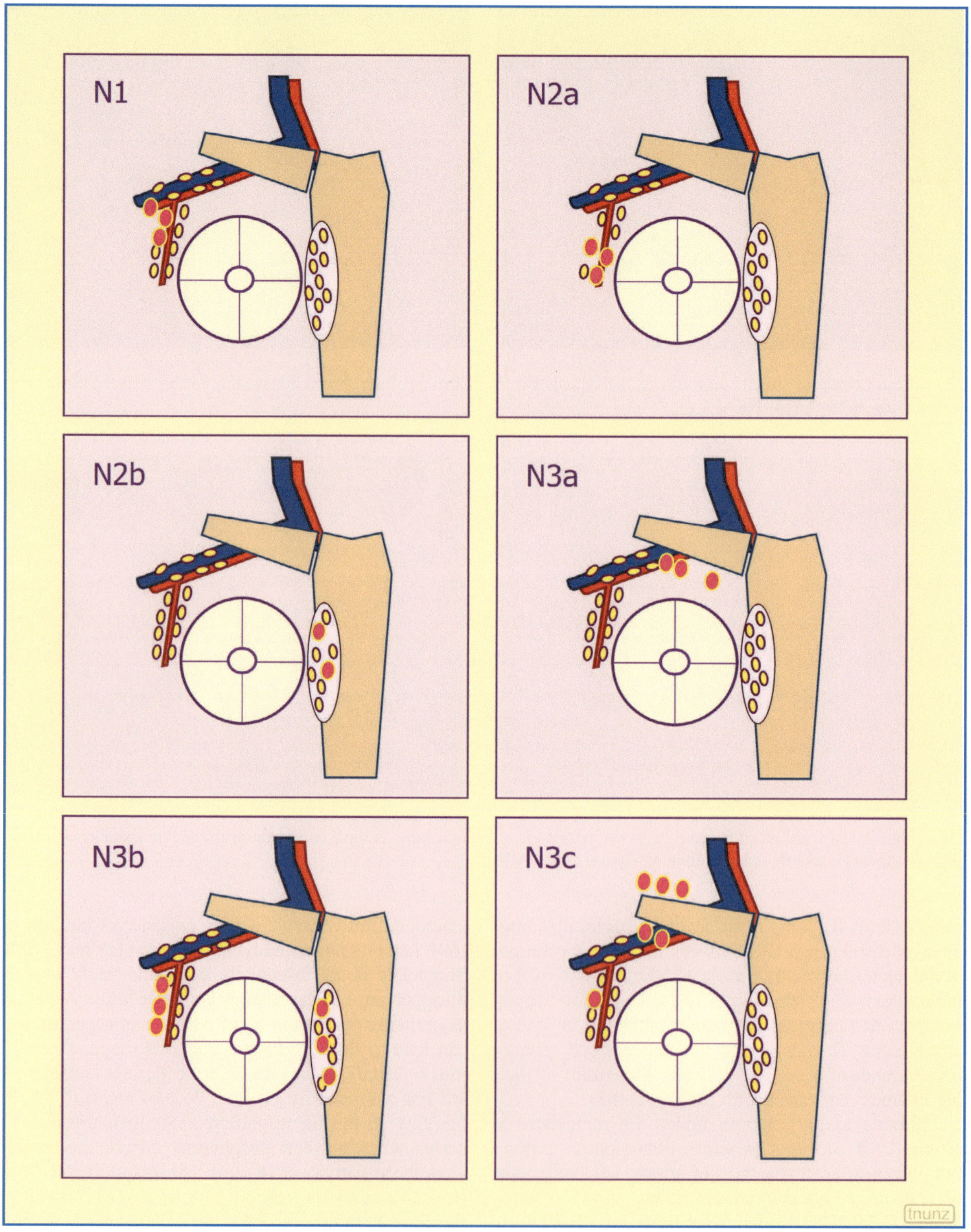

Fig. 4.74 N parameter for breast cancer. Regional lymph nodes include axillary, infraclavicular, internal mammary and supraclavicular, all only if ipsilateral. *N1*, single or multiple metastases to movable ipsilateral axillary lymph node(s); *N2a*, axillary metastases fixed to one another or to other structures; *N2b*, metastasis only in the internal mammary lymph nodes identified with imaging; *N3a*, subclavicular metastases; *N3b*, associated internal mammary and axillary metastases; *N3c*, supraclavicular metastases. Modified from [43]

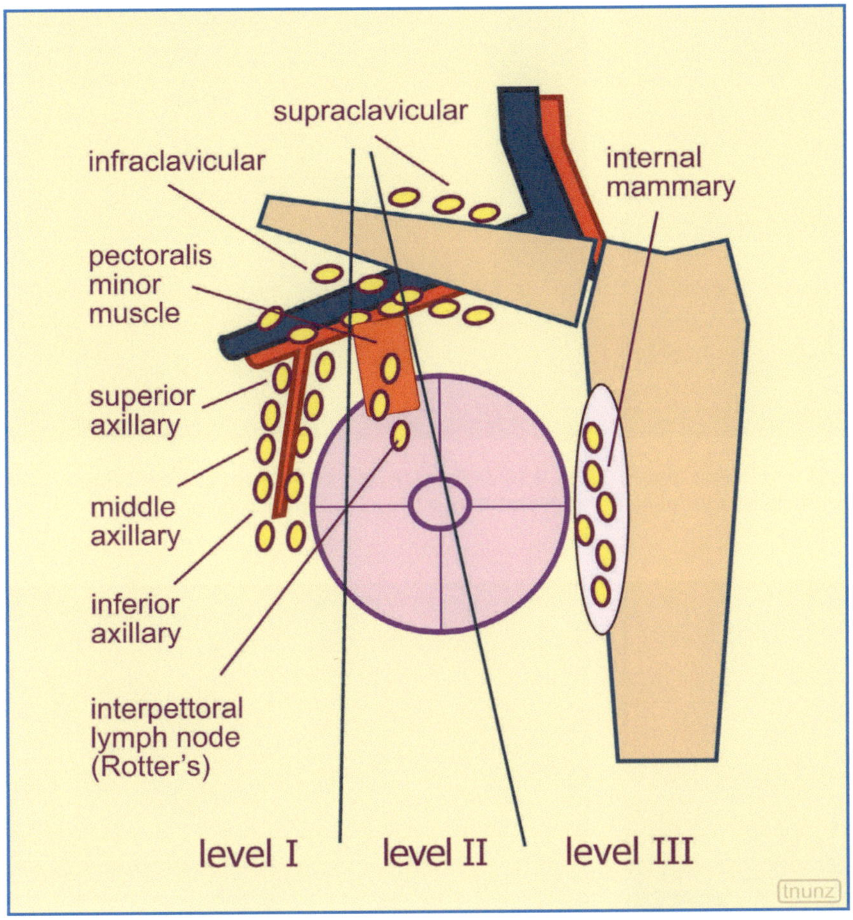

Fig. 4.75 Levels of axillary lymph nodes. *Level I*, inferior axilla, lymph nodes lateral with respect to the lateral margin of the pectoralis minor; *Level II*, middle axilla, lymph nodes between the lateral and medial margins of the pectoralis minor and interpectoral lymph nodes; *Level III*, axillary apex, lymph nodes medial to the medial border of the pectoralis minor (excluding the supraclavicular). Modified from [43]

investigation of lymph nodes with a conserved hilum but with diffusely or focally thickened cortex, if the thickness is >2 mm [70]. In an in vitro study the most specific patterns were the presence of focal lobulations of the lymph node cortex and the absence of an echogenic hilum [71].

In cases where the axillary lymph nodes appear suspicious or indeterminate, an integration with FNAC may be useful. This has shown a sensitivity of 31–100% and a specificity of 100% in identifying axillary metastases [61,69,71,73]. The sensitivity of FNAC, which is performed on the most suspicious or the largest lymph node, is correlated with the size of the primary tumor [74]. In terms of cost/benefit, the best option is routine axillary US with FNAC of the suspicious lymph nodes identified and surgical dissection only in cases with positive cytology. An alternative to FNAC, still with the aim of avoiding unnecessary sentinel lymph node procedures, is core biopsy, which is more invasive but more reliable [73] (Figs. 4.76–4.81).

Internal mammary lymphadenopathies are located in the anterior mediastinum immediately posterolateral to the sternum. This region is generally not examined, because it is a relatively infrequent site of lymph node metastasis at the time of the presentation of the primary tumor (the same holds true even for

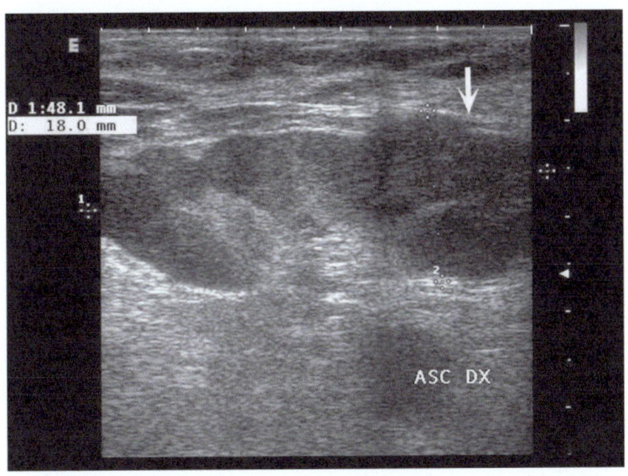

Fig. 4.76 Axillary lymph node metastasis from breast cancer. Large lymphadenopathy with asymmetric cortical thickening which displays a hypoechoic nodule at one end (*arrow*)

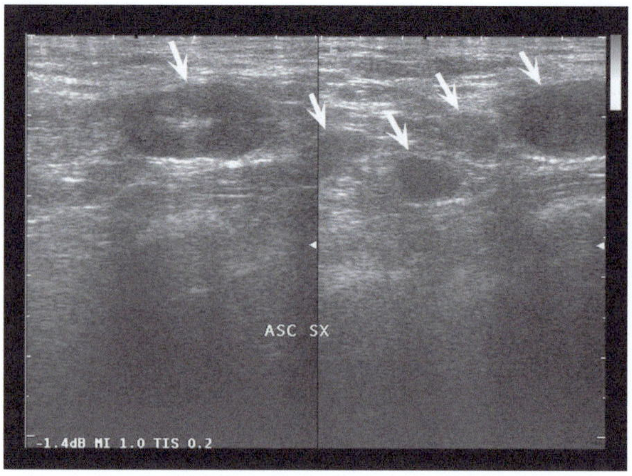

Fig. 4.77 Axillary lymph node metastasis from breast cancer. Multiple homogeneous hypoechoic adenopathies with partial conservation of the central echogenic hilum (*arrows*)

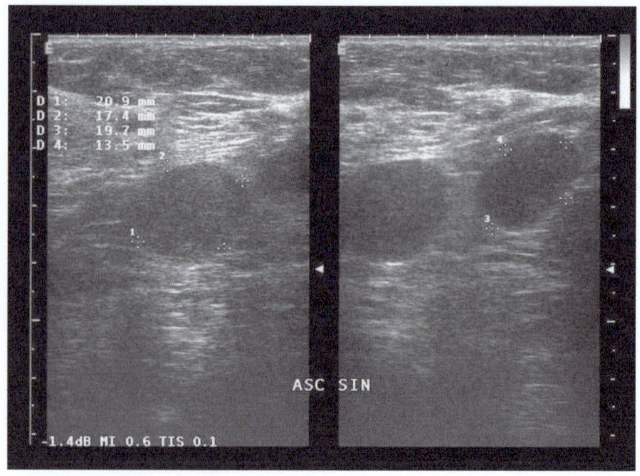

Fig. 4.78 Axillary lymph node metastasis from breast cancer. Multiple rounded hypoechoic adenopathies

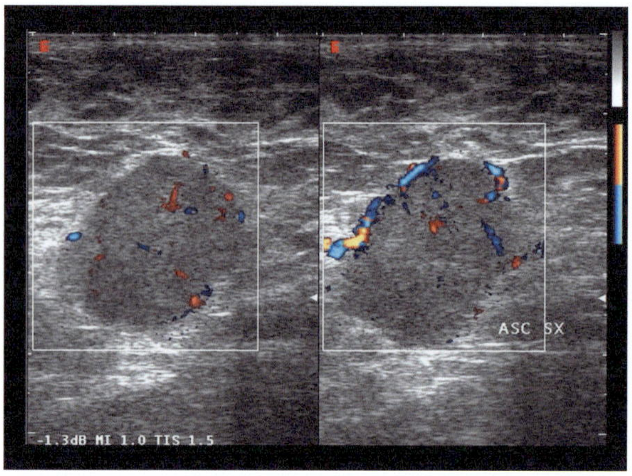

Fig. 4.79 Axillary lymph node metastasis from breast cancer. Two large oval hypoechoic adenopathies with capsular vascularity at directional PD

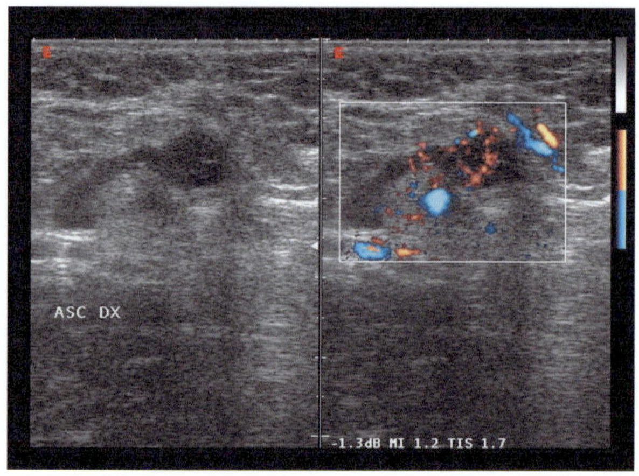

Fig. 4.80 Partial axillary lymph node metastasis from breast cancer. The lymph node displays nodular thickening of the cortex with increased and capsular vascularity at directional PD

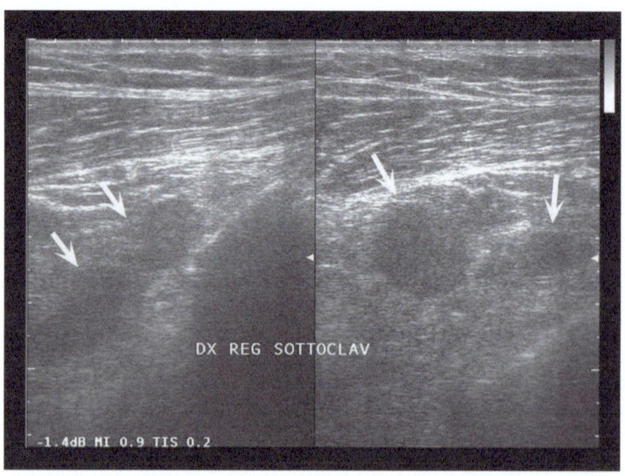

Fig. 4.81 Subclavicular lymph node metastasis from breast cancer. Multiple rounded hypoechoic adenopathies in the upper pectoral and subclavicular region (*arrows*)

tumors of the internal quadrants which favor axillary lymphatic spread), and also because US is only able to identify the larger lymphadenopathies in this site, regardless of the use of a superficial and/or abdominal transducer.

Supraclavicular lymphadenopathies are currently staged N3, although until not long ago they were classified M1 (as those contralateral to the abnormal breast still are). These are rather rare at the time of presentation of the disease. The lymph nodes microscopically identifiable at US exploration in this site are practically always pathologic. However, their characterization is based on the known imaging signs of enlarged malignant lymph nodes and possibly cytologic biopsy (Fig. 4.82).

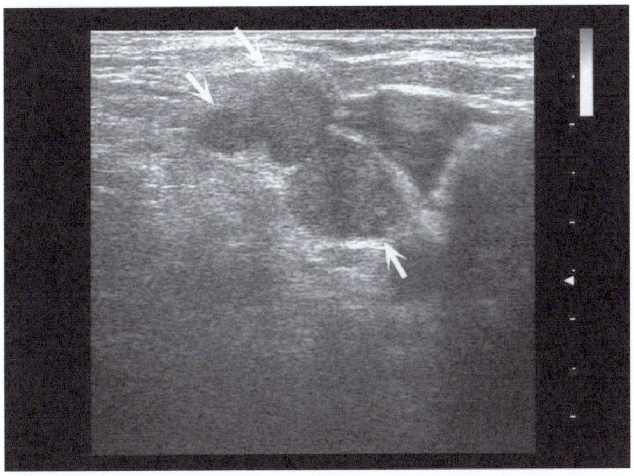

Fig. 4.82 Supraclavicular lymph node metastasis from breast cancer. Multiple confluent hypoechoic adenopathies in the upper supraclavicular regions (*arrows*) immediately external to the jugular vein

4.4 Locoregional Recurrence of Breast Cancer

The **monitoring** of women operated on for breast cancer is based on the clinical evaluation and a series of laboratory examinations, diagnostic imaging and possibly cytology-biopsy. The role of imaging at the locoregional level is played by annual mammography (bilateral except in cases of radical mastectomy), bilateral US and in select cases MR and PET. Undoubtedly PET, PET-CT and MR are more panoramic and sensitive methods than US, particularly in the evaluation of the axillary-supraclavicular regions [75], but they are generally indicated as second-line procedures, in the presence of a mammographic and/or US finding requiring further study or persistent clinical-laboratory findings despite negative US/mammography. One study demonstrated the utility of US breast and lymph node follow-up, while at the same time a routine evaluation of the abdomen was not recommended [76]. The frequency of the examinations, which should be correlated with the level of risk, needs to be higher (e.g. six monthly between the 2nd and 5th years) in the early years after surgery (60–80% of recurrences occur in the first three years and the median time from surgery is 2.3 years), in cases treated with breast-sparing surgery, in young women and in women with stage II disease. These parameters are all indicators of increased risk of local recurrence. Subsequently the frequency of monitoring can be reduced (e.g. annually from the 5th year on) [77,78].

Locoregional recurrence of breast cancer (1–2% per year) is a common and complex condition [2]. If isolated, it is still curable with a five-year survival rate of 41% after local recurrence (residual ipsilateral breast or thoracic wall after mastectomy) and 20% after lymph node recurrence (ipsilateral axillary or supraclavicular lymph nodes), whereas in cases of distant metastasis it is 13% [78]. This underlines the importance of an early diagnosis of locoregional recurrence.

A clear distinction needs to be made between radical surgery and breast-sparing surgery. After **radical or modified radical mastectomy** (today reserved mainly for multifocal forms, forms located within 2 cm of the nipple, large forms with respect to the overall size of the breast and/or forms associated with an extensive in situ component), possibly followed by radiation therapy, locoregional recurrence occurs in 50–70% of cases at the level of the thoracic wall alone, 10–15% at the level of the wall and the lymph node stations and 10–25% at the supraclavicular level. More rare are axillary and internal mammary recurrences. The known risk factors are size of the tumor, presence and extent of axillary lymph node involvement, histologic grade, edema, cutaneous infiltration and involvement of the pectoral muscle and fascia. The role of young age, histologic type and hormone receptor status is instead questionable [77]. Exploration should include not only the surgical scar, which should be evaluated with particular attention, but also the entire ipsilateral anterior and lateral thoracic wall, since almost half of parietal recurrences occur in a site other than the surgical scar. The investigation should also include the axillary region, the pectoral muscle planes (with level II and III lymph node stations) and the supraclavicular region. Study of the axilla can prove difficult given the irregularity in the skin surface for supporting the transducer and the postoperative accentuation of the axillary concavity. The internal mammary region is generally not examined, because it is rarely the site of recurrence and because US is only able to identify the larger lymphadenopathies regardless of the use of a superficial and/or abdominal transducer. **Parietal recurrences** after radical mastectomy can be cutaneous and identifiable clinically or, more frequently, subcutaneous. The latter generally presents as a single, heterogeneous, hypoechoic nodule with irregular margins and possible posterior acoustic shadowing. Recurrences in the intercostal spaces are rare. After mastectomy, but also after breast-sparing surgery, the presence of a generally submuscular prosthetic implant can create difficulty for US study (but even more for mammography), especially with regard to the detection of deep periprosthetic recurrences. Similar considerations are valid for cases of reconstruction with transposition of myocutaneous flaps, because in this case the frequent fatty-necrotic phenomena at the

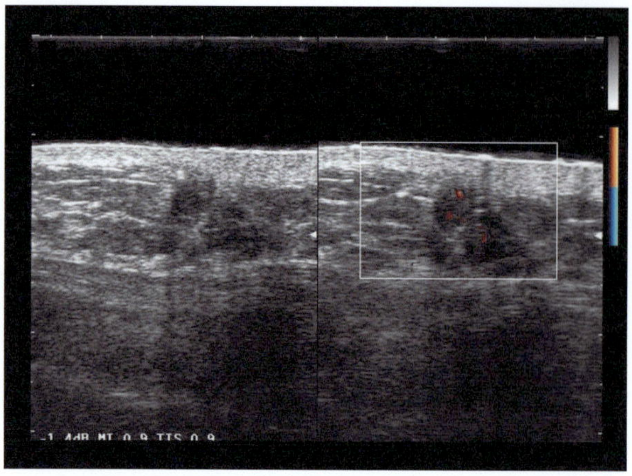

Fig. 4.83 Local recurrence after mastectomy. An ill-defined hypoechoic nodule with some internal vascular signals at directional PD can be seen at the level of the thoracic wall

periphery of the flap can create problems for the differential diagnosis (Fig. 4.83).

Breast-sparing surgery, which is generally followed by external irradiation, consists of simple lumpectomy, ample excision (at least 1–2 cm of healthy perilesional tissue) and quadrantectomy. The latter involves the resection of the entire involved quadrant, together with the overlying skin and the underlying portion of the superficial fascia of the pectoral muscle. If the technique is associated with axillary dissection and postoperative radiation therapy, the procedure is known as QUART, which today is the most widespread form of breast-sparing treatment. Recurrence after breast-sparing treatment occurs in 3–19% of cases. A distinction needs to be made between recurrences proper (70–80% of cases), which appear in the surgical scar due to the growth of microscopic residual tumor tissue, and "second tumors" (20–30% of cases) which manifest in other breast quadrants as a sign of metachronous multicentricity. The main risk factors for locoregional recurrence after breast-sparing treatment are positive resection margins, broad extension of the intraductal component and young age at the time of diagnosis [77].

Intramammary recurrence is relatively rare in the first year, but occurs in 5–10% of cases at 5 years and in 15% at 10 years from surgery. In particular, between the 2nd and 7th years true recurrences predominate, whereas the incidence of second tumors, which are rare in the first 4–5 years, progressively increases. The main risk factors are central site (<2 cm from the nipple-areola complex), macroscopic multifocality and extensive intraductal spread. Other factors, such as young age, tumor size, involvement of resection margins (role of radiation therapy!), histologic type and grade (bearing in mind however the greater incidence of multicentric forms in lobular tumors), lymphatic or vascular invasion, presence of necrosis or inflammatory infiltrate, involvement of axillary lymph nodes and hormone receptor status, are debatable. **Axillary-supraclavicular recurrence** is less frequent and can be difficult to identify because the symptoms are often subtle and usually overlap with those related to the collateral effects of surgery and radiation therapy [75]. Locoregional recurrence after QUART is preceded by or associated with distant metastases only in 10% of cases and therefore its early identification is important because it is still open to effective treatment. The US study needs to be panoramic, with particular attention paid to the surgical scar but also with exploration of the other quadrants, the pectoral-muscle plane, the contralateral breast and the axillas.

In order to perform US monitoring of the conservatively operated breast, an understanding of the **physiologic** and paraphysiologic **findings** at the level of the residual breast in general and the excision site in particular is required [79]. These changes are more evident in women who have undergone axillary lymph node dissection and been treated with radiation therapy, especially in the first year from treatment when edematous phenomena prevail. The skin tends to thicken, with a widening of the two hyperechoic lines which characterize it, and the development of an interposed hypoechoic edematous band. Subcutaneous edema appears as hypoechoic strips and bands (which should be distinguished from dilated ducts, which display a definite wall). Subsequently the subcutaneous fat becomes thickened and hypoechoic, possibly concealing or even enhancing Cooper's ligaments, which may appear hyperechoic with posterior acoustic shadowing. The residual corpus mammae takes on a heterogeneous hypoechoic appearance in the edematous phase, as do the breast ridges which radiate from the parenchyma towards the skin. The ridges also tend to be concealed in the hypoechogenicity of the subcutaneous fat they travel through. With increasing time from treatment, the residual parenchyma begins to show a variable appearance, with echogenic fibrous patches being evident and generally diffuse (with respect to which the surgical scar and any possible recurrences are rather easy to identify). Both axillary and intramammary fluid collections are common in the early phase and their detection, with possible aspiration, can be useful in the preliminary phase of adjuvant radiation therapy. In general, these seromas and lymphoceles do not create problems for differential diagnosis, and finding fluid-filled collections even years after surgery should come as no surprise. At the excision site the surgical procedure and consequent hyperdose of radiation therapy produce changes even more evident than in the rest of the breast. The superficial thickening is more marked, with possible deformation of the skin profile, whereas in the deep tissues a poorly defined hypoechoic image can be seen with a vaguely triangular shape with the apex oriented towards the deep tissues, which is an expression of the surgical focus. This area may contain more-or-less homogeneous anechoic fluid collections which tend to be reabsorbed over time, but may persist with limited size for years. With increasing time from surgery the excision site begins to take on a variable appearance in line with the intensity of intraparenchymal fibrous scarring. Generally the scar becomes smaller and sharper, with a hypoechoic appearance, although less marked and with possible posterior acoustic shadowing and amorphous calcifications. The scar can be visualized in 90% of cases one year after breast-sparing surgery, whereas with increasing time it becomes less and less identifiable at US (Figs. 4.84–4.86).

The surgical scar should be differentiated from **recurrence** in or near the **scar-line** (50% of cases). However, this is not always easy because the two events have a similar appearance, especially when the scar takes on a hypertrophic characteristic. The demonstration of stability over time – in practice, a US image similar to a previous control – is clearly crucial. Unlike recurrence, the surgical scar does not have a nodular appearance in all the scan planes, in that it appears thin when appropriate rotation of the transducer makes its visualization possible in the longitudinal sense. In addition, the scar is at least in part deformable with compression, often has a hypoechoic finger-like projection at the apex, which reaches the subcutaneous planes, and appears more as an attenuation of the beam without an associated nodule than a nodule producing posterior acoustic shadowing. The identification of vascular signals within the scar tissue is suspicious for recurrence, since the scar is relatively avascular, and should prompt and also guide cytologic biopsy. In addition, it should be borne in mind that a "young" scar (first 18 months from surgery) can also display some vascular signals [35]. The appearance of recurrence not in the scar also depends on the surrounding fibrous reaction. If this is marked (30% of cases), the recurrent nodule displays an irregular shape with infiltrated margins and significant acoustic shadowing, whereas if the reaction is poor (20% of cases), the nodule appears rounded with less-well-defined margins (Figs. 4.87–4.93). Second tumors have an appearance similar to that of malignant breast nodules in general, which is described elsewhere in this book.

Axillary recurrences can arise from the axillary tail or more commonly from the lymph nodes of the

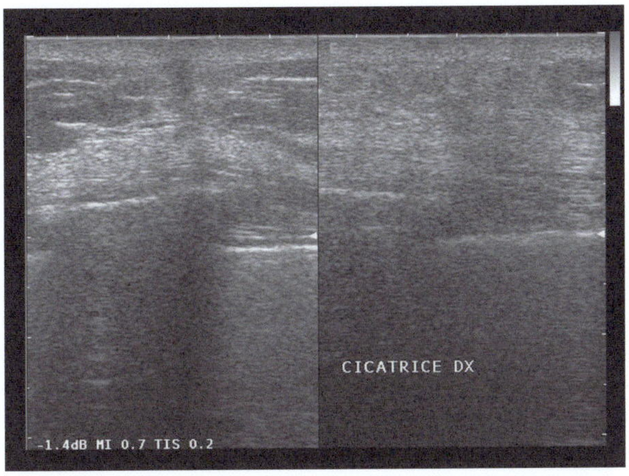

Fig. 4.84 Normal appearance of surgical scar after QUART. Thin hypoechoic band with posterior acoustic shadowing, sectioned transversely and longitudinally

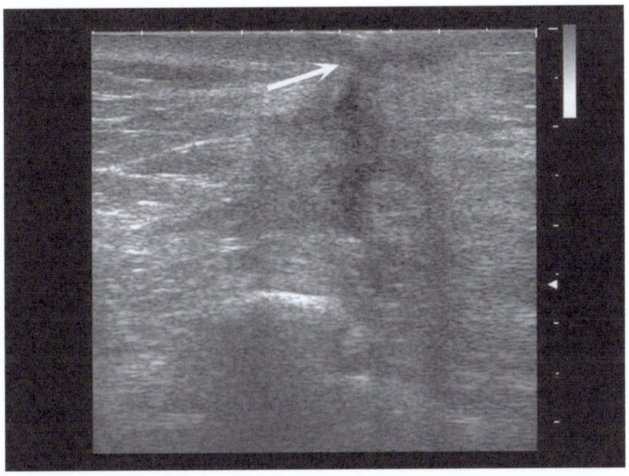

Fig. 4.85 Extensive scarring after QUART. Large and ill-defined hypoechoic area with mild enhanced through-transmission. This image was taken immediately deep to the cutaneous scar (*arrow*)

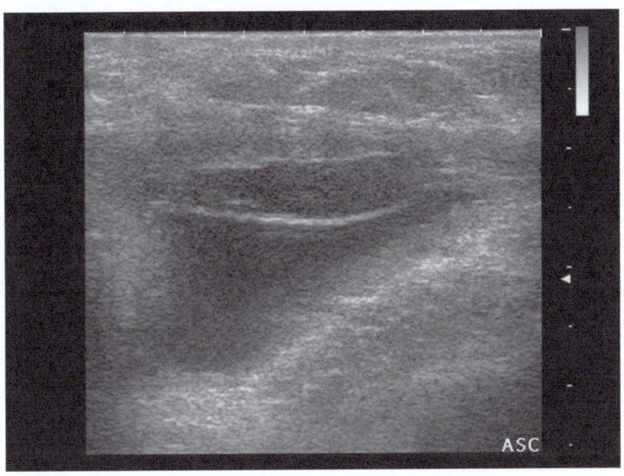

Fig. 4.86 Axillary lymphocele after lymphadenectomy. Fluid collection between the axilla and breast

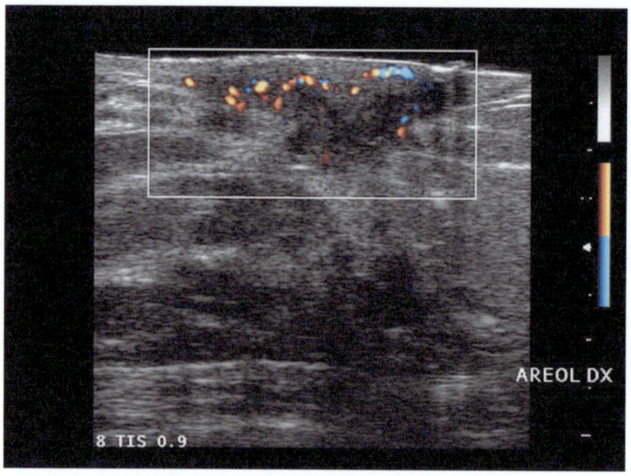

Fig. 4.87 Retroareolar cutaneous recurrence of breast cancer. Hypoechoic thickening of the areolar region with moderate and irregular vascularity at directional PD

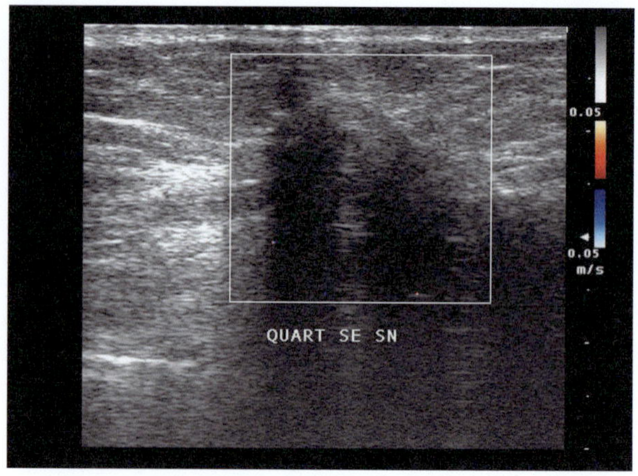

Fig. 4.88 Recurrence in surgical scar after QUART. Large solid nodulation with hypovascular appearance at CD

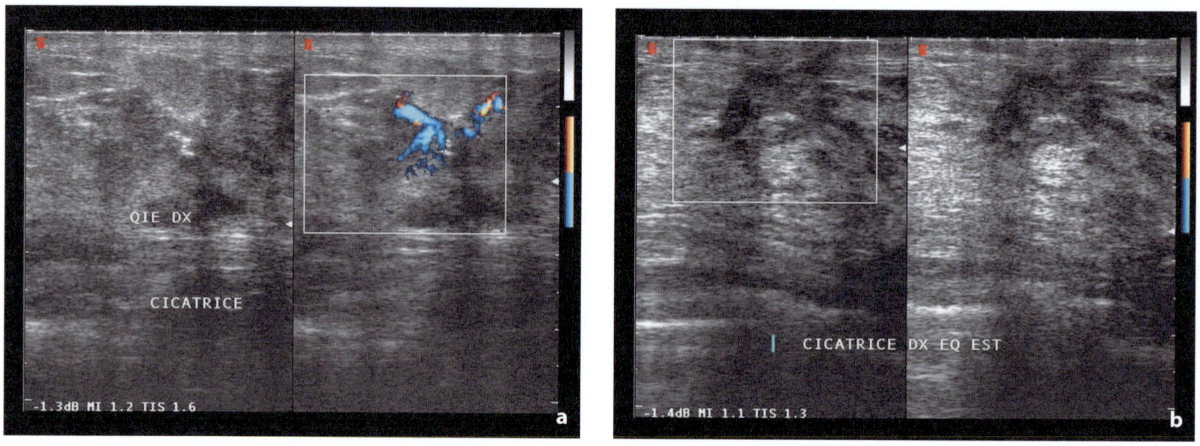

Fig. 4.89a,b Recurrence in surgical scar after QUART, with follow-up after chemotherapy. Infiltrating hypoechoic nodulation with calcifications and hypervascularity at directional PD (a). After chemotherapy the lesion appears slightly reduced in size and most of all shows poor flow signals (b)

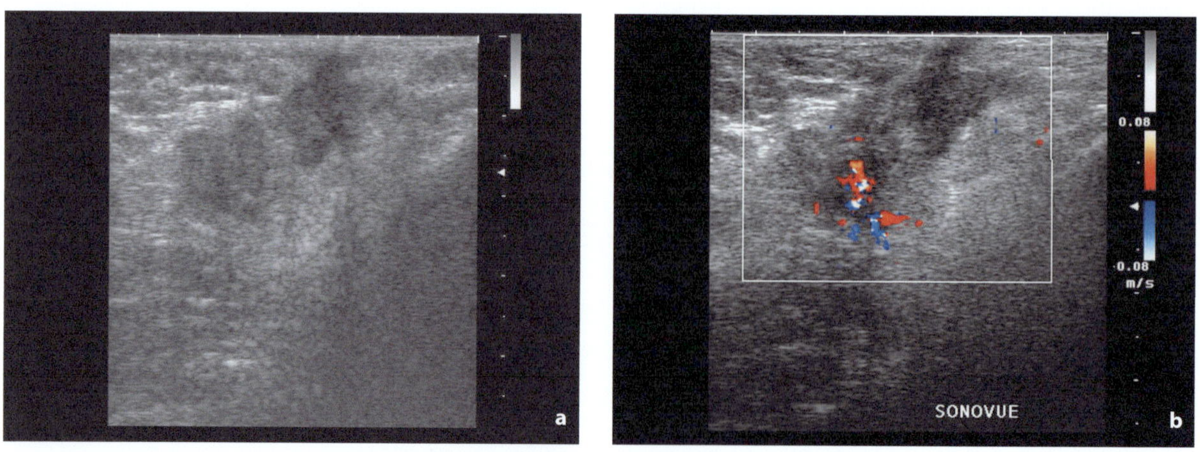

Fig. 4.90a,b Recurrence in surgical scar after QUART. Two ill-defined hypoechoic nodulations with similar appearance can be seen at the site of the surgical scar (a). CD with intravenous contrast medium however shows moderate vascularity of the deeper nodule, identifying it as local recurrence (b). In the absence of the CD finding, FNAC would probably have been targeted at the superficial lesion with a consequent false negative

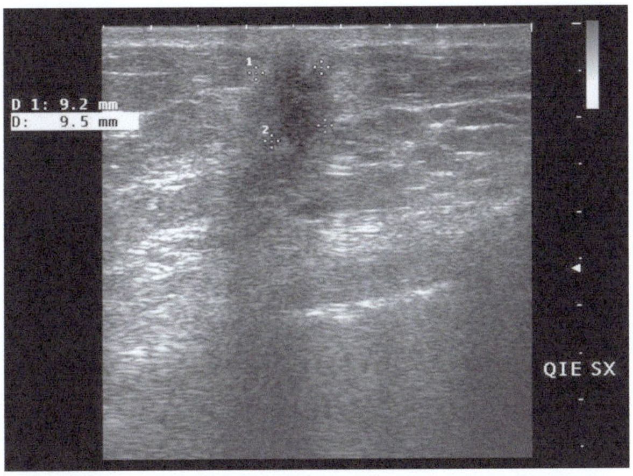

Fig. 4.91 Recurrence in surgical scar after QUART. Solid lesion with irregular margins and posterior acoustic shadowing

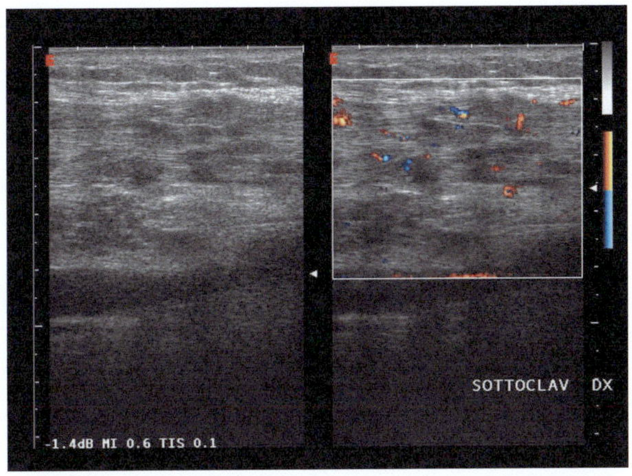

Fig. 4.92 High pectoral recurrence after QUART. Multiple hypoechoic areas in subclavicular site of the pectoral muscle. Increased regional vascularity at directional PD

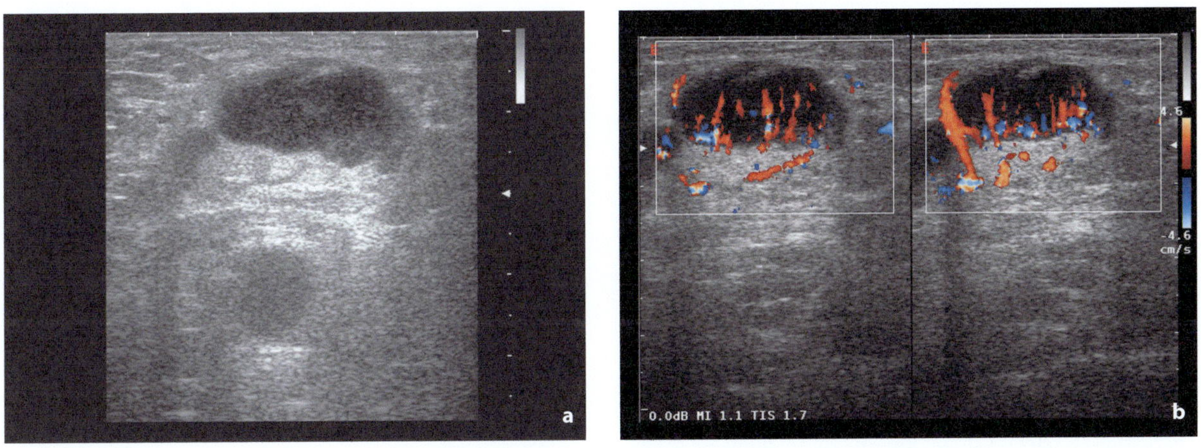

Fig. 4.93a,b High pectoral recurrence after QUART. Two subclavicular lymph nodes (**a**) with multiple capsular vessels seen at CD (**b**)

axilla, including those between the pectoral muscles and those located medial or inferior to the pectoralis minor muscle (if originally spared from dissection). Clearly it is important not to consider the residual lymph nodes from axillary dissection pathologic, but only those with suspicious characteristics. US can, however, have difficulty in identifying a recurrence of the apical lymph nodes. In doubtful cases, such as in the presence of edema of the upper limb (possible expression of level III lymphadenopathy) or neurologic symptoms (possible expression of invasion of the brachial plexus) a CT or MR study is indicated.

Supraclavicular recurrences are generally detected at palpation, although confirmation is still required. In this site almost all identified lymph nodes are pathologic, even though the characterization of small lymphadenopathies may require microscopic confirmation.

Internal mammary recurrences are visualized at US firstly as an intercostal hypoechoic nodulation and then as a heterogeneous retro-parasternal mass which grows through the intercostal space towards the surface. In advanced cases an irregularity of the sternal cortex may be seen.

References

1. Griff SK et al (2002) Breast cancer. In: Bragg DG et al (eds) Oncologic imaging. WB Saunders Company, Philadelphia, 265-294
2. Bartella L et al (2006) Imaging breast cancer. Radiol Clin North Am 45:45-67

3. Kronemer KA et al (2001) Gray scale sonography of breast masses in adolescent girls. J Ultrasound Med 20:491-496
4. Shetty MK (2003) Prospective evaluation of the value of combined mammographic and sonographic assessment in patients with palpable abnormalities of the breast. J Ultrasound Med 22:263-268
5. Shetty M et al (2002) Prospective evaluation of the value of negative sonographic and mammographic findings in patients with palpable abnormalities of the breast. J Ultrasound Med 21:1211-1216
6. Warner E (2001) Comparison of breast magnetic resonance imaging, mammography, and ultrasound surveillance of women at high risk for hereditary breast cancer. J Clin Oncol 19:3524-3531
7. Berg WA (2004) Supplemental screening sonography in dense breasts. Radiol Clin North Am 42:845-851
8. Leconte I et al (2003) Mammography and subsequent whole-breast sonography of nonpalpable breast cancers: the importance of radiologic breast density. AJR Am J Roentgenol 180:1675-1679
9. Ciatto S et al (2005) Role of multimedial diagnosis of breast cancer in women below 36 years of age. Radiol Med 109:321-329
10. Houssani N et al (2002) Accuracy of combined breast imaging in young women. Breast 11:36-40
11. Bonifacino A et al (2005) Accuracy rates of US-guided vacuum-assisted breast biopsy. Anticancer Res 25:2465-2470
12. Graf O et al (2007) Probably benign breast masses at US: is follow-up an acceptable alternative to biopsy? Radiology 244:87-93
13. Steyaert L (2001) The breast. In: Meire H et al (eds) Abdominal and general ultrasound, II Edition. Churchill Livingstone, London, 751-806
14. Szopinski KT et al (2003) Tissue harmonic imaging. Utility in breast sonography. J Ultrasound Med 22:479-487
15. Cha JH et al (2007) Characterization of benign and malignant solid breast masses: comparison of conventional US and tissue harmonic imaging. Radiology 242:63-69
16. Mehta TS (2003) Current uses of ultrasound in the evaluation of the breast. Radiol Clin North Am 41:841-856
17. Özdemir A et al (2001) Differential diagnosis of solid breast lesions. J Ultrasound Med 20:1091-1101
18. Kim MJ et al (2006a) Application of power Doppler vocal fremitus sonography in breast lesions. J Ultrasound Med 25:879-906
19. American College of Radiology (2003) Breast imaging reporting and data system: ultrasound. IV ed. American College of Radiology, Reston VA
20. Costantini M et al (2006) Characterization of solid breast masses. Use of sonographic breast imaging reporting and data system lexicon. J Ultrasound Med 25:649-659
21. Stavros AT et al (1995) Solid breast nodules: use of sonography to distinguish between benign and malignant lesions. Radiology 196:123-134
22. Del Frate C et al (2006) Sonographic criteria for differentiating of benign and malignant solid breast lesions: size is of value. Radiol Med 111:783-796
23. Stavros AT (2004) Breast ultrasound. Lippincott Williams & Wilkins, Philadelphia
24. Chao T-C et al (2002) Sonographic features of phyllodes tumors of the breast. Ultrasound Obstet Gynecol 20:64-71
25. Satake H et al (2000) Role of ultrasonography in the detection of intraductal spread of breast cancer: correlation with pathologic findings, mammography, and MR imaging. Eur Radiol 10:176-1732
26. Rotten D et al (1999) Analysis of normal breast tissue and of solid breast masses using three-dimensional ultrasound mammography. Ultrasound Obstet Gynecol 14:114-124
27. Ohlinger R et al (2003) Ultrasound of the breast – value of sonographic criteria for differential diagnosis of solid lesions. Ultraschall in Med 25:48-53
28. Soo MS et al (2003) Sonographic detection and sonographically guided biopsy of breast microcalcifications. AJR Am J Roentgenol 180:941-948
29. Yang WT et al (1997) In vivo demonstration of microcalcification in breast cancer using high resolution ultrasound. Br J Radiol 70:685-690
30. Hashimoto BE et al (2001) High detection rate of breast ductal carcinoma in situ calcifications on mammographically directed high-resolution sonography. J Ultrasound Med 20:501-508
31. Lamb PM et al (2000) Correlation between ultrasound characteristics, mammographic findings and histological grade in patients with invasive ductal carcinoma of the breast. Clin Radiol 55:40-44
32. Dogan BE et al (2005) Ductal dilatation as the manifesting sign of invasive ductal carcinoma. J Ultrasound Med 24:1413-1417
33. Huber S et al (1998) Effects of a microbubble contrast agent on breast tumors: computer assisted quantitative assessment with color Doppler US. Early experience. Radiology 208:485-489
34. Reinikainen H et al (2001) B-mode, power Doppler and contrast-enhanced power-Doppler ultrasonography in the diagnosis of breast tumors. Acta Radiol 42:106-113
35. Schroeder RJ et al (2003) Role of power Doppler techniques and ultrasound contrast enhancement in the differential diagnosis of focal breast lesions. Eur Radiol 13:68-79
36. Germer U (2002) Strong impact of estrogen environment on Doppler variables used for differentiation between benign and malignant breast lesions. Ultrasound Obstet Gynecol 19:380-385
37. del Cura JL et al (2005) The use of unenhanced Doppler sonography in the evaluation of solid breast lesions. AJR Am J Roentgenol 184:1788-1794
38. Peters-Engl C et al (1999) Tumor flow in malignant breast tumors measured by Doppler ultrasound: an independent predictor of survival. Breast Cancer Res Treat 54:65-71
39. Zhi H et al (2007) Comparison of ultrasound elastography, mammography, and sonography in the diagnosis of solid breast lesions. J Ultrasound Med 26:807-815
40. Du J et al (2008) Correlation of real-time gray scale contrast-enhanced ultrasonography with microvessel density and vascular endothelial growth factor expression for assessment of angiogenesis in breast lesions. J Ultrasound Med 27:821-831
41. Caumo F et al (2006) Angiosonography in suspicious breast lesions with non-diagnostic FNAC: comparison with power Doppler US. Radiol Med 111:61-72
42. Stavros AT (2004) Breast ultrasound. Lippincott Williams & Wilkins, Philadelphia
43. Witteking Ch et al (2005) TNM Atlas. Springer-Verlag, Berlin
44. Kim SJ et al (2008) Application of sonographic BI-RADS to synchronous breast nodules detected in patients with breast cancer. AJR Am J Roentgenol 191:653-658

45. Chao T-C et al (2003) Phyllodes tumors of the breast. Eur Radiol 13:88-93
46. Chang Y-W et al (2007) Sonographic differentiation of benign and malignant cystic lesions of the breast. J Ultrasound Med 26:47-53
47. Fornage BD (2000b) Breast sonography. In: Shirkhoda A (ed) Variants and pitfalls in body imaging. Lippincott Williams & Wilkins, Philadelphia, pp 153-169
48. Kim MJ et al (2006b) Galactocele mimicking suspicious solid masses on sonography. J Ultrasound Med 25:145-151
49. Stevens K et al (1997) The ultrasound appearances of galactocoeles. Br J Radiol 70:239-241
50. Sumkin JH et al (1998) Lactating adenoma: US features and literature review. Radiology 206:271-274
51. Ballesio L et al (2007) Adjunctive diagnostic value of ultrasonography evaluation in patients with suspected ductal breast disease. Radiol Med 112:354-365
52. Irshad A et al (2008) Characterization of sonographic and mammographic features of granular cell tumors of the breast and estimation of their incidence. J Ultrasound Med 27:467-475
53. Yang WT et al (2006) Sonographic and mammographic appearances of granular cell tumors of the breast with pathological correlation. J Clin Ultrasound 34:153-160
54. Mesurolle B et al (2008) Sonographic and mammographic appearances of breast hemangioma. AJR Am J Roentgenol 191:W17-W22
55. Soo MS et al (1998) Fat necrosis in the breast: sonographic features. Radiology 206:261-269
56. Youk JK et al (2005) Focal fibrosis of the breast diagnosed by a sonographically guided core biopsy of nonpalpable lesions. Imaging findings and clinical relevance. J Ultrasound Med 24:1377-1384
57. Reznek RH et al (2004b) Lymphoma. In: Husband JE et al (eds) Imaging in oncology, II Edition. Taylor & Francis, London, 817-874
58. Yang WT et al (2007) Breast lymphoma: imaging findings of 32 tumors in 27 patients. Radiology 245:692-702
59. Cariati M et al (2005) "Inflammatory" breast cancer. Surg Oncol 14:133-143
60. Caumo F et al (2005) Occult inflammatory breast cancer: review of clinical, mammographic, US and pathologic signs. Radiol Med 109:308-3202
61. Oruwari JU et al (2002) Axillary staging using ultrasound-guided fine needle aspiration biopsy in locally advanced breast cancer. Am J Surg 184:307-309
62. Ollivier L (2005) Imaging in evaluation of response to neoadjuvant breast cancer treatment. Cancer Imaging 5:27-31
63. Loehberg CR et al (2005) Neoadjuvant chemotherapy in breast cancer: which diagnostic procedures can be used? Anticancer Res 25:2519-2526
64. Tardivon AA et al (2006) Monitoring therapeutic efficacy in breast carcinomas. Eur Radiol 16:2549-2558
65. Balu-Maestro et al (2002) Imaging in evaluation of response to neoadjuvant breast cancer treatment benefits in MRI. Breast Cancer Res Treat 72:145-152
66. Powles TJ et al (1995) Randomised trial of chemoendocrine therapy started before or after surgery for treatment of primary breast cancer. J Clin Oncol 13:547-552
67. Vallone P et al (2005) Color-Doppler using contrast medium in evaluating the response to neoadjuvant treatment in patients with locally advanced breast carcinoma. Anticancer Res 25:595-599
68. Allan SM et al (1994) Color Doppler ultrasound for axillary lymphnode staging in breast cancer. Breast 3:94-96
69. Alvarez S et al (2006) Role of sonography in the diagnosis of axillary lymph node metastases in breast cancer: a systematic review. AJR Am J Roentgenol 186:1342-1348
70. Duchesne N et al (2005) Redefining ultrasound appearance criteria of positive axillary lymph nodes. Can Assoc Radiol J 56:289-296
71. Bedi DG et al (2008) Cortical morphologic features of axillary lymph nodes as a predictor of metastasis in breast cancer: in vitro sonographic study. AJR Am J Roentgenol 191:646-652
72. Krishnamurthy S et al (2002) Role of ultrasound-guided fine-needle aspiration of indeterminate and suspicious axillary lymph nodes in the initial staging of breast carcinoma. Cancer 95:982-988
73. Nori J et al (2005) Role of axillary lymph node ultrasound and large core biopsy in the preoperative assessment of patients selected for sentinel node biopsy. Radiol Med 109:330-344
74. Koelliker SL et al (2008) Axillary lymph nodes: US-guided fine-needle aspiration for initial staging of breast cancer - Correlation with primary tumor size. Radiology 246:81-89
75. Hathaway PB (1999) Value of combined FDG PET and MR imaging in the evaluation of suspected recurrent local-regional breast cancer: preliminary experience. Radiology 210:807-814
76. Kauczor H-U et al (1994) Value of routine abdominal and lymph node sonography in the follow-up of breast cancer patients. Eur J Radiol 18:104-108
77. de Bock et al (2006) Isolated loco-regional recurrence of breast cancer is more common in young patients and following breast conserving therapy: long-term results of European Organisation for Research and Treatment of Cancer studies. Eur J Cancer 42:351-356
78. Elder E et al (2006) Patterns of breast cancer relapse. Eur J Surg Oncol 32:922-927
79. Calkins AR et al (1988) The sonographic appearance of the irradiated breast. J Clin Ultrasound 16:427-429

The Abdomen

5

5.1 Abdominal Masses

The initial approach to the patient with a presumed palpable mass is to ensure that there effectively is a mass corresponding to the palpated finding, which in fact is not the case in around 20% of cases (e.g. pseudomass produced by cecum filled with fecal material). Moreover, the "mass" may be located within the abdominal wall (hematoma, abscess, hernia, tumor, etc.).

US is the first-choice imaging modality in most of these events, although in some cases it does require the integration of a more panoramic and accurate technique such as CT. While it is true that US is more effective in the study of certain abdominal regions and CT in others, it is also true that the mass may be, as stated above, not really present or of little significance, such as a large renal cyst. This therefore suggests an initial US study in all cases combined with the selective use of CT [1]. Retrospectively US has demonstrated a high positive predictive value (99%) and negative predictive value (97%) in the study of palpable abdominal masses. The organ of origin is correctly defined in 87% of cases, and the histologic diagnosis is precisely hypothesized in 77% [2]. US is not generally able to identify the different fasciae bounding the different retroperitoneal spaces and can therefore have difficulty in defining the exact site of retroperitoneal lesions, having to base itself solely on the spatial relations between these and the adjacent structures. In addition, for particularly large masses US may have difficulty defining the organ of origin and the anatomic relations (also for the purposes of surgical planning), even if panoramic reconstructions are used.

Solid masses may be the result of enlarged organs (e.g. significantly myomatous uterus) or neoformations proper. The exact nature can be hypothesized, based not only on the location of the lesion, but also on the presence of adipose components, calcifications, necrotic areas or signs of vascularity. The adipose nature of the mass, even though suspicious on the basis of a hyperechoic appearance, cannot always be well defined, at least not with the immediacy offered by CT and MR (Figs. 5.1–5.18).

The differential diagnosis of "**cystic masses**" includes abscesses, locular effusion, pseudocysts of the pancreas, cysts and tumor cysts of the ovary, lymphoceles, cystic lymphangiomas, massive hydronephrosis and acute urinary retention (Figs. 5.19–5.21).

Vascular masses (aortic aneurysms, iliac aneurysms, aneurysms of the visceral branches) are easily recognized due to the presence of an aneurysmal lumen with flow signals or in the event of partial or complete luminal thrombosis due to parietal calcifications (Fig. 5.22).

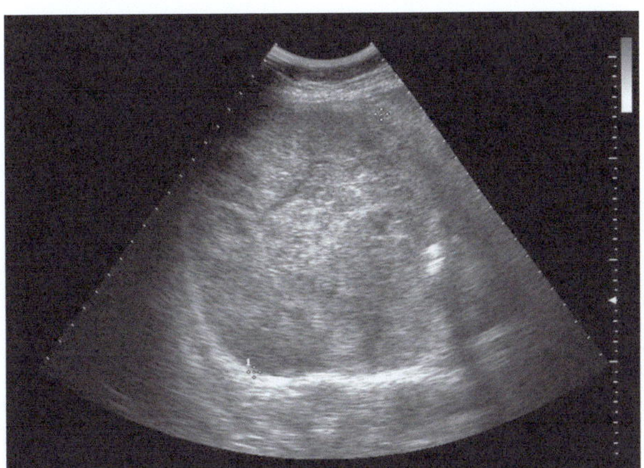

Fig. 5.1 Peritoneal metastasis from breast cancer. Large, solid, rounded mass with heterogeneous echogenic appearance at the pelvic level

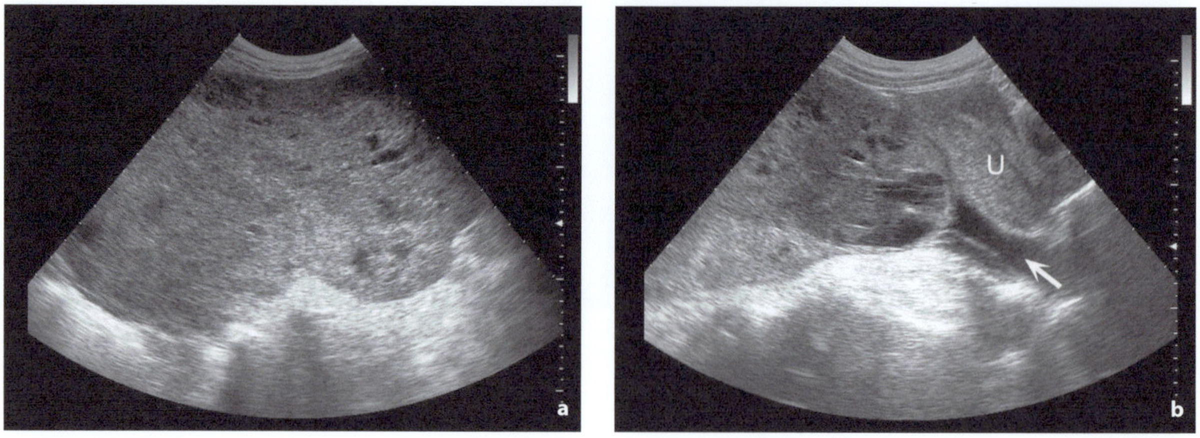

Fig. 5.2a,b Abdominal fibrosarcoma. Prevalently solid hypogastric mass with anechoic areas seen in transverse and longitudinal sections. Pelvic fluid layer (*arrow*). *U*, uterus

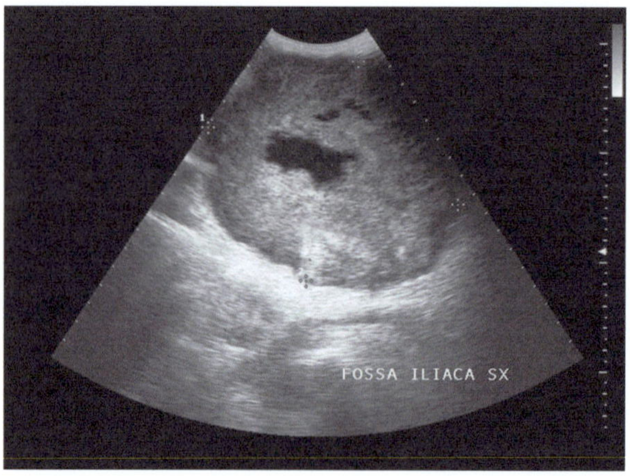

Fig 5.3 Recurrence of pelvic sarcoma. Solid mass with necrotic center

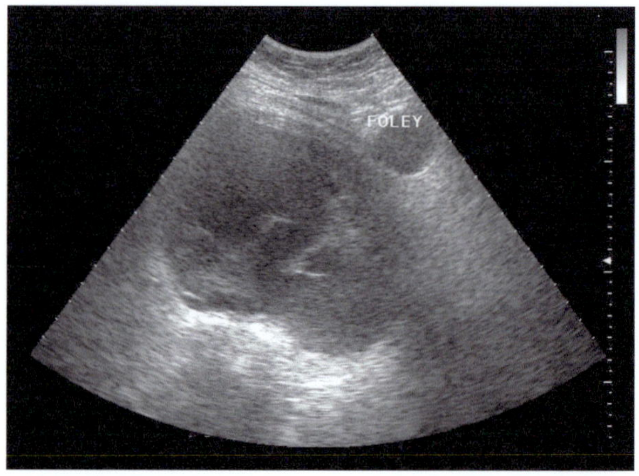

Fig. 5.4 Recurrence of pelvic stromal sarcoma. Retrovesical mass with complex structure

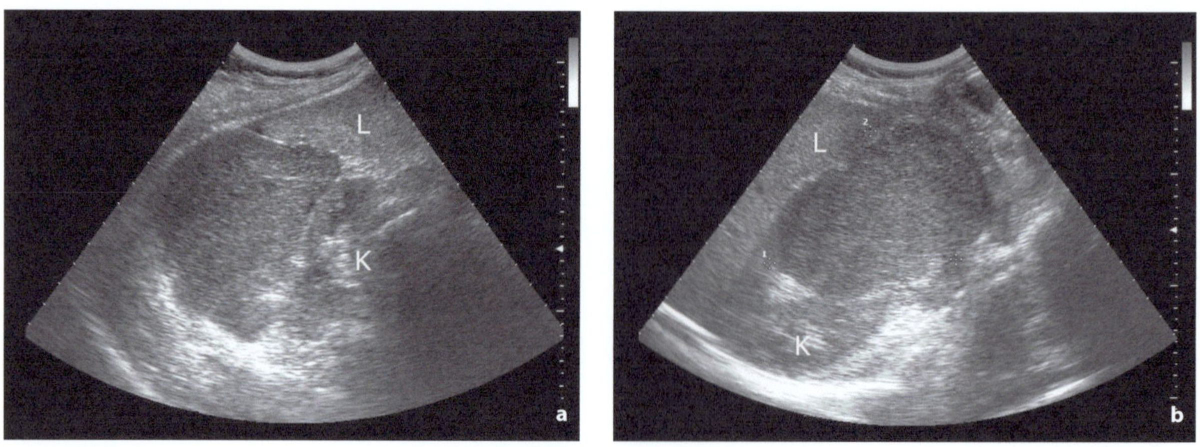

Fig. 5.5a,b Retroperitoneal liposarcoma. Relatively homogenous hypoechoic mass located external to the right kidney and posterior to the liver. *K*, kidney; *L*, liver

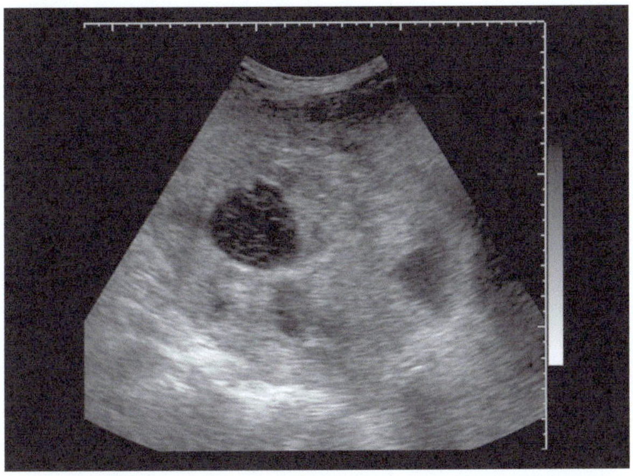

Fig. 5.6 Retroperitoneal liposarcoma. Large solid mass with some anechoic areas

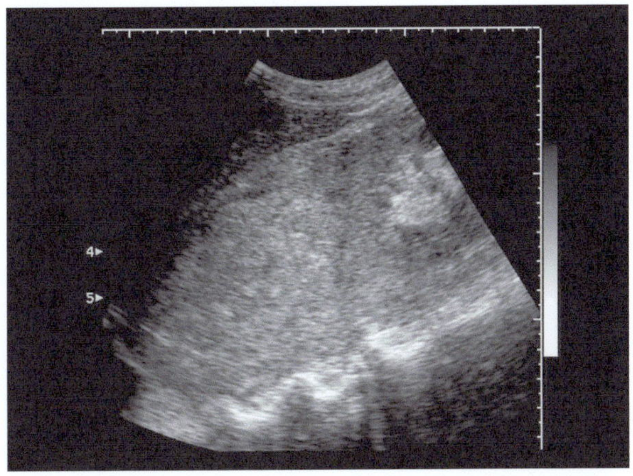

Fig. 5.7 Retroperitoneal sarcoma. Echogenic mass invading the upper pole of the left kidney

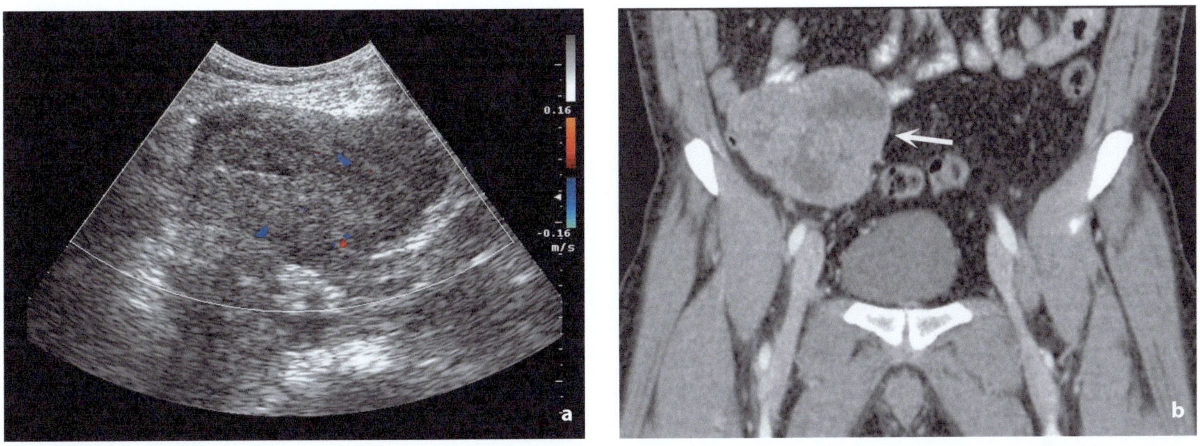

Fig. 5.8a,b Malignant abdominal schwannoma. In a patient with neurofibromatosis, the study of the right iliac fossa reveals a heterogeneous hypoechoic mass with some vascular signals at CD (**a**). Coronal CT reconstruction confirms the mass in the ileocecal region (**b**, *arrow*)

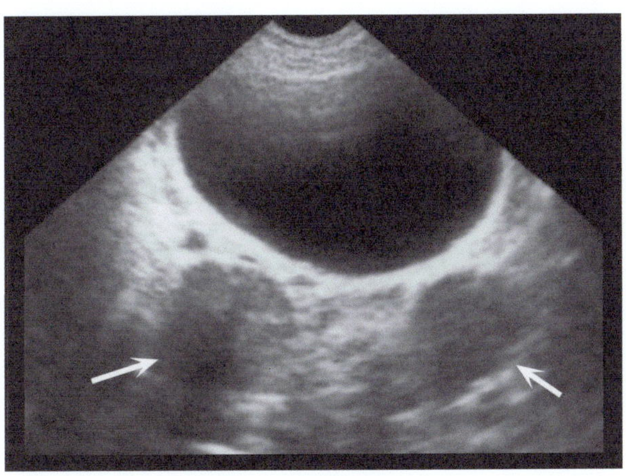

Fig. 5.9 Pelvic neurofibromatosis. Retrovesical hypoechoic nodulations (*arrows*) in a patient with neurofibromatosis

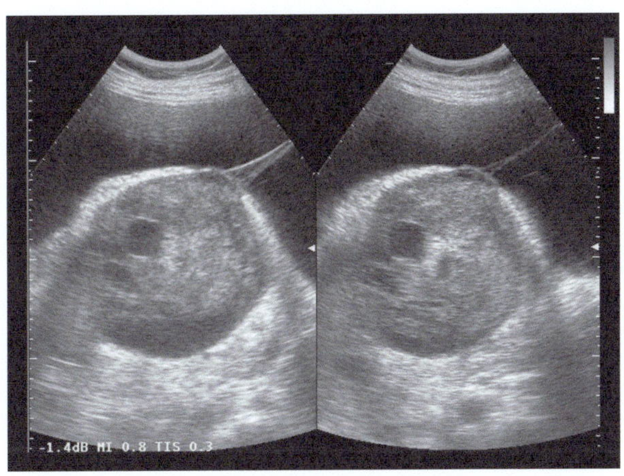

Fig. 5.10 Recurrence of peritoneal sarcoma. Rounded solid mass with some necrotic-liquefactive areas. Peritoneal effusion is associated

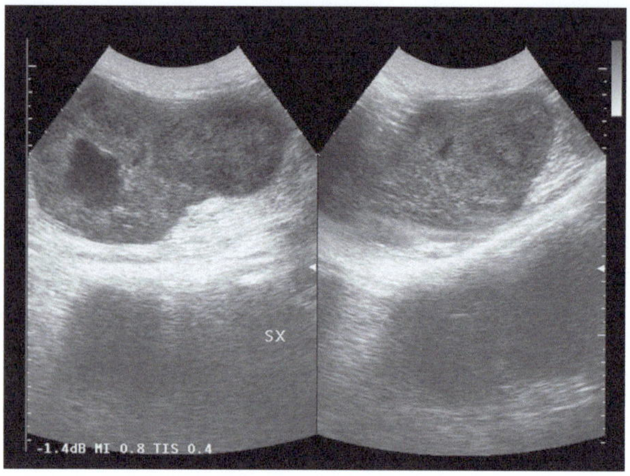

Fig. 5.11 GIST. Solid, lobulated, hypoechoic mass with internal necrotic-liquefactive areas located in the left iliac fossa

Palpable masses are very common findings in **children**, related primarily to age. In the neonate the nature of abdominal-pelvic masses is generally benign and the appearance is often cystic. The most frequent origin is the kidney (55% of cases) or at least retroperitoneal. The most common finding is high-grade hydronephrosis, either obstructive or nonobstructive, although other conditions include multicystic dysplastic kidney, polycystic kidney disease, nephroblastoma, hydrometrocolpos, ovarian cysts (generally unilocular, homogeneous and with a thin wall), cystic and solid ovarian tumors, urachal cysts (median supravesical cystic mass, with debris in the event of overlying infection), intestinal duplication cysts (digestive-tract-like layered wall), cysts of the mesentery and omentum (lymphatic masses), giant meconium pseudocyst (thick and echogenic wall and viscous echogenic content, occasionally pseudosolid),

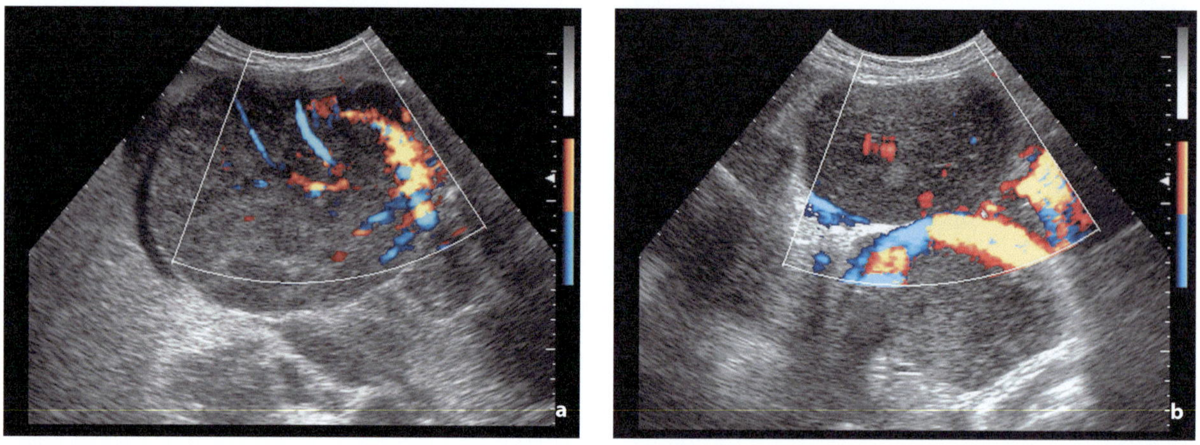

Fig. 5.12a,b Abdominal lymphoma. Large, solid, mesenteric mass with large surrounding vessels and limited internal flow signals at directional PD

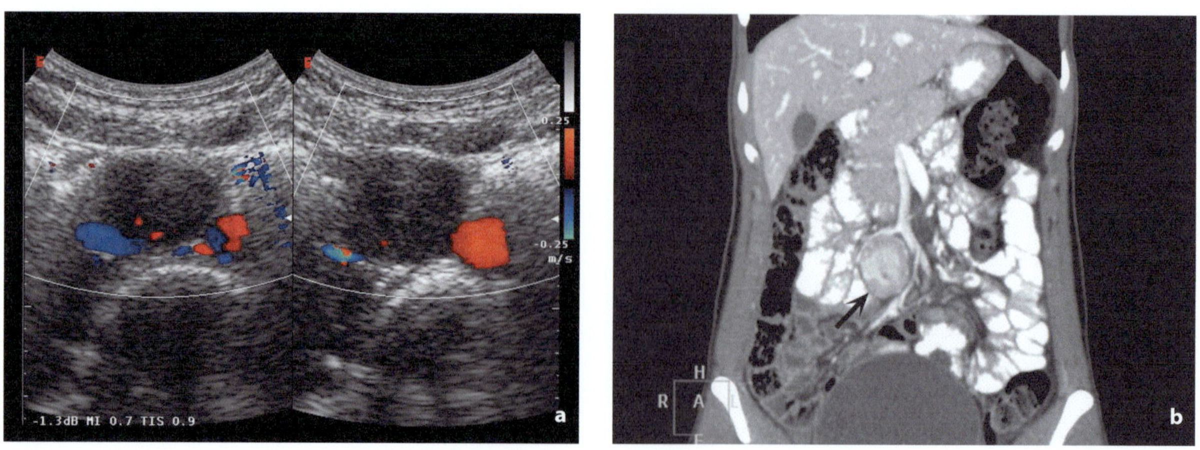

Fig. 5.13a,b Extra-adrenal pheochromocytoma. Para-aortic hypoechoic mass with poor vascular signals at CD (**a**). Coronal CT reconstruction shows moderate contrast enhancement of the mass (**b**, *arrow*)

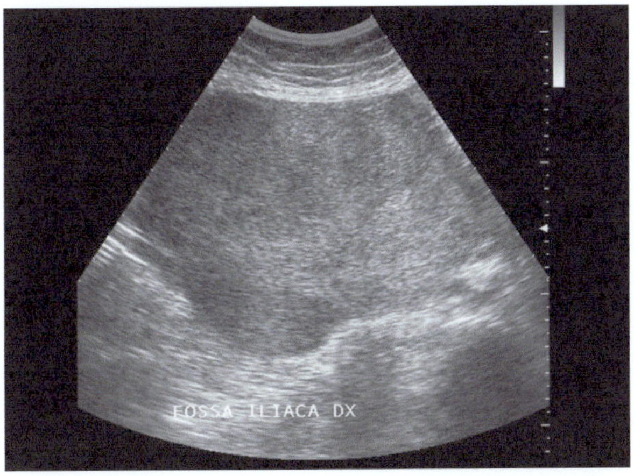

Fig. 5.14 Peritoneal metastasis from melanoma. Large pelvic mass with relatively homogeneous echogenic appearance

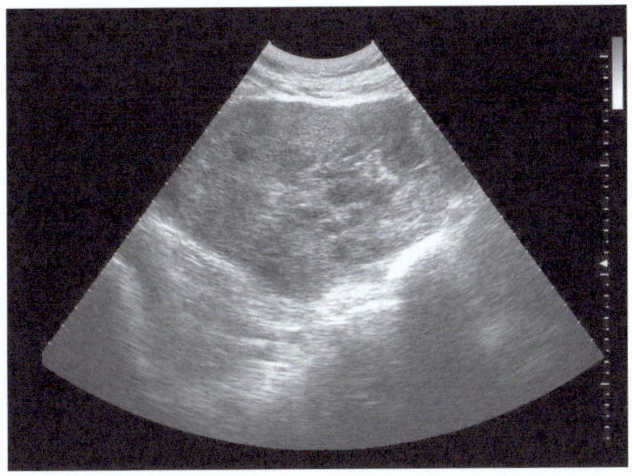

Fig. 5.15 Pelvic recurrence of colon cancer. Heterogeneous echogenic mass occupying large part of the pelvis

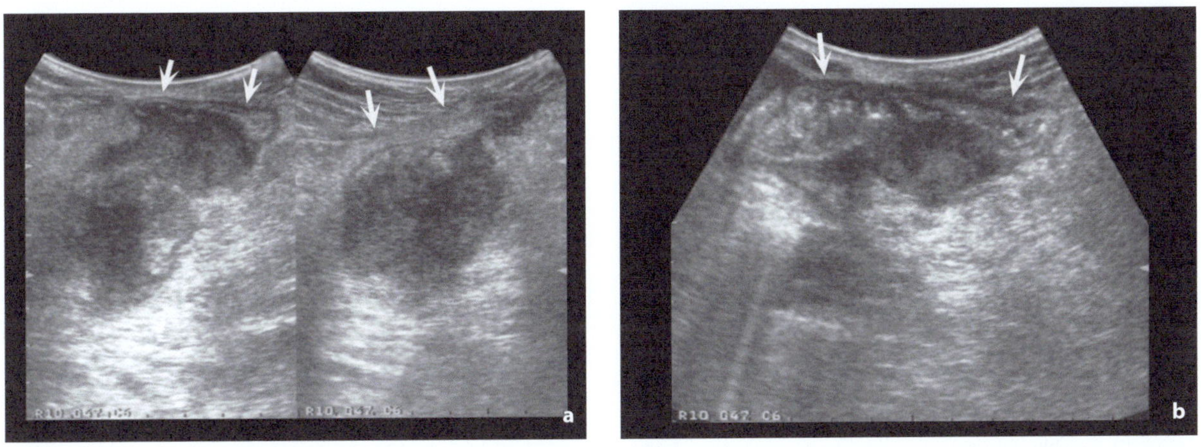

Fig. 5.16a,b Paracolostomy recurrence of colon cancer. Solid heterogeneous hypoechoic masses in direct relation with the anastomotic bowel loop (*arrows*)

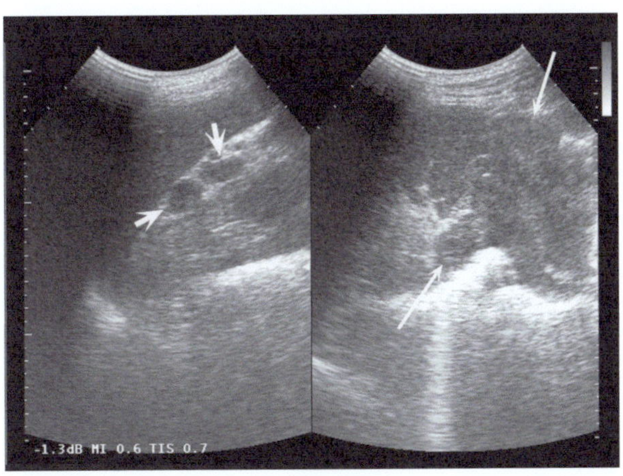

Fig. 5.17 Recurrence of colon cancer. Para-anastomotic mass (*long arrows*) associated with splenic hilar lymphadenopathies (*short arrows*)

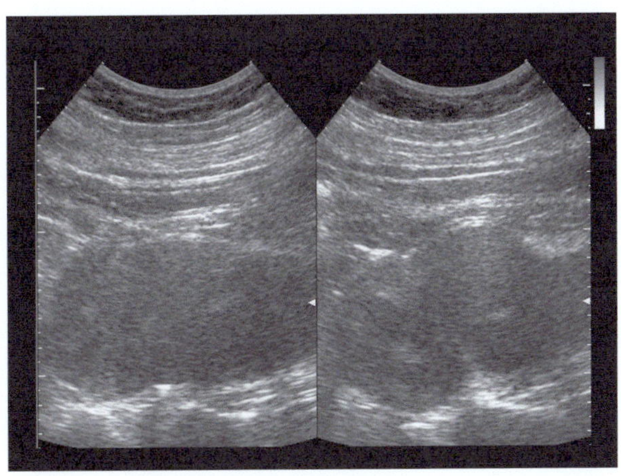

Fig. 5.18 Retroperitoneal neurofibroma in patient with type I neurofibromatosis. Paravertebral, macrolobulated, heterogeneous, hypoechoic mass

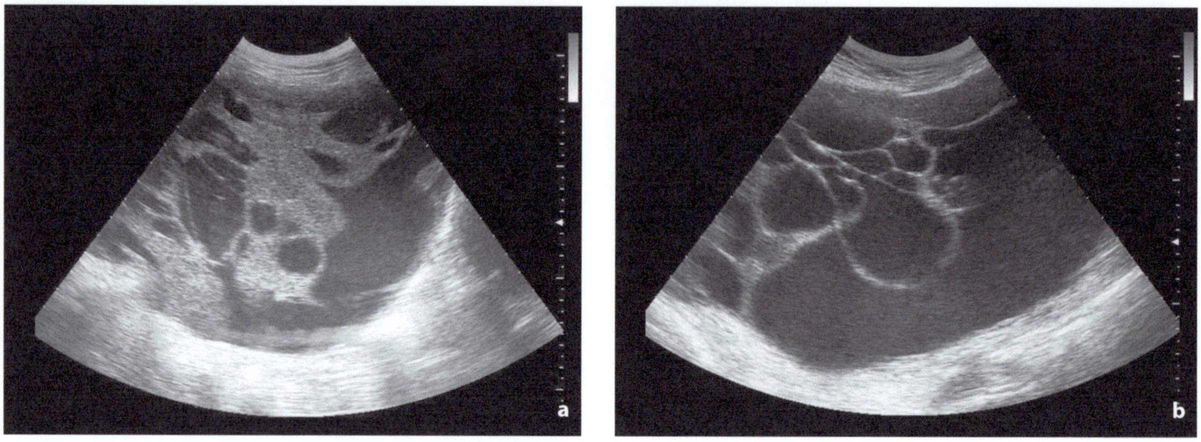

Fig. 5.19a,b Ovarian cancer. Extensive mass with complex structure, irregular septations and solid areas

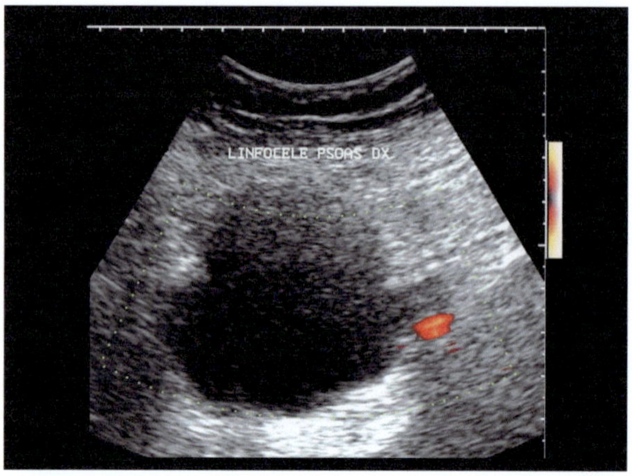

Fig. 5.20 Lumbar lymphocele. Significant unilocular homogeneous fluid collection with avascular appearance at PD after retroperitoneal lymphadenectomy

Hutch's diverticulum (ureterovesical junction), giant prostatic utricle, fetus in fetu, anterior sacral meningocele, adrenal hemorrhage, neuroblastoma, cystic teratomas, bile duct cysts (cystic dilatation of the bile duct, often with a "tear drop" appearance, associated with biliary atresia in 44% of cases), hepatoblastoma, etc. [3,4] (Fig. 5.23). Even in older children the origin is often retroperitoneal, especially renal (55% of cases), although there is a slight increase in the risk of malignancy: hydronephrosis, nephroblastoma, hepatoblastoma, fibrolamellar HCC, hepatic adenoma, cystic papillary tumor of the pancreas, retroperitoneal lymphangioma, gallbladder hydrops, megacolon, intestinal intussusception, hydrometrocolpos, ovarian teratomas, tumor or torsion of undescended testicle [3]. In particular, giant cystic masses in pediatric subjects may be due to gallbladder cysts, splenic cysts, gallbladder hydrops, pancreatic cysts

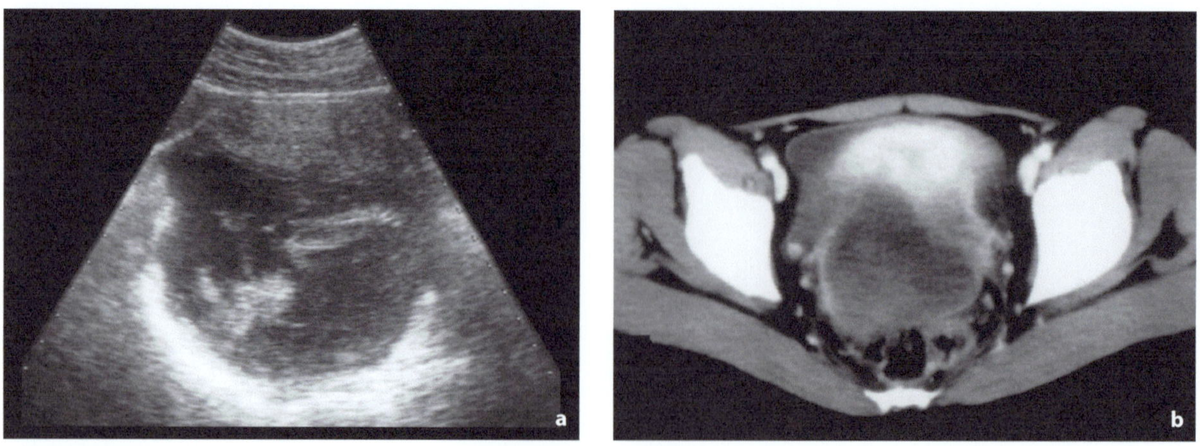

Fig. 5.21a,b Tuboovarian abscess. Heterogeneous hypoechoic fluid collection in retrouterine location (**a**). CT less clearly shows the heterogeneity of the internal content, but better defines the walls and the topographic relations of the mass (**b**)

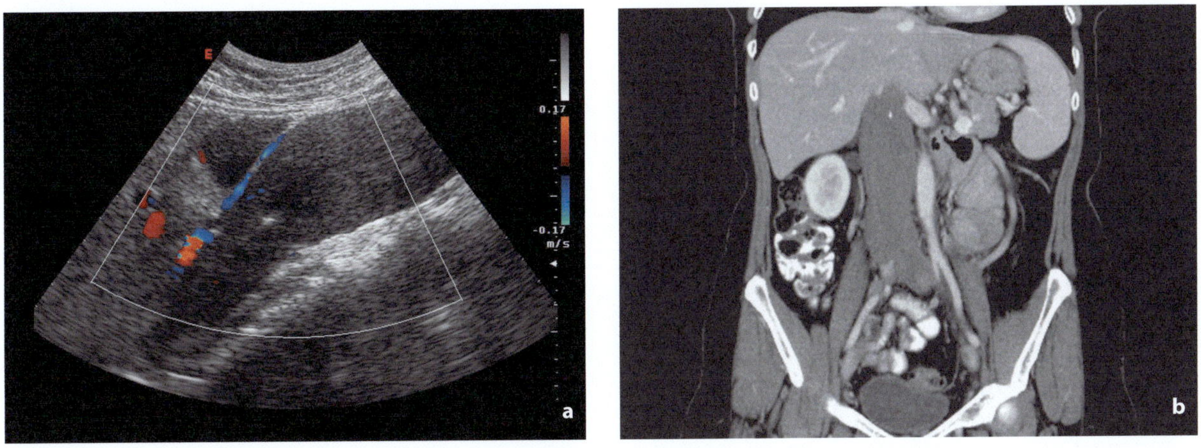

Fig. 5.22a,b Thrombosis of the inferior vena cava from recurring uterine leiomyosarcoma. Both the CD image and the CT scan show the massive widening of the vein caused by the neoplastic tissue

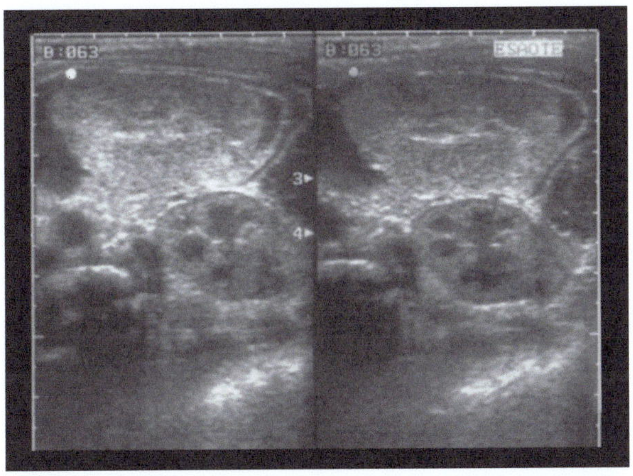

Fig. 5.23 Neonatal abdominal mass (intestinal duplication cyst). Mass with the stratified digestive wall and heterogeneous internal content can be seen in the left flank anterior to the kidney

and pseudocysts, cystadenomas of the pancreas, hydronephrosis, multicystic dysplastic kidney, multilocular cystic nephroma, a resolving process of adrenal hemorrhage, cystic neuroblastoma, cysts of the mesentery and omentum, intestinal duplication cysts, meconium pseudocysts, cysts and cystic tumors of the ovary, hematocolpus, urachal cysts, appendicular abscesses, sacrococcygeal teratomas and spinal fluid pseudocysts (subjects with ventricular-peritoneal shunt) [5].

In **adolescents** pelvic masses mostly arise from the adnexa and may be associated with pain due to expansive growth, torsion or internal bleeding. The masses include simple follicular cysts, corpus luteum cysts, mature teratomas, hemorrhagic cysts and, more rarely, ovarian torsion cysts, tubo-ovarian abscesses, ectopic pregnancies and malignant tumors (especially dysgerminoma and yolk sac tumors) [6]. The differential diagnosis of pelvic tumors, particularly in females, also includes masses of inflammatory origin, such as those resulting from complications of appendicitis, diverticulitis and Crohn's disease.

Persistent gynecologic **masses** are found at US in 1–2% of **pregnant** women, although only 1–3% of these are malignant. The most common findings include follicular or hemorrhagic ovarian cysts, uterine leiomyomas and ovarian hyperstimulation syndrome. The latter, which is linked to induction of ovulation as part of assisted conception techniques, appears as a marked enlargement of the ovary, with multiple, large, thin-walled, peripheral cysts. Given the possible presence of peritoneal effusion, there is the theoretical risk of suspecting an expansive lesion, although the US presentation is rather characteristic (not to mention the patient history). Rare findings include ovarian teratomas, hydrosalpinx, endometriomas, ovarian cystadenomas and cystadenocarcinomas, massive hydronephrosis, mesenteric lipomas and renal ectopia. Endometriosis, which usually involves infertility, may undergo a process of decidualization during pregnancy and mimic a malignant lesion due to its complex appearance and hypervascularity at CD [7]. Relatively infrequent conditions that are directly related to pregnancy include hyperreactio luteinalis not correlated with pharmacologic induction of ovulation, theca lutein cysts (with complete hydatidiform mole in 14–30% of cases) and luteomas [8].

A particular problem regards the **complicated abdominal** mass. The finding of masses in a patient who presents in emergency clinical conditions is not a rare event, whether they are effectively responsible for the symptoms or simply an incidental finding already known to the patient or unrecognized. Symptomatic masses may cause intrinsic or extrinsic obstruction of the bile ducts (jaundice), the collecting system (hydronephrosis) or the intestine (occlusion), or they may cause bleeding (intraparenchymal, retroperitoneal, intraperitoneal and intraluminal bleeding in hollow organs) (Figs. 5.24–5.26).

Bleeding (rupture) of a mass is not a very common event but should be considered in patients with nontraumatic acute/subacute anemia [9]. Bleeding creates a number of diagnostic and therapeutic problems because it may lead to spread of the tumor cells [10]. The task of the diagnosing physician should first of all be to suspect that an expansive lesion may be the cause of the hemorrhage, define the type of expansive lesion and provide information relevant for the choice between surgery or embolization (site and severity of the bleeding, presence of active source of hemorrhage, etc.) and for treatment planning (identification of the afferent vessels at the hemorrhage site, etc.). The

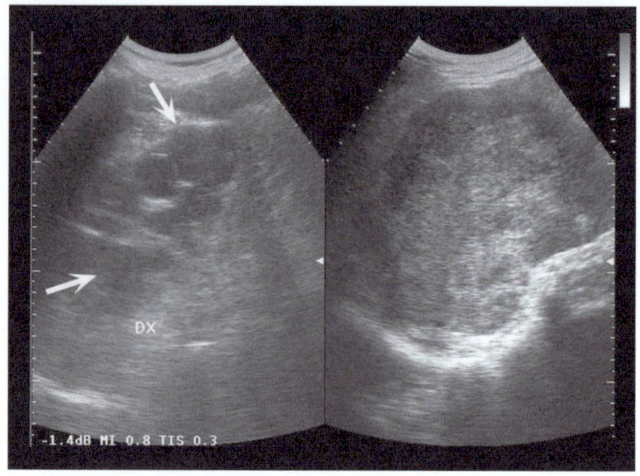

Fig. 5.24 Pelvic recurrence of bladder cancer with hydronephrosis. Solid mass in the pelvis associated with moderate pelvicaliceal dilatation and parenchymal thinning (*arrows*)

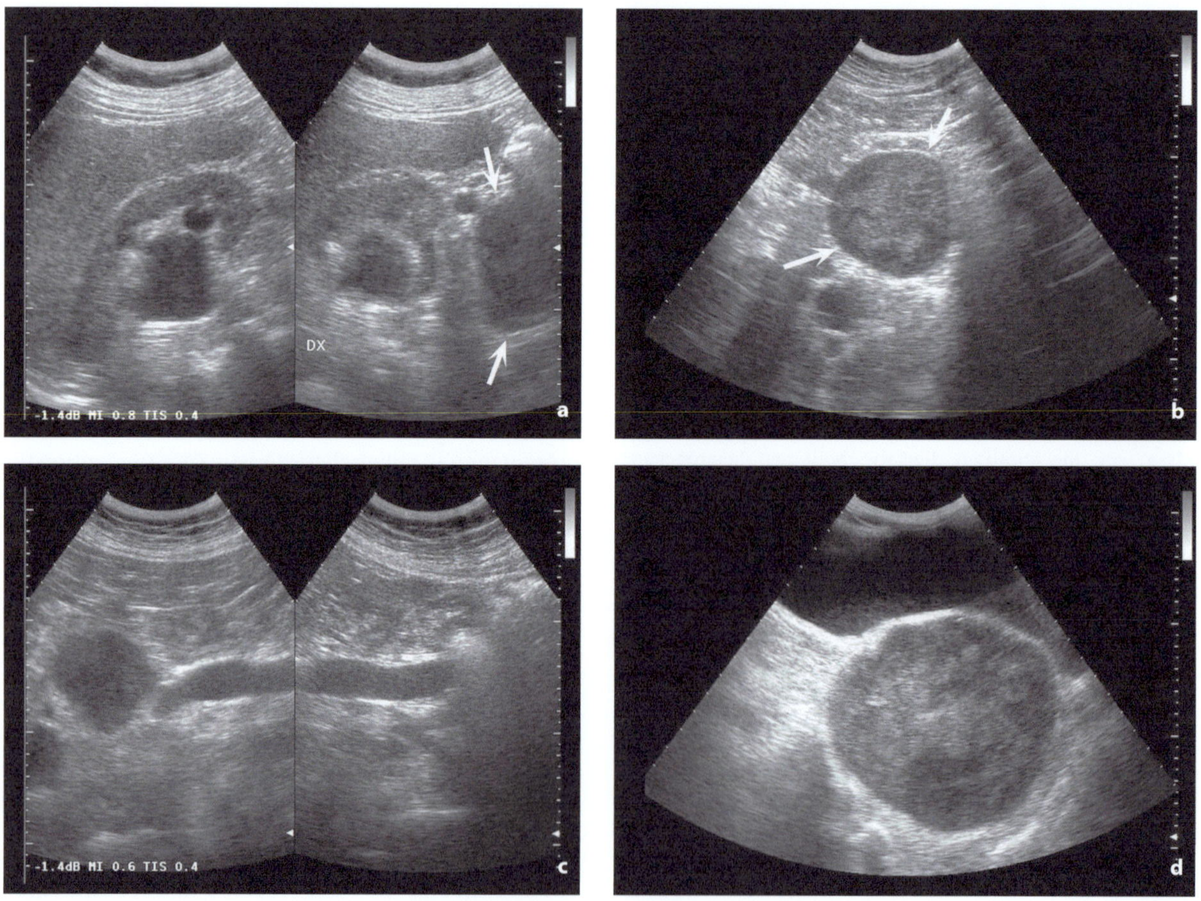

Fig. 5.25a-d Double recurrence of uterine leiomyosarcoma with hydronephrosis. Moderate pelvicaliceal dilatation on the right, associated with a solid lumbar mass (**a**,**b**, *arrows*) is a possible cause of the obstruction. However, distally a marked lumbar ureteric stricture can be seen (**c**) and in fact a second obstructive mass is present at the retrovesical level (**d**)

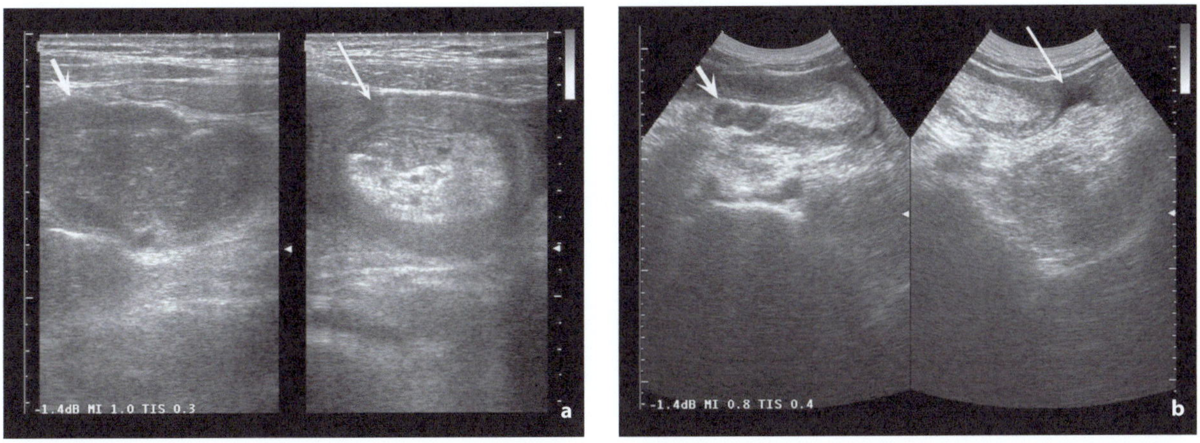

Fig. 5.26a,b Obstructive intestinal intussusception due to mesenteric lymph node metastasis from melanoma. High-resolution study (**a**) shows the dilated loops with corpuscular content proximal to the obstruction (*short arrow*) and the characteristic appearance of a loop in a loop (*long arrow*), also with the eccentric echogenic mesentery invaginated. The panoramic study with the abdominal transducer (**b**) identifies the invaginated hypoechoic lymph nodes (*short arrow*) and peritoneal effusion a sign of "decompensated" occlusion (*long arrow*)

hemorrhage can arise from non-neoplastic lesions such as complicated cysts, from benign tumors, from malignant tumors or from metastases. The most common causes of bleeding in the liver are HCC and adenomas, whereas rare etiologies include FNH (very rarely), metastasis (melanoma), large cavernous hemangiomas, lymphomatous lesions, angiomyolipomas and angiosarcomas. Rupture of the spleen is rather infrequent and may be caused by hemangiomas, teratomas, sarcomas, lymphomas or metastases. Adrenal hemorrhage in the adult is associated with carcinomas, metastases or myelolipomas, but it is rare. Renal hemorrhage is definitely more common and is principally caused by clear-cell carcinomas and especially angiomyolipomas, whereas less common causes include cysts, sarcomas and metastases. Gynecologic bleeding, in addition to ectopic pregnancy, is principally caused by the rupture of cysts [11–15].

Regardless of the histotype of the lesion, some masses have a greater tendency to hemorrhage. Characteristics include large size, rapid growth, invasiveness, hypervascularity, location adjacent to relatively large vessels, internal development of pseudoaneurysms, peripheral location and protrusion from the surface of an organ or peduncular morphology [16]. It should also be recalled that rupture can occur in the absence of a mass, when an organ is made fragile by a diffuse neoplastic process, e.g. in splenomegaly resulting from leukemia or lymphoma, with the development of subcapsular and/or perisplenic hematomas. Hemorrhage can develop within the mass, at the subcapsular level, or towards the outside in the peritoneal cavity, the retroperitoneal spaces or the adjacent ductal and visceral structures. The rupture of a mass may be spontaneous or induced by even mild trauma, or by biopsy, embolization or surgery. Cancer patients are often characterized by predisposing factors such as vessel fragility and a reduction in platelet count induced by chemotherapy. Patients with HCC and cirrhosis have the added burden of portal hypertension, increased PT and reduced platelet count associated with liver disease. In some cases antiplatelet therapy may play an aggravating role. The clinical presentation is variable, with some subjects presenting progressive anemia and vague soreness in the quadrant involved, while others may present sudden-onset acute abdomen and even hypovolemic shock. The US appearance of hemoperitoneum varies over time and depends on the velocity of production, the exploration site and the baseline coagulative state of the patient [17–20]. As a general rule it appears anechoic, although it may be slightly corpuscular with fine or even coarse echoes which move in the fluid. The appearance may be more echogenic, even stratified, near to the source of hemorrhage, particularly in cases which develop in a few hours [21]. Lastly, when the hemorrhage occurs in subjects with ascites, blood-fluid levels may be created, with an echogenic sedimentary component and an overlying anechoic layer (hematocrit effect). When present, blood clots appear echogenic and can be identified in sloping sites in close proximity to the bleeding mass (sentinel clot sign), and possibly stratified on its surface. These should not be confused with collapsed bowel loops or epiploic appendages floating in the effusion. The mass itself is modified in appearance by the hemorrhage and may even be concealed – occasionally the presence of a bleeding lesion is an intraoperative surprise when the procedure is

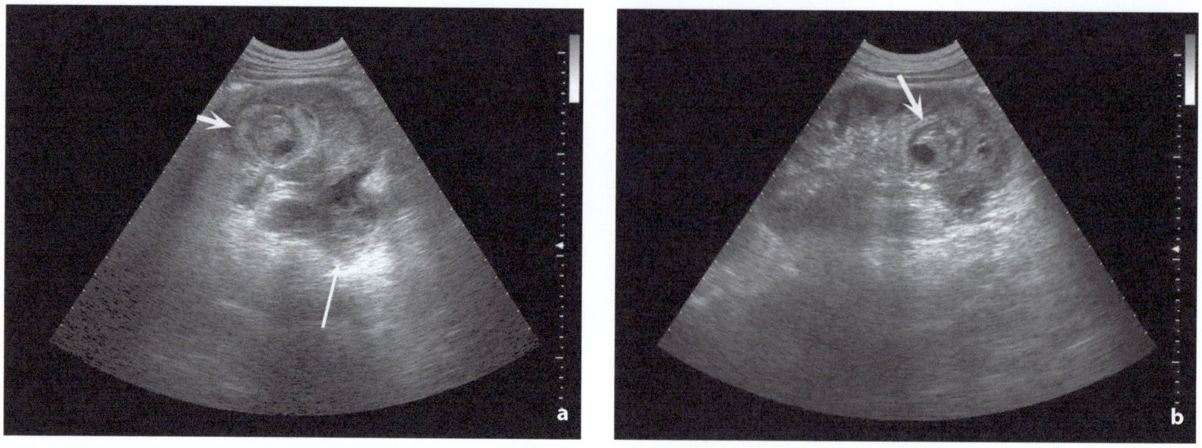

Fig. 5.27a,b Rupture of a pseudoaneurysm within an angiomyolipoma. Posterior perirenal blood collection (*long arrow*) associated with a heterogeneous echogenic renal mass (*short arrows*), with a small internal anechoic area indicating the intralesional pseudoaneurysm

performed for a hemorrhagic focus. The mass becomes heterogeneous internally, particularly in the part with the hemorrhage, with an irregular or patently interrupted surface and possible evidence of internal pseudoaneurysms, fluid-fluid levels or subcapsular collections [11,16,19]. Pseudoaneurysms, which are produced by the vascular erosion of the mass, appear anechoic at US, with a "come and go" signal at spectral analysis and eddying vascular signal at CD [16,22]. CEUS may be able to identify the effusion of contrast medium as a sign of hemorrhage in progress [23,24] (Fig. 5.27, Video 5.1).

In cases of **torsion** of a mass along the axis of the peduncle – a characteristic occurrence particularly in adnexal neoformations (2.7% of gynecologic emergencies) – the mass itself can be identified, solid or more often cystic or complex, with possible signs of infarction. The convoluted appearance of the vascular peduncle is then identified, which at CD has a typical spiral shape (whirlpool sign) [25–27]. Avascularity may be demonstrated within the convoluted peduncle or the mass itself, indicative of strangulation. In addition to the total absence of flows, the lesion may present only reduced arterial flows or reduced arterial and venous flows, and both of these presentations are suspicious for ovarian devascularization [27,28]. A frequent sign is a small amount of effusion in the rectouterine pouch.

5.2 Focal Lesions in Patients without Chronic Liver Disease

US plays a role in the identification of focal hepatic lesions, both in patients with a known extrahepatic malignancy (prior or in course) and in subjects where the finding is incidental. Once identified, hepatic lesions need to be characterized, first of all in terms of benignity or malignancy. Malignant metastatic lesions need to be adequately defined in number, site (segmental attribution), size, morphostructural characteristics and vascular relations. This is required for the purposes of preoperative planning and for a possible comparison after chemotherapy. Although throughout all of these phases there is a significant role for more accurate and panoramic modalities such as CT, MR and PET, US still has an important task to perform, albeit one of integration [29]. There is no doubt that the sensitivity of US, which ranges from 63% to 85% in the most recent studies, is lower than that of CT, MR and PET. Particularly in obese subjects, deep lesions (posterior segments of the right lobe and segment I) can be hard to identify, in part due to beam attenuation. However, even superficial lesions such as those on the anterior profile of the liver – especially segments IV and V – can go unrecognized due to the compression of the superficial layers in the field of insonation. This underlines the importance of modifying the transmit frequency, focal zone depth and gains throughout the examination.

CD can be of some help in identifying lesions. First of all it is able to rule out the vascular nature of a hypo-anechoic image, such as in the case of a transversally sectioned vessel, but also in the eventuality of a vascular disease such as an aneurysm, as well as being able to confirm the nonvascular nature of a finding, such as cystic masses adjacent to vessels. In addition hypo-anechoic lesions can stand out better with respect to the vascular structures "colored" by the Doppler signal, while hypervascular lesions (HCC, FNH, some metastases) become more evident thanks to the greater concentration of color signal [30].

Even **spectral Doppler** of the **hepatic artery** has been suggested for the identification of focal lesions, especially in patients with suspected occult metastases. Indeed, in these cases both dynamic CT and spectral Doppler have suggested the presence of hemodynamic modifications to the extent of increasing the risk or the suspicion of occult metastasization, which then appeared macroscopically in subsequent controls. In fact, CT has quantitatively demonstrated greater parenchymal enhancement in the arterial phase in subjects who then go on to develop hepatic lesions or who have occult lesions, than in healthy subjects. In the subject with metastasis there appears to be a generalized increase in arterial hepatic flow, perhaps in response to a reduction in portal supply (induced by tumor mediators) [31–33]. A number of Doppler parameters can be recorded. These include V_{max} and RI of the hepatic artery, flow volume in the hepatic artery, flow volume in the portal vein, total flow volume in the liver (flow volume in the artery + flow volume in the portal vein, normally in the proportions of around 1/4 and 3/4) and Doppler perfusion index (DPI, arterial flow volume/total hepatic flow volume, normally around 0.25). Factors that definitely influence the Doppler spectrum are the postprandial state (examination should be performed on an empty stomach) and possible underlying chronic liver disease. Spectral evaluation of the hepatic artery has also been proposed as a prognostic indicator in patients with liver metastases and the selection of subjects to undergo adjuvant chemotherapy [34,35].

CEUS can undoubtedly increase the sensitivity (as well as the specificity) of US in the identification of liver metastases, since those that are sought after appear as enhancement defects (not due to cysts) in the opacified parenchyma during the portal-sinusoidal phase. The patient search for “enhancement defects” in the several minutes of the portal-sinusoidal vascular phase with second-generation contrast medium, or even in the postvascular parenchymal phase with first-generation contrast medium, makes identification of a significant number of small lesions not visible at the initial US examination possible. Since the liver can be well explored in all of its sites, the sensitivity of CEUS is practically comparable with CT and MR [36,37]. Studies on transit times of contrast media have suggested faster wash-in and wash-out times in subjects with liver metastases than in healthy controls, but these functional findings need to be confirmed [38].

An adequate **characterization** of the focal lesions found is fundamental, especially when this is relevant for the staging of a cancer patient, or when it occurs in a phase preliminary to surgical resection of the liver. However, despite the diagnostic techniques available today, differential diagnosis is still difficult. In a large patient population with hepatic lesions considered to be malignant [39], the diagnosis was found to be benign at resection in 7% of total cases (but as high as 24% in the subcategory with diagnosis of hilar cholangiocarcinoma). The alternative is cytologic or histologic evaluation of all lesions that are candidates for hepatic resection, but this opens the door to complications and also produces the opposite problem of false negatives. In general, in a subject without chronic liver disease, the likelihood of the lesion being benign rather than malignant is greater, regardless of whether it is a single focus or a multifocal (<4) lesion and whether the patient has an extrahepatic malignancy. The prevalence of lesions such as cysts and hemangiomas is so high as to reduce the likelihood of finding a malignant lesion [40]. This is particularly true, at least in CT, for small lesions (<15 mm), which are malignant only in 5% of cases (but in 19% if 2–4 lesions are present and 76% if >4) [41].

A frequent problem is posed by **subcentimeter lesions** identified at CT (up to 17% of outpatients studied with conventional CT) and MR and not adequately characterized [41]. While in most cases these are small cysts, it is also true that they can be solid lesions, especially in cancer patients, in whom 12% of subcentimeter lesions identified at CT prove to be metastatic [42]. With the current multislice CT scanners this situation is unlikely to change a great deal, because although many small lesions are better characterized, the scanners also identify a much larger number of microlesions. In these cases then, a US correlation is advisable, and should be possibly performed immediately [43,44]. In a study [44] in patients with extrahepatic tumors and hepatic lesions <15 mm found to be indeterminate at CT, US was able to identify 48% of the lesions. Factors influencing the rate of detection were the morphotype of the patient, the size of the CT finding (if >5 mm) and the availability of direct evaluation of the reference CT images. The site of the lesion did not prove to be influential. US was able to characterize 93% of the lesions identified (33 cysts, 18 solid lesions/metastases and 5 hemangiomas). In the cases where US was unable to characterize the finding and a definitive diagnosis was important from the clinical point of view, a further study with CEUS, MR or needle aspirate may be appropriate. The latter has proven feasible and effective even in small lesions [45,46] (Fig. 5.28).

Anechoic focal lesions can be the expression of congenital cysts, acquired cysts (trauma, abscess, etc.), segmental dilatation of the bile ducts, polycystic kidney syndromes, cystic dilatation of the bile ducts, cystic hydatidosis, abscesses, hematomas (acute phase), bilomas (acute phase), cystic metastases,

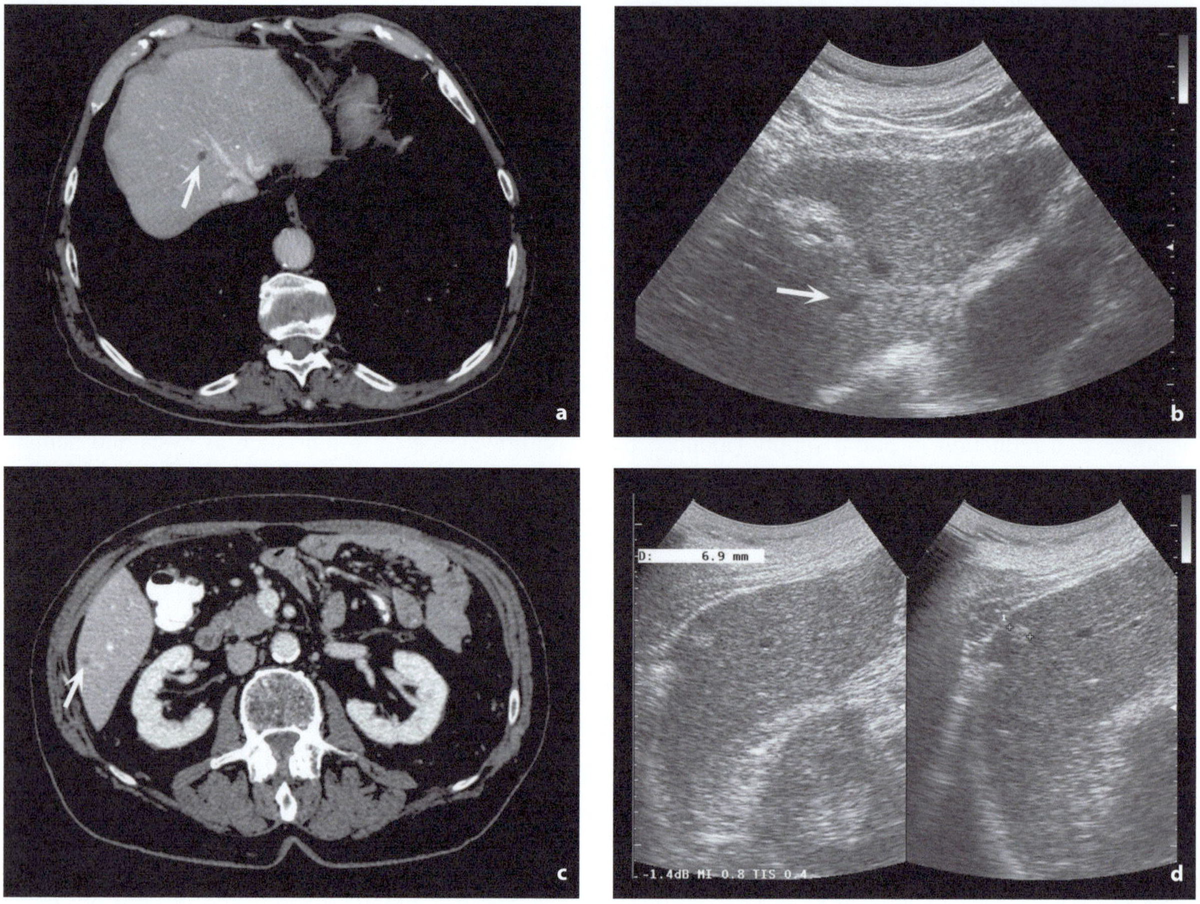

Fig. 5.28a-d Extemporaneous US study after CT. CT finding of two hypoattenuating, subcentimeter, nonspecific areas (**a**, **c**, *arrows*) which at US are found to be a microcyst (**b**, *arrow*), and a small hemangioma (**d**, *between the calipers*)

biliary cystadenomas, intrahepatic gallbladder, arterial aneurysms, arterial pseudoaneurysms or venous aneurysms. Simple cysts (at least 1% of individuals <60 years of age and at least 3% of those >60 years) are predominant in females (F/M 4:1) and most commonly found in the left lobe [40]. They appear as single, or more often multiple, homogeneous anechoic lesions with enhanced through-transmission and sharp margins but no walls. Marginal calcification may be present, as well as possible partial internal septations with an overall multilobulated appearance [40] (Fig. 5.29). The finding of heterogeneous content, solid components, thick and irregular septations or internal vascular signs suggests the need for further diagnostic procedures due to the risk of biliary cystadenomas or metastases.

Solid lesions to include in the differential diagnosis are HCC on a healthy liver (see next section), hemangioma, adenoma, FNH, metastasis, intrahepatic cholangiocarcinoma and rare lesions. Hepatic

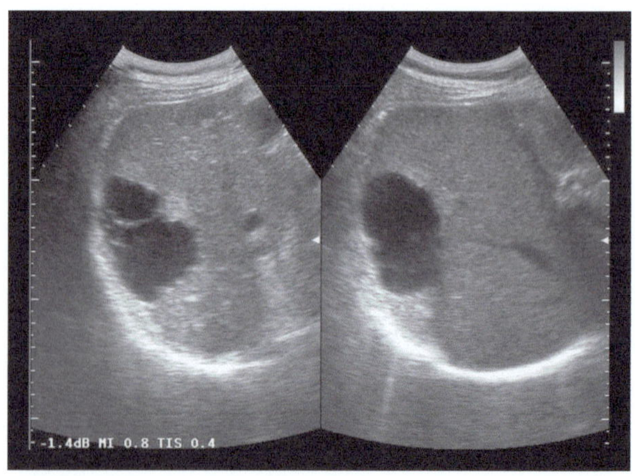

Fig. 5.29 Atypical hepatic cysts. Substantially unilocular anechoic mass with sharp lobulated margins and mildly heterogeneous hyperechoic appearance of the adjacent parenchyma

pseudolesions should also be borne in mind, such as areas of healthy parenchyma in a fatty liver ("focal sparing") and areas of focal steatosis (skip areas).

Liver metastases are found at postmortem in 25–50% of patients with extrahepatic carcinoma, and their identification is important both for staging and the choice of treatment. The liver is fertile ground for the development of metastases, because it receives 25% of cardiac output, because it is the site of venous return from most digestive organs, because its sinusoid are wide and have a basal fenestrated membrane, and because the local hormonal mechanisms stimulate the growth of cell colonies [47]. Metastases most commonly originate from tumors of the lung, colon, pancreas, breast and stomach. Some 25–40% of patients with gastrointestinal cancer or small-cell lung cancer have metastases at presentation. The highest prevalence is in patients with carcinoma of the lung (small cell), gallbladder, pancreas, colon, stomach and esophagus, as well as in patients with carcinoid. Prostate cancer, together with renal, cervical and head and neck (squamous cell) cancers have the lowest rates of liver metastases [30,40,47]. The tumors which most frequently metastasize to the liver are colon (~40%), stomach (>20%), pancreas (~20%), breast and lung (~10%). There are multiple spread patterns of metastases which may occasionally coexist: (1) portal hematogenous, from the abdominal viscera; (2) arterial hematogenous, from the lungs and other organs of the systemic circulation; (3) retrograde lymphatic, from tumors of the stomach, pancreas, gallbladder, etc.; (4) by contiguity, from adjacent organs such as the gallbladder, colon, stomach; (5) peritoneal, from ovarian tumors or from other intraperitoneal organs. Growth times are extremely variable and depend on many factors, which are only in part predictable: the doubling time for metastases from colorectal cancer varies from 1 to 36 months [47]. Traditionally, these lesions have been differentiated as hypervascular, with hyperattenuation/hyperintensity in the arterial phase of dynamic CT/MR (endocrine tumors, sarcomas, clear-cell renal carcinomas, etc.) and hypovascular, which are more frequent and without hyperattenuation/hyperintensity in the arterial phase of CT/MR. In reality, with real-time CEUS it has been possible to observe how nearly all these histotypes display at least some form of enhancement in the arterial phase, occasionally lasting only a few seconds and therefore not always "interceptable" in CT/MR multiphase acquisitions.

Today the diagnostic imaging modalities still tend to underestimate the presence of liver metastases, especially with regard to subcentimeter lesions. The accuracy of conventional US is approximately 64–85%, being limited with respect to CT and MR as it is markedly influenced by the experience of the sonographer and the build of the patient. CEUS is able to significantly increase diagnostic accuracy with respect to the baseline examination, but due to the additional costs and greater complexity of the study it does not appear to be feasible on a routine basis and is indicated only in patients with extrahepatic tumors with an elevated prevalence of liver metastases, or in patients evaluated with US in the preoperative phase. CEUS can perform a more precise measurement of metastases than US, but this needs to be done in the relatively early phase of enhancement because in the sinusoidal phase the lesion may appear reduced in size [48]. IOUS has very high sensitivity (97–98%), being able to identify lesions as small as 2 mm, and is therefore particularly useful in the choice of surgical technique [40].

Liver metastases are multiple in 90% of cases and prevalent in the right lobe, although they often present in both lobes. Their appearance varies considerably in relation to the histologic and bioevolutionary characteristics of the primary tumor, its degree of vascularity, its size and its site, although often in an unpredictable way [40]. They may be isolated or confluent. The shape largely depends on their size – when the metastases are <3 cm they tend to be round, but as they grow they tend to take on a different shape, often becoming irregular. The margins of small lesions are generally regular and well circumscribed with respect to the surrounding hepatic tissue, but as they grow the margins become poorly defined, and in some cases identifying a line of demarcation with the surrounding tissue becomes impossible. Invasive growth can occasionally occur in metastases from breast or lung cancer, as well as from melanoma. The most frequent US pattern is hypoechogenicity, especially in small lesions, followed by hyperechogenicity and lastly isoechogenicity. Moreover, no precise correlation has been found between the US appearance of the metastases and their origin. In general, rapidly growing metastases, such as those from lung and pancreas cancer or from melanoma, have a hypoecoic appearance and also tend to be hypervascular. Metastases from breast cancer also tend to be hypoechoic, whereas secondary lesions from neuroendocrine tumors, renal cell carcinomas and choriocarcinomas tend to be hyperechoic [29]. A frequent finding in liver metastases, especially in larger forms and above all from lung cancer, is the peripheral hypoechoic halo, mostly due to compression and reactive edema, which gives the lesion an overall target appearance. The halo is not specific, because it may also be seen in FNH, fungal abscess, hemangioma, adenoma, lymphoma, HCC and peripheral cholangiocarcinoma [49]. A frank target appearance with a variable number of rings of differing echogenicity is found particularly in metastases from neuroendocrine tumors. In other cases the appearance is poorly defined, with tenuous areas and ill-defined hypoechogenicity or hyperechogenicity. In the case of a background of steatosis, which is not a rare occurrence since many of these patients are undergoing chemotherapy at the time of examination, the appearance is usually hypoechoic. In other circumstances the metastases may take on a hemangiomatous, generally homogeneous hyperechoic appearance, such as in the case of lesions originating from the colon. Malignancies which most often give rise to calcified metastases, possibly with posterior acoustic shadowing, are mucinous adenocarcinoma (colon, stomach, ovary), neuroblastoma, chondrosarcoma, osteosarcoma, endocrine pancreas, melanoma, mesothelioma, medullary thyroid carcinoma, and pulmonary carcinoma. In the presence of ovarian tumors, the metastases may be found within the parenchyma, as well as in the capsule and often arise after chemotherapy [50]. The pseudocystic appearance due to necrotic phenomena is typical of the histotypes (colon cancer, breast or ovarian cancer, squamous cell tumors, sarcomas, melanomas, etc.) characterized by a marked cellular proliferation not associated with a similar angiogenesis and therefore sufficient blood supply. Alternatively, the pseudocystic appearance is the result of treatment, e.g. GIST after therapy with imatinib. Internal septations are possible, whereas fluid-fluid levels due to necrotic hemorrhage are much more rare [40]. The patently cystic appearance is characteristic of primary histotypes (ovarian cystadenocarcinoma, pancreatic macrocystic mucinous adenocarcinoma, etc.) whose specific neoplastic cellular differentiation produces a cystic structure regardless of overlying necrosis. Abscess degeneration (colon cancer) is possible, with gaseous microbubbles in the form of echogenic nuclei with reverberation artifacts (Figs. 5.30–5.50, Video 5.2–5.7).

At CD the metastases may appear with no vascular signals, display a displacement of adjacent vessels (detouring pattern, 40% of cases) or present more-or-less significant internal vascularity (1/3 of metastases against 3/4 of HCC) [51,52]. The internal vessels may be prevalently peripheral or uniformly distributed with variable spectral profiles, in terms both of venous and especially arterial flow. The absence or the barest representation of the diastolic component, with an elevated RI, is highly suggestive of malignancy, although relatively infrequent. In general the vascularity of metastases is limited and not sufficient to be a significant help in terms of characterization. CD may be able to identify vascular invasion at the level of the portal branches or the suprahepatic veins, although this is rather uncommon in metastatic lesions, especially

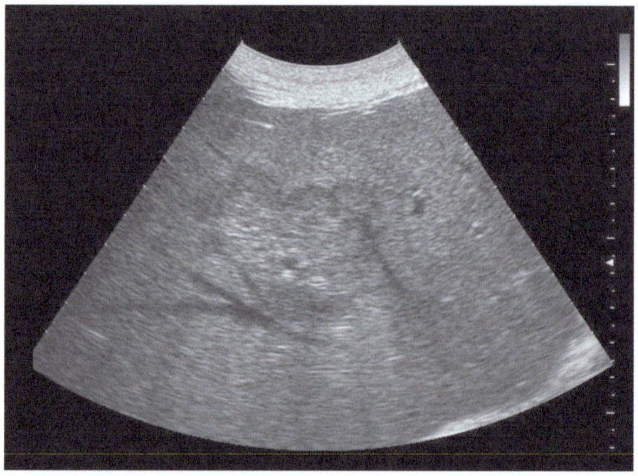

Fig. 5.30 Hepatic metastasis from stomach cancer. Irregularly shaped, heterogeneous, iso-hypoechoic lesion with a thin peripheral hypoechoic halo

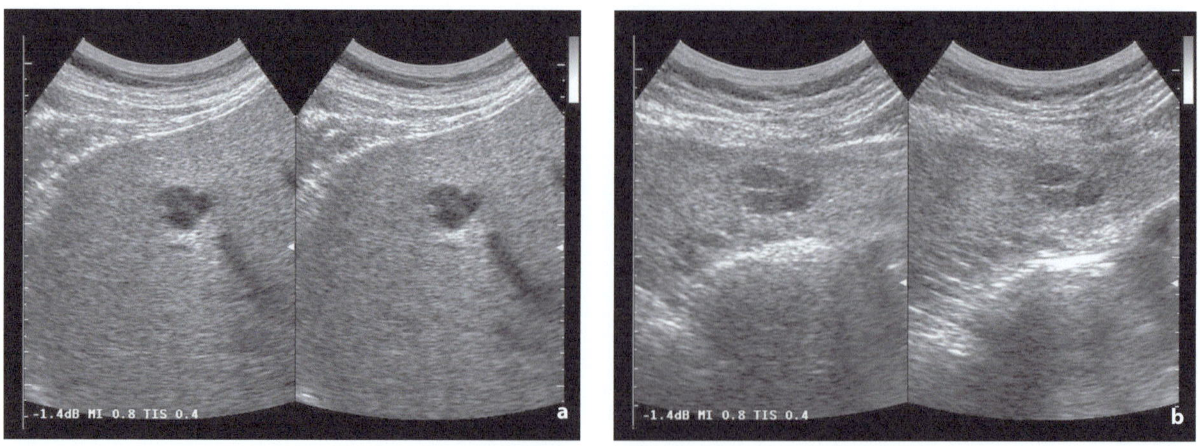

Fig. 5.31a,b Cystic-like hepatic metastasis from melanoma. Two hypo-anechoic masses, in the right hepatic lobe (**a**) and the other in the left hepatic lobe (**b**)

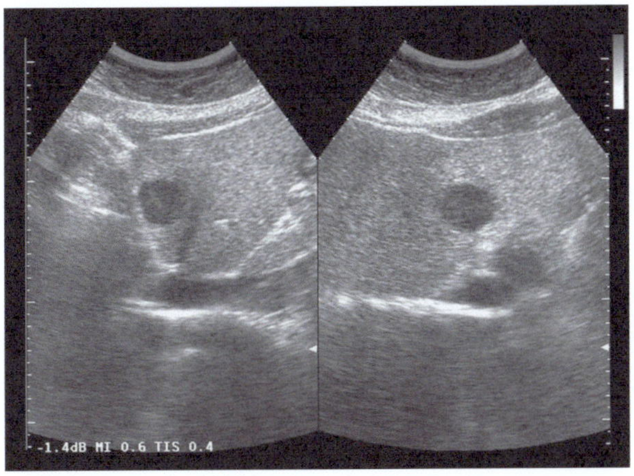

Fig. 5.32 Liver metastasis from breast cancer in steatosis. Markedly hypoechoic lesion with respect to the parenchymal background

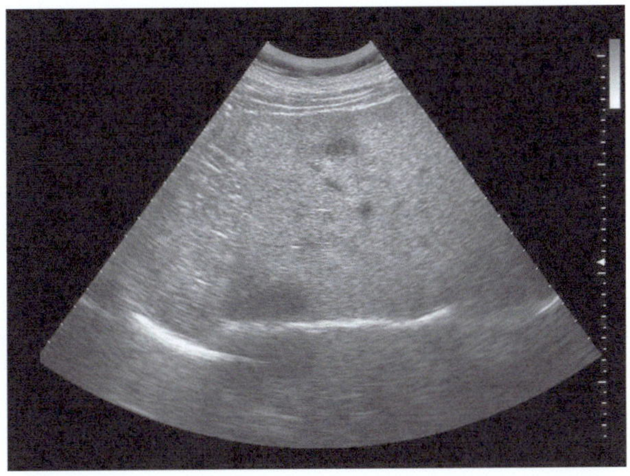

Fig. 5.33 Liver metastases from breast cancer in steatosis. Hypoechoic lesions with respect to the parenchymal background, with ill-defined margins

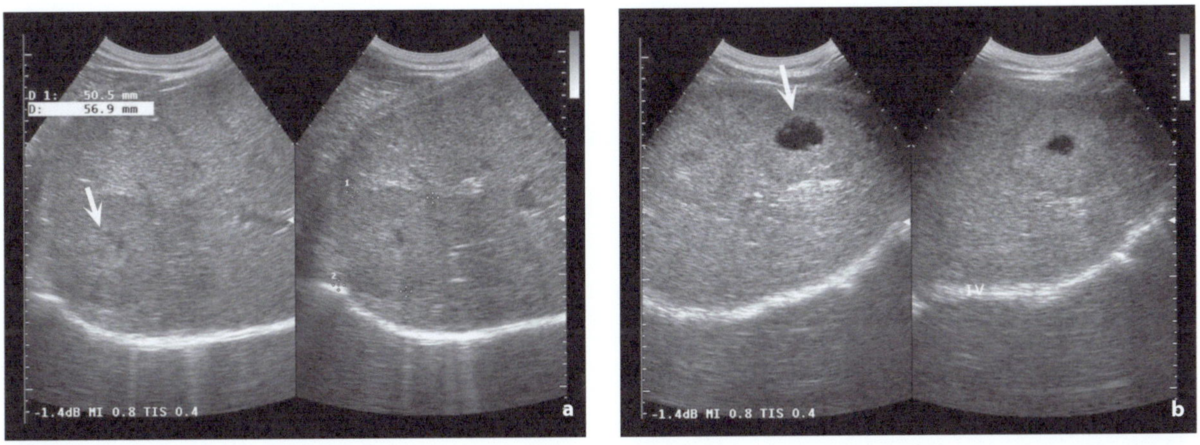

Fig. 5.34a,b Liver metastasis from colon cancer. Mildly hypoechoic masses with slight (**a**, *arrow*) or marked (**b**, *arrow*) central liquefaction

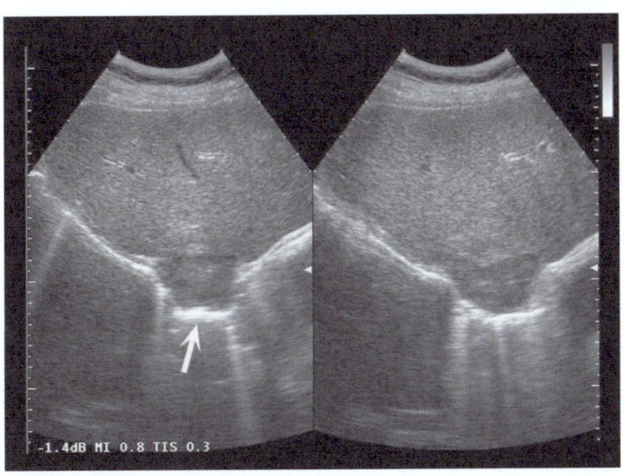

Fig. 5.35 Liver metastasis from ovarian cancer. Hypoechoic lesion bulging from the hepatic dome (*arrow*)

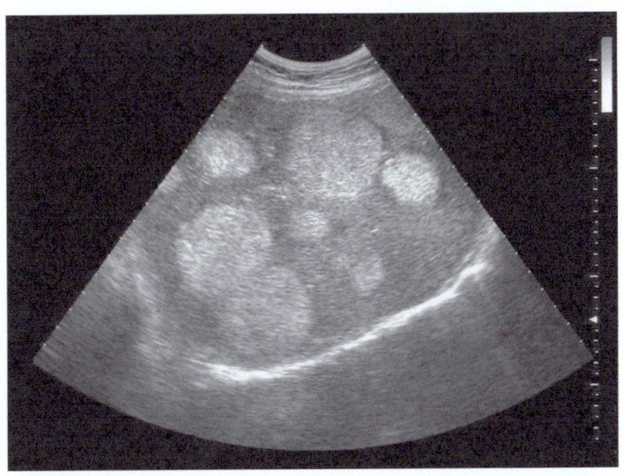

Fig. 5.36 Liver metastasis from melanoma. Multiple well-defined, relatively homogeneous, hyperechoic lesions with a slight peripheral hypoechoic halo

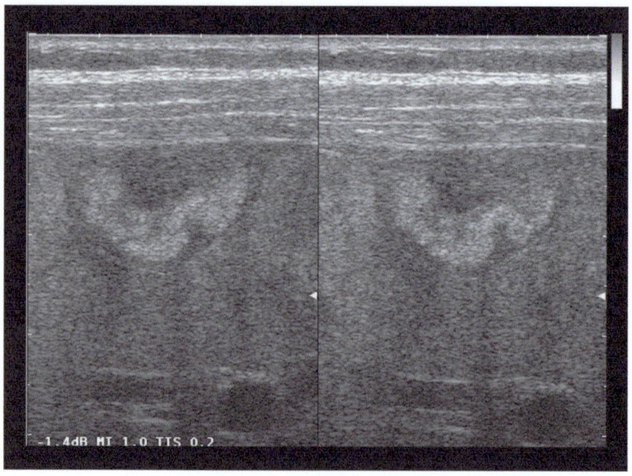

Fig. 5.37 Capsular liver metastasis from ovarian cancer. Use of the superficial transducer makes accurate definition of the echogenic area possible, which produces a marked retraction and scalloping of the surface of the left hepatic lobe

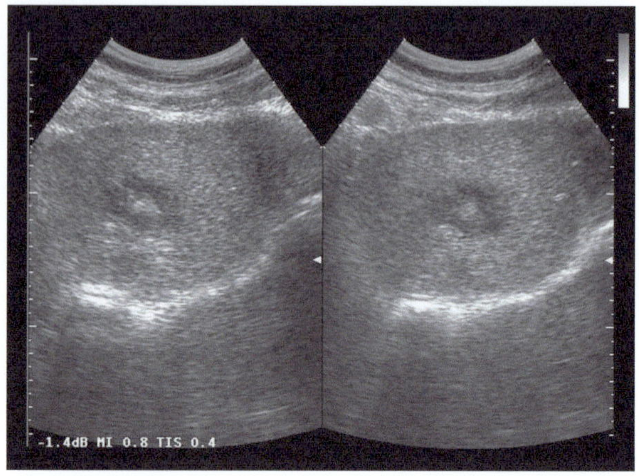

Fig. 5.38 Liver metastasis from breast cancer. Hypoechoic mass with echogenic center

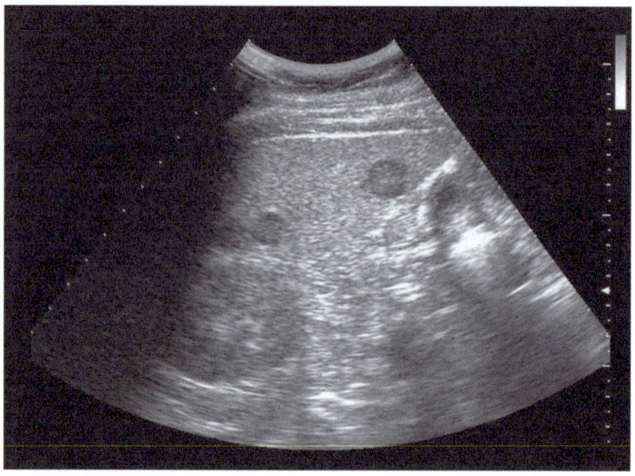

Fig. 5.39 Liver metastasis from breast cancer in steatosis. Macronodular lesions appearing markedly hypoechoic against the parenchymal background

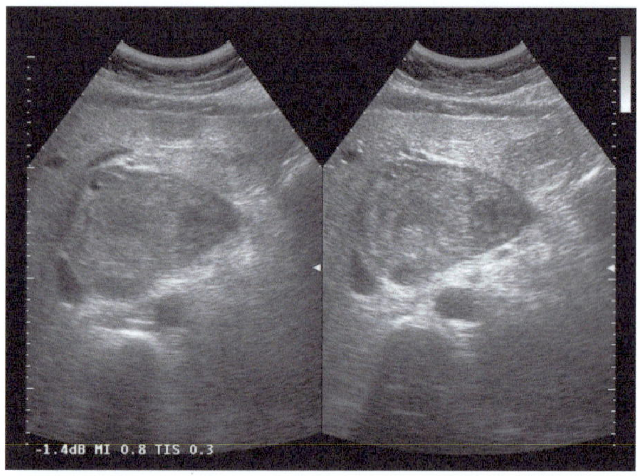

Fig. 5.40 Liver metastasis from angiosarcoma of the breast. Large, heterogeneous, hypoechoic lesion at the level of the caudate lobe

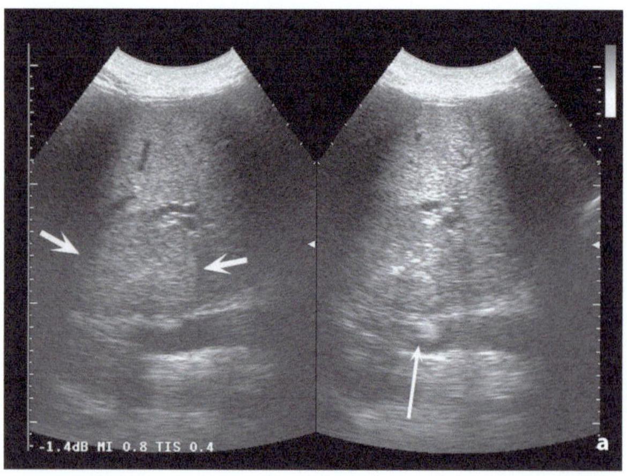

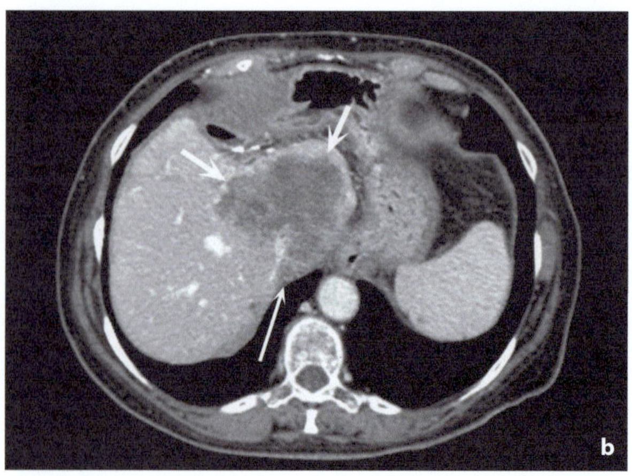

Fig. 5.41a,b Liver metastasis from colon cancer, with infiltration of the vena cava. Heterogeneous and mildly hypoechoic hepatic lesion (**a**, *short arrows*) with echogenic areas in the inferior vena cava (*long arrow*). CT correlation in the venous phase (**b**)

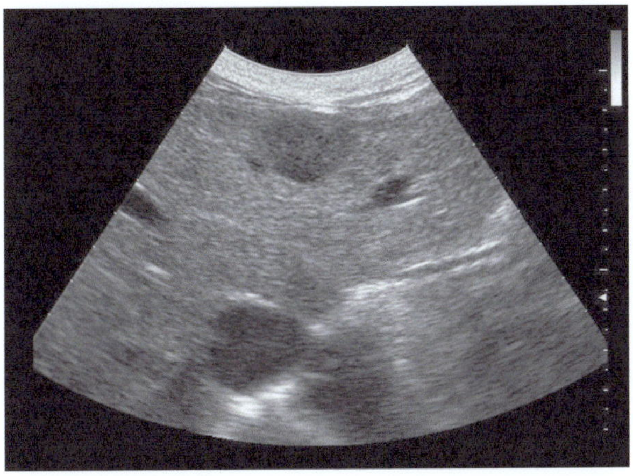

Fig. 5.42 Liver metastasis from neuroendocrine tumor of the pancreas. Markedly hypoechoic macronodular lesion

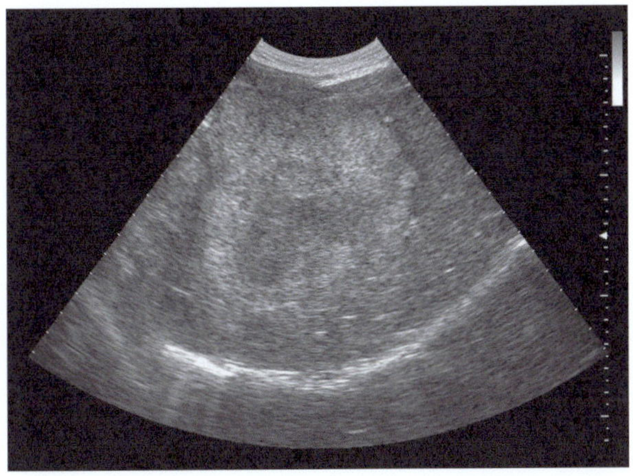

Fig. 5.43 Liver metastasis from stomach cancer. Heterogeneous echogenic mass with tendency to central hypoechogenicity and slight peripheral hypoechoic halo

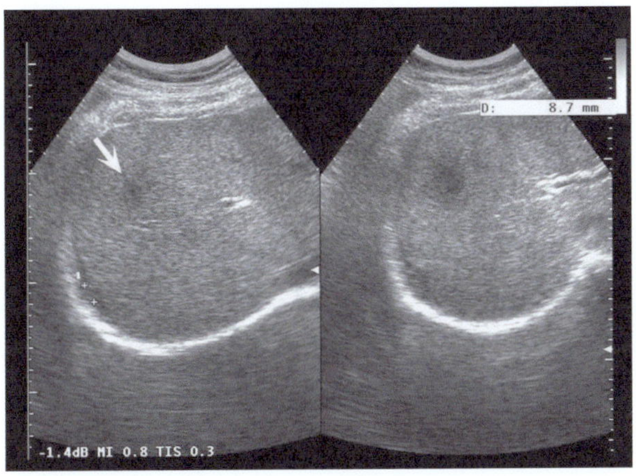

Fig. 5.44 Parenchymal and capsular liver metastases from ovarian cancer. Two heterogeneous hypoechoic areas can be identified, one inside the liver (*arrow*) and the other on the surface (*between the calipers*)

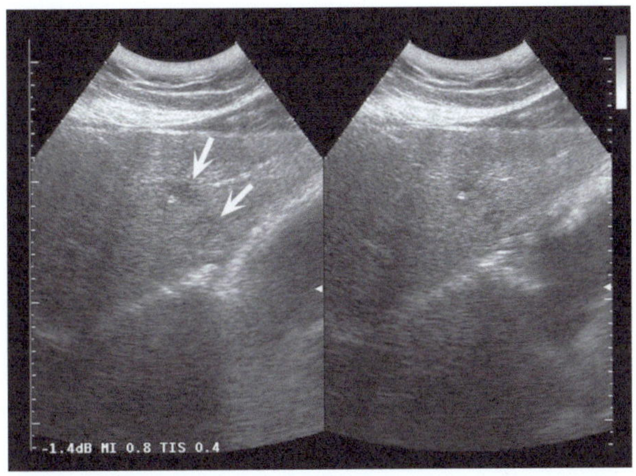

Fig. 5.45 Liver metastasis from pancreatic cancer. Ill-defined and irregular hypoechoic areas in the left hepatic lobe (*arrows*)

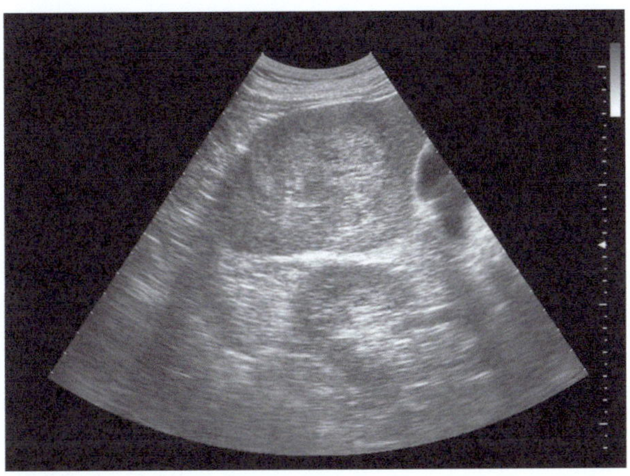

Fig. 5.46 Hepatic metastasis from rectal cancer. Large heterogeneous echogenic lesion in hepatic segment V

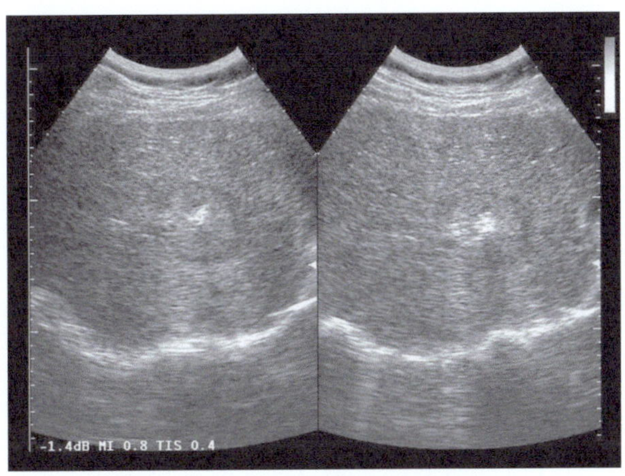

Fig. 5.47 Calcified liver metastasis from pancreatic cancer. Target lesion with isoechoic appearance, thin peripheral hypoechoic halo and central calcified echogenic nucleus

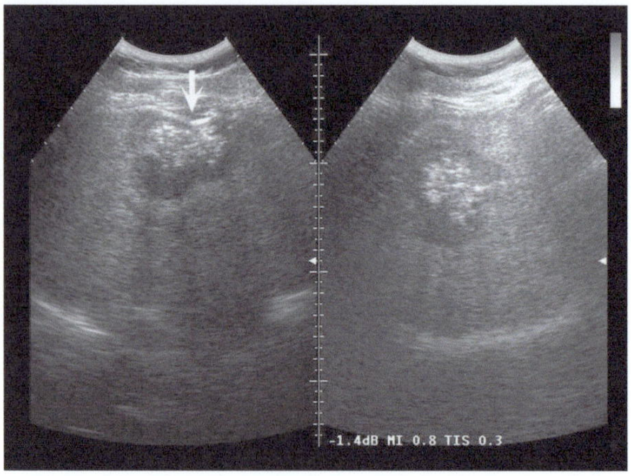

Fig. 5.48 Calcified liver metastasis from ovarian cancer. Hypoechoic mass with multiple and especially central calcifications and retraction of the capsular hepatic surface (*arrow*)

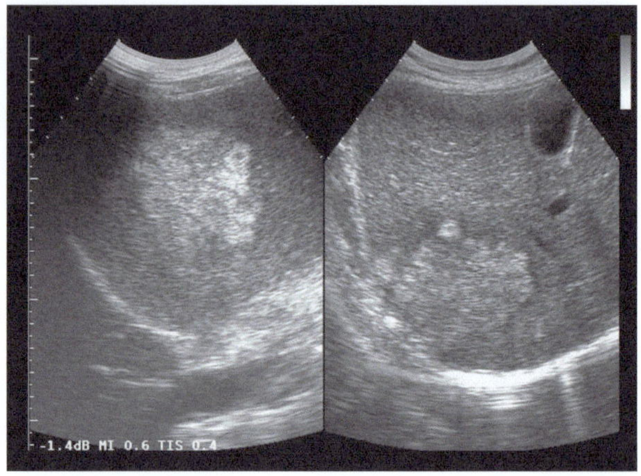

Fig. 5.49 Liver metastasis from rectal cancer. Heterogeneous hyperechoic lesion with peripheral hypoechoic halo

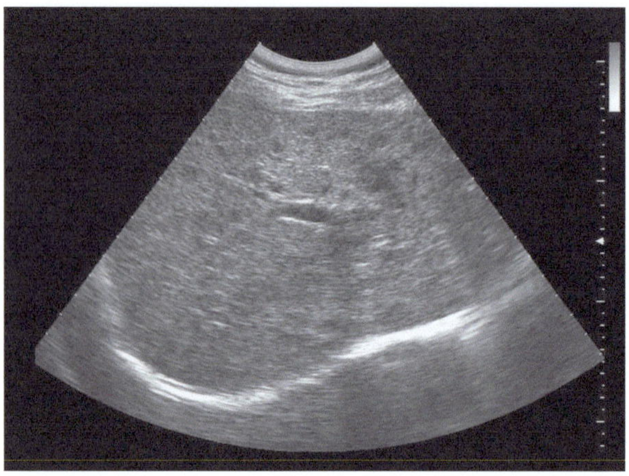

Fig. 5.50 Liver metastasis from melanoma. Multiple miliary hypoechoic lesions

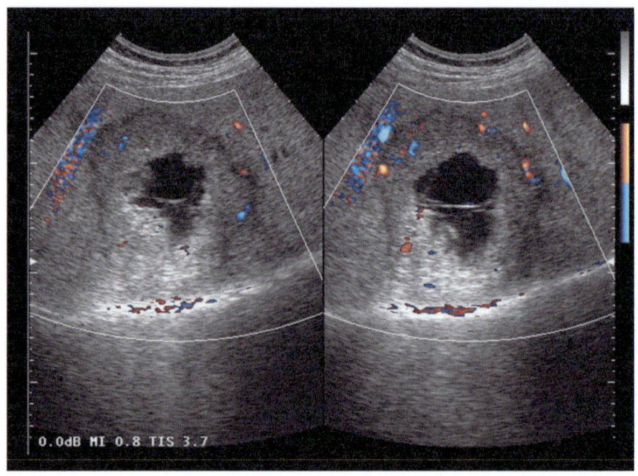

Fig. 5.51 Abscessed liver metastasis from colon cancer. Large lesion with necrotic-liquefactive center and some peripheral vascular signals at directional PD

with regard to portal invasion (<5% of cases) [40]. However, CD is unable to show whether and when hypovascularity within liver metastases is an expression of necrosis, an element which is generally indicative of malignancy (Figs. 5.51–5.53).

CEUS evaluation has proven to be particularly useful in the characterization of metastases. Regardless of the appearance in the arterial phase, a hypoechoic hepatic lesion in the portal-sinusoidal phase should be considered malignant (metastatic) until proven otherwise, both in cases of cancer patients and when the lesion is an incidental finding [36,37,53]. In the arterial phase, the metastases display different levels of enhancement and can appear hypervascular, albeit very briefly, even when not considering those histotypes that have classically been considered hypervascular (endocrine tumors of the pancreas, sarcomas, RCC, transitional cell carcinomas, etc.). The typical pattern of arterial enhancement is annular, with a generally thick and continuous hyperechoic ring, whereas diffuse, homogeneous or heterogeneous enhancement is much rarer. In the portal-sinusoidal phase some generally sharply hypoechoic areas can be seen, characterized internally by teeming echoes in real time, which are an expression of the "microcirculation" and indicative of lesion activity [53] (Fig. 5.54).

Monitoring of known hepatic lesion in patients undergoing **systemic therapy** is usually performed with US and/or CT. Of course the latter is in general preferable, since it provides a more complete hepatic and extrahepatic picture, with better definition of the

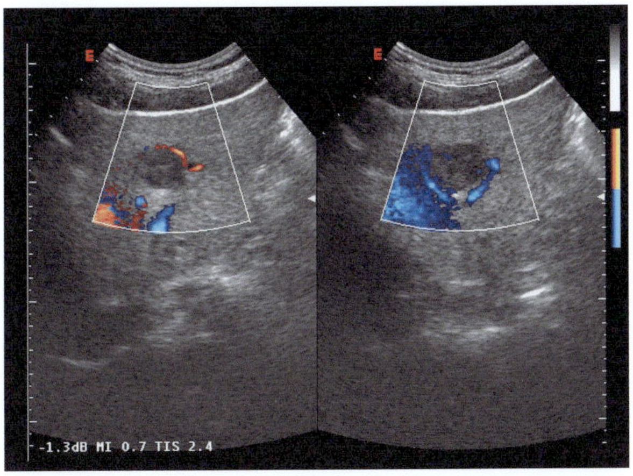

Fig. 5.52 Liver metastasis from breast cancer. Heterogeneous hypoechoic lesion on a background of fatty liver, which at PD shows some internal flow but above all a pattern of displacement of an adjacent vessel

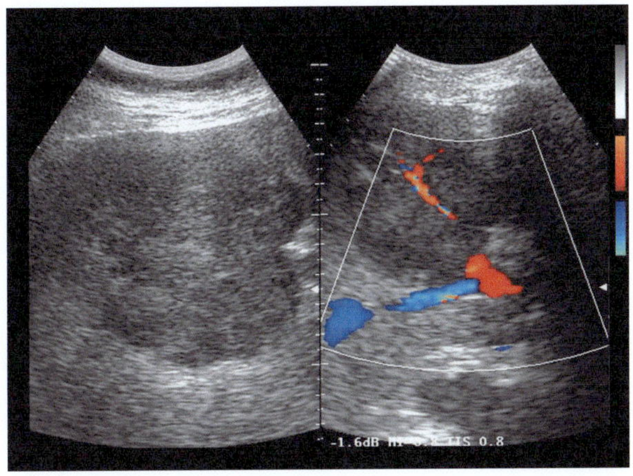

Fig. 5.53 Liver metastasis from endometrial cancer. Large parahilar invasive hypoechoic lesion which encircles a hepatic arterial branch at CD

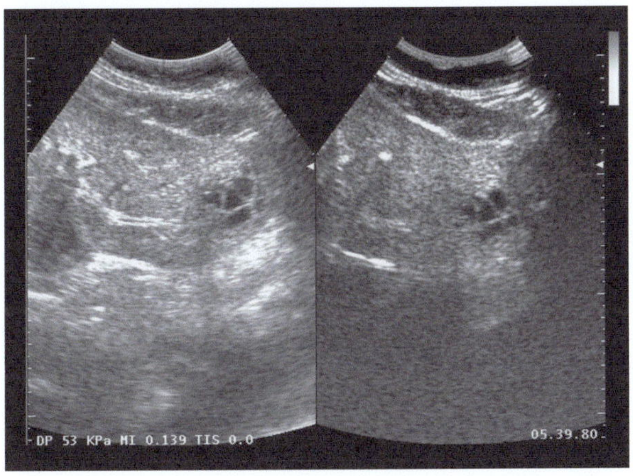

Fig. 5.54 Cystic metastasis from lung cancer. Multiseptated mass of the left lobe, which at CEUS (*right*) shows clear septal enhancement

number and size of liver metastases and some additional information regarding the internal modifications the lesions undergo during treatment. Given its simple repeatability, US can nonetheless be useful between the different rounds of chemotherapy, thus making it possible to lengthen the interval between scheduled CT examinations. The routine use of CEUS, obviously with the exclusion of patients who already show evident progression at the baseline US study, could go a long way towards bridging the gap between US and CT.

In patients who are also monitored with US, adequate knowledge of the pretreatment baseline conditions of metastatic liver disease is required in order to be able to evaluate the changes. US study of the hepatic parenchyma after chemotherapy is in fact challenging, especially due to fibrofatty liver which is created and which tends to increase the risk of underestimating the number and/or size of the lesions present. In subjects with diffuse metastasization, an assessment of the response to treatment is often difficult and risks becoming rather subjective. In patients with diffuse hepatic involvement where the measurement of the individual lesions often becomes unfeasible, measurement of the dimensions of the liver can be of some use (at least the longitudinal diameter of the right lobe, which should always be measured) or, at least in theory, spectral analysis of the hepatic artery [47] (Figs. 5.55–5.57).

CD has limited applications, since metastatic lesions generally have limited color signals and therefore offer little possibility of documenting a response to treatment in terms of reduced angiogenesis. However, the finding of intralesional vascular signals can be considered a sign of greater lesion activity, and in histotypes with a hypervascular appearance of liver metastases, a subjective or objective decrease in the Doppler vascular signals may be considered a criterion for the evaluation of response. In a recent study using a Doppler technique – dynamic flow – and with the injection of US contrast medium, quantitative monitoring of the response to specific treatment with imatinib was performed in subjects with liver metastases from GIST. In patients who responded to treatment, there was an evident and very early reduction in intralesional vascularity [54].

CEUS appears to be much more promising, since it is able to study lesion perfusion in the form of contrast enhancement in real time. The populations of the studies published to date, however, have been rather

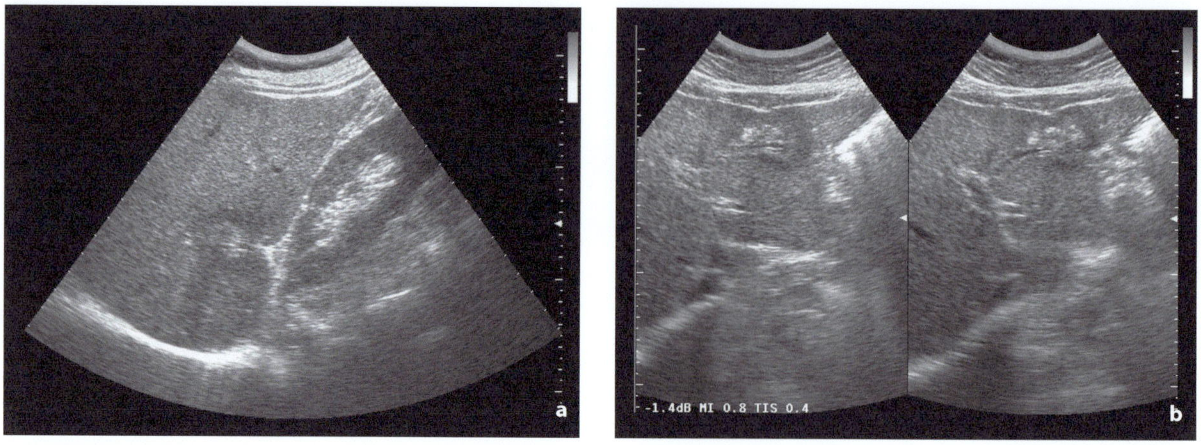

Fig. 5.55a,b Liver metastasis from ovarian cancer being treated with chemotherapy. Lesions with calcified echogenic center and adjacent capsular retraction

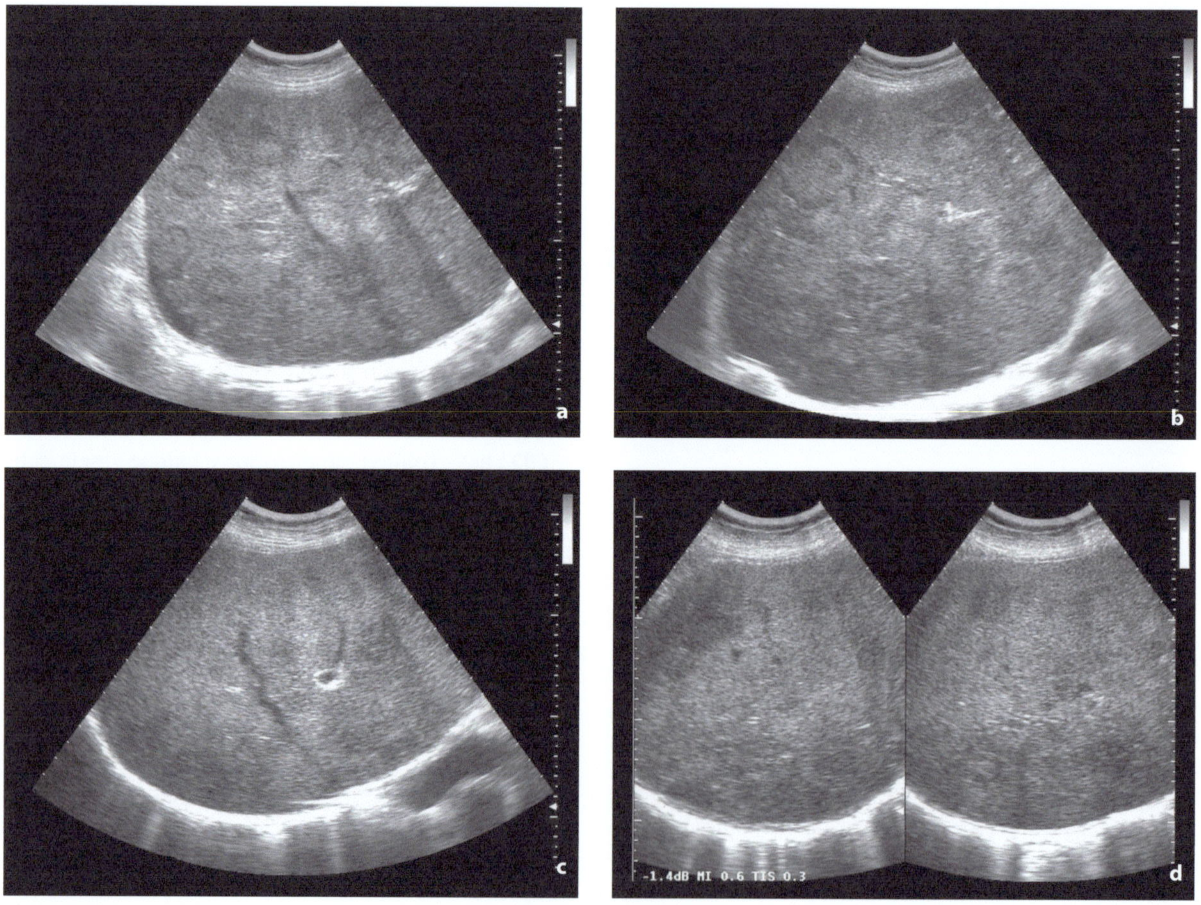

Fig. 5.56a-d Liver metastases from breast cancer, before and after treatment. The initial study (**a**,**b**) shows diffuse disruption of the liver structure, with micronodules and macronodules. After eight weeks (**c**,**d**) from the start of chemotherapy, the hepatic lesions appear ill defined. The images suggest good response to treatment, although defining and quantifying the number and size of residual lesions is challenging

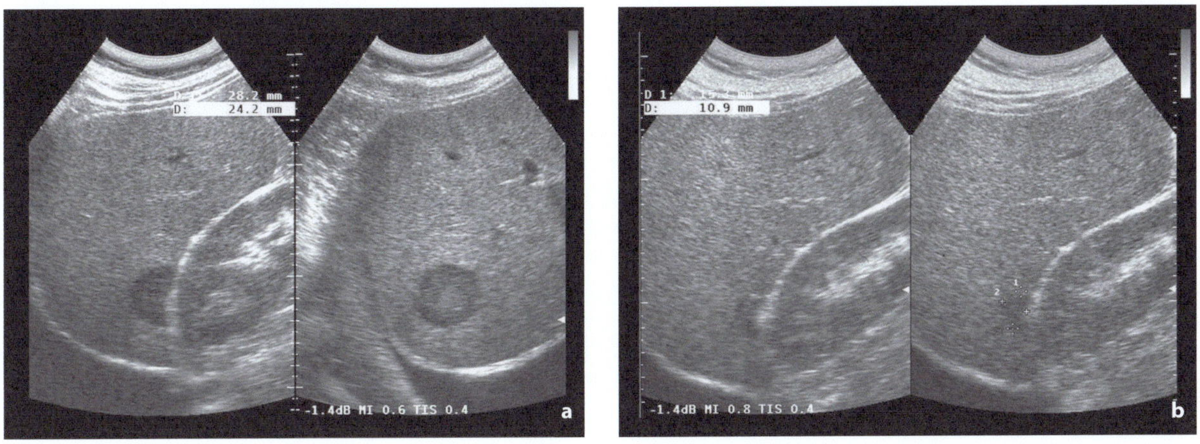

Fig. 5.57a,b Liver metastasis from breast cancer, before and after treatment. Subcapsular hepatic nodule (**a**) associated with pleural effusion. After twelve weeks of treatment the lesion appears markedly reduced in size (**b**)

limited, especially due to the poor availability of systems for perfusion quantification. There is also a need to evaluate whether the parameter to be considered is lesion enhancement in the arterial phase or the microcirculation in the portal-sinusoidal phase. In patients with liver metastases from GIST, the effectiveness of CEUS in monitoring the response to treatment with imatinib and in identifying intralesional recurrences has been demonstrated, although only qualitatively. In responsive cases, the treated lesions may even increase in size or remain stable for lengthy periods of time, but they do show marked devascularization, taking on a cystic-like appearance in which the residual or recurrent tissue appear well circumscribed by the contrast enhancement [55]. It has been seen in liver metastases treated with chemotherapy that the contrast enhancement of the lesion in the arterial phase of pretreatment CEUS is greater than in late responders, whereas during treatment it decreases in responders and remains unchanged in the non-responders [56,57]. Moreover, in an anecdotal case a progression in disease treated with systemic chemotherapy was observed despite the reduction in hypervascularity in the arterial phase [58].

Hemangioma is the most frequent solid lesion of the liver, with a prevalence in adults of up to 20%, and a predominance among females. Hemangioma is a vascular tumor with spaces lined with endothelium and interposed between fibrous septa. Multiple lesions appear in 10–80% of cases. Hemangiomas are asymptomatic, although in exceptional circumstances they may undergo spontaneous rupture, mass-effect symptoms or disseminated intravascular coagulation in cases of thrombosis of multiple and large lesions [30]. Small hemangiomas (<3 cm in 60–70% of cases) appear as markedly hyperechoic and occasionally

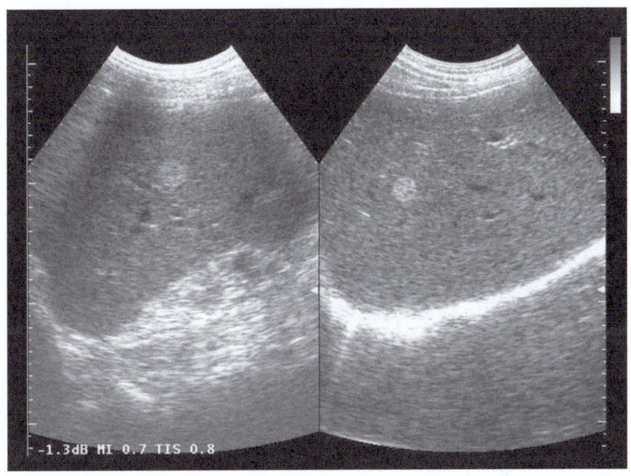

Fig. 5.58 Hemangioma of the liver. Rounded, relatively well-defined and homogeneous echogenic patch visualized with an intercostal (*left*) and subcostal (*right*) approach

"brilliant" masses (when the distance from the transducer is greatly reduced, as in the case of intercostals access to lateral hemangiomas of the right lobe), and possibly multilobular with homogenous echotexture and well-defined margins. They appear with no perifocal hypoechoic halo, possibly with enhanced through-transmission, and are often located beside a vessel or spanning a vessel (typically in a corner of the hepatic veins) or in a peripheral or subcapsular site (Figs. 5.58–5.61). However, these hemangiomas do not create problems for differential diagnosis. Instead problems arise with "atypical" hemangiomas (around 20% of cases). These may appear as hypoechoic lesions (intrinsically or because there is an echogenic background of steatosis), heterogeneous echogenic

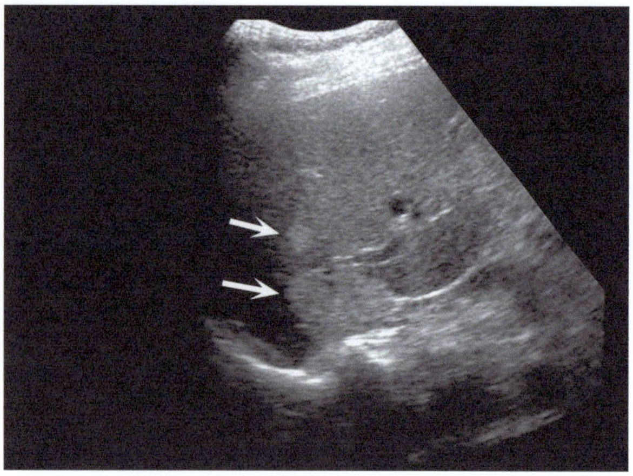

Fig. 5.59 Hemangiomas of the liver. Two relatively well-defined and homogeneous echogenic masses (*arrows*)

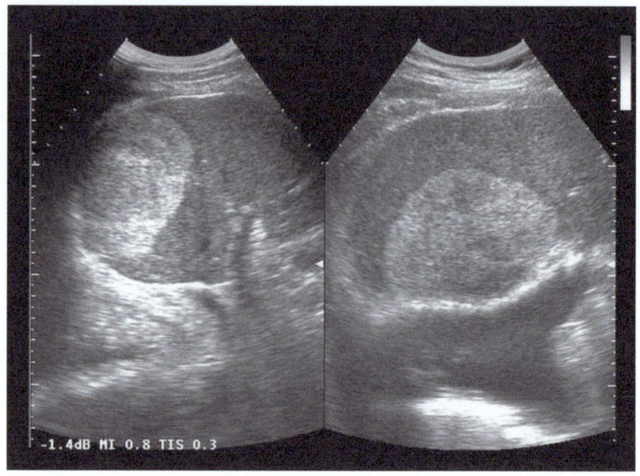

Fig. 5.60 Hemangiomas of the liver. Two large, relatively well-defined and homogenous echogenic masses

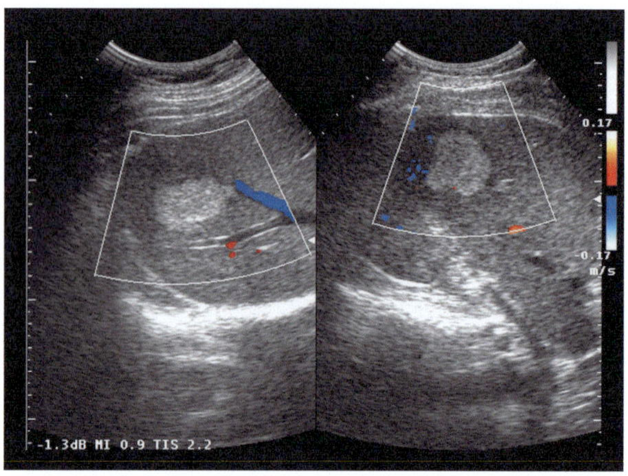

Fig. 5.61 Hemangioma of the liver. Relatively well-defined and heterogeneous echogenic mass with mildly enhanced through-transmission and no vascular signals at CD

masses (with possible posterior acoustic shadowing or the presence of some calcifications or heterogeneous areas due to necrosis or fibrosis), lesions with a more-or-less evident peripheral hypoechoic halo, and masses with some sign of growth with respect to a previous examination [59] (Figs. 5.62–5.67, Video 5.8–5.10). The atypical forms are often characterized by a generally thin peripheral echogenic portion and a hypoechoic center with no peripheral hypoechoic halo. Studies in children have shown that liver hemangiomas can be hypoechoic, disorganizing and with internal flows at CD mimicking a metastases [50]. A characteristic element that can be identified is a thin echoic rim which clearly circumscribes the lesion with respect to the surrounding parenchyma, which may also be seen in FNH, granulomas and intrahepatic splenosis [60]. High-flow hemangiomas often appear hypoechoic and may produce arteriovenous fistulas in the surrounding parenchyma. These can create ill-defined and occasionally wedge-shaped hypoechoic areas in B-mode and may also cause an incorrect measurement of the size of the hemangioma itself. Over time, hemangiomas may slightly increase or decrease in size, as well as decrease in echogenicity. At CD, hemangiomas, and especially hyperechoic hemangiomas, may appear with no vascular signal at all, since they are more-or-less vascular lesions but generally with slow flows below the threshold of identification. Alternatively, hypoechoic forms or medium-large sized lesions in particular may display a spot-like pattern of internal color signals (10–30% of cases), especially in the periphery. In these lesions the flow pattern may be continuous (venous) or, more rarely, pulsed (arteriolar), but always with low velocity and good representation of the diastolic component (when the spectrum can be sampled). In contrast to what was thought in the past, therefore, the finding of arterial flows does not rule out hemangioma, even in the case of small lesions, although a truly hypervascular appearance of hemangioma is rare [51,52,62]. The surrounding parenchyma may appear particularly rich with vascular signals, due to the presence of compressed vessels produced by the expansive growth of the hemangioma and the frequent development of local perfusion changes. The CD finding, therefore, is not absolutely specific, because there are atypical hemangiomas which display vascular signals, and there are malignant lesions, especially metastases, which show no flow signals in a manner similar to typical hemangiomas. CD can nonetheless be of practical relevance: masses with a hemangioma-like appearance in B-mode and with no vascular signals at

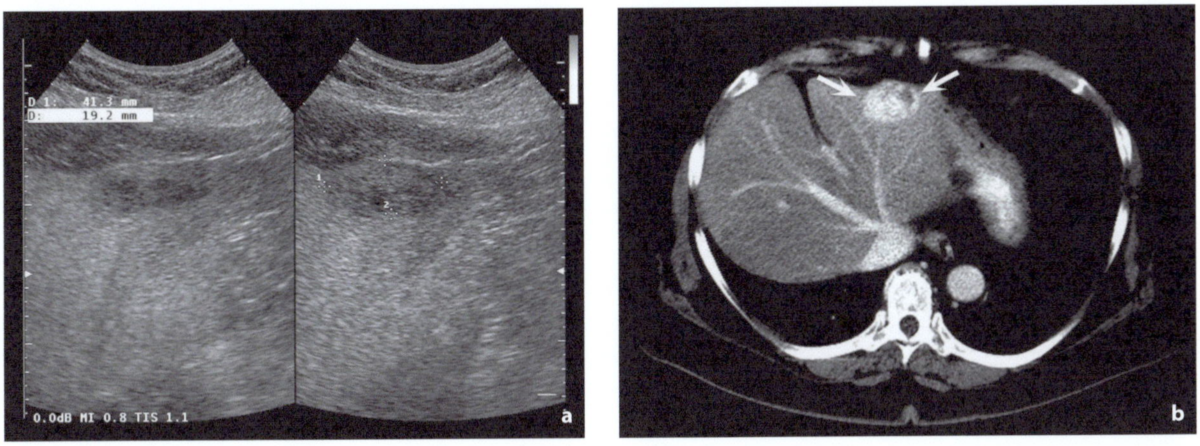

Fig. 5.62a,b Hemangioma of the liver. Heterogeneous hypo-anechoic mass (**a**). The appearance is nonspecific but the axial CT scan in the portal phase shows progressive centripetal opacification of the lesion (**b**, *arrows*)

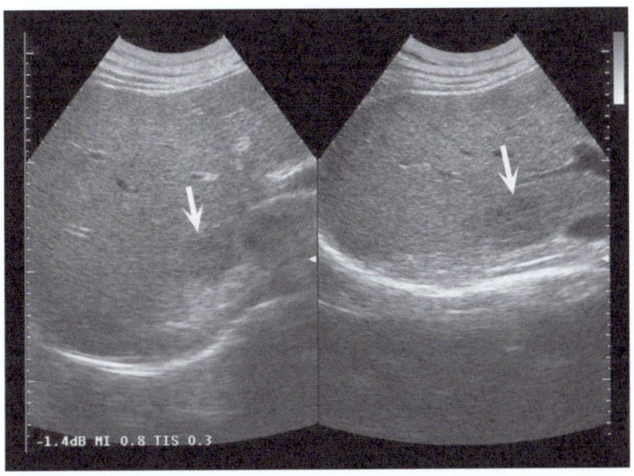

Fig. 5.63 Hemangioma of the liver. Poorly defined and mildly hypoechoic lesion (*arrow*)

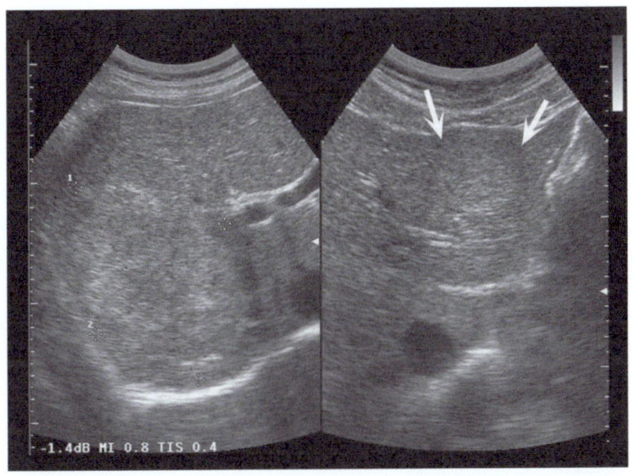

Fig. 5.64 Hemangiomas of the liver. Two heterogeneous and mildly echogenic masses in the right hepatic lobe (*between the calipers*) and in the left hepatic lobe (*arrows*)

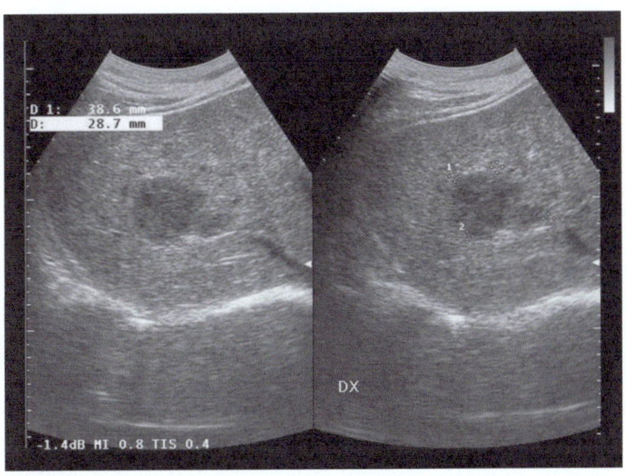

Fig. 5.65 Atypical hemangioma of the liver. Lobulated, slightly heterogeneous hypoechoic mass in the right hepatic lobe

CD may be scheduled for follow-up, at least in patients without a known extrahepatic neoplasm, whereas masses with vascular signals and/or those identified in cancer patients may require further investigation [30]. In the typical forms, CEUS shows peripheral enhancement in the arterial phase in the form of hyperechoic globules, followed by centripetal and persistent enhancement with progressive increase in size of the globules and with a total or subtotal hyperechogenicity (sparing the most central part) in the portal-sinusoidal phase. The identification of globular centripetal enhancement is important because this is not seen in malignant lesions. There are, however, a number of atypical characteristics related most of all to the intralesional flow velocity. These include annular or homogeneous enhancement in the arterial phase in small high-flow hemangiomas, very slow and late

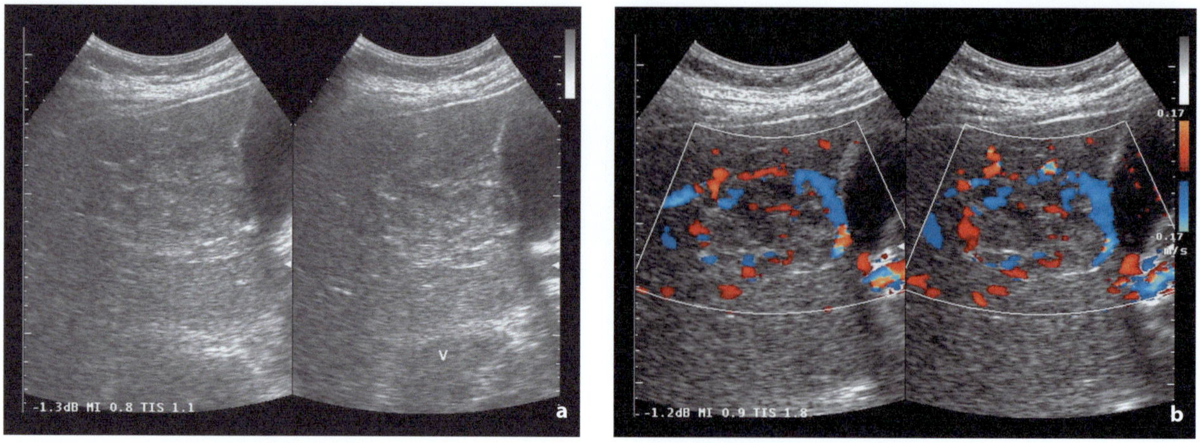

Fig. 5.66a,b Atypical hemangioma of the liver. Ill-defined heterogeneous echogenic mass located adjacent to the gallbladder (**a**). CD shows moderate vascularity diffusely distributed both centrally and peripherally (**b**)

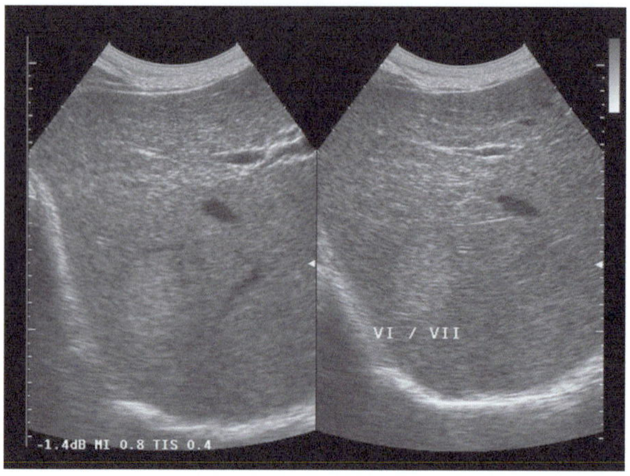

Figs 5.67 Atypical hemangioma of the liver. Ill-defined, heterogeneous and mildly hyperechoic mass

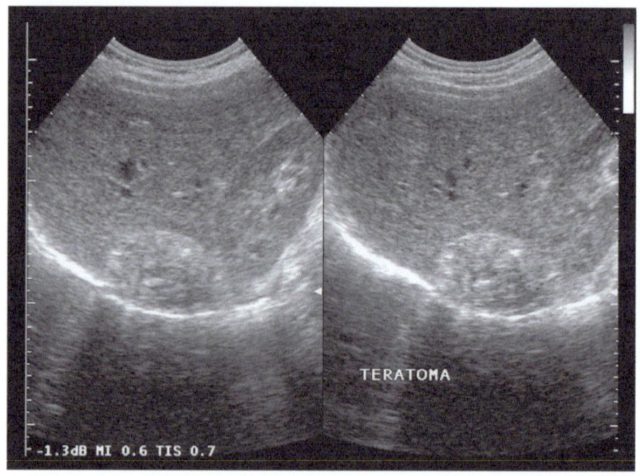

Fig. 5.68 Mesenchymal hamartoma of the liver. Prevalently solid mass characterized by a heterogeneous echogenic appearance with well-defined margins and several internal calcifications

enhancement, substantial isoechogenicity in all vascular phases (small hemangiomas), isoechogenicity or even hypoechogenicity in the portal-sinusoidal phase, etc. [53]. Biopsy puncture is generally ill-advised due to the risk of hemorrhage, particularly in peripheral hemangiomas, and because it can be inconclusive for diagnostic purposes. With appropriate caution, however, FNAC may be performed even in hemangiomas, usually with 22 G needles [40].

Hepatic hamartoma is a rare mesenchymal tumor with solid and cystic components, which is generally identified between 4 months and 2 years of age and which can reach a considerable size. The appearance may vary from multiple small cysts within a solid mass to a more-or-less septated prevalently cystic lesion (Fig. 5.68). In the latter case the appearance is similar to hydatidosis and biliary cystadenoma/adenocarcinoma [62,63].

Biliary hamartomas (von Meyenburg complexes) are biliary malformations composed of disorganized ducts and fibrous stroma associated with hepatic and/or renal cystic anomalies. Numerous subcentimeter foci distributed uniformly in the hepatic parenchyma may be seen which appear hyperechoic when small or hypoechoic especially when larger, with possible comet tail signs [64].

Angiomyolipomas, which may be associated with tuberous sclerosis and therefore with similar lesions in the kidneys, consist of various amounts of thin-walled vessels, smooth muscle cells and fat. The fat content varies from 10% to 90% and influences the echogenicity and therefore the possibility of diagnosis

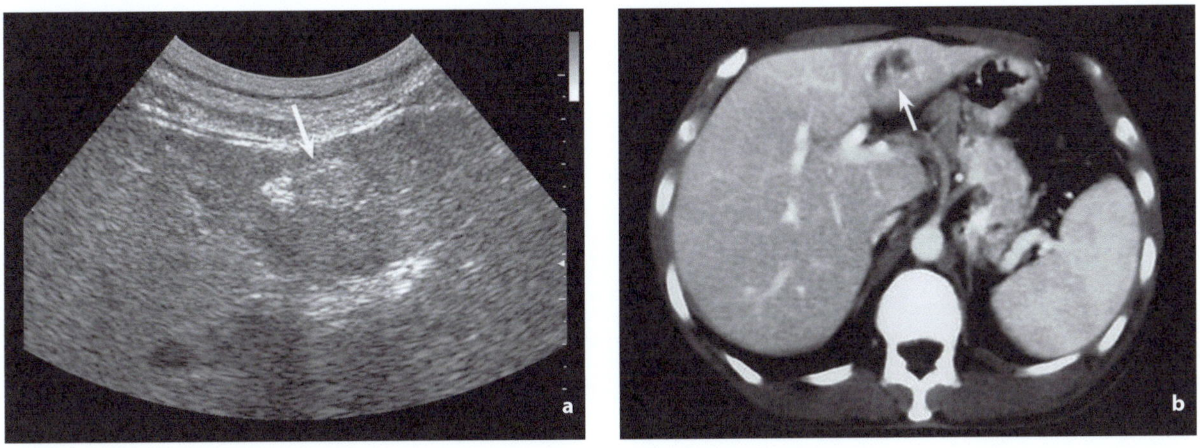

Fig. 5.69a,b Angiomyolipoma of the liver. Relatively well-defined and homogeneous hyperechoic mass (**a**, *arrow*) immediately medial to the round ligament. Axial CT scan in the portal phase shows the prevalent fat density of the lesion (**b**, *arrow*)

or at least the US suspicion. A markedly hyperechoic lesion with generally homogeneous echotexture and mild posterior acoustic shadowing can be suspicious for angiomyolipoma [62]. Similar considerations hold for lipoma, which however appears markedly and homogeneously hyperechoic. At CD, angiomyolipoma displays variable vascularity, particularly peripheral or at least not in the more echogenic portions in lesions with heterogeneous echotexture (Fig. 5.69).

Myofibroblastoma (inflammatory pseudotumor) is a rare lesion predominantly found in males (M/F ratio 8:1), which is multiple in 19% of cases. It usually appears as a complex and prevalently cystic mass, with solid components in the form of septations or peripheral portions [62].

Focal nodular hyperplasia (FNH) has a prevalence of up to 3%, is more common among females (generally between 20 and 50 years of age, with F/M ratio of 8:1) and appears to be associated with the use of oral contraceptives. FNH is generally treated conservatively, except for particularly large or pedunculated lesions, with treatment generally limited to periodic follow-up. The lesion consists of regenerative hyperplastic nodules and fibrous septations containing vessels, bile ducts and inflammatory cells. It may be capsulated or not and tends to be found peripherally, producing a bulge in the surface of the liver, or with exophytic development. FNH is multiple in 10–20% of cases and is often associated with hemangiomas. It appears as a relatively circumscribed mass, occasionally with lobulated margins, homogeneous echotexture and echogenicity equal to or slighter higher than the surrounding parenchyma, but also mildly hypoechoic, especially in cases of fatty liver. The size is generally limited, <50 mm in 65% of cases. In around 20% of cases, especially in large lesions, a central echogenic band of scar tissue may be seen, from which thin echogenic strips irradiate towards the periphery. However, a scar may also be seen in adenomas and fibrolamellar HCC. In some cases, identifying FNH is challenging due to its isoechoic appearance, although it may be perceived due to its mass effect on surrounding vessels and the presence of a thin capsular echogenic rim. In 15% of cases a peripheral hypoechoic halo is present. At CD and especially at PD the appearance is usually notably hypervascular, at both the perilesional and intralesional level. In typical forms (80%), pulsating vessels irradiating from a central afferent vessel ("wheel" pattern) can be seen. The central artery displays high systolic velocity as well as good representation of the diastolic component and a low RI (mean 0.51, lower than that of the hepatic artery and the intralesional arterioles). Venous flow with a peripheral and above all perinodular distribution may also be detected [65]. In the absence of a central scar, however, FNH displays intense vascularity, although not distributed in a radial pattern but rather irregular and poorly specific. Diagnosis is easy in the presence of an isoechoic mass with central scarring and wheel vascular pattern, but becomes more challenging in smaller lesions, which may mimic hemangiomas or even metastases. The CEUS appearance is characterized by very intense and early arterial enhancement, preceded by initial opacification of the central artery and then the vessels irradiating from it. There follows a slow wash-out of contrast medium, with hyperechogenicity or, more often, isoechogenicity in the portal-sinusoidal phase and eventual identification of the hypoechoic central scar [53] (Figs. 5.70–5.73).

Hepatocellular adenoma is most common in women of childbearing age and is associated primarily

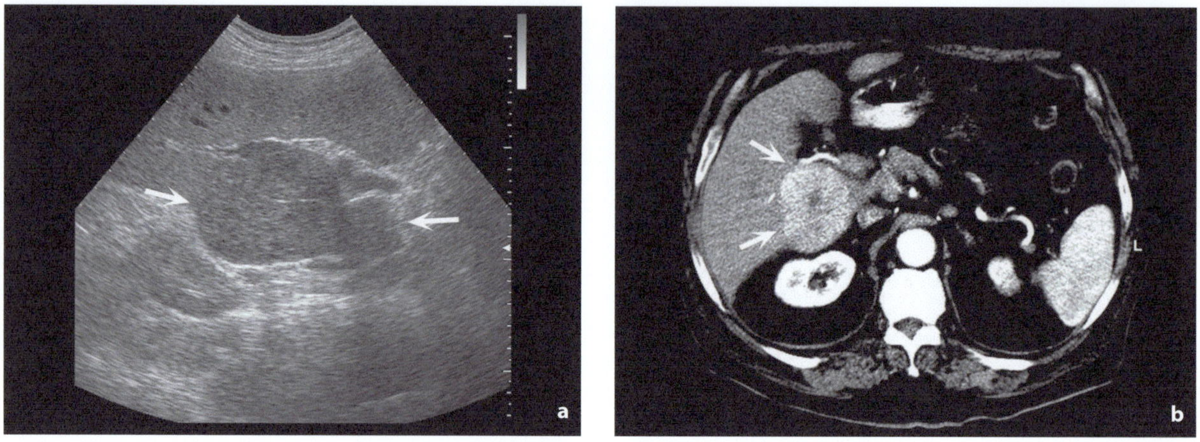

Fig. 5.70a,b FNH. Oval, exophytic, mildly hypoechoic lesion located at the base of the caudate lobe (**a**, *arrows*). Axial CT scan in the arterial phase shows a hypervascular lesion with a central hypoattenuating scar (**b**, *arrows*)

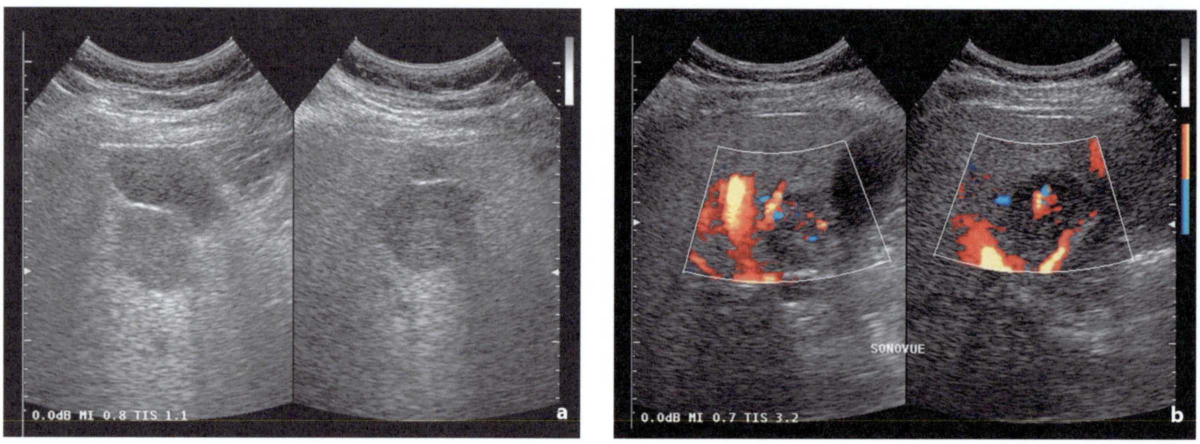

Fig. 5.71a,b FNH in steatosis in a patient with pectoral recurrence from breast cancer. Nonspecific hypoechoic mass located adjacent to the gallbladder (**a**). Study with directional PD and US contrast medium shows marked central arterial vascularity (**b**)

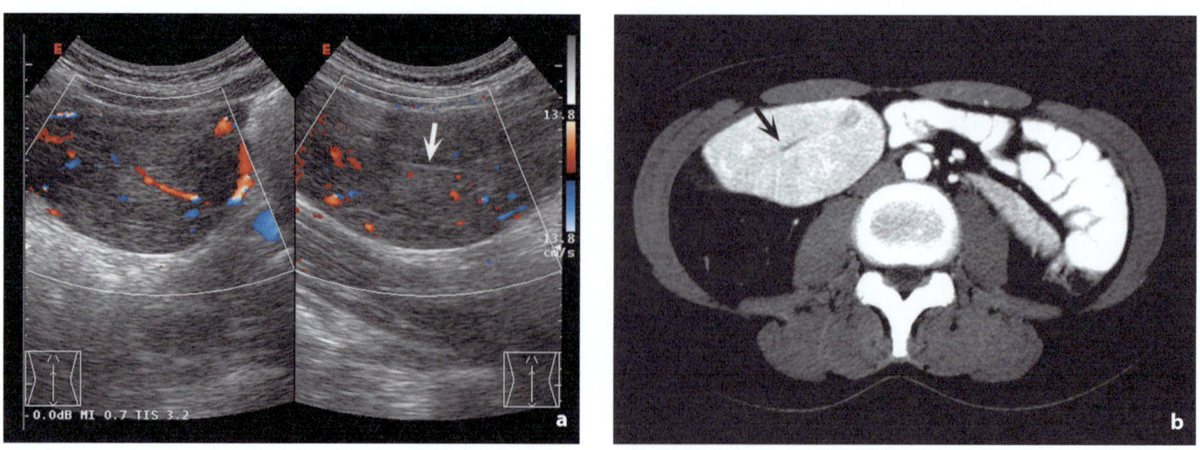

Fig. 5.72a,b FNH. Exophytic homogeneous isoechoic mass with central scar (*arrow*) and irradiating vessels at CD (**a**). Axial CT image in the arterial phase shows intense contrast enhancement and the hypoattenuating scar (**b**, *arrow*)

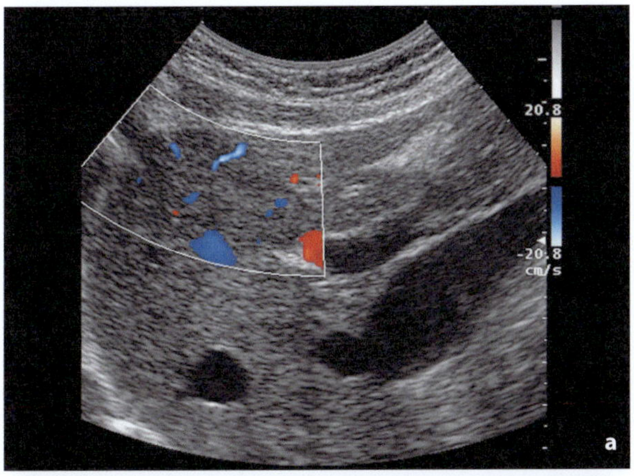

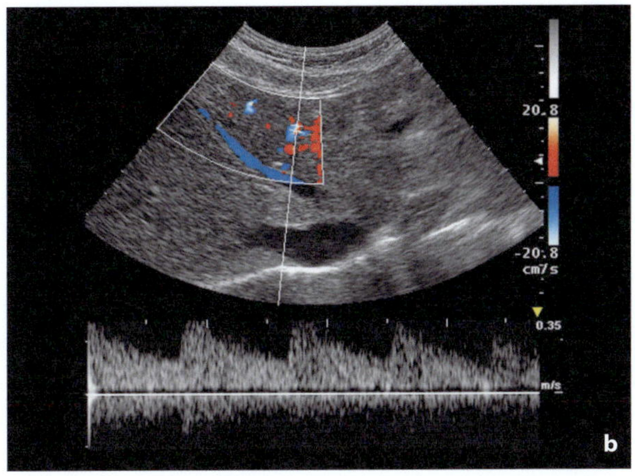

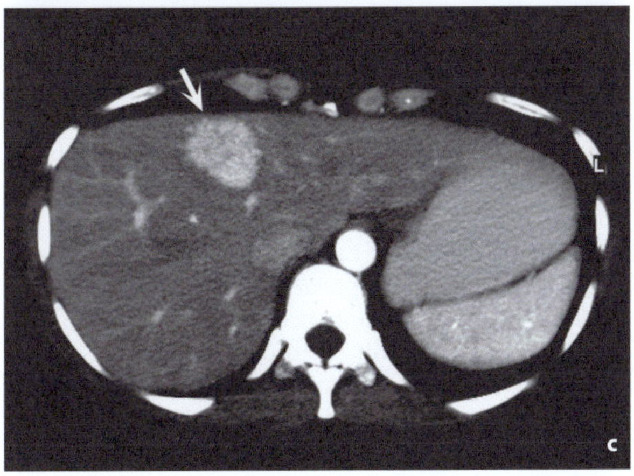

Fig. 5.73a-c FNH. Substantially isoechoic mass with some internal irradiating arterial branches at CD (**a**). Spectral Doppler confirms the low-resistance intralesional arterial flow (**b**). Axial CT scan in the arterial phase shows a hypervascular lesion (**c**, *arrow*)

with the use of oral contraceptives as well as conditions such as type I glycogenosis (up to 50% of patients with this disease), use of androgen steroid therapy, tyrosinemia, galactosemia, diabetes and cirrhosis. It is 4–7 times less common than FNH [66]. Given the risk of hemorrhagic complications and malignant degeneration, as well as the difficult differentiation from well-differentiated HCC, the adenoma is usually treated surgically. It is composed of pleomorphic hepatocytes with a loss of normal structure and without bile ducts, and generally appears capsulated. The appearance is of a rounded, well-defined, solitary lesion (80–90% of cases) with heterogeneous iso-hypoechoic appearance, possible perilesional hypoechoic halo and the presence of internal anechoic (necrotic-hemorrhagic) or echogenic (adipose deposits) areas or calcifications [67]. At diagnosis the size is often notable. CD reveals large arterial and venous vessels at the periphery, especially in subcapsular location and veins located centrally. In general, however, the overall appearance is of a moderately vascular lesion, with both perinodular and intranodular distribution but without particular morphologic signs and especially without the cartwheel appearance typical of FNH, with a prevalence of continuous flows over pulsed flows. The CEUS appearance is characterized by a generally rapid and intense enhancement in the arterial phase with peripheral and capsular macrovessels and possible internal heterogeneity. The prevalent echogenicity is progressively reduced, with mild hyperechogenicity at the beginning of the portal-sinusoidal phase tending to progressive isoechogenicity [53].

Nodular regenerative hyperplasia is a rare disorder characterized by regeneration of the hepatic parenchyma in the absence of cirrhosis. Single or multiple nodules may be found. The appearance is generally hypoechoic or isoechoic and only exceptionally hyperechoic. The echotexture may be heterogeneous and the lesions can mimic metastases [68].

Intrahepatic extramedullary hematopoiesis is a compensatory process which arises in the event of a reduction in erythrocyte production due to a disturbance of the normal function of bone marrow. The rare focal forms have a variable appearance, from homogeneous echogenic foci to heterogeneous hypoechoic masses with possible peripheral hypoechoic halo and deformed vessels crossing it seen at CD [69] (Fig. 5.74).

In **eosinophilic necrosis**, focal eosinophilic infiltration of the liver occurs, leading to tissue damage (granuloma or abscess), in association with conditions such as hypereosinophilic syndrome, parasitic infestations, allergies and neoplasms. The US presentation closely mimics metastases (also in the CT and MR study) due to the presence of multiple, rounded or oval, homogeneous, hypoechoic lesions with ill-defined margins and no posterior acoustic shadowing but possible enhanced through-transmission [70]. Although the diagnosis may be hypothesized on the basis of a possible peripheral hypereosinophilia, biopsy is fundamental. Serial US examinations show progressive regression (Fig. 5.75).

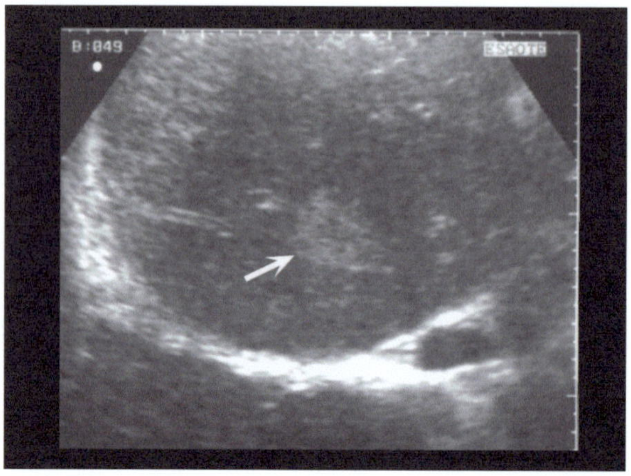

Fig. 5.74 Hepatic extramedullary hematopoiesis. Heterogeneous echogenic area in the right lobe (*arrow*)

Tuberculoma appears as a poorly defined hypoechoic lesion caused by the confluence of smaller areas, or as hypoechoic lesions with a hyperechoic rim and possible internal abscessed liquefaction.

Liver **abscesses** can be of bacterial or amebic origin and present as single or multiple masses with no capsule and irregular, ill-defined margins and generally evident enhanced through-transmission. They are usually hypoechoic but can have irregular echogenic areas or contain gas or internal air-fluid levels. Diffuse microabscesses create an appearance of parenchymal heterogeneity which is not always easy to characterize if not in the appropriate clinical setting [40]. During abscess formation, CD is able to demonstrate perifocal hyperemia, but once it has been formed the collection shows no vascular signals. CEUS identifies perfusion of the walls and septa, avascularity of the necrotic-liquefactive components and possible perifocal reactive hyperemia [71]. The appearance of the abscess, however, varies with its evolution, and especially in the pre-liquefactive phase it may mimic a malignancy (Fig. 5.76).

Hydatid cysts are caused by the larval stage of *E. granulosus* and appear as fluid-filled masses with thick walls and enhanced through-transmission (Figs. 5.77, 5.78). Wall calcifications, internal loculations and daughter cysts may be present. CD and CEUS show the constant absence of vascular flow. The dead cysts appear as heterogeneous calcified areas. The rare forms of multilocular echinococcosis can have an invasive, tumor-like appearance.

Splenosis is a post-traumatic or postoperative autotransplant of splenic tissue occasionally on the surface of the liver or immediately subcapsular. US displays a homogenous, mildly hypoechoic mass occasionally separated from the remaining parenchyma by a thin

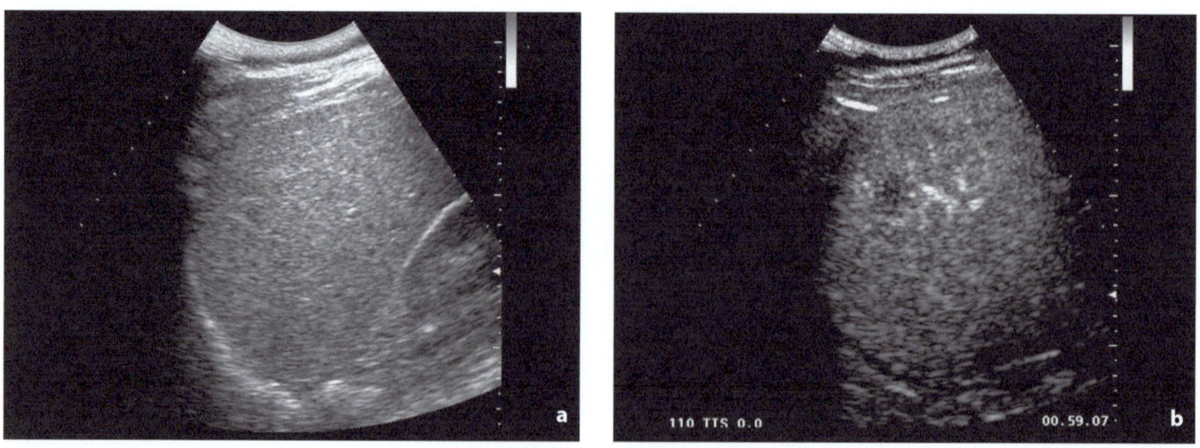

Fig. 5.75a,b Hepatic eosinophilic necrosis (patient with history of breast cancer). Small hypoechoic mass with evidence of an echogenic rim (**a**). CEUS shows poor vascularity in the portal phase, which alone is insufficient to differentiate the lesion from metastasis (**b**)

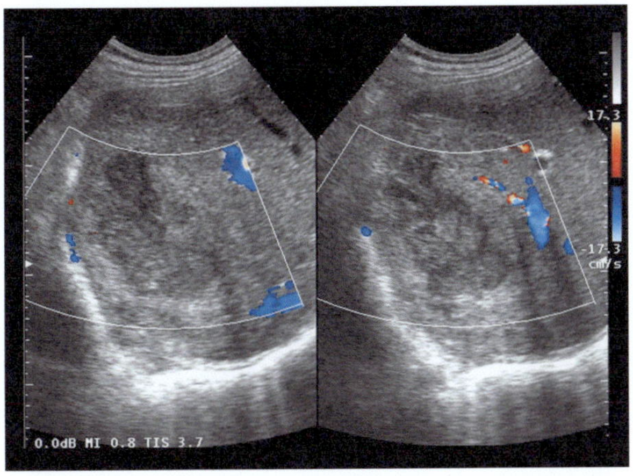

Fig. 5.76 Pyogenic abscess of the liver. Oval heterogeneous hypoechoic mass with tendency to internal liquefaction and substantial avascularity at CD

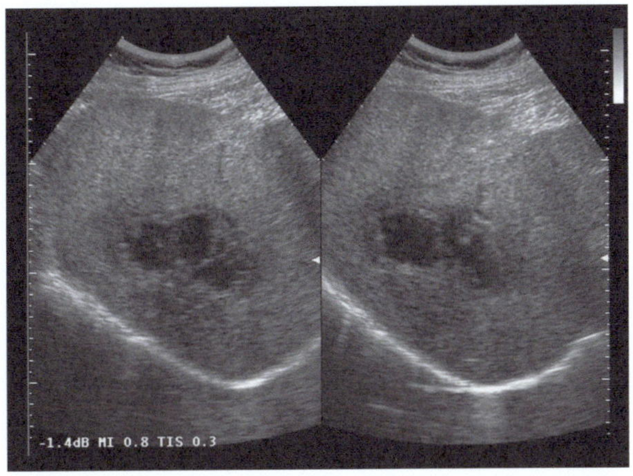

Fig. 5.77 Hepatic hydatidosis. Irregularly shaped cystic mass with internal fluid components

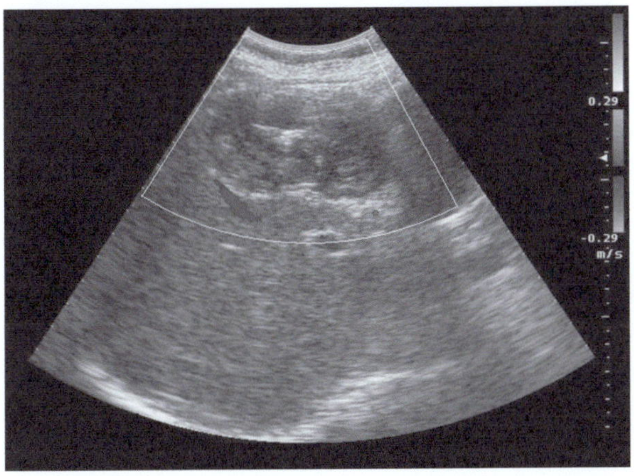

Fig. 5.78 Hepatic hydatidosis. Heterogeneous cystic mass located adjacent to the gallbladder with marginal and internal calcification and avascular appearance at CD

echogenic rim, with some vascular signals at CD and especially with hypervascularity in the arterial phase of CEUS, which can mimic HCC (Fig. 5.79).

Hepatic porphyria manifests as multiple heterogeneous areas of variable size containing blood.

Intrahepatic cholangiocarcinoma develops from the bile ducts, accounts for around 10% of primary malignant tumors of the liver and may be associated with hemochromatosis, Caroli disease, congenital cystic dilatation of the bile ducts, sclerosing cholangitis, clonorchiasis or ulcerous rectocolitis. The intrahepatic form is more common than the hilar form known as Klatskin tumor, at least in Western countries. Peripheral intrahepatic cholangiocarcinoma manifests generally as a solitary mass (95% of cases) often moderate in size, with poorly defined margins

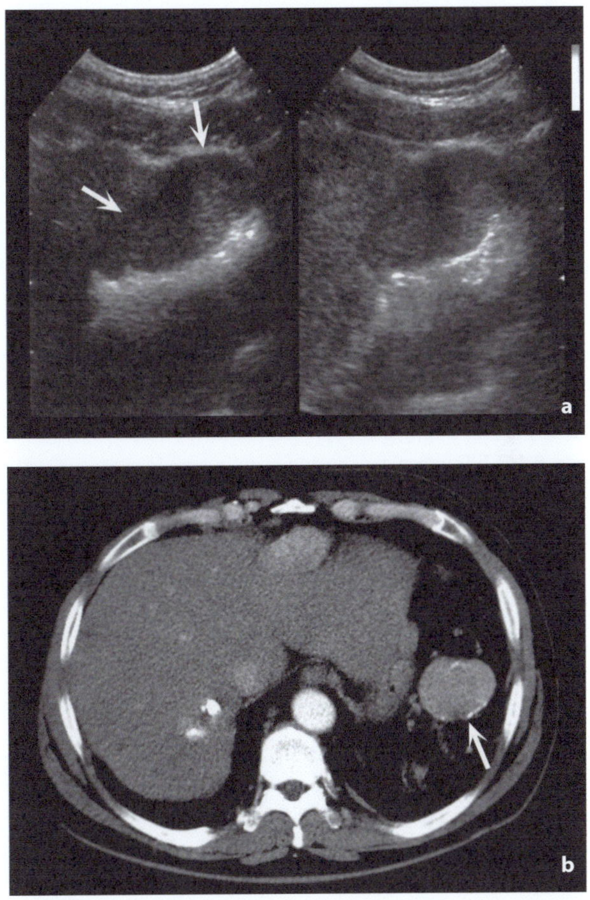

Fig. 5.79a,b Intrahepatic splenosis. Well-defined hypoechoic mass on the anterior surface of the hepatic capsule (**a**, *arrows*). Corresponding CT in the arterial phase (**b**) with enhancement similar to the normal enhancement of the spleen and to the enhancement of another similar area in the splenic area (*arrow*)

and heterogeneous, prevalently hypoechoic or hyperechoic appearance. A perifocal halo may be present and occasionally the lesion is located adjacent to a hepatic vein. Calcifications are very rare. Proximally the bile ducts may appear dilated or show a frank intraluminal growth. Vascular signals at CD are usually scarce and peripheral, whereas CEUS can identify a variable degree of generally heterogeneous enhancement in the arterial phase and a substantial hypoechogenicity in the portal sinusoidal phase [53] (Figs. 5.80, 5.81, Video 5.11).

Biliary cystadenoma and **cystadenocarcinoma**, which can only be differentiated histologically, are prevalent in middle-aged females and manifest with jaundice and soreness in the right upper quadrant. They appear as multilocular cystic masses of significant size, with possible intraluminal papillary projections and calcifications in the solid areas.

Primary and secondary hepatic **lymphomas** may involve the liver diffusely, with relatively homogeneous hepatomegaly, or present as focal lesions (6–8% of focal hepatic lesions). Liver involvement is seen in 50% of subjects with lymphoma, although it takes on a focal character in only 8%, generally of the NHL type. Abdominal lymphadenopathies or splenomegaly are often associated. The appearance of the nodules is variable. Generally they appear hypo-anechoic, though they can be hyperechoic, heterogeneous or with a target appearance, and the margins can be sharp or even infiltrating. The generally multiple lesions can be micronodular or macronodular and even confluent [72,73]. CEUS shows a variable degree of enhancement in the arterial phase and, above all, a hypoechoic appearance in the portal-sinusoidal phase [53]. The lymph nodes at the hepatic hilum appear enlarged, deformed and hypoechoic (Figs. 5.82, 5.83).

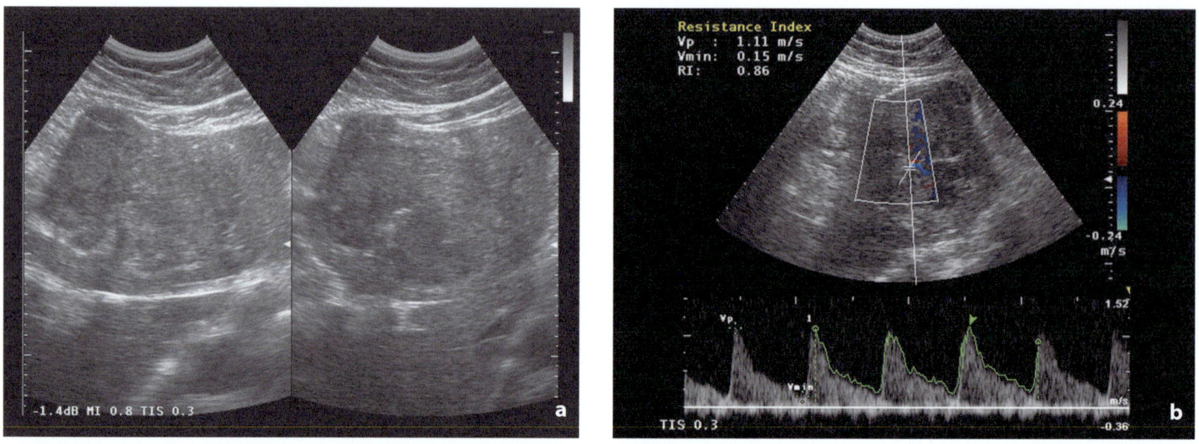

Fig. 5.80a,b Intrahepatic cholangiocarcinoma. Hypo-isoechoic lesion of the left hepatic lobe (**a**). Spectral Doppler of the left branch of the hepatic artery which is encircled by the mass (**b**)

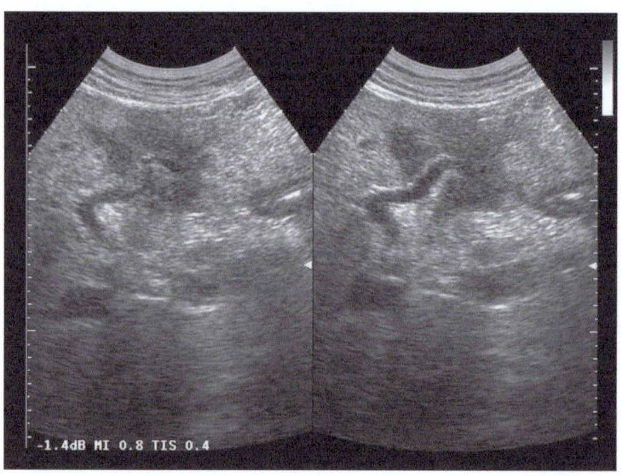

Fig. 5.81 Intrahepatic cholangiocarcinoma. Hypoechoic lesion with infiltrating margins can be seen encircling the left portal branch. Steatosis

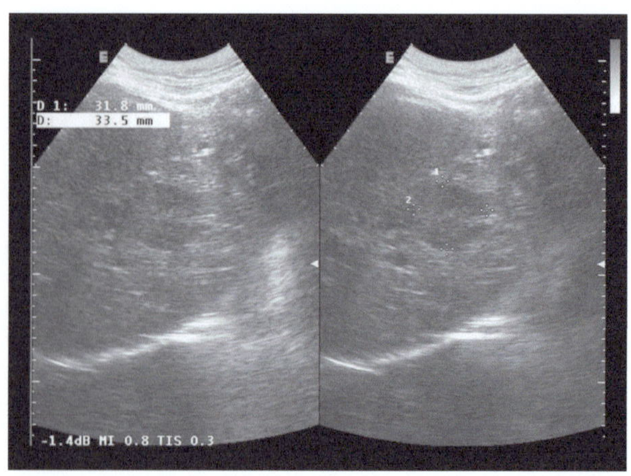

Fig. 5.82 Hepatic lymphoma. Heterogeneous hypoechoic nodule of the liver (*calipers*)

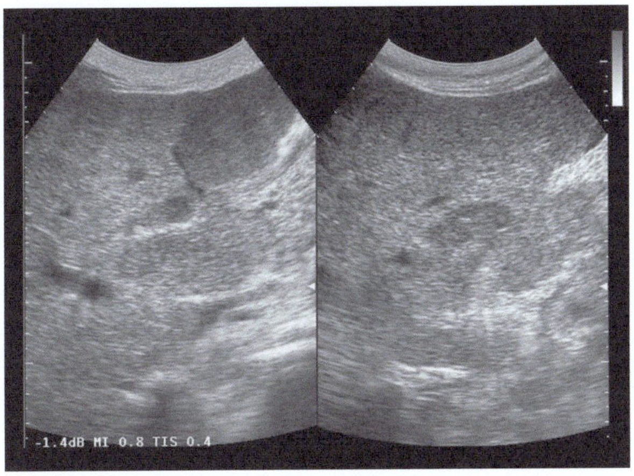

Fig. 5.83 Hepatic lymphoma. Multiple hypoechoic lesions varying in size in the hepatic parenchyma

Epithelioid hemangioendothelioma is a rare vascular tumor with middle-to-low malignancy. The appearance is generally hypoechoic, diffuse or with multiple confluent nodules. Intralesional calcifications are possible. The healthy liver undergoes a process of hypertrophy and the organ can therefore be enlarged and deformed due to the incorporation of healthy portions with portions in heterogeneous cystic transformation [40,62].

Angiosarcoma is prevalent in males (M/F ratio 4:1) and can be correlated with exposure to substances such as Thorotrast, arsenic, androgen steroids and vinyl chloride. The tumor manifests as single or multiple heterogeneous hypoechoic lesions, or diffuse hepatic disruption. Synchronous metastases can be found in the spleen [30,62].

Nondifferentiated embryonic sarcoma is very rare and is predominantly found in children (mean age 12 years). It appears as a large heterogeneous mass with well-defined margins and multiple internal cystic areas [62].

Hepatoblastoma is an aggressive tumor typically found in infants (<3 years), which presents as heterogeneous and prevalently hyperechoic masses but with hypoechoic and anechoic portions. CD displays hypervascularity. Internal calcifications and posterior acoustic shadowing may be seen [30].

Fibrolamellar HCC should also be considered in this setting. It is a rather rare form of hepatocellular carcinoma (2% of cases) which originates in a healthy liver, particularly in young women. It manifests as single nodules with well-defined and lobulated margins, and variable echogenicity, ranging from hypoechoic to hyperechoic [40]. The growth is slow and expansive and its size is often considerable at diagnosis. A central echogenic "scar" and calcifications may be seen. CD reveals a hypervascular appearance and CEUS a moderate but heterogeneous enhancement, tending to hypoechogenicity in the portal-sinusoidal phase [53].

Focal sparing in steatosis are parenchymal portions where the infiltration of fat is reduced or absent, such that they appear as single or multiple hypoechoic defects which are evident against a steatosis-induced hyperechoic parenchymal background. These areas can simulate focal lesions, especially when located centrally in the parenchyma, and are rounded or oval in shape. However, CD shows normal vessels which cross the pseudonodular area without displacement or other modifications, while CEUS reveals the substantial isoechogenicity (isovascularity) to the surrounding parenchyma in all the phases of contrast enhancement, thus making a definitive diagnosis possible [53] (Figs. 5.84–5.87, Video 5.12, 5.13).

Focal steatosis is due to a non-uniform deposit of fat with the liver, thus leading to the creation of one or more areas of fatty liver, which may have a rounded and focal appearance. These areas appear hyperechoic (although usually less markedly than with hemangiomas, lipomas and angiolipomas), with irregular or angular margins and a prevalence in segments IV and V (whereas they are never found in the caudate lobe). CD only reveals normal vessels, which cross the lesion with no sign of a mass effect, with distribution and branching similar to the other parenchymal areas. CEUS shows a perfusion of these areas similar to the adjacent parenchymal areas and therefore makes definitive diagnosis possible [53].

Overall, the causes of **hypoechoic lesions** in the liver include metastases, hemangiomas, lymphomas,

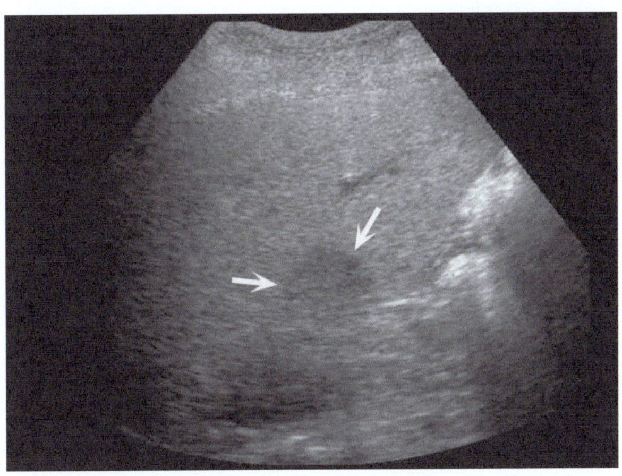

Fig. 5.84 Focal sparing in steatosis. Rounded image (*arrows*) appearing hypoechoic with respect to the moderately hyperechogenicity of the fatty liver background

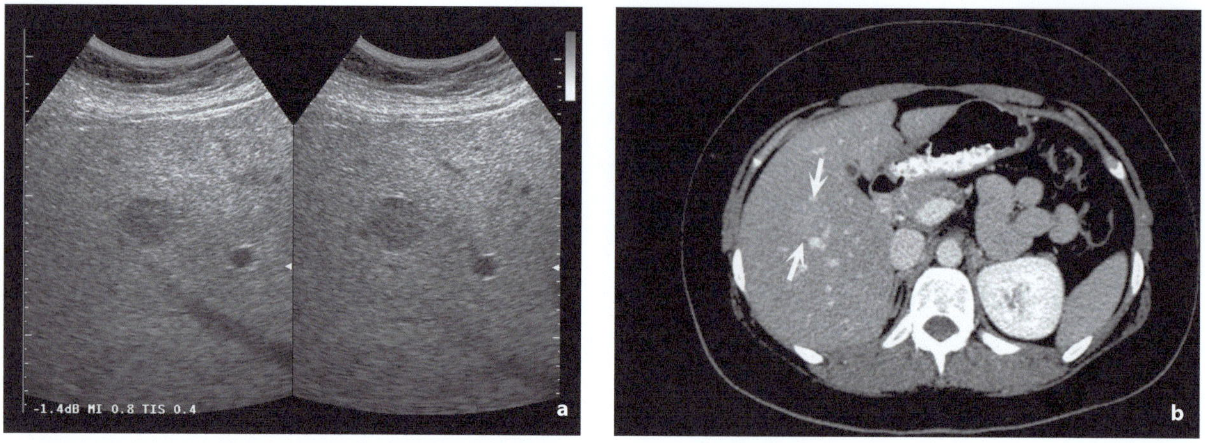

Fig. 5.85a,b Focal sparing in steatosis. Patently nodular image with relatively well-defined margins and homogeneous hypoechoic appearance (**a**). CT scan in the venous phase shows mild hyperattenuation of the lesion, thus ruling out metastasis (**b**, *arrows*)

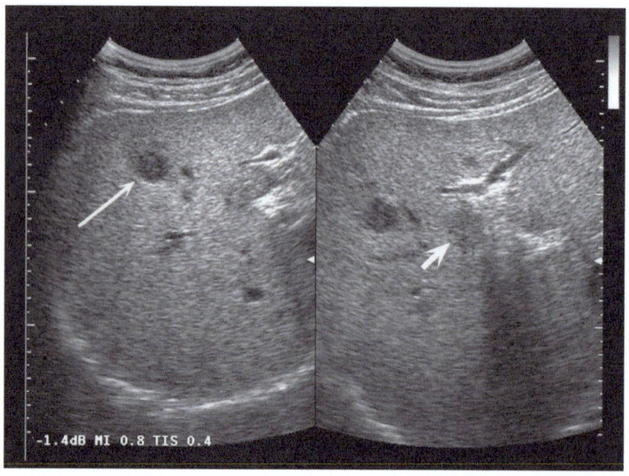

Fig. 5.86 Association of focal sparing in steatosis and liver metastasis. The metastasis from melanoma appears more markedly hypoechoic (*long arrow*), whereas the skip area appears more tenuous (*short arrow*)

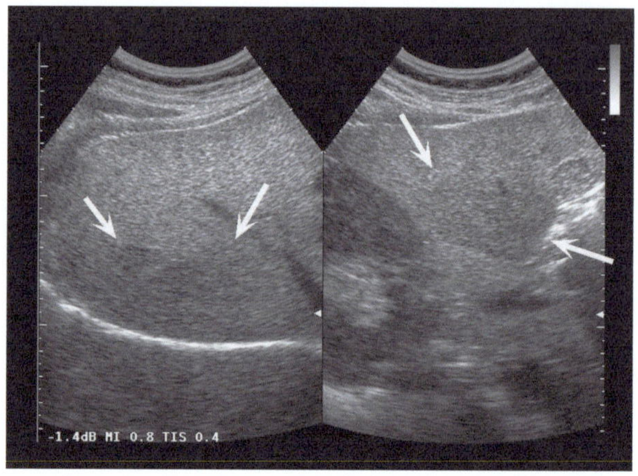

Fig. 5.87 Focal sparing in steatosis. Multiple, generally tenuous hypoechoic areas

abscesses, complicated cysts, adenomas, FNH, HCC and focal sparing in steatosis. **Isoechoic lesions** instead include adenomas, FNH, HCC, hemangiomas, metastases, hematomas and hepatization of the gallbladder. Lastly, **hyperechoic lesions** include hemangiomas, regenerative nodules, HCC, FNH, metastases, abscesses, necrosis, biliary hamartomas, focal steatosis and porphyria [59]. Multiple lesions, which are generally echogenic and associated with hepatomegaly, may be found in patients with glycogenosis.

In the setting of a **fatty liver**, hepatic lesions more often tend to appear more hypoechoic against the hyperechoic background than they generally are (e.g. 81% of hemangiomas appear hypoechoic), with margins more commonly ill-defined and a more evident presence of enhanced through-transmission (whereas normally posterior enhancement is found in hemangiomas and HCC but not in metastases). All these features tend to render the characterization of lesions more complex. In addition, the echogenic rim which can characterize hypo-isoechoic hemangiomas is barely identifiable [74].

False images of focal hepatic lesions can be produced by a number of anatomic and pathologic conditions. The main fissure or the accessory fissures can partially circumscribe a parenchymal area and therefore mimic the echogenic rim of an isoechoic lesion. The echogenic area with possible posterior acoustic shadowing of the round ligament in transverse section can mimic a lesion, although this can be recog-

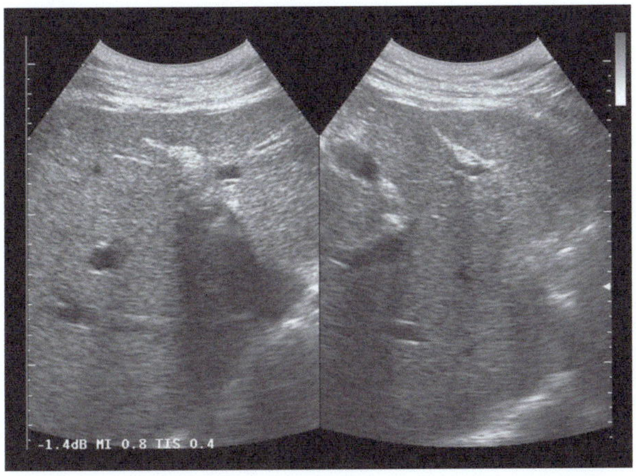

Fig. 5.88 Hepatic pseudolesion created by the round ligament. Elongated hyperechoic "mass" with posterior acoustic shadowing (*left*), which upon rotation of the transducer extends longitudinally (*right*)

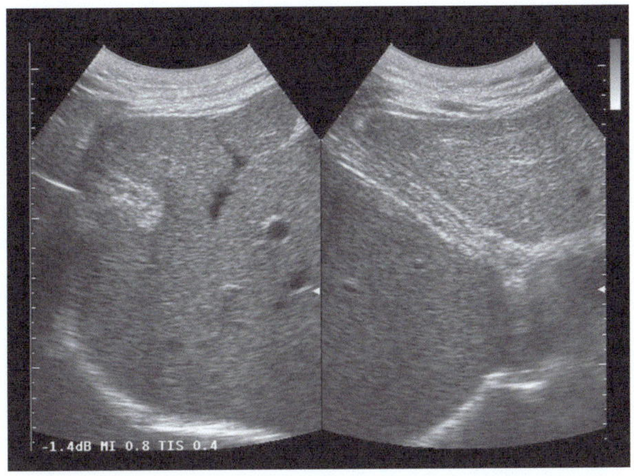

Fig. 5.89 Hepatic pseudolesion caused by a diaphragmatic slip. Ill-defined, heterogeneous, echogenic nodulation with partial posterior acoustic shadowing (*left*) which upon rotation of the transducer extends longitudinally (*right*) and takes on a multilayered and fibrillar appearance

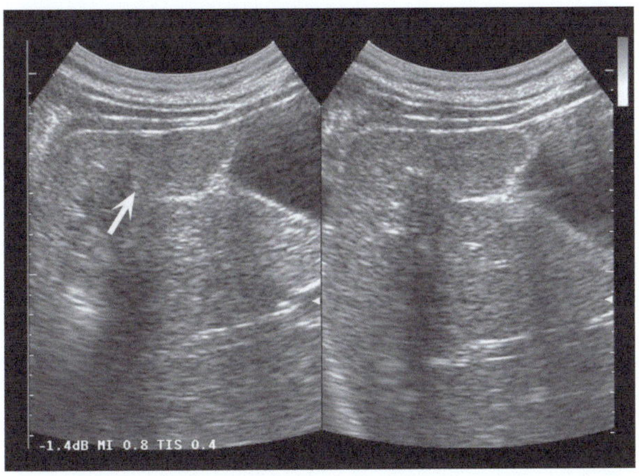

Fig. 5.90 Hepatic pseudonodulation. The image of the fissure which extends to the bed of the gallbladder circumscribes an area of (apparent) mild hypoechogenicity adjacent to the gallbladder (*arrow*)

nized by rotating the transducer and detecting the longitudinal unfolding of the echogenic image. The diaphragmatic slips c,an mimic peripheral echogenic lesions of the liver, although these tend to move with respiration and can be followed in the various scan planes external to the hepatic surface. The transmission of ultrasound through the hepatic vessels, and in particular the suprahepatic vein, can distally create a false image of an echogenic lesion. The hypoechoic perfusion alterations produced by fistulas can mimic a focal lesion, although they are usually characterized by a wedge-shaped appearance and at any rate can be differentiated with CEUS [50,75,76] (Figs. 5.88–5.90).

5.3 Focal Lesions in Patients with Chronic Liver Disease

Hepatocellular carcinoma (HCC) is one of the most common tumors, although its incidence varies in different countries with peak incidence in Asia. HCCs in a healthy liver tend to present in a young age as well-defined monofocal lesions. The most common conditions of liver disease are virus, alcohol and hemochromatosis related. A lesion identified only in the symptomatic phase is associated with an absolutely negative prognosis, in part also due to progression of the underlying liver disease, with a five-year survival rate of 0–10%. In contrast, the forms identified early have a greater possibility for treatment, with a five-year survival rate >50% for both surgical resection and transplant [77].

HCC can develop de novo, but generally **hepatocarcinogenesis** is a progressive process which begins with a regeneration nodule and evolves in the subsequent phases of low-grade dysplastic nodule (ordinary adenomatoid hyperplasia), high-grade dysplastic nodule (adenomatoid hyperplasia with atypia), early HCC nodule, early-advanced HCC nodule (nodule in nodule) and lastly overt HCC. During this process the portal vascular supply, which is the main supply of the hepatic parenchyma, is progressively reduced and eventually disappears, whereas the arterial supply becomes predominant and then exclusive.

The serum **alpha-fetoprotein** assay can identify increased levels in patients with HCC, although it is often normal in subjects with small nodules of recent onset, such that the test is more useful for monitoring and prognosis than for an early diagnosis. Using a threshold of 20 ng/mL produces a sensitivity of 60%, which falls to 22% with a threshold of 200 ng/mL. In the latter case the probability that the lesion identified is a HCC becomes very high [77]. When utilized as a screening option, **US** has shown a sensitivity of 65–80% but a specificity >90% [77]. Conceptually, a lesion identified in a patient with chronic liver disease should be considered a HCC until proven otherwise, even though nearly half of the nodules <2 cm and most nodules <1 cm are benign (focal steatosis, dysplasia, hemangiomas, etc.) [77,78]. US is the most utilized technique for the identification and initial characterization of HCC, which is completed by extemporary CEUS and/or second-level modalities such as dynamic MSCT and MR which are also able to perform adequate staging [77]. For the definitive diagnosis of HCC, standard criteria are used which were initially formulated for dynamic CT and MR, but which are also valid for CEUS and have the aim of reducing the need for biopsy. For lesions >2 cm identified during monitoring, the **Barcelona criteria** consider diagnostic the presence of an AFP >200 ng/mL or a hypervascularity of the lesion in the arterial phase demonstrated by two imaging modalities (angiography, CT, MR and CEUS) or by a single modality if there is also hypovascularity in the portal phase. In this case there is no need for biopsy confirmation, unless the AFP is <200 ng/mL or the imaging findings are uncharacteristic or the nodule is in a cirrhotic liver. With regard to lesions of 1–2 cm, biopsy is indicated, unless two imaging modalities coincidentally reveal characteristic findings. Lastly, for lesions <1 cm, short-term follow-up alone is advised even in the presence of suggestive radiologic findings – no growth over a two-year period rules out a tumor [77,79].

Dysplasia is a precancerous nodular lesion produced by the evolution of regenerative nodules. Its identification increases the probability of developing a HCC [78]. These are small lesions with isoechoic or hypoechoic appearance and possible thin echogenic rim. In addition, in a minority of cases the dysplastic nodule appears hyperechoic in relation to the intralesional accumulation of fat. However, there is no definite relationship between echogenicity and degree of dysplasia [80]. The identification of dysplastic nodules can be challenging, as can be its differentiation from a regenerative nodule on the one hand or a small HCC on the other. Indeed all of these lesions display variable echogenicity – lower than, equal to or greater than that of the surrounding parenchyma (Figs. 5.91, 5.92). This leads to limitations in not only sensitivity (1.6% in a study on explanted livers) but also specificity of US with respect to CT and MR. In some cases,

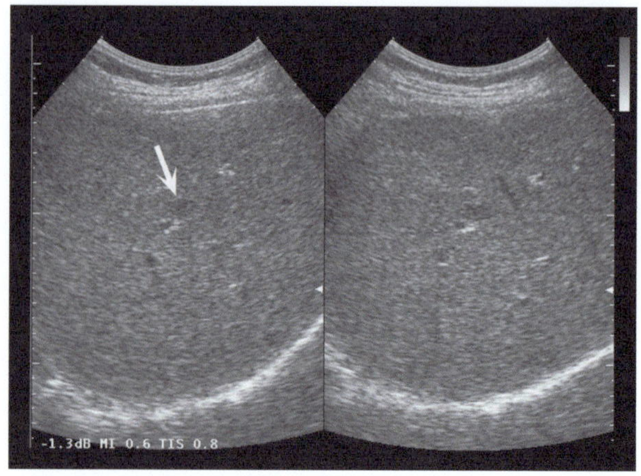

Fig. 5.91 Dysplastic nodule. Hypoechoic area (*arrow*) in the heterogeneous liver resulting from chronic hepatitis

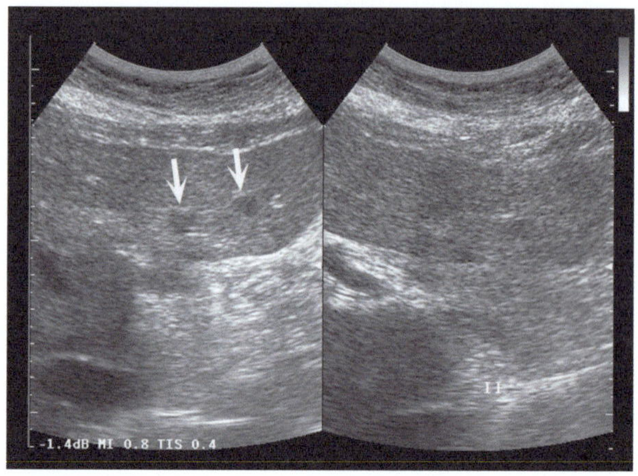

Fig. 5.92 Dysplastic nodules. Hypoechoic areas (*arrows*) in the left hepatic lobe

compatibly with the reduced size of the lesions, CD can be useful as it shows arterial signals and high flow in HCC (although present in <50% of cases) or possibly also continuous signals, which are absent in precancerous lesions [81]. Alternatively, CEUS can be used, which in most HCC nodules shows contrast enhancement in the arterial phase, whereas in most dysplastic nodules substantial hypovascularity with the surrounding parenchyma can be seen (although high-grade dysplasias can appear mildly hyperechoic in the arterial phase and hypoechoic in the portal-sinusoidal phase) [53].

In most patients with compensated liver disease, at least in those undergoing periodic monitoring, HCC is identified in the monofocal form, especially if a single etiologic factor is responsible for the underlying liver disease. The size of the lesion at diagnosis, however, is not a reliable predictor of the subsequent course of the disease [82]. The echogenicity of a small lesion is not very specific, as it may range from a hypoechoic to a hyperechoic appearance in both HCC and benign lesions [78].

Small HCCs (<2 cm) generally have a nodular appearance and can be classified into four types: nodular, nodular with extranodular growth, confluent multinodular and with irregular margins. These lesions tend to present a homogeneous echotexture and are hypoechoic in as many as 75% of cases. As they grow, HCC nodules at first tend to appear hypoechoic, then to develop greater central echogenicity and finally to become diffusely echogenic, although heterogeneously so. It also appears that nodules with a peripheral hypoechoic halo grow faster than those that are homogeneously hypoechoic. Occasionally, a hypoechoic area may be seen in a broader echogenic lesion, a characteristic of the development of a "nodule in nodule" [50]. There are, however, small HCCs which may have an echogenic appearance, especially due to adipose metaplasia, fibrosis and/or sinusoidal dilatation, and thus mimic hemangiomas. Statistically, however, it is more likely that a hyperechoic lesion in a subject with chronic liver disease is a HCC than a hemangioma and as such the new nodule should be considered suspicious until proven otherwise [83]. In a screening study on 2341 cirrhotic patients, US found 46 pre-existing hyperechoic lesions, of which 24 were HCC and 22 hemangiomas, and 38 new lesions found during follow-up, of which 31 were HCC nodules and 7 dysplastic nodules [84]. In terms of differential diagnosis it should be borne in mind that metastases on a cirrhotic liver are rare (Figs. 5.93–5.105, Videos 5.14–5.18).

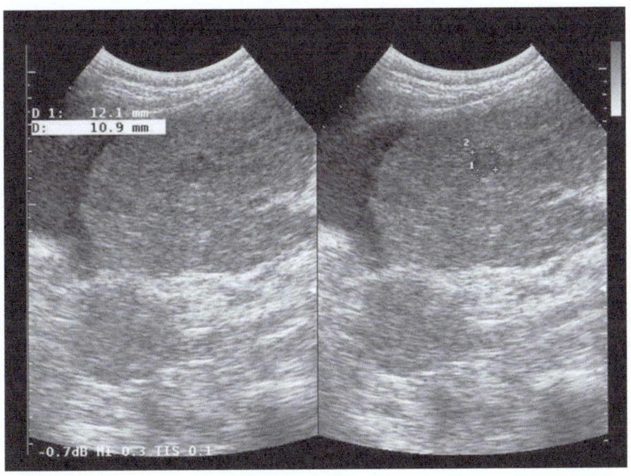

Fig. 5.93 HCC. Small heterogeneous hypoechoic nodule. Peritoneal effusion is associated

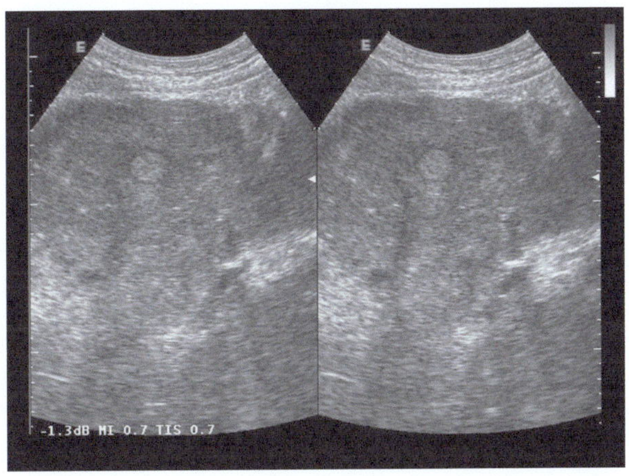

Fig. 5.94 HCC. Small echogenic nodule with peripheral hypoechoic halo

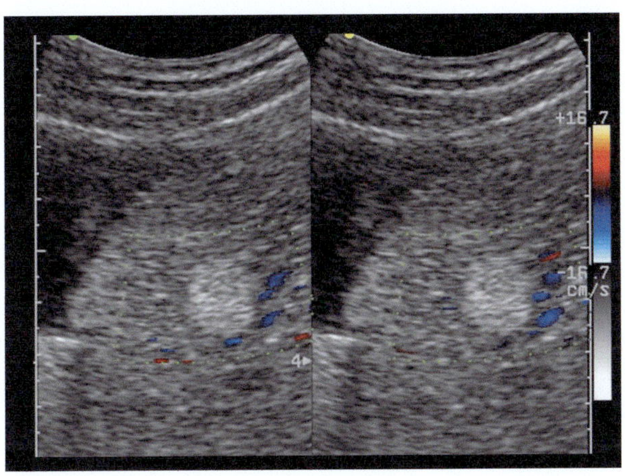

Fig. 5.95 HCC. Small heterogeneous echogenic nodule with no internal signals at CD

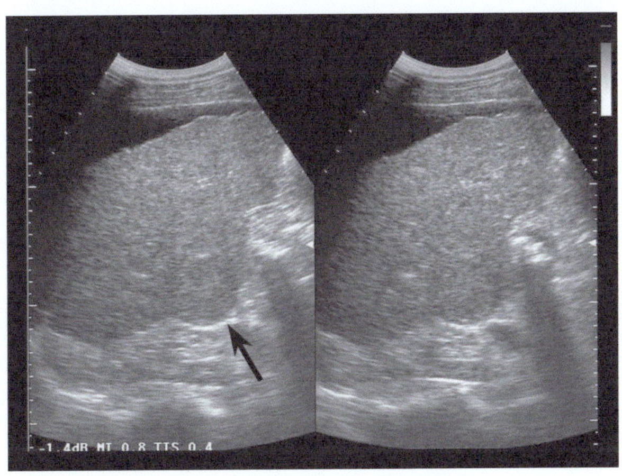

Fig. 5.96 HCC. Mildly hypoechoic nodule producing a bulge in the deep hepatic profile (*arrow*)

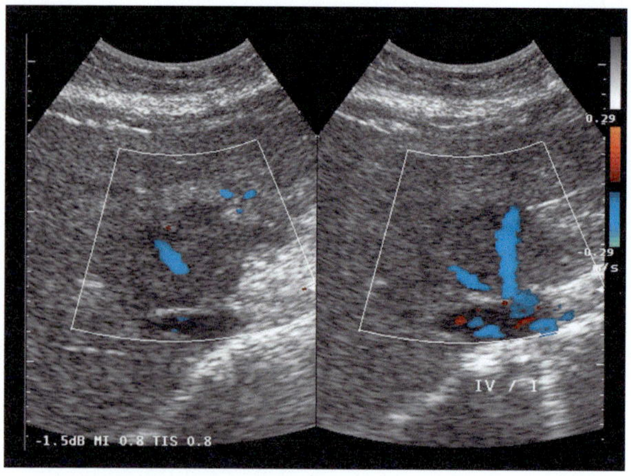

Fig. 5.97 HCC. Hypoechoic nodule located around the confluence of the middle and left hepatic veins which are patent at CD

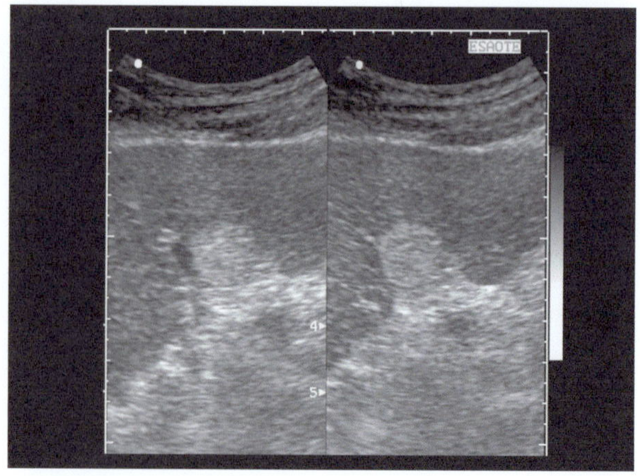

Fig. 5.98 HCC. Homogeneous hyperechoic nodule in the left lobe

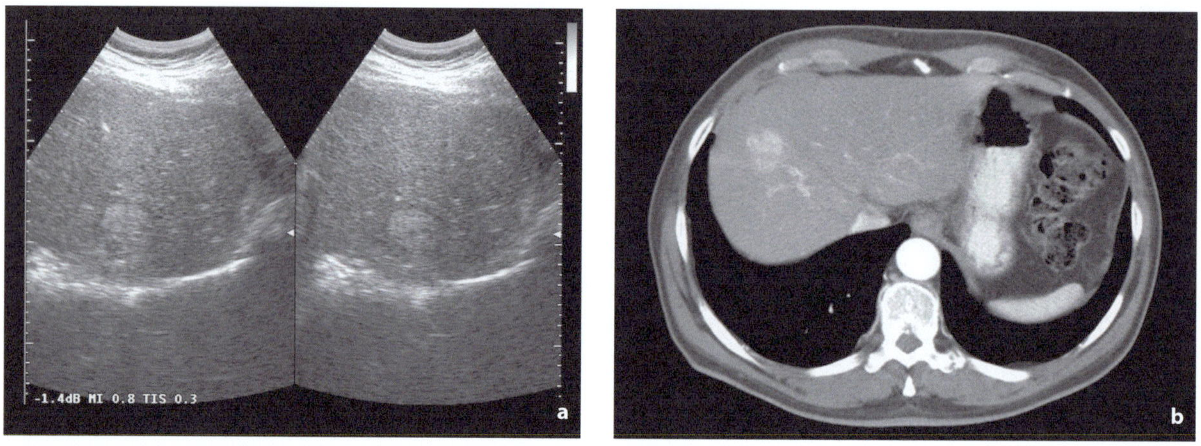

Fig. 5.99a,b HCC. Relatively well-defined and homogeneous echogenic nodule (**a**). CT scan in the arterial phase shows the hypervascular nature of the lesion (**b**)

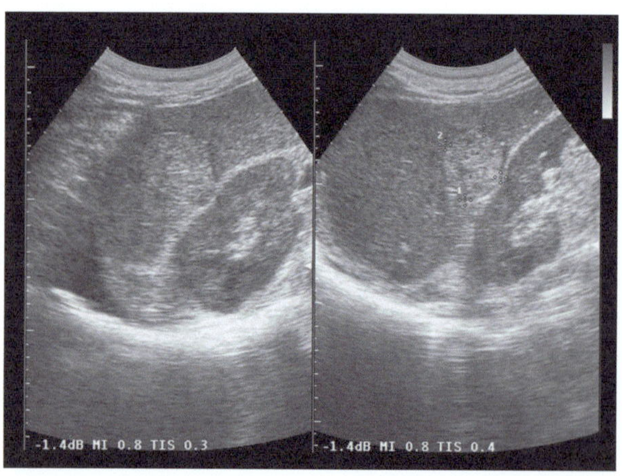

Fig. 5.100 HCC Relatively well-defined and homogeneous echogenic nodule producing a slight bulge in the deep hepatic profile

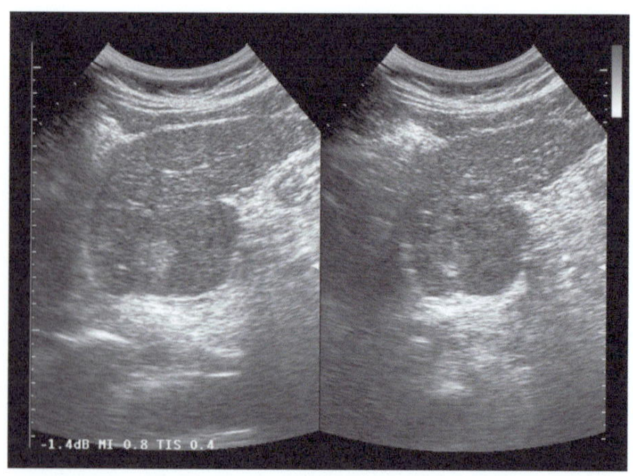

Fig. 5.101 HCC. Nodule with mixed structure due to the presence of a hyperechoic area in the context of a iso-hypoechoic mass which bulges from the dorsal profile of the left hepatic lobe

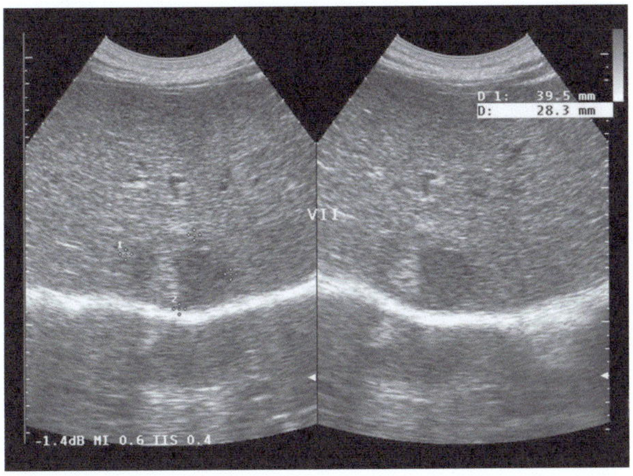

Fig. 5.102 HCC. Nodule with mixed structure due to the presence of hypoechoic and hyperechoic components

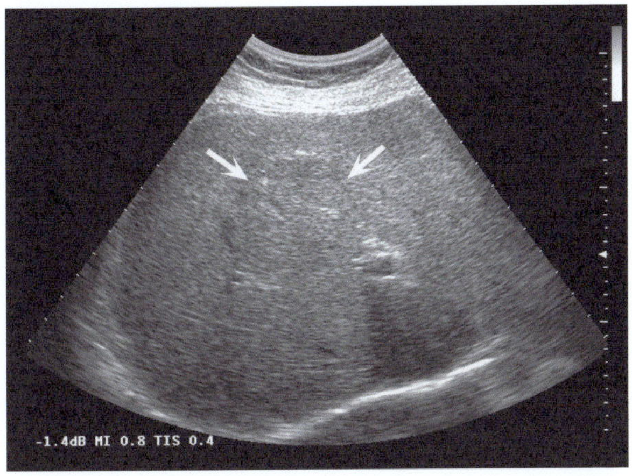

Fig. 5.103 HCC. Substantially isoechoic nodule is identifiable only as a result of presence of a hyperechoic rim (*arrows*)

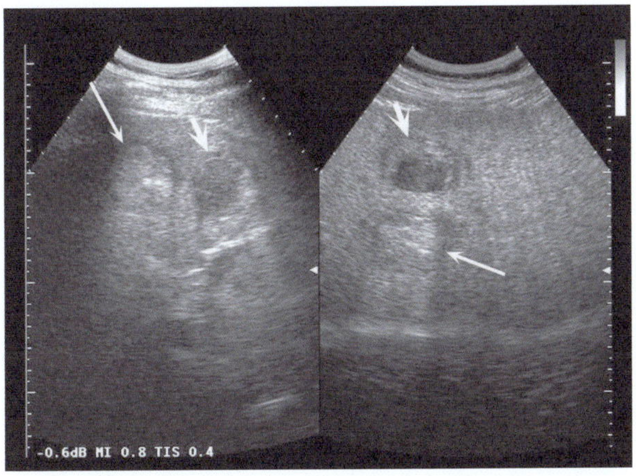

Fig. 5.104 HCC in a healthy liver. Two adjacent nodules with different appearances, one relatively homogeneous and echogenic with a thin peripheral hypoechoic halo (*long arrow*) and the other heterogeneous hypoechoic with hyperechoic margins (*short arrow*)

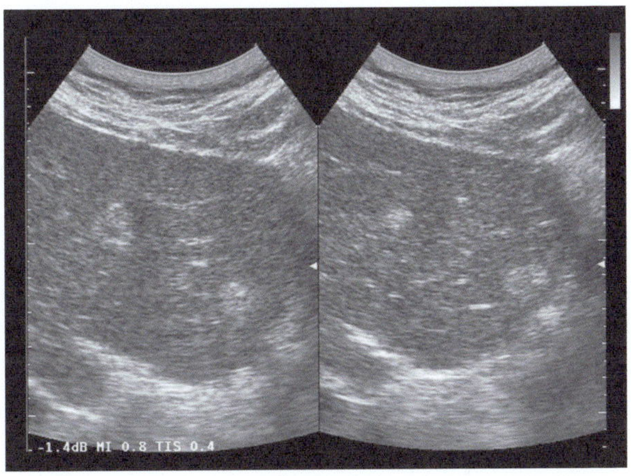

Fig. 5.105 HCC. Two heterogeneous echogenic nodules

The identification of small HCCs is made more challenging by the presence of a generally heterogeneous parenchymal background as a consequence of chronic liver disease, although in some studies on explanted livers the degree of parenchymal heterogeneity did not prove to be a determining factor [85]. HCCs that may more easily be missed at US evaluation tend to be small, isoechoic, superficial (especially if rounded) and characterized by diffuse invasive growth [18]. The use of contrast medium can notably increase the detection of color signals in these lesions, from 33% to 92%, thus facilitating the identification of arterial hypervascularity [86]. In the past the sensitivity reported for US has been very variable, from 33% to 96%, but more recent studies performed on explanted livers have indicated lower values (20–27%), with marked dependence on the size of the lesions [81,85]. However, one of the important features of US is its ability, in the presence of an area of greater heterogeneity, to arouse suspicion of the presence of a lesion, which in many cases will subsequently be confirmed by CEUS, CT or MR. In some cases the small lesion can cause a focal bulge in the hepatic surface, especially but not exclusively identifiable in the presence of associated ascites (particularly if the US study is performed with a thorough exploration of the surface of the organ using different frequencies) [50].

Medium-sized (2–5 cm) and **large** (>5 cm) **HCCs** can be classified as nodular, massive or diffuse. The

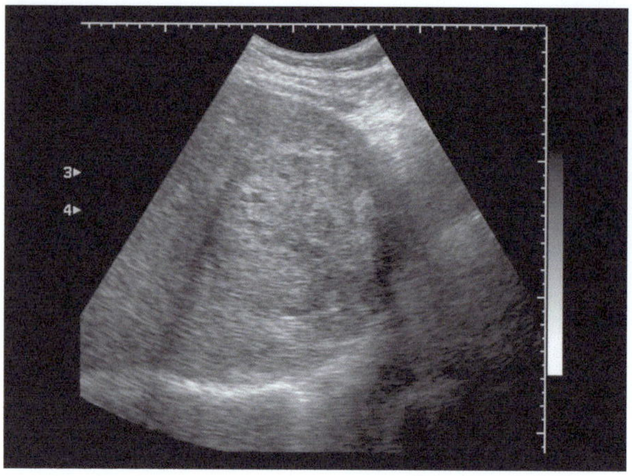

Fig. 5.106 HCC. Large nodular lesion with heterogeneous echogenic appearance (mosaic) and marginal hypoechoic halo

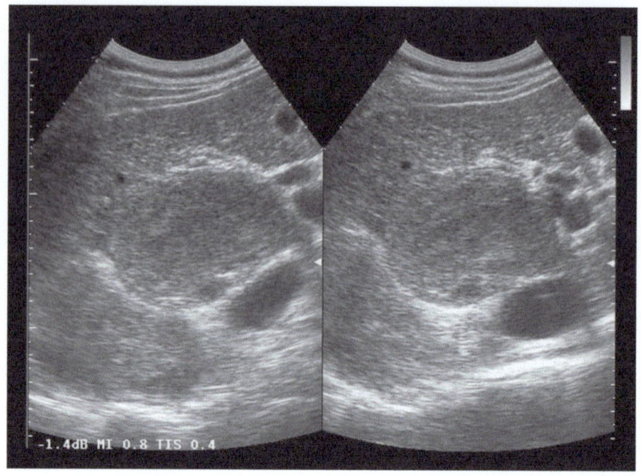

Fig. 5.107 Exophytic HCC. Large heterogeneous hypoechoic nodule protruding towards the posterior subhepatic space

lesions tend to present a peripheral hypoechoic capsular-like rim and have an echogenic appearance as a consequence in particular of fibrosis. One or more central echogenic areas tend to form with the growth of hypoechoic lesions, and around 50% of large HCCs have a heterogeneous echogenic appearance. In particular, a "mosaic" appearance may be seen with areas of differing echogenicity separated by thin septa (Figs. 5.106, 5.107). Calcifications are rather infrequent except in fibrillar HCC, whereas internal liquefactive necrosis may be seen in the larger masses. The invasive forms display irregular and ill-defined margins and signs of invasion of the adjacent structures, especially the portal branches. The diffuse form appears with nodular and heterogeneous disruption of the echostructure of the hepatic parenchyma, contributing to which are the underlying cirrhotic disease and perfusion alterations secondary to venous obstruction and fistulas [40]. In the multifocal forms, multiple nodules can be seen of different size, the morphostructural appearance of which is often heterogeneous, with the larger lesions appearing more echogenic and inhomogeneous.

At **CD** HCC generally appears more vascular than the surrounding parenchyma, with hypertrophic arterial vessels reaching the periphery of the nodule, surrounding it and penetrating inside, occasionally with the typical "basket" pattern [51,52]. Alternatively the "vessel within the tumor" pattern may be identified, whereby color signals branching at the center of the nodule, or a dotted pattern with multiple punctate and non-branching signals, may be seen [86]. The forms without significant intranodular signals have become infrequent findings and are limited to small lesions. The intranodular vessels are prevalently arterial, tortuous, and irregularly distributed, with sharp angles or interruptions. They show high systolic flow (with measured velocities even higher than those of the aorta) and elevated RI values as a consequence of arteriovenous fistulas and low resistance to flow. The diastolic component is variable and in blind vessels may even be absent. In large HCCs the vascular appearance is rather heterogeneous with signals of both arterial and venous flow. PD is better than CD for the study of HCC located more superficially or intermediate in depth, whereas it provides little useful information for lesions located in the left lobe, the study of which is often hampered by cardiac artifacts to which PD is more sensitive, and for lesions located deep within the right lobe, due to the poorer penetration of PD with respect to CD [87]. The use of contrast medium can notably increase the number of lesions that display vascular signals and better define the vascular pattern [86]. Indubitably the CD findings are not in themselves conclusive, but it can be stated that a lesion with internal vascular signals in a subject with chronic liver disease is highly likely to be a HCC, whereas a lesion with no vascular signals has a moderate probability of not being a HCC (Figs. 5.108–5.110).

At **CEUS** early HCC can appear substantially isoechoic in all the vascular phases or it may show mild hyperechogenicity in the arterial phase and/or hypoechogenicity in the portal-sinusoidal phase, thus making it difficult to distinguish from a high-grade dysplastic nodule. When an initial-advanced HCC is formed, the appearance of a hypervascular nodule within the iso-hypovascular nodule may be seen, which is characteristic. Advanced HCC is generally characterized by early enhancement in the arterial

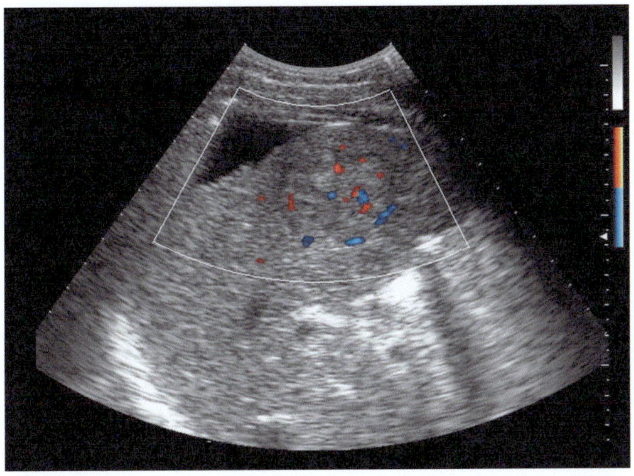

Fig. 5.108 HCC. Mildly hypoechoic nodule with some internal arterial flows at directional PD. Perihepatic effusion can also be distinguished

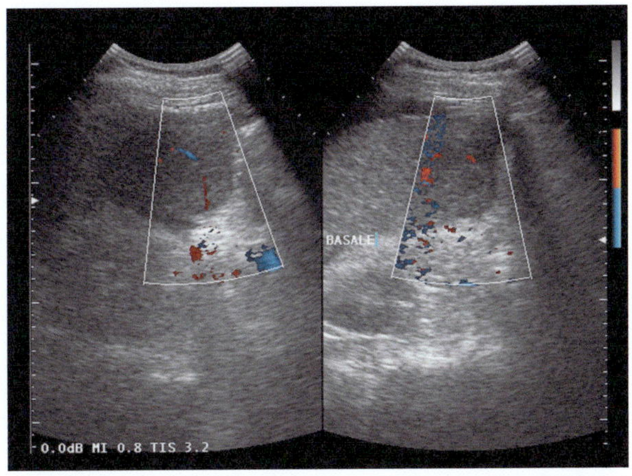

Fig. 5.109 HCC. Heterogeneous hypoechoic nodule, with some scattered internal arterial flows at directional PD. Perihepatic effusion can also be distinguished

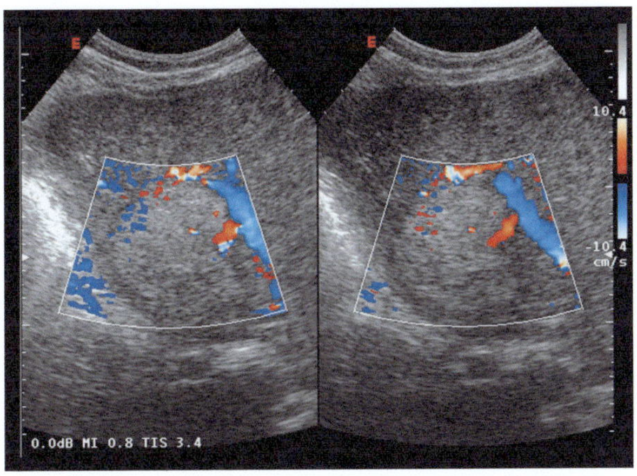

Fig. 5.110 HCC. Relatively well-defined and homogeneous echogenic macronodular lesion with some afferent arteries seen at CD

phase, which becomes iso- or more often hypoechoic in the portal-sinusoidal phase [53,88] (Fig. 5.111). Isoechogenicity in the portal-sinusoidal phase can create difficulties for differential diagnosis with respect to other hypervascular lesions with high flow, especially hemangiomatous lesions, whereas portal and sinusoidal hypoechogenicity in association with arterial hypervascularity is practically diagnostic in the setting of chronic liver disease. There is also the possibility of hypovascular HCC, which is usually well differentiated with little enhancement in all the phases. The arterial phase may also reveal one or more hypertrophic feeding vessels which feed one or more poles and then penetrate within the nodule forming a macrovascular network with a "basket" pattern or chaotic distribution. Large HCCs have a CEUS

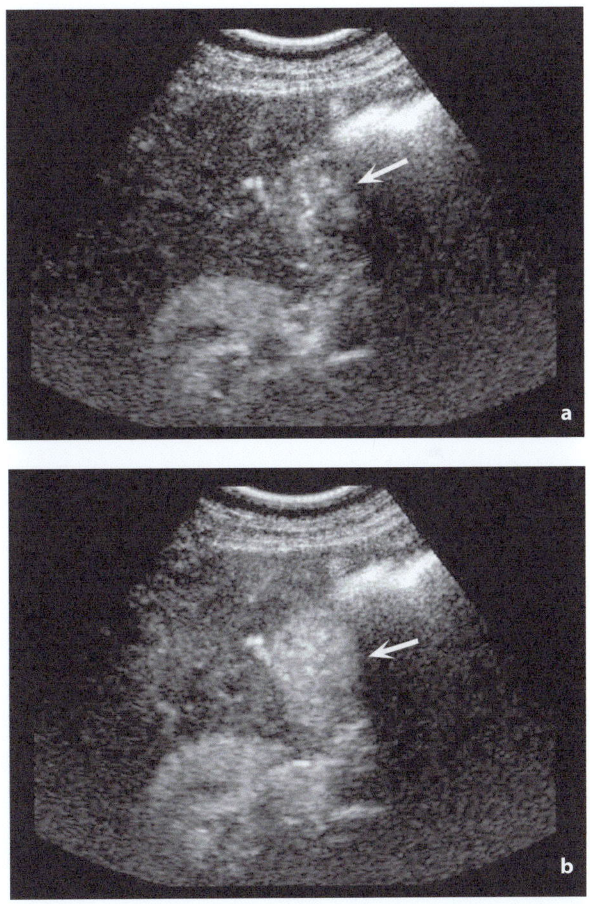

Fig. 5.111a,b HCC. The two CEUS scans in the arterial phase show the rapid and intense enhancement of the lesion (*arrow*)

appearance similar to that indicated above but are more likely to display areas of hypoperfusion or no perfusion due to necrosis, especially in the center of the lesion, as well as venous lakes.

Vascular involvement of the portal vein, or more rarely, the hepatic veins is relatively common, especially in the invasive forms, and characterizes HCC with respect to other hepatic lesions such as metastases. The probability of the neoplastic nature of a thrombus increases with increasing size of the lesion. Unlike benign thrombi, which are also not uncommon in subjects with chronic liver disease, malignant thrombi appear more echogenic and heterogeneous, they tend to widen the vessel and they can show internal arterial signals at CD (recanalized benign thrombi may show internal but exclusively venous flows) or an enhancement in the arterial phase at CEUS. Extensive masses can also invade the inferior vena cava, occasionally reaching the right atrium, or the bile duct. HCC is second only to renal cell carcinoma in its frequency of caval invasion [30,50] (Figs. 5.112–5.115, Videos 5.19, 5.20).

Apart from the cases that at presentation are already in an advanced stage, with decompensated cirrhosis, extensive or diffuse HCC and portal thrombosis, US, even when integrated with CEUS, is generally unable to provide a sufficiently accurate **evaluation of the disease**, which is fundamental for treatment planning (number and size of lesions, vascular involvement, extrahepatic spread of the disease, etc.) (Figs. 5.116, 5.117). In these cases, dynamic CT or MR are needed (possibly with the use of liver-specific contrast media), whereas oily agent CT is no longer used for the purposes of staging. CEUS cannot be used for the systematic study of all the parenchyma in the arterial phase, and therefore even with the use of multiple

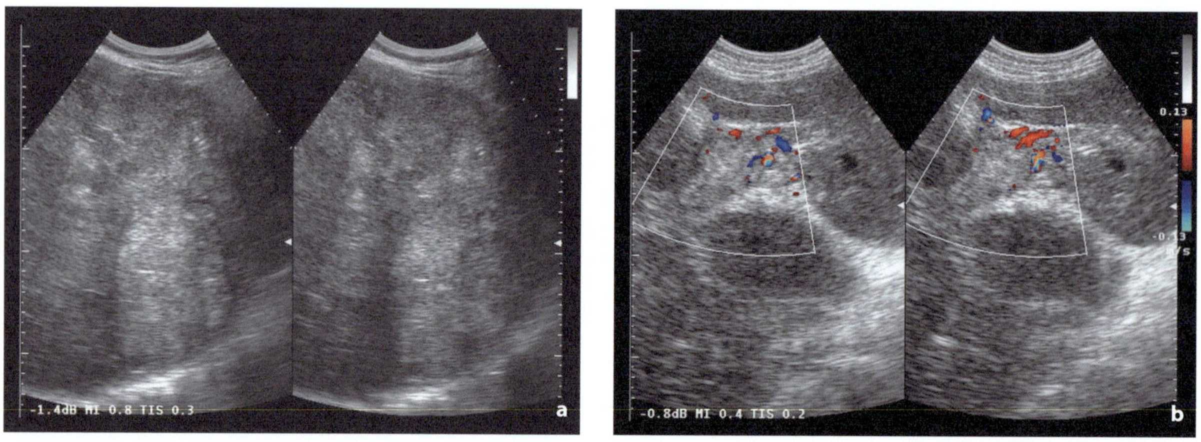

Fig. 5.112a,b Invasive HCC with malignant portal thrombosis. Diffuse structural disruption of the right lobe (**a**). Heterogeneous echogenic material can be seen at CD in the portal bifurcation with some internal arterioles (**b**)

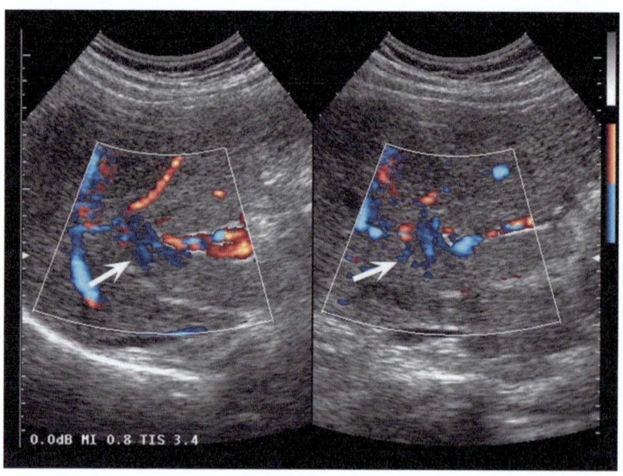

Fig. 5.113 Benign portal thrombosis. Complete obstruction of the proximal venous tract, with recanalized venule instead in the distal tract (*arrows*) seen at directional PD

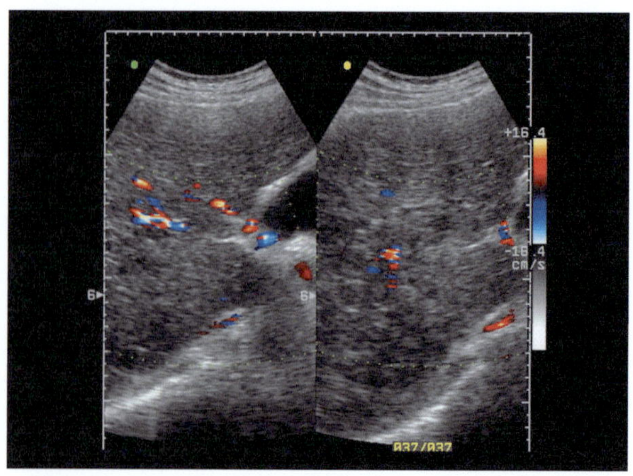

Fig. 5.114 Malignant portal thrombosis. Arterial signals can be distinguished within the thrombus

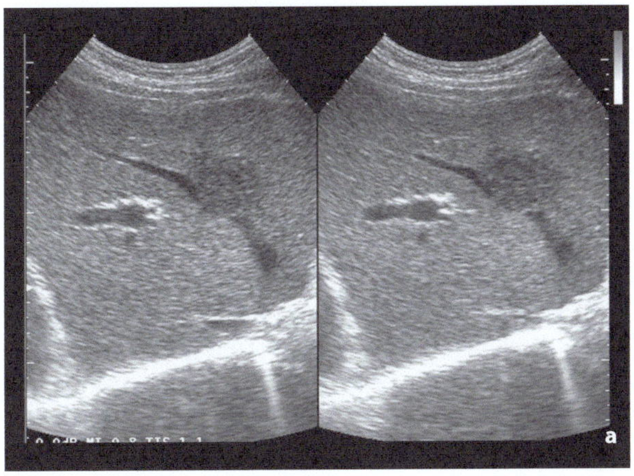
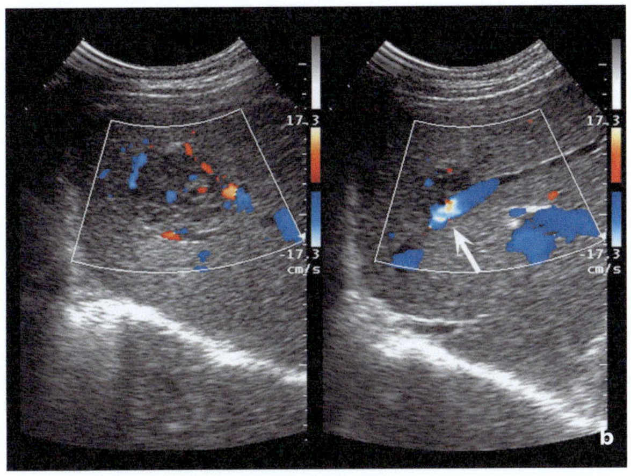

Fig. 5.115a,b HCC with venous involvement. Extensive heterogeneous hypoechoic nodule located at the middle hepatic vein (**a**). CD shows the arterial hypervascularity of the nodule and the stenosis of the vein (**b**, aliasing artifact, *arrow*)

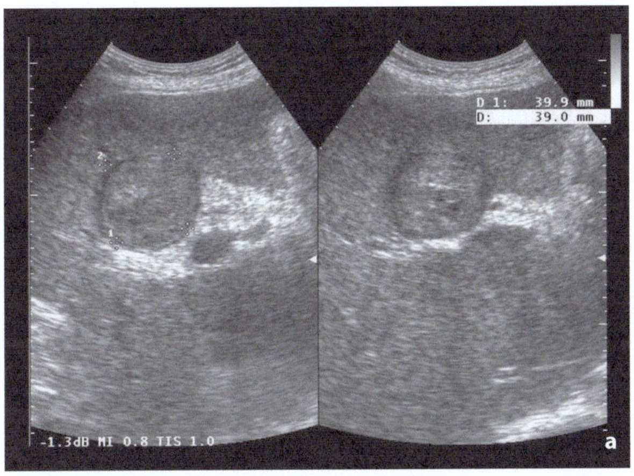
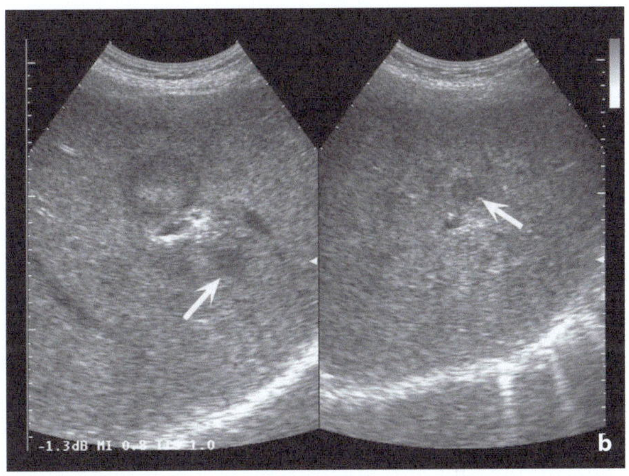

Fig. 5.116a,b HCC with satellite nodules. Within the larger nodule (**a**) at least two "daughter" hypoechoic areas can be seen (**b**, *arrows*)

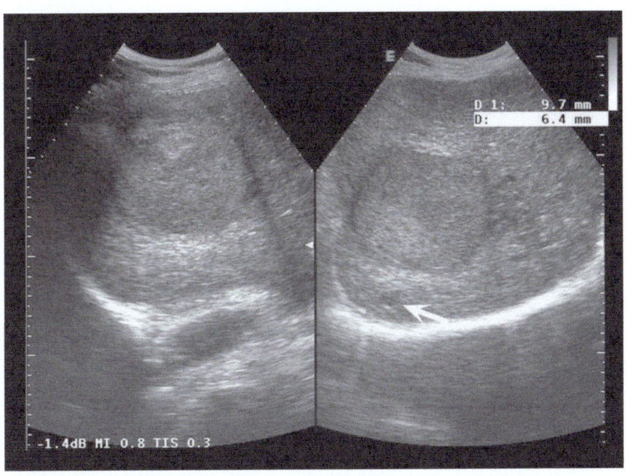

Fig. 5.117 HCC with "daughter" lesion. Large relatively homogeneous echogenic HCC with peripheral hypoechoic halo. A small hypoechoic satellite nodule is associated (*arrow*)

injections of contrast medium cannot rule out the presence of other nodules, which is clearly fundamental for treatment planning.

The **Barcelona Clinic Liver Cancer** (BCLC) staging classification [89] classifies HCC into various stages important for therapeutic management and is today preferable to both the TNM and Okuda systems. In the early stage the patient has a WHO performance status of 0, conserved liver function (Child A or B), a single tumor >5 cm or up to 3 lesions <3 cm with no signs of macroscopic vascular invasion or extrahepatic spread (with Child A and single lesion >2 cm the term very early stage is used). In these subjects a variety of treatments may be used, such as transplant, resection or percutaneous ablation, with good probability of response. In the intermediate stage the performance status is still 0 and the Child is still A or B, but the HCC is larger or multifocal, without signs of

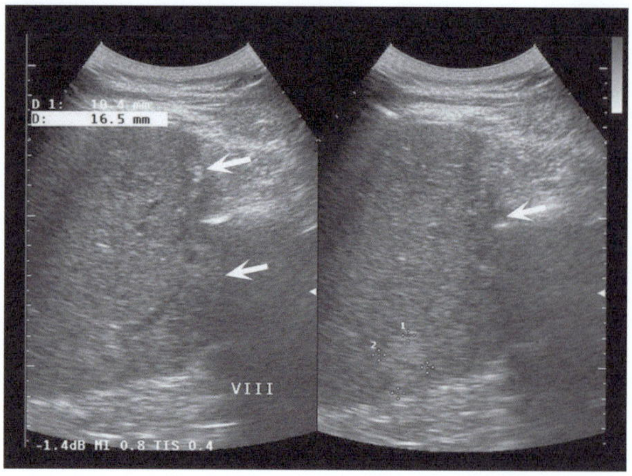

Fig. 5.118 HCC, postoperative recurrence. Echogenic nodule (*between the calipers*) adjacent to the wedge resection (*arrows*)

macroscopic vascular invasion or extrahepatic spread and without symptoms linked to the tumor itself. These patients are candidates for TACE. Advanced-stage HCC is present in patients with a performance status of 1 or 2, Child A or B and symptoms linked to the tumor, which causes vascular invasion or extrahepatic spread. These patients are candidates for TACE or TACE + percutaneous ablation, but with overridingly palliative aims. Lastly, the terminal stage includes subjects with a performance status of 3 or 4, Child C and nodules of any number or size. These patients only receive supportive medical therapy.

Lastly, the US techniques also have an important role to play in the identification of postoperative **recurrence** (Fig. 5.118, Video 5.21).

5.4 Gallbladder Wall Lesions

US is the imaging modality of choice in the study of the gallbladder. Wall lesions are a relatively common, generally incidental and asymptomatic finding during US hepatobiliary study, so it is important to be aware of the differential diagnostic appearances in order to identify cases that require follow-up or diagnostic work-up. As a general rule, polypoid lesions >10 mm tend to be treated surgically due to the risk of their malignant nature, whereas lesions between 5 mm and 9 mm tend to receive US monitoring, even if the interval is not particularly brief. Growth >5 mm or the presence of wall thickening are other possible indications for surgery. Micropolypoid wall lesions generally require no further study [30,90]. In different patient populations, the sensitivity of US has been reported to be 36–90% in identification of these lesions, which peaks if there are no associated calculi in the gallbladder and if the lesion in question is polypoid [90].

Around 95–99% of gallbladder polyps are cholesterol polyps. The remaining cases are made up of hyperplastic, adenomyomatous, adenomatous and malignant polyps (around 1%, primary and secondary) or are even due to ectopic gastric mucosa. Cholesterolosis is a form of hyperplastic cholecystosis caused by the deposit of lipid-containing macrophages and esters in the lamina propria of the gallbladder. The mucosa becomes hyperemic with numerous small and yellowish polypoid deposits. Adenomyomatosis is a form of hyperplastic cholecystosis characterized by diverticular outpouchings of the mucosa of the muscle layer (Rokitansky–Aschoff sinuses). It may be localized or diffuse and can cause luminal stricture at the site involved. Adenoma ("true polyp") can be single or multiple and tends to be prevalent in the infundibulum.

The lesions that may be missed at US are small intraluminal polyps, especially when located in an angulated area of the gallbladder such as at the level of the proximal third, or wall thickening not associated with significant intraluminal alterations or evident alterations of the adjacent hepatic parenchyma. The **differential diagnosis** of **polypoid lesions** includes blood clots (hemobilia), compacted debris and of course poorly calcified calculi. Fixity with changing patient posture is a requirement for a correct differentiation from the latter, although gallstones firmly adhering to the wall of the gallbladder are possible. A distinction needs to be made with respect to deposits of biliary sludge, which can mimic a wall lesion when very dense. However, the integrity of the underlying wall, the absence of vascular signals and partial regression at an examination subsequent to litholytic medical therapy usually makes an appropriate differential diagnosis possible [30, 91].

Once the solid nature of the lesion has been determined, the evaluation needs to consider its size, shape, surface, base (sessile or pedunculated) and the internal texture. **Cholesterol polyps** are often multiple and present as pedunculated lesions with a granular surface and fine echotexture with no posterior acoustic shadowing (Fig. 5.119). **Localized adenomatosis** appears with sessile wall thickening, often located in the fundus, containing multiple microcystic pseudo-diverticular images, small calculi and/or small crystals of cholesterol with comet tail artifacts (Figs. 5.120, 5.121). Neoplastic polyps (**adenomas** and stage T1 **adenocarcinomas**) appear as rounded and either sessile or pedunculated masses with nodular and irregular surfaces (anemone-like) and a hypo-isoechoic structure. The lesion tends to involve all the wall layers and is associated with wall thickening which

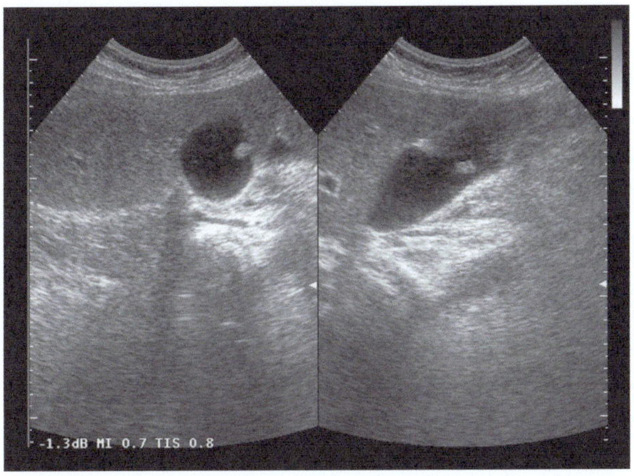

Fig. 5.119 Cholesterol polyp of the gallbladder. Small echogenic formation with thin peduncle in the gallbladder lumen

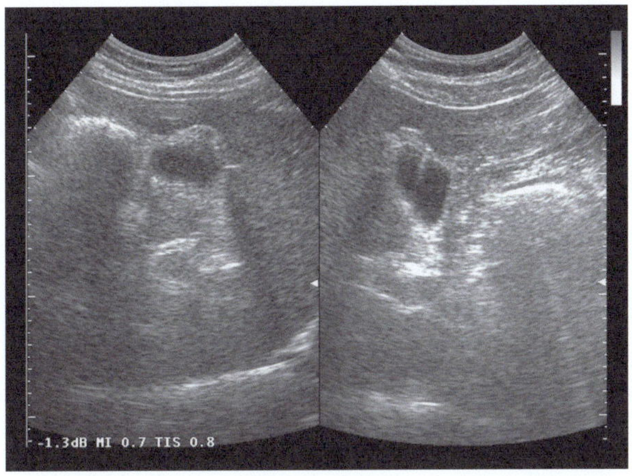

Fig. 5.120 Adenomyosis in the gallbladder fundus. Outpouching of the gallbladder wall containing biliary sand and microcalculi, with reverberation artifacts

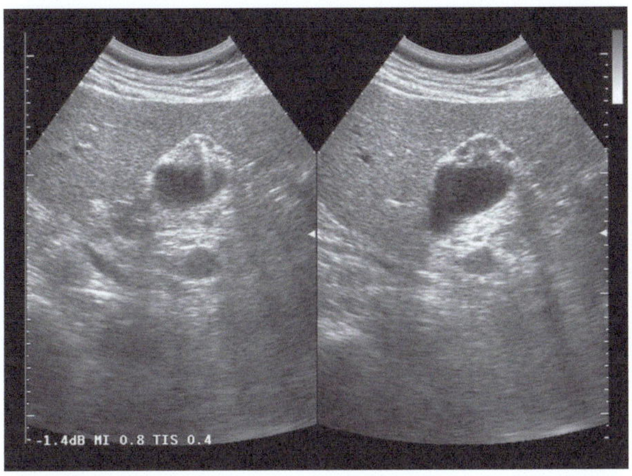

Fig. 5.121 Adenomyosis in the gallbladder fundus. Outpouching of the gallbladder wall containing biliary sand and microcalculi, with reverberation artifacts

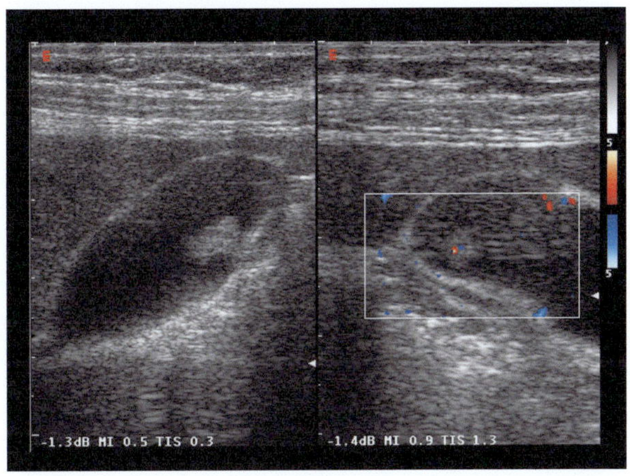

Fig. 5.122 Adenomatous polyp of the gallbladder. Polypoid lesion with a thin base and some internal vascular signals at CD located on the posterior wall of the gallbladder

extends laterally [59, 92, 93] (Fig. 5.122). Some additional information can be obtained with 3D study, which can demonstrate the granular surface of the polypoid lesions (82% of cases against 45.5% of 2D US) and the pedunculated appearance of the base of the lesions (86% of cases against 14% of 2D US), as well as being able to correctly differentiate a neoplastic polyp from a non-neoplastic one (91% of cases against 54.5% of 2D US) [93]. CD displays vascular signals only in adenomas, and above all in carcinomas (where relatively high flows are recorded, >20–30 cm/s, but with RI values similar to those of benign lesions), and therefore is useful when positive in characterizing gallbladder "polyps" and in the choice of surgical treatment (as well as in the distinction between carcinoma and masses of biliary sludge) [90,91]. The distinction with transabdominal US between benign and malignant polyps is not always easy, especially when the lesions are relatively small. EUS offers a good representation of the various lesions of the gallbladder wall [92], but it evidently cannot be used in a routine fashion. However, the polypoid lesions identified with EUS can be adequately monitored with transabdominal US.

Carcinoma of the gallbladder is the fifth gastrointestinal tumor in order of frequency in the United States (8570 new cases/year with an estimated 3260 deaths), with a peak incidence in elderly women (mean age 72 years) [30]. It may be associated with colon polyposis, inflammatory intestinal disease and porcelain gallbladder (carcinoma is present in 25% of the latter patients). US has reported an accuracy of 80% in the identification of gallbladder cancer [90]. Three forms may be seen: intraluminal polypoid (15–30% of cases), intramural with circumferential, segmental or diffuse thickening (5–30%), and massive lesions, with total or near-total replacement of the gallbladder itself (40–65%) [91,94]. A very common finding (44–100% of cases) is cholelithiasis. In the advanced forms of carcinoma it is often only the identification of a minimum residual central lumen containing calculi that at US enables the attribution of the mass to the gallbladder (of course in addition to the site and the failure to visualize a normal gallbladder) (Figs. 5.123–5.126).

The **differential diagnosis** of **gallbladder cancer**, especially in its variant of diffuse wall thickening, includes chronic cholecystitis and in particular the xanthogranulomatous form. This is a rare inflammatory process characterized by infiltration of the gallbladder walls by lipid-containing histiocytes and multinucleated giant cells. The inflammation causes marked and irregular wall thickening which can mimic carcinoma [30]. Porcelain gallbladder appears as a massive process of partial or complete calcification of the gallbladder walls with intense posterior acoustic shadowing and difficulty in evaluating the luminal content of the organ (not to mention a possible neoplastic degeneration within the lumen). Since this is a precancerous condition, it is often indicated for cholecystectomy, even when asymptomatic. The neoplastic forms with abundant luminal polypoid tissue can be mistaken

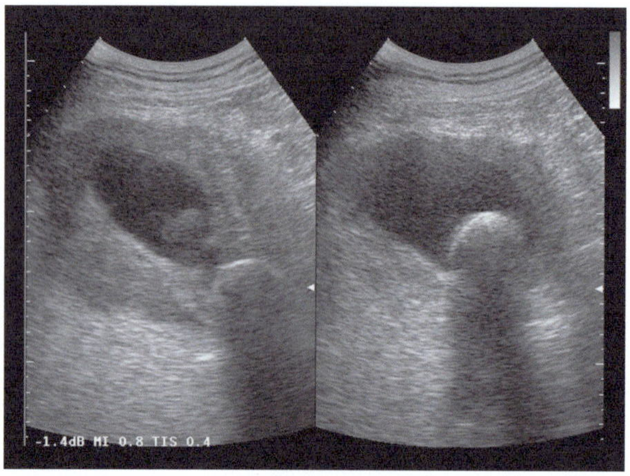

Fig. 5.123 Gallbladder cancer. Diffuse marked thickening of the gallbladder wall. Cholelithiasis is associated

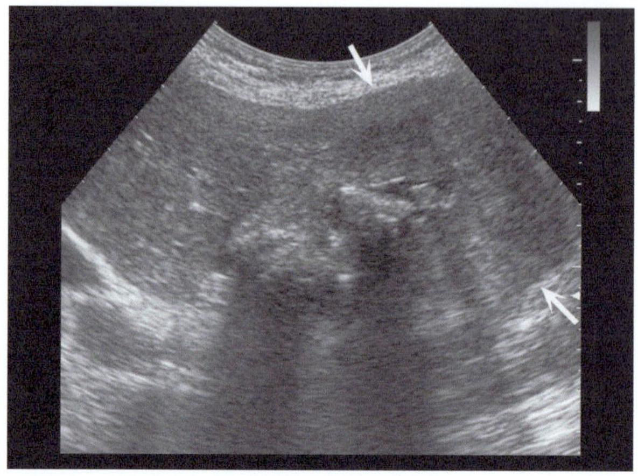

Fig. 5.124 Gallbladder cancer. Diffuse and evident hypoechoic thickening of the gallbladder wall (*arrows*). The small residual lumen of the organ is occupied by calculi

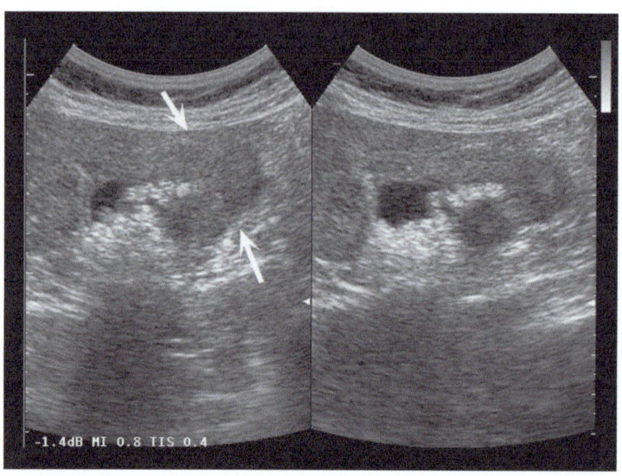

Fig. 5.125 Gallbladder cancer. Notable wall thickening of the gallbladder fundus (*arrows*). Microlithiasis is associated

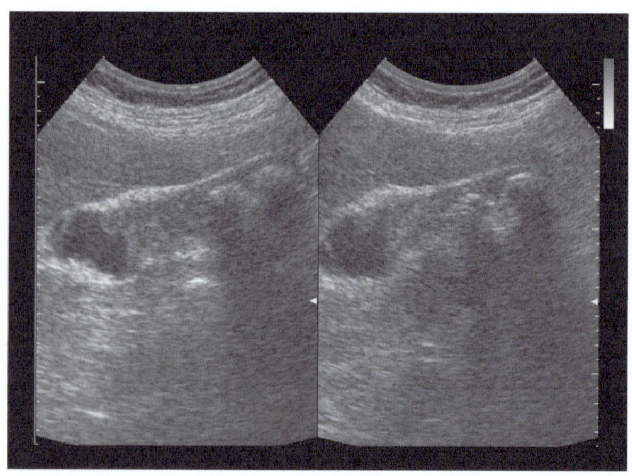

Fig. 5.126 Gallbladder cancer. Hypoechoic tissue with intraluminal development. Cholelithiasis is associated

for or mimicked by masses of biliary sludge, a gallbladder empyema or a luminal blood collection (Figs. 5.127–5.130).

In most cases gallbladder cancer is identified in a relatively advanced phase and the various appearances therefore tend to be combined. The lesion appears as a heterogeneous, hypoechoic, diffuse and irregular thickening of the gallbladder wall, with luminal vegetations and hypoechoic infiltrations in the adjacent hepatic parenchyma (segments IV and/or V) (Fig. 5.131). Hepatic invasion occurs relatively early: in the presence of a hypoechoic mass invading the gallbladder bed and is associated with wall thickening of the gallbladder, distinguishing it from a primary carcinoma and an invasive hepatic lesion, especially a metastatic one, can be challenging. In many cases this spread to the liver by direct extension is associated with more distant liver metastases, apparently on a hematogenous basis. US tends to understage the extension of carcinoma and at any rate patients need to undergo a second-level diagnostic examination, with CT or MR. The study should search for signs of invasion in the portal vein and the bile ducts, involvement of the adjacent hepatic parenchyma, non-contiguous hepatic metastases and lymphadenopathies of the cystic duct, the hepatic hilum and the lumbar region (Figs. 5.132, 5.133). The absence of capsular separation, and the presence of lobulations of the margins and irregularities of the margins themselves can suggest invasion of the adjacent hepatic parenchyma. The 3D images can be useful for precisely locating and evaluating the extension of carcinoma of the gallbladder [93].

One last cause of neoplastic alterations of the

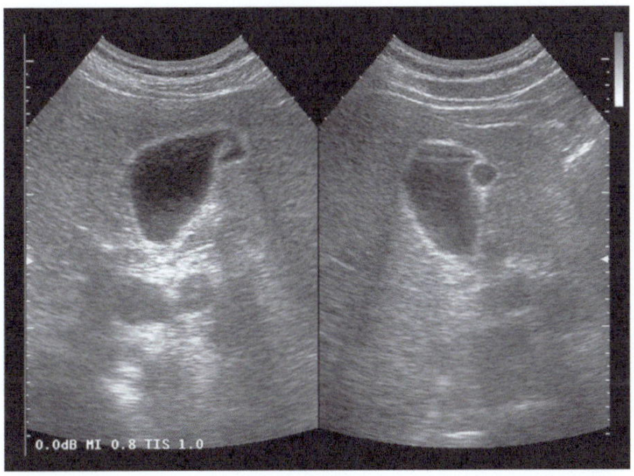

Fig. 5.127 "Phrygian cap" gallbladder. Folding of the fundus of the gallbladder on its body mimics a wall alteration, seen as polypoid (*left*) or intramural (*right*), according to the scan plane

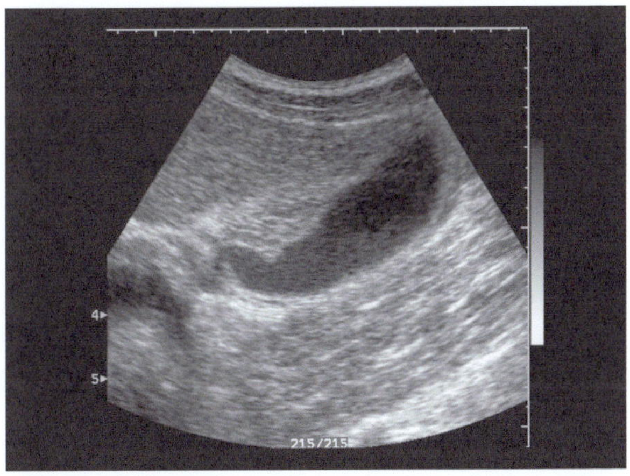

Fig. 5.128 Chronic cholecystitis. Diffuse but asymmetrical thickening of the gallbladder wall mimicking a tumor

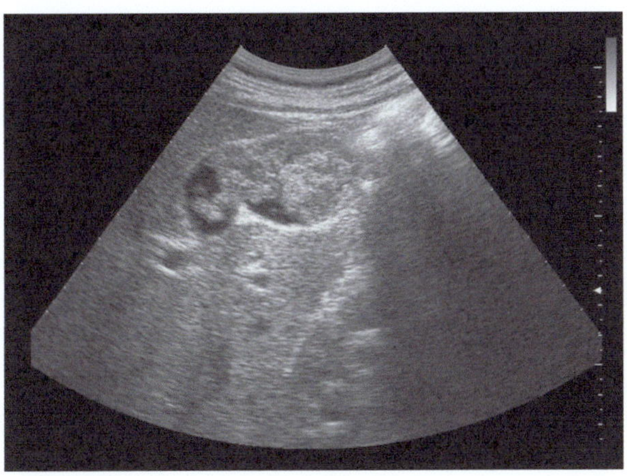

Fig. 5.129 Biliary sludge mimicking a gallbladder tumor. Dense and heterogeneous material in the gallbladder lumen

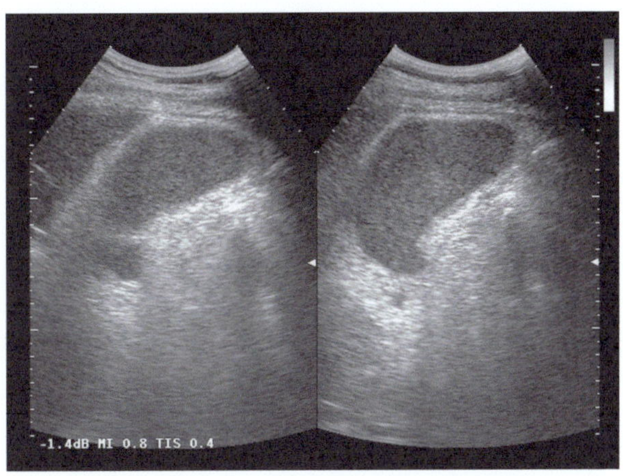

Fig. 5.130 Biliary sludge. Complete obliteration of the lumen due to muddy biliary material which mimics neoplastic tissue. The gallbladder walls are visible and appear thin

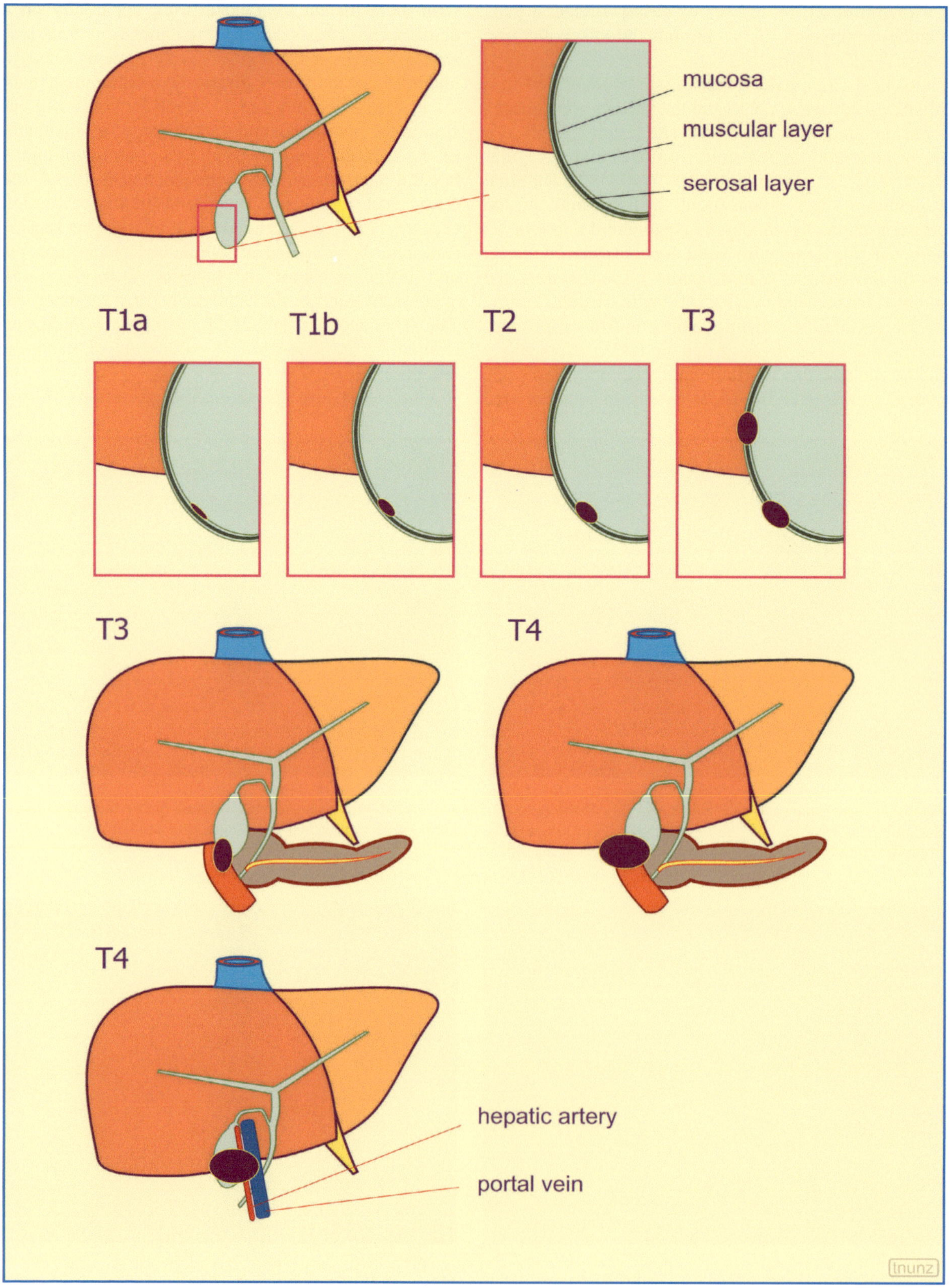

Fig. 5.131 Staging of gallbladder cancer. *T1a*, invasion of the lamina propria; *T1b*, invasion of the muscle layer; *T2*, invasion of the perimuscular fibrous tissue but not through the serosa or into the liver; *T3*, invasion through the peritoneal serosa and/or into the adjacent hepatic parenchyma and/or into the adjacent structures (stomach, duodenum, colon, pancreas, omentum, bile duct); *T4*, vascular invasion (portal vein or hepatic artery) or invasion of at least two extrahepatic structures and organs. Modified from [95]

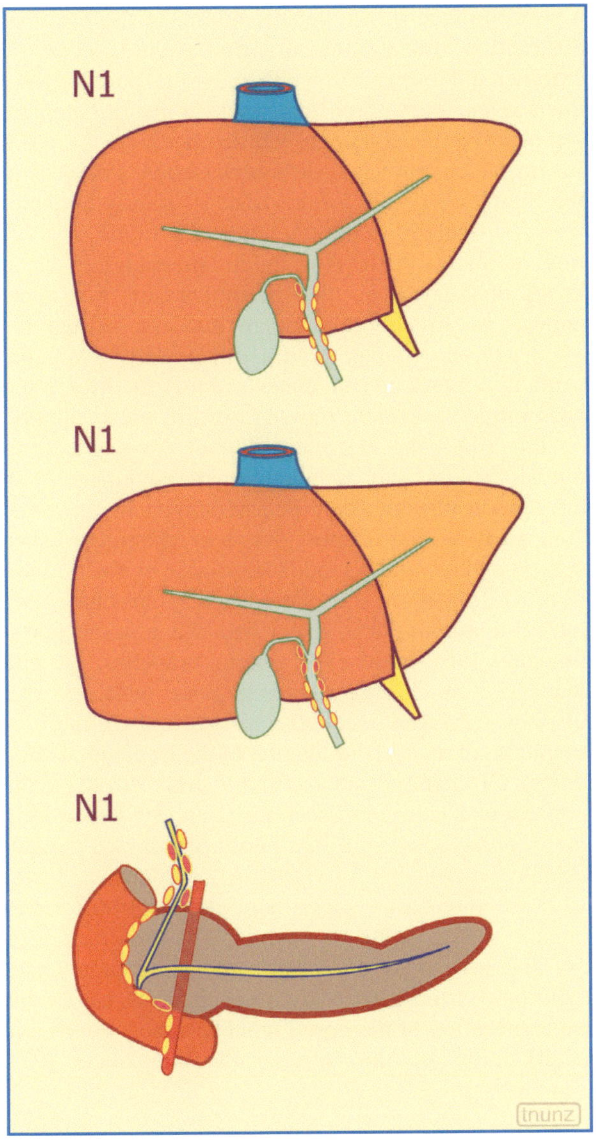

Fig. 5.132 N parameter for gallbladder cancer. Regional lymph nodes include cystic duct, pericholedocal, hepatic hilar, peripancreatic, periduodenal, periportal, celiac and superior mesenteric lymph nodes. *N1* refers to metastasis in one or more of the listed lymph node stations. Modified from [95]

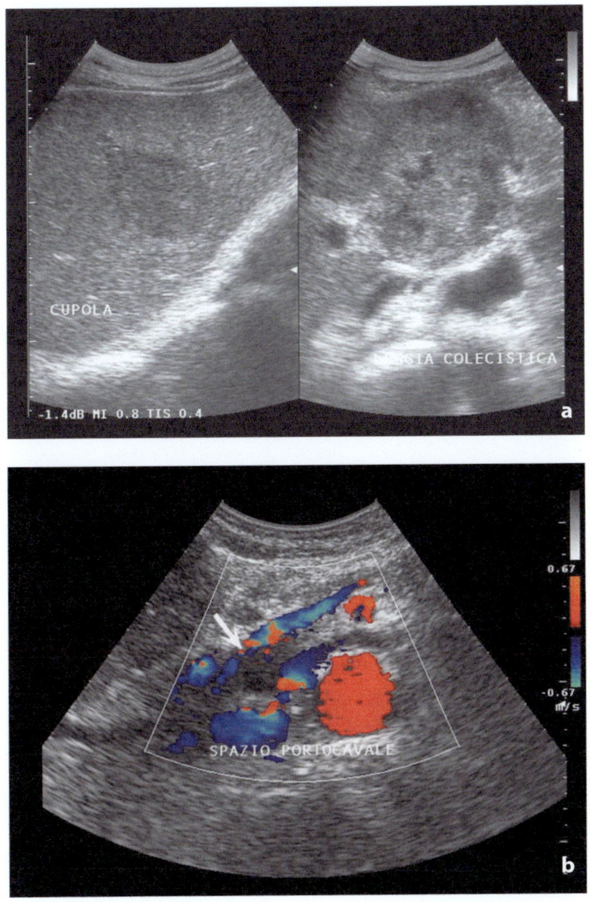

Fig. 5.133a,b Gallbladder cancer with hepatic and lymph node metastases. Mass occupying the gallbladder fossa (**a**) associated with a hypoechoic hepatic lesion and a lymphadenopathy of the portacaval space (**b**, *arrow*)

gallbladder wall is given by **metastases**. These are relatively infrequent but possible, especially in patients with melanoma, lung cancer or breast cancer. The general appearance is of one or more polypoid masses protruding into the lumen, with irregular surfaces and which tend to thicken the wall of the organ (Figs. 5.134, 5.135, Video 5.22).

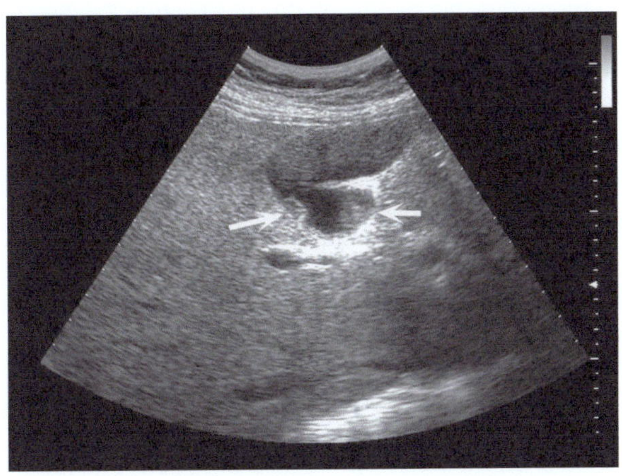

Fig. 5.134 Gallbladder metastasis from melanoma. Hypoechoic polypoid lesion protruding into the gallbladder lumen (*arrows*)

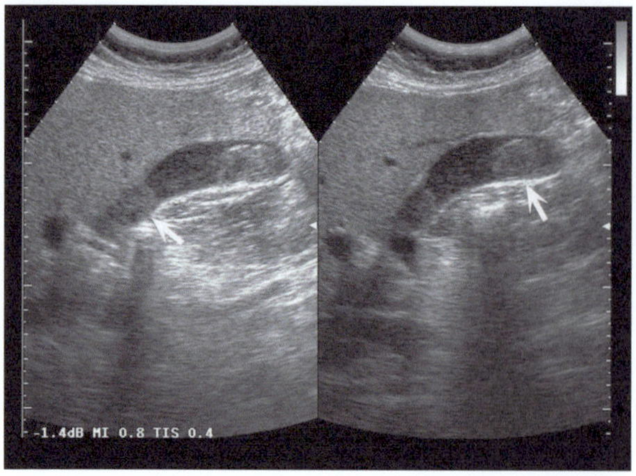

Fig. 5.135 Gallbladder metastasis from melanoma. Intraluminal polypoid hypoechoic lesions (*arrows*). Diffuse, mild heterogeneity of the intraluminal bile is associated

5.5 Malignant Obstructive Jaundice

Obstructive jaundice is caused by a blockage to the passage of conjugated bilirubin from the liver to the hepatopancreatic ampulla. In particular, "surgical" jaundice is defined as jaundice caused by a mechanical obstruction at some level of the extrahepatic bile passage. Tumors are responsible for 30–35% of the total cases of obstructive jaundice. In the cancer patient there is often a differential diagnostic problem of verifying whether the increase in bilirubin is caused by lesions to the hepatic parenchyma or by lesions which produce an obstruction of the biliary tract.

US is the undisputed first choice modality in the study of obstructive jaundice, and is able to confirm a dilatation of the biliary tract (accuracy 85–95%), demonstrate the height of the obstruction (accuracy >90%) and possibly clarify the cause (1/3 of cases) (Fig. 5.136). A detailed definition of the obstructive lesion can be obtained with EUS or intraductal US (high-frequency mini-transducer introduced with an endoscopic retrograde approach or a percutaneous descending approach). In addition, the accurate etiologic definition often requires further investigations such as MRCP.

The obstruction can be at a number of levels: intrapancreatic (at the level of the distal bile duct, 90% of cases of obstructive jaundice), suprapancreatic (between the hepatic hilum and the head of the pancreas, 5%) or hilar (at the hepatic hilum, 5%). Of course a lesion can only cause obstructive jaundice when the common bile duct is involved.

Under normal conditions, the **intrahepatic bile ducts** have a diameter <2 mm and are barely if at all perceptible. They may be identifiable when adjacent to a portal branch or the hepatic hilum. In the event of obstruction, dilatation occurs, first at the level of the extrahepatic bile passage, then in the parenchymal ducts adjacent to the hilum, then in the intrahepatic segmental branches on the left and lastly on the right. In chronic obstructions, such as caused by a neoplasm, the dilatation of the biliary tract is usually conspicuous, particularly in the tract proximal to the obstruction but also at the level of the intrahepatic bile ducts. When obstruction occurs, the intrahepatic bile ducts appear as branching tubular anechoic structures >2–3 mm in diameter, with moderately echogenic walls and increasing diameter towards the hilum and becoming less evident moving towards the periphery. At the hilum the confluent dilated ducts create an overall "spider web" or "caput medusae" image, with the general appearance of the parenchyma being one of "too many tubular images" due to overlapping of both vessels and bile ducts made identifiable by their dilatation. The tortuous and dilated biliary structures can have a diameter >40% larger than the adjacent portal branches [96]. Unlike the venous branches, the bile ducts present an irregular echogenic wall and can display enhanced through-transmission. If there is suspicion of an initial dilatation of the intrahepatic bile ducts, CD can prove useful by demonstrating the nonvascular nature of these ducts and by confirming their course adjacent to the portal branches ("parallel channel" sign) (Fig. 5.137). This is particularly useful in those rare cases where a dilatation of the intrahepatic vessels (due to vascular abnormalities such as arteriovenous malformations in Rendu–Osler syndrome, arterial hypertrophy in cirrhosis, cavernous transformation of the portal branches, etc.) can mimic a dilatation of the intrahepatic bile ducts [97].

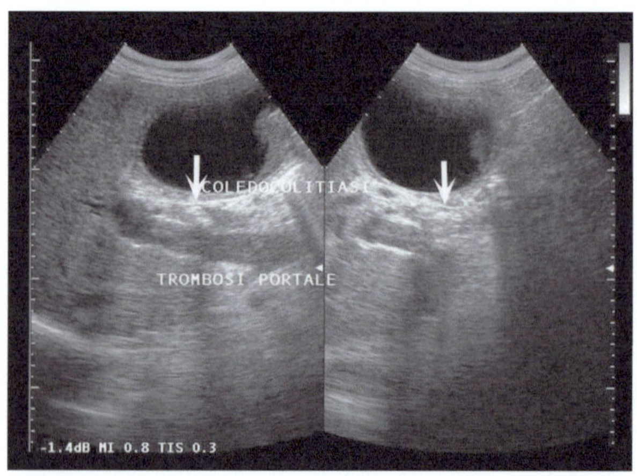

Fig. 5.136 Association of choledocholithiasis and portal thrombosis. Echogenic nuclei in the lumen of the dilated bile duct (*arrows*), associated with mild hypoechogenicity of the portal lumen

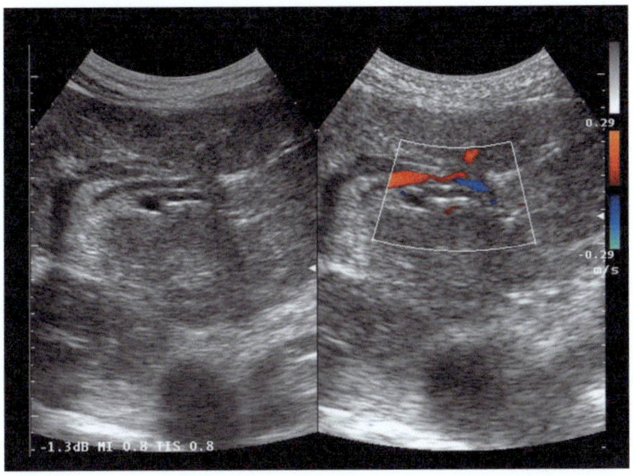

Fig. 5.137 Double duct sign. Two parallel ductal images in the left hepatic lobe, which at CD are shown to correspond to the left portal branch with signs of vascular flow, and the dilated and avascular bile duct

In particular, on the left the "shotgun" sign may be seen, composed of the left portal branch ventrally and the left hepatic duct lying immediately dorsal to this. It should, however, also be borne in mind that the biliary tract can be obstructed without dilatation proximal to the obstruction. This is the case of a recent obstruction (although an event which more commonly concerns choledocholithiasis than neoplasms), cirrhosis, massive hepatic metastasization and some forms of cholangitis (sclerosing and AIDS-related). In these cases the intrahepatic bile ducts are unable to dilate or they do so to a lesser extent than would normally happen in other individuals with a similar obstruction [30]. In cases of hemobilia or pneumobilia, the dilatation of the intrahepatic bile ducts may pass unrecognized because in the former the ducts become isoechoic to the hepatic parenchyma and in the latter they may be concealed by reverberation artifacts. It should also be noted that an obstructive neoplasm can cause the proximal formation of biliary sand and even calculi, with the consequent risk that the identification of the latter findings leads to satisfaction of discovery and consequent misdiagnosis of the underlying neoplasm.

The **common bile duct**, lying ventrally and laterally to the portal vein, normally has an internal diameter no greater than 5 mm, with a slight progressive increase in the distal direction with an increase that is dependent on age (1 mm extra per decade after 50 years). More debatable is the effect of a prior cholecystectomy, but in these patients there is a tendency to consider a bile duct with a diameter of 6–7 mm normal, regardless of the subject's age [30]. Diameters of 6–9 mm are considered thresholds for biliary dilatation in general, whereas a diameter >10 mm is considered pathologic and indicative of an obstruction: in this case the typical "shotgun" sign may be seen, composed of the portal vein lying dorsally and the dilated bile duct with a diameter similar to the vein lying ventrally. Another element of suspicion is given by a diameter of the distal bile duct that is markedly greater than that of the proximal tract. This can be found in the very early phase of obstruction, in patients with the recent removal of the obstruction or in patients with an obstruction present but little possibility of proximal dilatation of the biliary tract (e.g. cirrhosis and occasionally massive metastasization). In these cases, if the diameter is measured too close to the hilum there is the risk of a false negative for biliary dilatation.

It may be useful in patients with a dilatation of the bile duct near the threshold to have them undergo a fatty meal test: after around half an hour a non-obstructed bile duct will decrease in diameter by 2 mm, whereas the lack of a decrease, or even an increase, in the diameter suggests a partial obstruction of the bile duct [98].

The **height** of the obstruction is usually identified by US with ease, on the basis of both indirect signs of the level of the dilatation of the biliary tract and direct identification of the obstruction. The latter can be sought after by performing transverse and longitudinal scans and following the dilated bile duct to the transition point. The use of CD can be useful for distinguishing the bile duct from the regional vessels, especially distally. In addition, distal obstructions of the bile duct may produce an overdistension of the gallbladder (>3 cm in width and >10 cm in length), which instead is absent in the case of obstructions proximal to the confluence of the cystic duct. The demonstration of an enlarged gallbladder in cases of malignant obstructive jaundice compared with no enlargement or scarring due to benign stenosis (Courvoisier sign) is, however, not a reliable criterion.

With regard to the diagnosis of the **cause** of the jaundice, the most common tumors that produce obstructive jaundice can have a distal, suprapancreatic or hilar location. They include extrahepatic cholangiocarcinoma (typically of the hepatic hilum or the common hepatic duct), gallbladder carcinoma invading the bile duct, ampullary carcinoma and carcinoma of the head of the pancreas. In addition, there are also other conditions that can cause obstructive jaundice, such as the extrinsic pressure exerted by subhepatic masses and particularly by lymph node metastases located between the hepatic hilum, the portal vein and the head of the pancreas. Alternatively, primary or secondary intrahepatic tumors may grow, causing compression of the hilum and thus obstruction of the

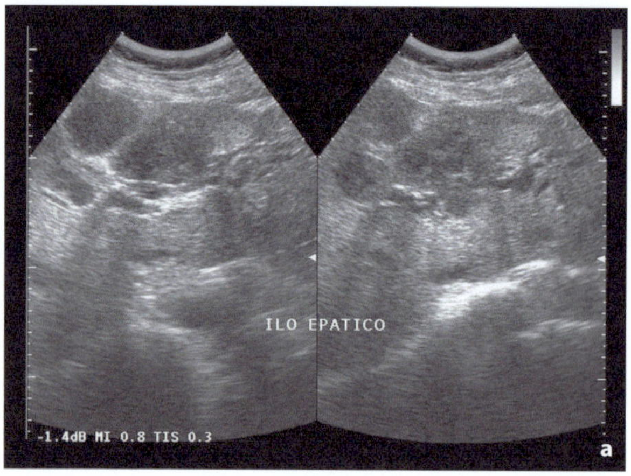

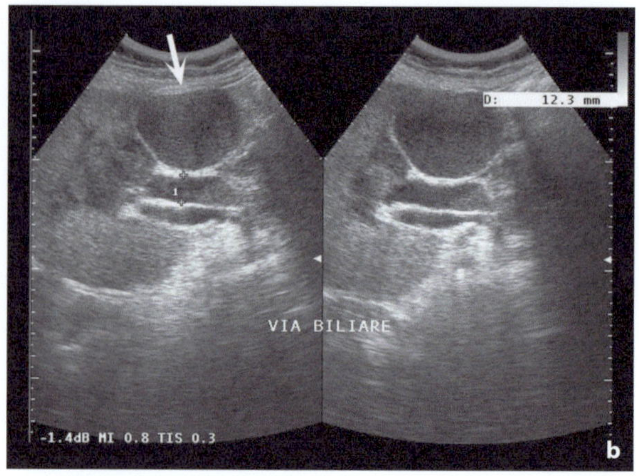

Fig. 5.138a,b Multifactorial presentation of jaundice in patient with metastasis from breast cancer. Multiple hypoechoic liver metastases, especially parahilar, associated with dilatation of the intrahepatic bile ducts (**a**). The common bile duct (*between the calipers*) appears dilated, with the presence of luminal sludge (**b**). An enlarged and also compressing hilar lymph node can also be distinguished (*arrow*)

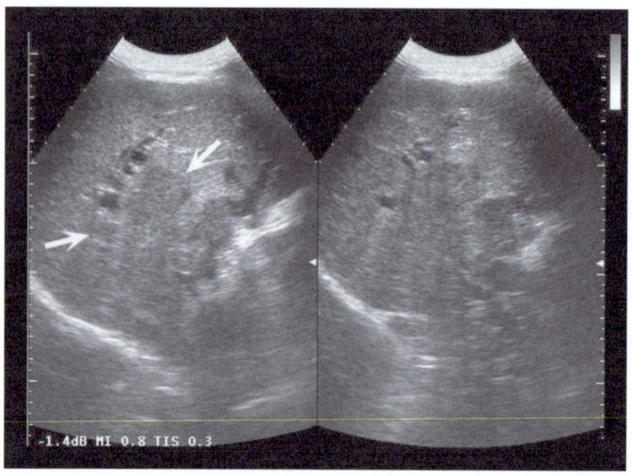

Fig. 5.139 Hepatic lymphoma causing jaundice. Hypoechoic infiltrate of the hepatic hilar region (*arrows*)

biliary tract. In lymphomas there is also the possibility of a paraneoplastic form of jaundice related to obstruction at the level of the bile canaliculi [50]. It should also be noted that in many cancer patients jaundice has a multifactorial nature, since the causes may include the obstructive primary tumor (e.g. carcinoma of the head of the pancreas), metastases from it to the regional lymph nodes, liver metastases (with a dual mechanism of compression on the hilum and functional disruption of the liver itself) and lastly the biliary sludge which accumulates in the bile duct proximal to the neoplastic stenosis (Figs. 5.138–5.142).

Hilar cholangiocarcinoma or Klatskin's tumor accounts for 20% of cholangiocarcinomas and has a five-year survival rate of 35% with tumor resection [39]. It is often difficult to identify directly, not only

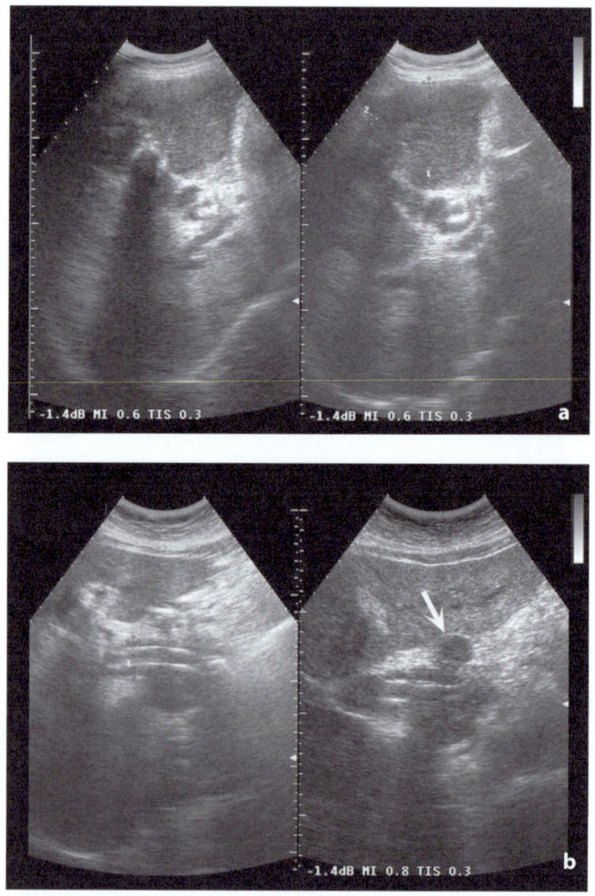

Fig. 5.140a,b Obstructive gallbladder cancer, treatment with biliary stent. Gallbladder mass (*between the calipers*) compressing the hilum (**a**). Presence of metallic stent and hilar lymphadenopathy (**b**, *arrow*)

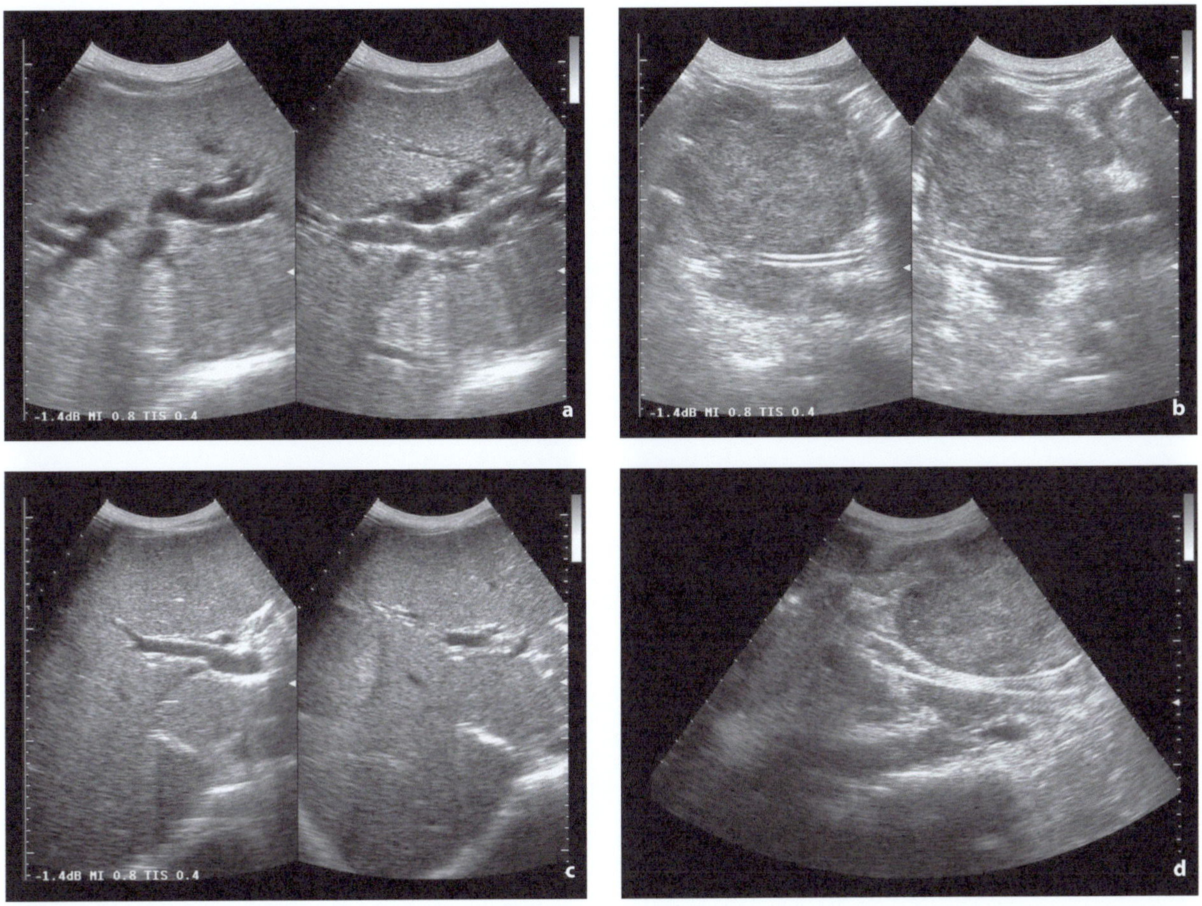

Fig. 5.141a-d Obstructive pancreatic carcinoma, treatment with biliary stent. Evident dilatation of the intrahepatic biliary ducts (**a**) in patient with large mass in the head of the pancreas (**b**) and presence of plastic biliary stent. The dilatation of the biliary ducts appears reduced (**c**) after placement of a metallic stent (**d**)

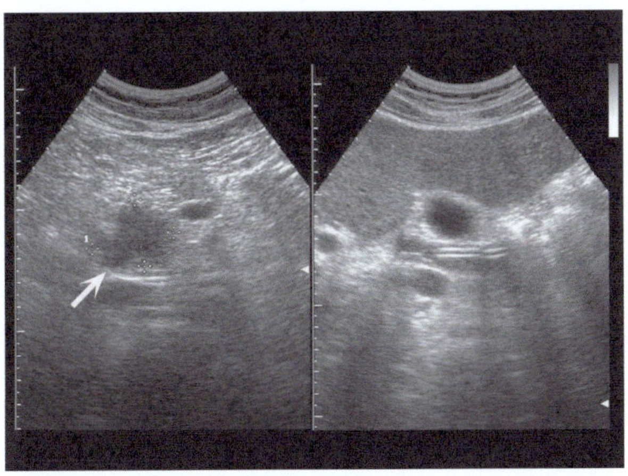

Fig. 5.142 Pancreatic carcinoma with biliary stenting. Hypoechoic lesion in the head of the pancreas (*arrow*), with proximal dilatation of the bile duct with deployed plastic stent

with US but also with CT, due to the limited extraductal component. Nonetheless, identifying the level of the obstruction is relatively easy due to the dilatation of the intrahepatic ducts alone. It may, however, at least be possible to identify an "empty space" between the dilated ducts at the hilum, i.e. an absent communication between the dilated bile ducts of the right lobe and those of the left lobe. In cases where it may be directly identified, extrahepatic cholangiocarcinoma appears as a focal thickening of the bile duct walls or solid nodulations protruding into the lumen of the dilated and suddenly amputated duct. Occasionally, invasion of the gallbladder may be seen, which may give rise to doubt about a primary gallbladder tumor with invasion of the hepatic hilum. The demonstration of invasion of the portal vein or the hepatic artery, as well as hepatic lesions (either by direct or distant

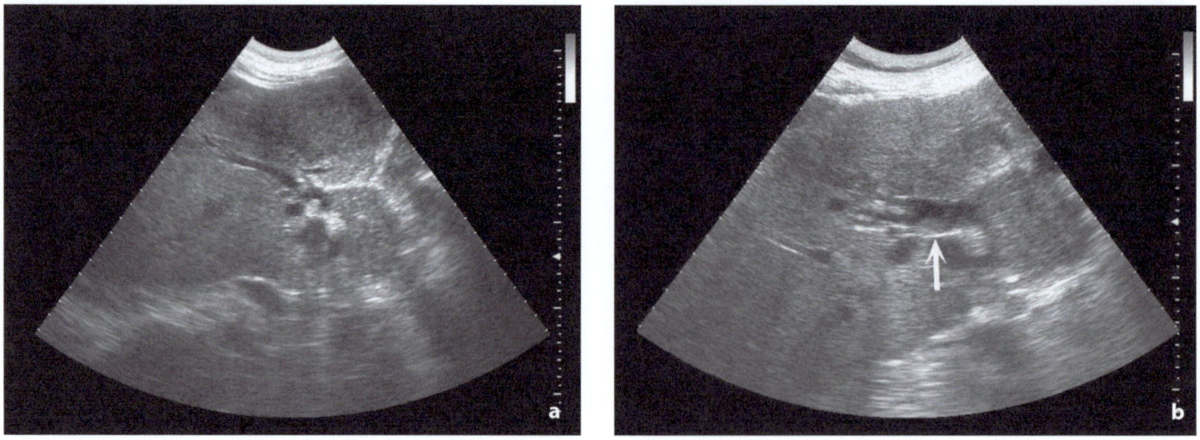

Fig. 5.143a,b Klatskin tumor. Hypoechoic invasion of the hepatic hilar region, associated with dilatation of the intrahepatic bile ducts and signs of intraluminal growth (*arrow*)

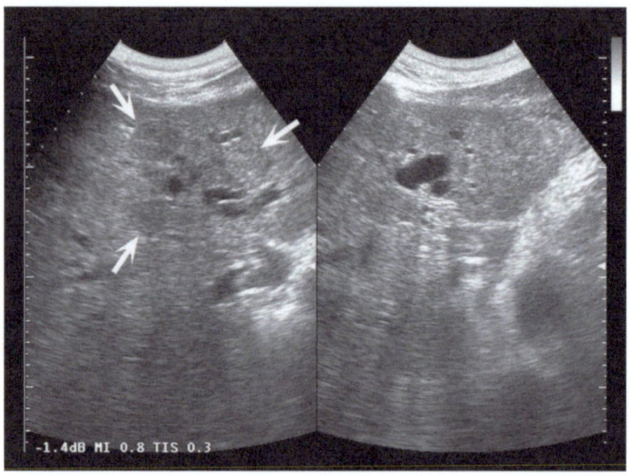

Fig. 5.144 Intrahepatic cholangiocarcinoma. Mildly hypoechoic parahilar nodule (*arrows*) causing dilatation of the left intrahepatic bile ducts

spread) or lymphadenopathies indicates that the mass in nonoperable (Figs. 5.143, 5.144).

In **ampullary carcinomas**, combined dilatation of the intrahepatic and extrahepatic bile ducts can be seen extending all the way to the hepatopancreatic ampulla. Occasionally dilatation of the pancreatic duct and peripancreatic lymphadenopathies may be associated. Ampullary carcinoma is in itself identifiable only when large, appearing as a hypoechoic mass similar to malignancies of the pancreas. Accurate staging of the tumor can be provided by EUS.

5.6 Pancreatic Tumors

Primary tumors of the pancreas can be classified as epithelial (exocrine and endocrine) and nonepithelial (sarcomas and lymphomas). The most common and relevant exocrine tumor is **ductal adenocarcinoma** (75–92% of all pancreatic tumors and 95% of pancreatic carcinomas), with onset in the 6th and 7th decade of life and a M/F ratio of 1.3:1. The lesion develops in the head of the pancreas in 60–70% of cases, in the body in 20% and in the tail in 5–10%. There is also a diffuse form characterized by global enlargement of the gland (5–15%). Risk factors include cystic fibrosis, Peutz–Jeghers syndrome and several rare familial syndromes. At the time of diagnosis, 40% of patients already have lymph node metastases, 35% peritoneal metastases and 50% liver metastases. Only 5–10% of cases are operable with radical criteria [99]. The tumors of the head of the pancreas, unlike those of the body, tail and uncinate process, are associated with jaundice and ductal dilatation (Figs. 5.145, 5.146).

US is often the first imaging modality which identifies a pancreatic tumor, being the option of choice in the study of jaundice and also the most commonly used technique in patients with painful or dyspeptic abdominal symptoms. The sensitivity for the identification of pancreatic carcinoma was in the early patient populations relatively limited, with an unsatisfying detection of neoplasms in 20–25% of cases. With the current US systems the evaluation possibilities have increased, with sensitivity and specificity >90% [100]. Nonetheless a thorough exploration of all the pancreatic segments from different anatomic approaches is still crucial to avoid misdiagnosing particularly deep lesions or lesions concealed by intestinal gas. The factors which influence sensitivity the most are the size (<2 cm vs. >2 cm), the site (head vs. body and above all tail) and the experience of the sonographer [90].

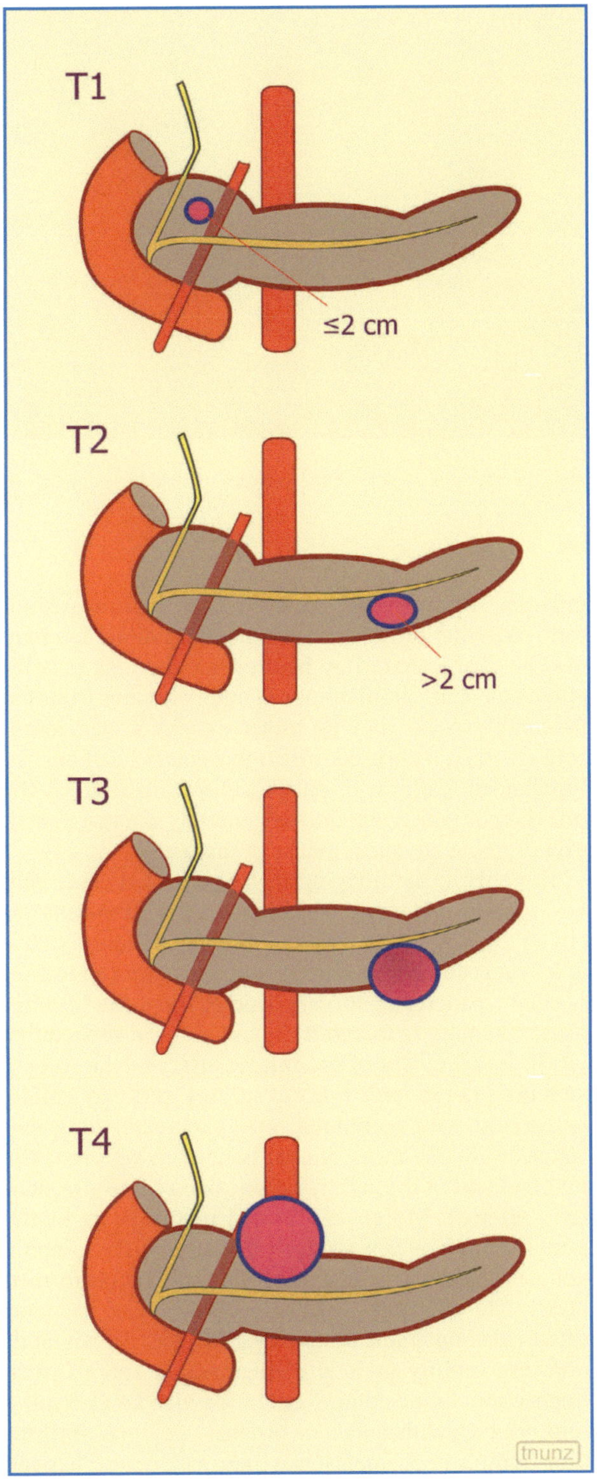

Fig. 5.145 Staging of pancreatic adenocarcinoma. *T1*, tumor limited to the pancreas (head, body or tail) and <2 cm; *T2*, tumor limited to the pancreas and >2 cm; *T3*, tumor of any size with extraglandular extension but without involvement of the celiac trunk or the superior mesentery artery; *T4*, tumor of any size with invasion of the celiac trunk or superior mesenteric artery. Modified from [95]

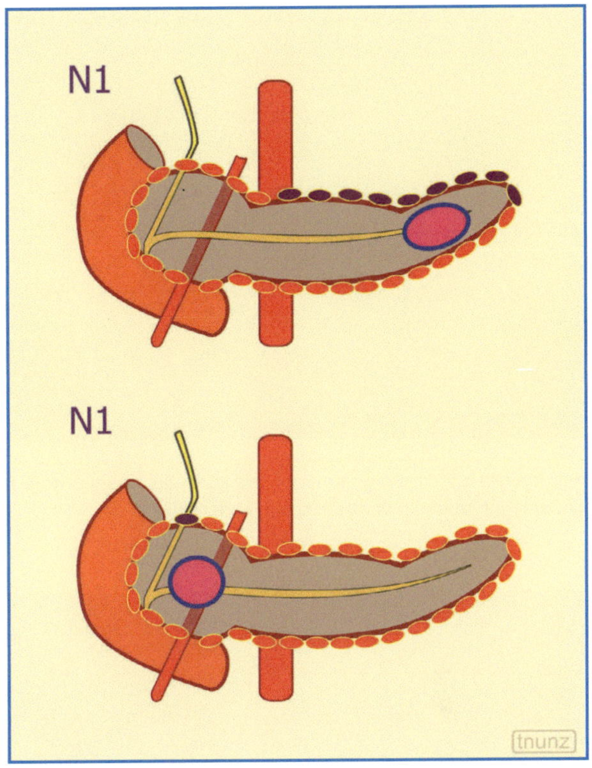

Fig. 5.146 N parameter for pancreatic carcinoma. Regional lymph nodes include the peripancreatic lymph nodes: superior to the head of the pancreas, inferior to the head and the body, anterior pancreaticoduodenal, pyloric (only for tumors of the head), proximal mesenteric, posterior pancreaticoduodenal, common hepatic duct, splenic hilar and pancreatic tail (only for tumors of the body and tail), celiac (only for tumors of the head). *N1* indicates involvement of one or more of the listed lymph node stations. Modified from [95]

In most cases, pancreatic carcinoma presents as an ill-defined hypoechoic lesion which deforms the profile of the gland. The appearance can be heterogeneous, echogenic and occasionally with amorphous calcifications (although calcifications are usually suggestive of a neuroendocrine form) (Figs. 5.147, 5.148). CD does not provide additional useful information for the identification and characterization of the malignancy, although at times it can be useful in differential diagnosis, in particular with regard to focal hypertrophic forms of chronic pancreatitis, which typically appear hypovascular.

The indirect signs of carcinoma include dilatation of the bile ducts, dilation of the pancreatic duct, obstructive pancreatitis with the formation of pseudocysts in the parenchyma distal to the tumor (up to 11% of cases), signs of vascular infiltration, lymph node metastases and liver metastases. A **dilatation of the pancreatic duct** can also be found in cases of carcinoma of the ampulla, the distal bile duct and the

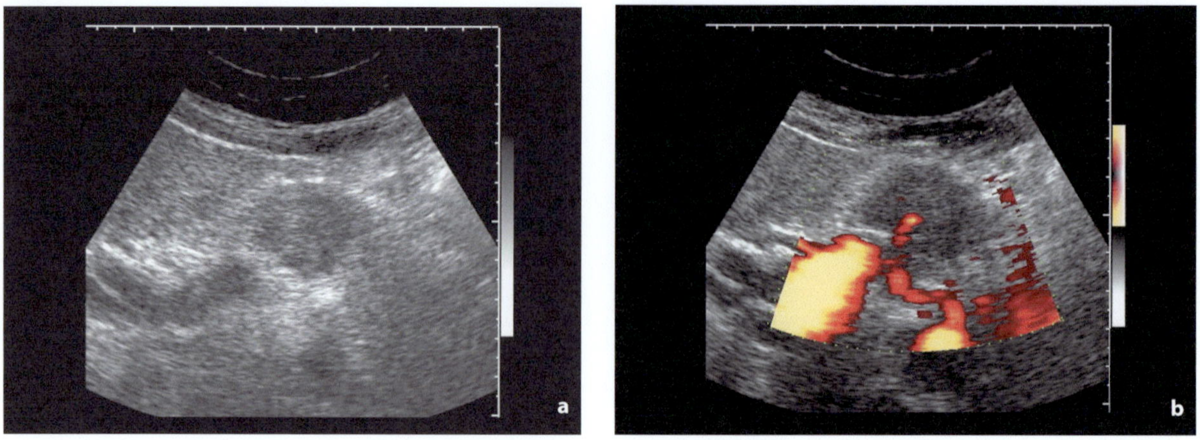

Fig. 5.147a,b Adenocarcinoma of the pancreas. Hypoechoic lesion of the isthmus region of the pancreas (**a**), which appears to encircle the initial tract of the splenic artery at PD (**b**)

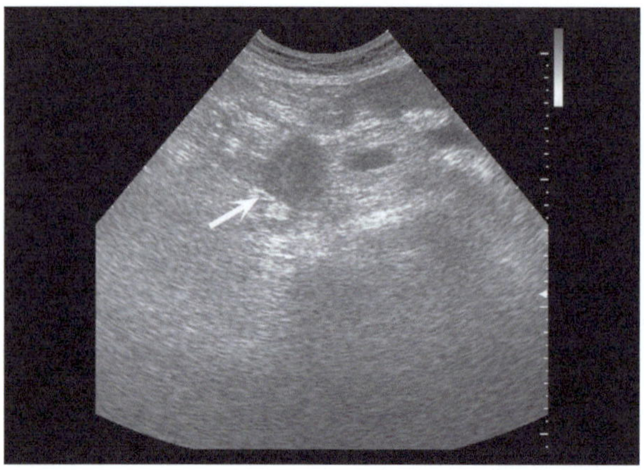

Fig. 5.148 Adenocarcinoma of the pancreas. Solid hypoechoic lesion of the head of the pancreas (*arrow*)

pancreas, as well as distal choledocholithiasis and chronic pancreatitis. The neoplastic nature of the lesion may be suspected when the dilatation is marked (>50% of the anteroposterior pancreatic diameter), sharp and regular, whereas inflammation should be considered when the dilatation is irregular and associated with intraluminal calculi. A tumor of the head of the pancreas is typically associated with combined dilation of the bile duct and pancreatic duct (**double duct sign**) with the two ducts appearing not only increased in diameter but also abnormally distant from each other. This finding is highly suspicious for carcinoma of the head of the pancreas or ampullary carcinoma, even when the latter cannot be directly visualized. However, alternative causes for combined ductal dilatation should be considered, such as cholangiocarcinoma with intrapancreatic development, lithiasis of the distal bile duct and chronic pancreatitis. Signs of **chronic inflammation due to obstruction** are not rare, such that the appearance of ductal dilatation may also be characterized by heterogeneity of the pancreatic tissue and calcifications. Tumors arising from the uncinate process may be rather exophytic and therefore readily confused with mesenteric lesions or lymphadenopathies, in part because dilatation of the bile duct or pancreatic duct is generally not associated, except in the advanced phase of disease.

In general, the imaging techniques, and especially US, tend to understage the local spread of the tumor. Given the low survival rate of resected patients (<10% at 5 years) and the morbidity and mortality (up to 5%) of major pancreatic surgery, one of the tasks of diagnostic imaging is to avoid useless surgical procedures [100]. Involvement of the splenic artery or the splenic vein does not in itself rule out surgery as it may still be performed with combined total pancreatectomy and splenectomy. What is crucial is demonstration of the involvement of the celiac, hepatic and superior mesenteric arteries. Moreover, limited involvement of the portal vein does not totally rule out surgery, since a venous resection with graft could still be performed [100]. The possible large size of the mass (>2 cm) often rules out radical surgery. The specific signs of non-resectability include extraglandular spread (with hypoechoic tissue coming out of the gland and coming into contact with adjacent organs), vascular infiltration, lymph node metastases (peripancreatic, hepatic hilar and lumbar) and hematogenous metastases. These are elements that are generally better identified with CT, but they should be sought with US since the demonstration of an inoperable pancreatic tumor and with liver metastases can render further diagnostic work-up unnecessary. In addition, precisely defining the baseline characteristics of the extension of disease is crucial in patients undergoing neoadjuvant treatment, in order to be able to monitor and identify operable cases (although the final judgment in these cases, is the domain of CT/MR). In advanced cases, peritoneal effusion and signs of carcinosis may also be seen. US and CD are able to identify the more evident cases of **vascular involvement**, with an accuracy greater than angiography, especially for the arteries, but nonetheless lower than CT, MR and EUS (Fig. 5.149). EUS is particularly useful in evaluation of the resectability of small tumors, being comparable with spiral CT in the diagnosis of involvement of the portal vein and mesenteric vein, but less reliable for the identification of invasion of the mesenteric artery [101]. The visualization of glandular tissue between the tumor and the vessel and evident integrity of the echogenic vessel wall are indicative of it being undamaged, although these findings are not always easy to demonstrate when the tumor is adjacent to the vessel. Vascular involvement is identifiable as significant contiguity between lesion and vessel (>2cm along the longitudinal axis of the vessel), significant perivascular spread of the neoplastic tissue (especially if >25% and even more so if >50% of the vessel circumference – encasement), vascular deformation with stenosis and turbulence of flow (aliasing artifact) and frank invasion of the vessel wall (which becomes irregular or no longer identifiable, with luminal thrombosis of peripancreatic arteries or veins which display structured internal echoes and color signal defects) [100]. Involvement of the mesenteric-portal axis occurs in 65% of tumors of the head of the pancreas and is classified in several grades: grade 1, vascular compression or absence of adipose cleavage plane with regular flow (10–20 cm/s); grade 2, irregularity and rigidity of the vessel wall at one point, with moderately accelerated flow; grade 3, concentric irregularity of the vessel wall with turbulent flow, grade 4, neoplastic thrombosis with completely absent flow, or partially conserved but turbulent. Pancreatic resection is possible only in grades 1–2 and in grade 3 where vascular infiltration is <35 mm lengthwise [102]. In general, CD has a sensitivity of 72% and a specificity of 45% in the diagnosis of venous involvement, which rises to 83% and 100%, respectively, with the use of contrast medium. Without distinguishing between arteries and veins, CD without contrast medium has demonstrated an overall sensitivity of 79% and a specificity of 89%. Here the risk is undoubtedly of false negatives, whereas false positives for vascular involvement are rare [100] (Figs. 5.150–5.152).

In the setting of the differential diagnosis, a not uncommon event is **chronic pancreatitis** and in particular the hypertrophic, massive variants (inflammatory pseudotumors). A focal pancreatic mass occurs

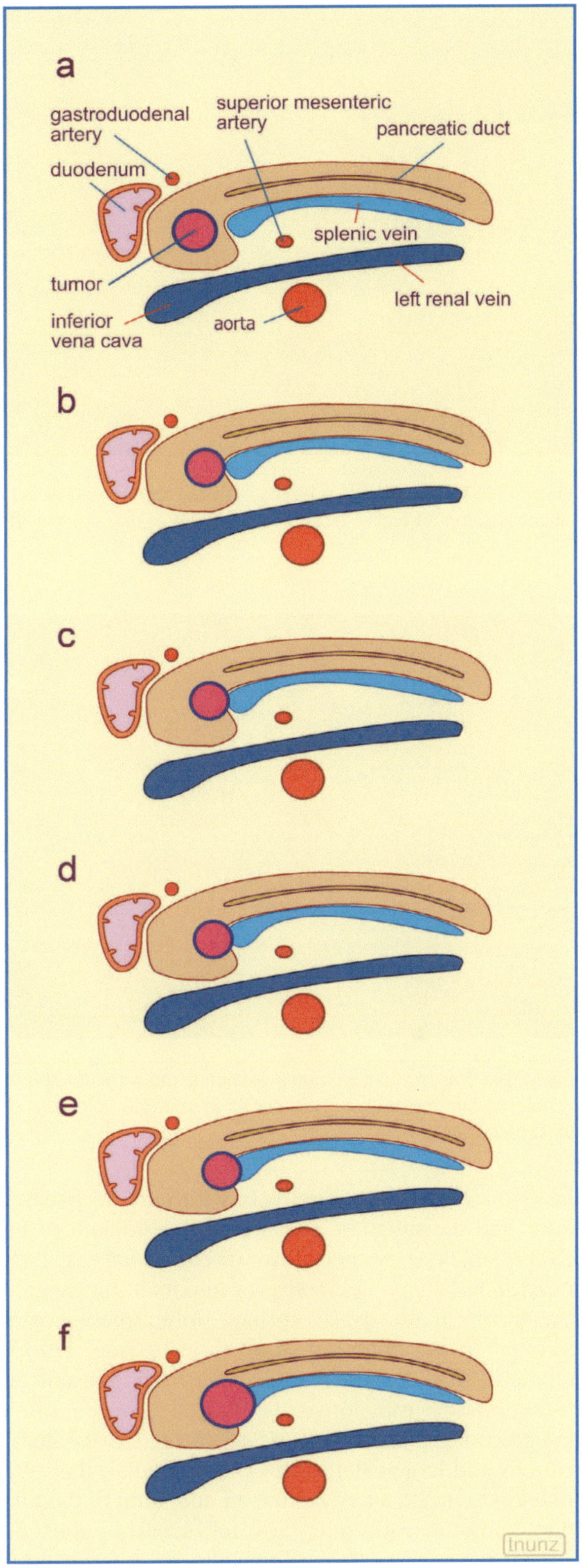

Fig. 5.149a-f Involvement of the portal system in pancreatic carcinoma. Normal anatomic finding (**a**) and varying degrees of venous involvement (**b-f**)

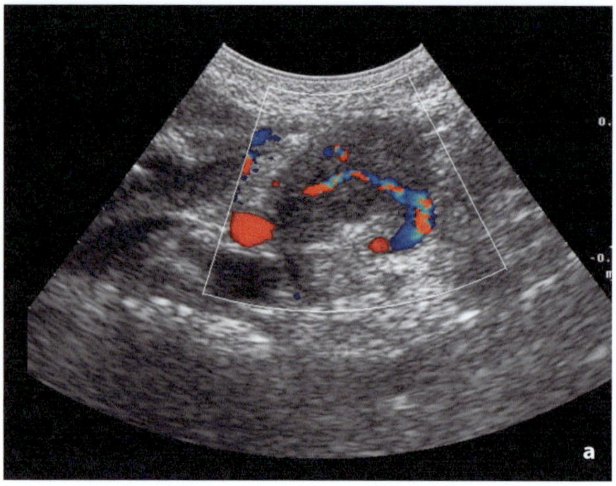

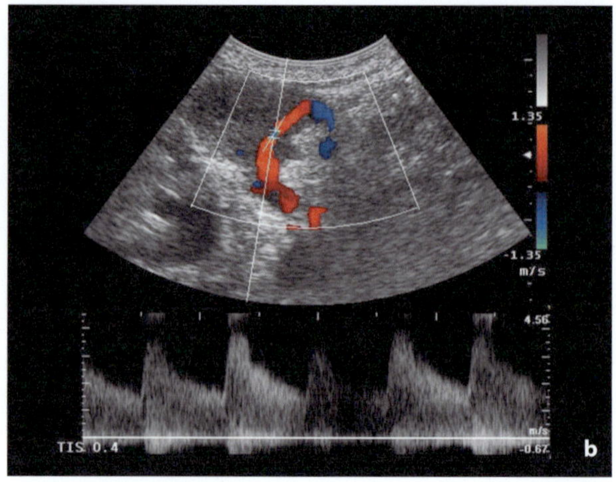

Fig. 5.150a,b Pancreatic carcinoma invading the vessels. Solid mass of the body of the pancreas seen encircling the splenic artery, site of aliasing artifacts (**a**). Spectral Doppler of the stenotic artery (**b**) identifies very high systolic peak velocities (>400 cm/s)

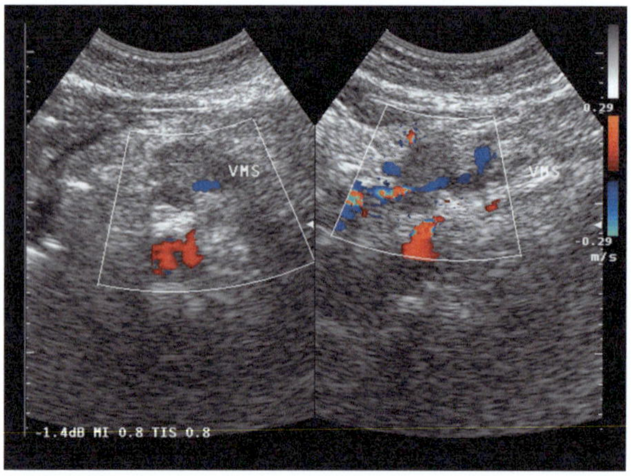

Fig. 5.151 Pancreatic carcinoma invading the vessels. Hypoechoic nodule encircling the superior mesenteric vein, site of aliasing artifacts

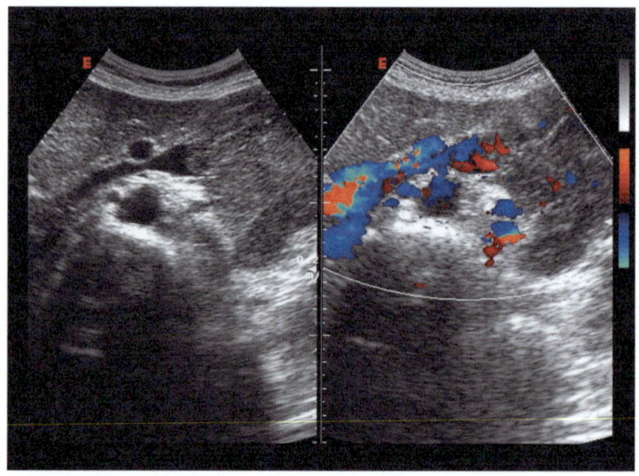

Fig. 5.152 Pancreatic carcinoma infiltrating the vessels. Heterogeneous hypoechoic tissue in the lumen of the splenic vein

in as many as 30% of patients with chronic pancreatitis and the situation is made more complicated by the possible coexistence of two diseases, since it is not rare for ampullary carcinomas or tumors of the head of the pancreas to cause chronic inflammation and atrophy of the body-tail due to obstruction. Useful elements for the differential diagnosis present in inflammatory pseudomasses include a more often hyperechoic appearance, a greater incidence of calcifications and large calcifications in particular, the relative lower incidence of combined dilatation of the bile duct and pancreatic duct. Several recently published studies have used CD and some also with intravenous contrast medium to evaluate the vascularity of the mass. They found a greater number of vessels and earlier enhancement in the presence of a tumor and a hypo-isovascularity in chronic pancreatitis. Moreover, in carcinoma, the vessels are often tortuous and penetrating, whereas in focal pancreatitis they are few and peripheral [103]. At EUS, instead, carcinoma has a hypovascular appearance and is characterized by the absence of internal vessels, which in contrast are present in inflammatory pseudotumors. In addition, evidence of collateral flow and signs of vascular infiltration can be elements that are indicative of malignancy, since these alterations are not seen in pancreatitis [104]. With regard to CEUS, preliminary studies have shown a hypovascularity in inflammatory pseudotumors and the absence of isoperfusion in tumors. The greater vascularity of pseudotumors with respect to carcinomas is explained by the presence in the former of inflammatory changes such as

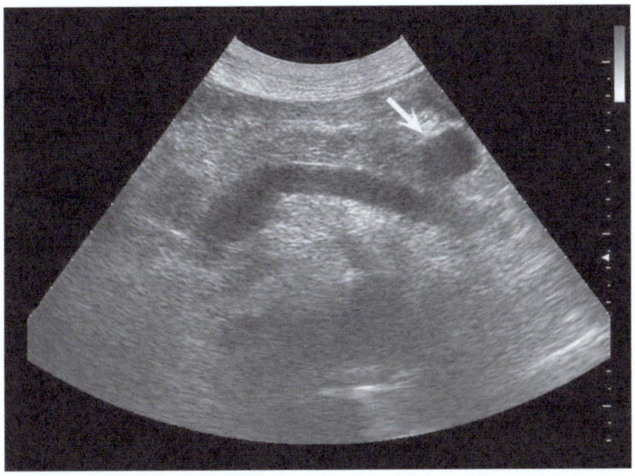

Fig. 5.153 Pancreatic cyst. Homogeneous anechoic mass on the anterior margin of the tail-body transition of the pancreas (*arrow*)

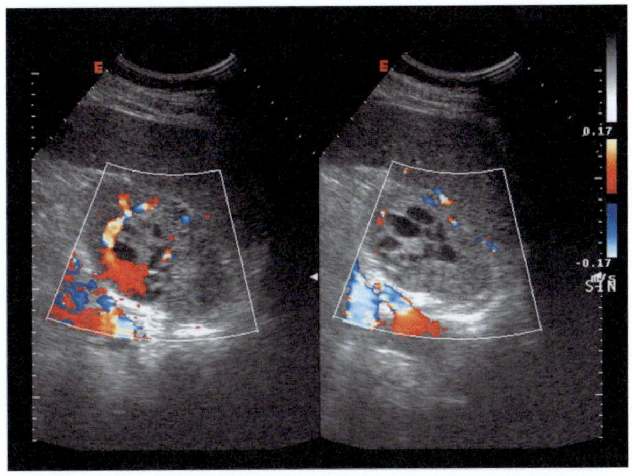

Fig. 5.154 Microcystic tumor of the pancreas. Echogenic mass with several internal macrocystic anechoic areas can be seen in the tail of the pancreas

interlobular fibrosis and the perilobular and sufficient periductal inflammatory infiltrate to require blood flow [105]. These are, however, relative elements which often require work-up with techniques such as CT, EUS or MRCP. US-guided biopsy has also been used in select cases, although with some less than satisfying results and not greater accuracy than 50%. There is also the need for microhistologic sampling, although FNAC has often proven unable to rule out malignancy in all cases [106,107]. However, the marked consistency of inflammatory pseudomasses often hinders adequate sampling. Better results have been obtained with EUS biopsy, although there is little agreement in the literature. Even a collapsed duodenum can mimic a mass at the level of the right or dorsal surface of the head of the pancreas.

With the increasing use of imaging modalities the finding of masses with a cystic appearance and generally limited in size at the level of the pancreas has become a less than rare event. **Cystic tumors** of the pancreas account for a minority of pancreatic malignancies (1–15%) and also a minority (<15%) of cystic masses arising from the pancreas, since around 80% of these masses are pseudocysts. The first risk therefore is to misdiagnose these tumors as pseudocysts [108] (Fig. 5.153). The detailed morphostructural appearance of these cystic masses is well visualized with CT and MR (especially MRCP with possible secretin stimulation), especially if CEUS is not used, which has proven to be very effective in showing enhancement of septations and intracystic solid components of cysts that are adequately accessible to the study [109]. The lesions have a variable malignant potential. In some cases the physical examination and patient history combined with the imaging findings are sufficiently characteristic if not pathognomonic to reach a definitive diagnosis, whereas in others a working diagnosis can be made which nonetheless requires histologic evaluation. In general, however, follow-up is preferable, with resection of those lesions which show signs of growth or changes in their internal structure [108].

From a practical point of view, these tumors can be subdivided into focal lesions (small in size, e.g. intraductal mucinous-papillary tumor of the collateral ducts, and large in size, e.g. microcystic serous cystadenoma, micro-macrocystic serous cystadenoma and mucinous cystadenoma) and diffuse lesions, such as the intraductal mucinous-papillary tumor of the main pancreatic duct and serous cystadenoma (microcystic or macrocystic, generally in the context of von Hippel–Lindau syndrome).

Serous cystadenoma (1–2% of pancreatic tumors) is prevalent in females >60 years of age, predominantly found in the head of the pancreas (70% of cases) and generally treated conservatively. The extension is variable, up to involving the entire gland. It is characterized by a honeycomb appearance, with numerous thin and vascular septations, possibly converging towards a sort of central fibrous or fibrocalcified scar which is found in around half of cases. The cystic loculations may be very small (<2 cm) in the microcystic variant, or mixed with both small and large occurrences. Very small and dense cysts, however, may paradoxically create echogenic areas. Aspiration reveals a high glycogenic content [90,110] (Figs. 5.154–5.156).

Mucinous cystadenoma (3% of pancreatic tumors) is usually treated surgically due to its malignant potential. It is prevalent among females (F/M ratio 10:1) in the 5th–6th decade of life, with the most common site being the body-tail (80–95% of cases) [108]. The appearance is usually nonspecific, uni- or multilocular,

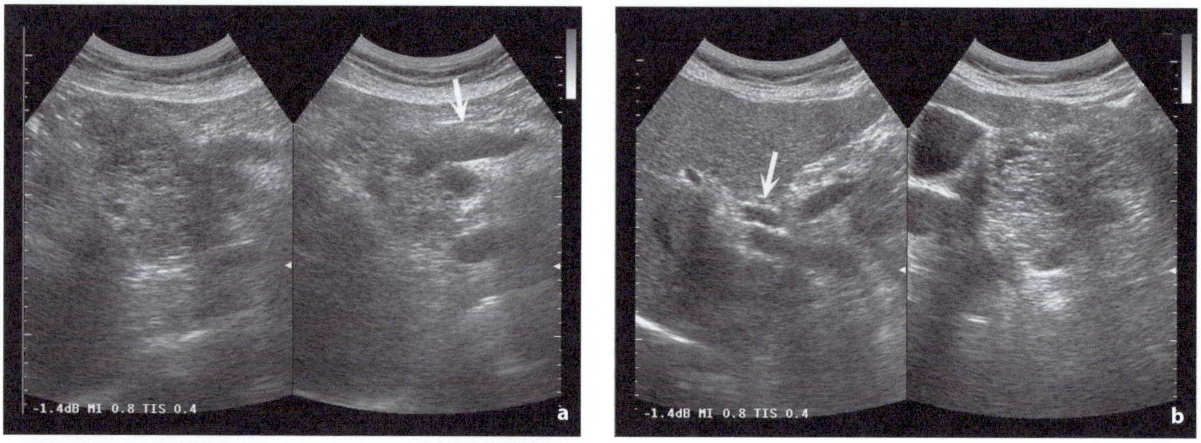

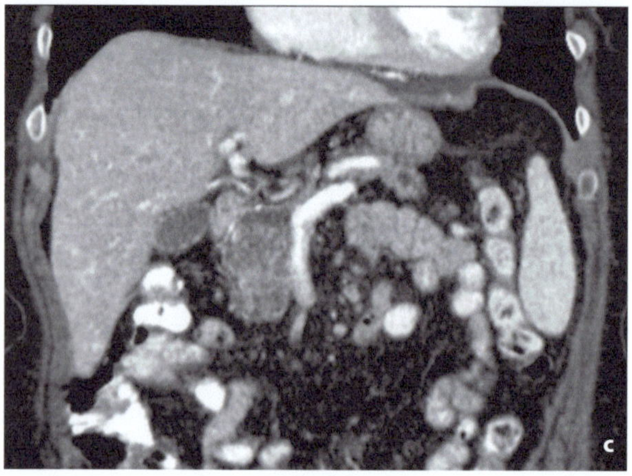

Fig. 5.155a-c Serous cystadenocarcinoma of the pancreas. The head of the pancreas is occupied by a large heterogeneous mass with several internal hypo-anechoic areas, which causes a dilatation of the pancreatic duct (**a**, *arrow*) but not the bile duct (**b**, *arrow*). Coronal CT reconstruction confirms the mass in the head of the pancreas (**c**) adjacent to the superior mesenteric vein

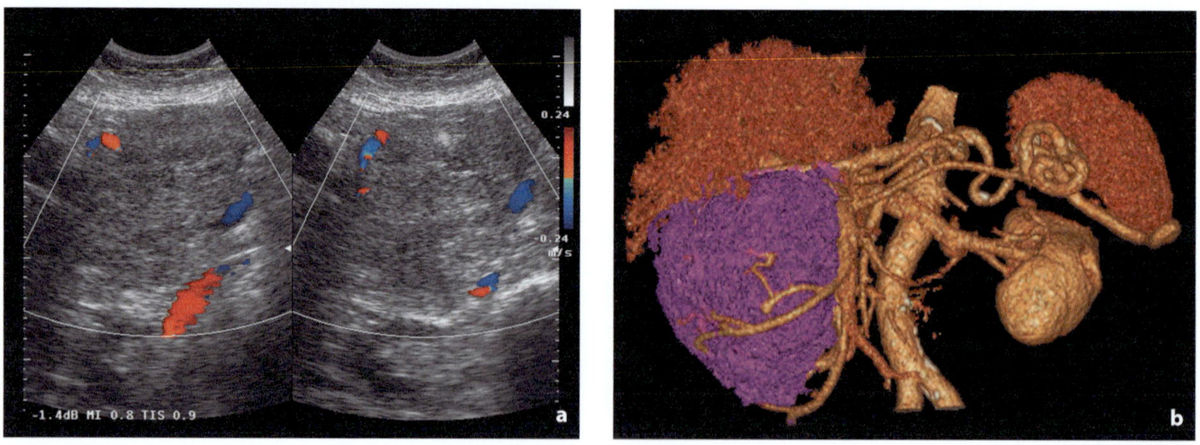

Fig. 5.156a,b Microcystic cystadenoma of the head of the pancreas. Finely septated, ill-defined, heterogeneous hyperechoic mass displacing without invading the adjacent vessels but which appears markedly hypovascular at CD (**a**). 3D CT reconstruction (**b**) shows the mass and its relations with the surrounding vascular structures

with loculations varying in size (usually each >20 mm and a maximum of five), with generally thick walls, few septations varying in thickness and possible mural calcifications and nodulations (20% of cases) [30,110]. In doubtful cases, imaging-guided aspiration may be performed. In addition to a high percentage of mucin, the malignant forms present elevated levels of the tumor markers CEA and CA-129, whereas the finding of elevated amylase levels indicates a pseudocyst (Figs. 5.157, 5.158).

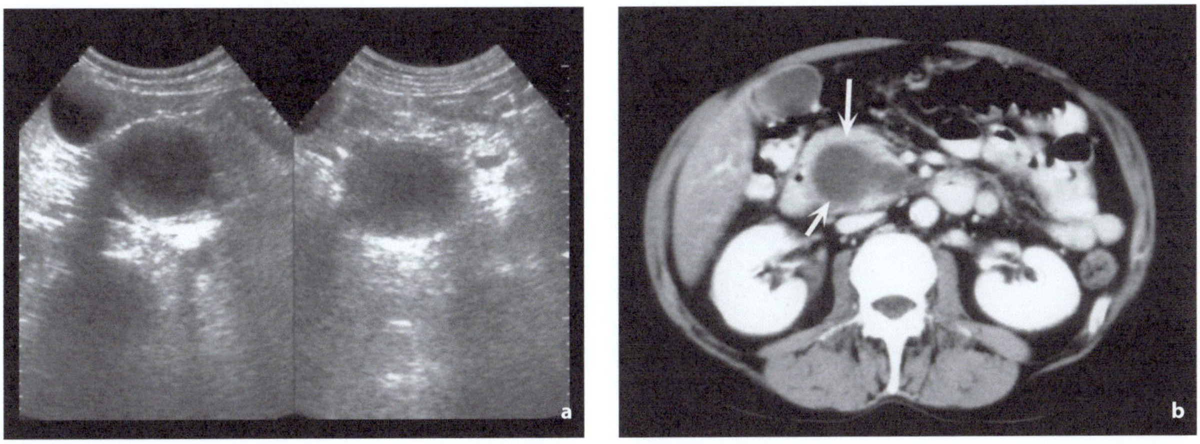

Fig. 5.157a,b Mucinous cystadenoma of the pancreas. Homogeneous anechoic mass is seen widening the head of the pancreas (**a**). CT correlation (**b**, *arrows*)

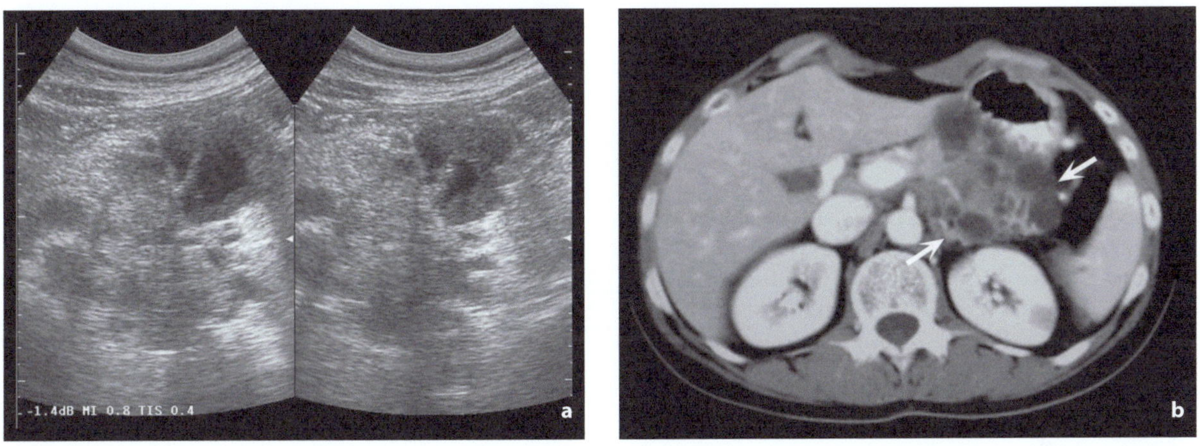

Fig. 5.158a,b Mucinous cystadenocarcinoma of the pancreas. Ill-defined complex structured tumor with heterogeneous solid areas and cystic components (**a**). CT correlation shows the cystic transformation of the body-tail of the pancreas (**b**, *arrows*)

Mucinous intraductal tumors are usually found incidentally in middle-aged to elderly subjects and may be benign or malignant. They present as septated cystic masses with varying appearance, with a size depending on whether it arises from the main pancreatic duct or the collateral ducts (the latter form is prevalent in the uncinate process). In the former case, with segmental or diffuse dilatation of the pancreatic duct, the appearance can be similar to that of chronic obstructive pancreatitis, although without the characteristic intraductal calculosis [90,111,112]. The walls of the loculations may show solid components. MSCT and MRCP are able to show the communication with the excretory system and therefore suggest the diagnosis, something which is rather unlikely with US.

Neuroendocrine tumors of the pancreas – or more precisely of the pancreatic area, since many of them arise from the duodenum or other structures adjacent to the pancreas – derive from the neural crest and can be functioning (insulinoma, gastrinoma, glucagonoma, VIPoma, somatostatinoma, carcinoid, etc.) or nonfunctioning [113]. Functioning tumors tend to become manifest due to the effects of hormone hypersecretion, whereas nonfunctioning tumors tend to be incidental findings. The malignancy potential is variable, being lower in insulinomas, which are often small and located principally in the body-tail, and higher in other forms, especially (90%) in nonfunctioning tumors, which are often large and located mainly in the head of the pancreas.

At the time of diagnosis, insulinomas have a mean diameter <20 mm, gastrinomas around 35 mm and nonfunctioning tumors >5 cm. These lesions tend to form a bulge in the profile of the pancreas, which is usually their only characteristic sign. The larger forms can have a variable appearance, with necrotic

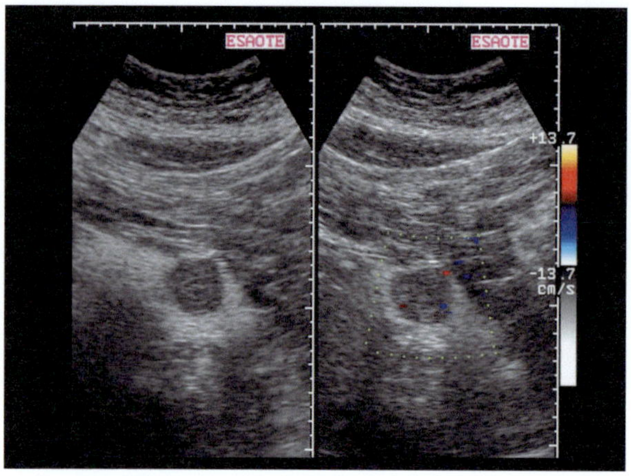

Fig. 5.159 Insulinoma of the pancreas. Heterogeneous hypoechoic nodule between the body and the tail of the pancreas. CD (*right*) shows some intranodular arterial flows

hypoechoic components and possible calcifications. Small tumors appear rounded or oval, homogeneous, hyperechoic or more often hypoechoic, with sharp, well-defined margins and occasional small calcifications [90,113]. CD performed with a transabdominal or endoscopic approach and CEUS can reveal the arterial hypervascularity of the lesions [114,115]. EUS may be useful as an alternative technique to CT or MR in the search for insulinomas [116]. Octreotide scintigraphy is especially useful for distinguishing these tumors from pancreatic carcinoma, which has a different prognosis and treatment plan. IOUS is feasible when the identification of a small insulinoma is not possible preoperatively [117]. Liver metastases from endocrine tumors may appear hypoechoic or hyperechoic with hypo-anechoic necrotic areas. Hyperechogenicity may be a distinctive element of the metastases from endocrine tumors with respect to metastases from pancreatic carcinoma (Figs. 5.159, 5.160).

The pancreas is rarely involved in **lymphomas**, and then usually with NHL forms. US is able to identify a hypoechoic mass with no enhanced through-transmission or diffuse, pancreatitis-like infiltration [118].

Pancreatic **metastases** are rare and in most cases they originate from melanoma, breast carcinoma, ovarian carcinoma, renal cell carcinoma or small-cell pulmonary carcinoma, often as the result of an advanced phase of neoplastic spread. One or more relatively well-defined hypoechoic nodular lesions may be seen, with varying vascularity. Unlike primary tumors, vascular infiltration is rare, whereas ductal involvement is possible and can cause jaundice or pancreatitis [90,119] (Fig. 5.161).

In summary, **anechoic lesions** of the pancreas may be due above all to cysts, pseudocysts, necrosis,

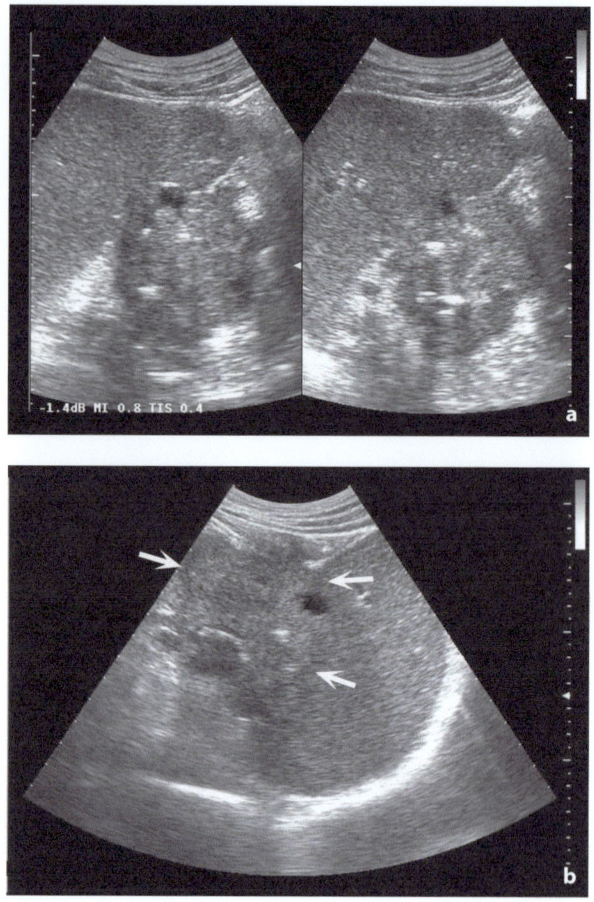

Fig. 5.160a,b Malignant non-functioning neuroendocrine tumor of the tail of the pancreas. Heterogeneous hypoechoic mass with amorphous calcifications (**a**) invading the splenic hilum (**b**, *arrows*)

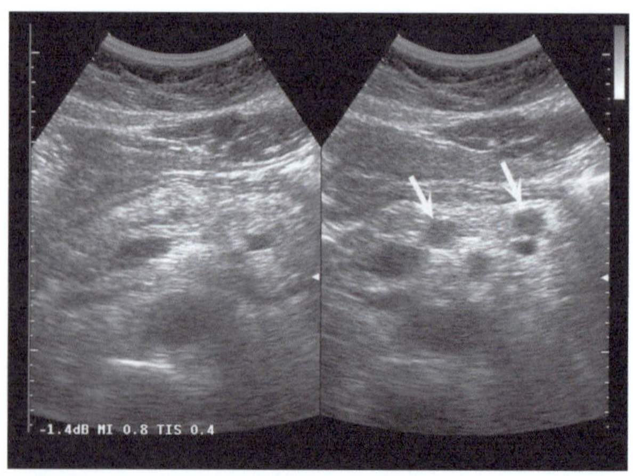

Fig. 5.161 Pancreatic metastasis from melanoma. Small hypoechoic nodules in the hyperechoic pancreas (*arrows*)

dilated or transverse sections of vascular structures, **hypoechoic lesions** due to carcinomas, ampullary carcinomas, neuroendocrine tumors, lymphomas, metastases, abscesses, cyst and complicated pseudocysts, focal pancreatitis, duodenal diverticula, **isoechoic lesions** due to carcinomas, lymphomas, focal pancreatitis, annular pancreas and pancreas divisum, and **hyperechoic lesions** due to hemangiomas, lipomas, calculi and calcifications [59].

5.7 Focal Splenic Lesions

The spleen is the largest lymphatic organ of the body. It rarely is the cause of symptoms, although there may be a palpable mass, pain/soreness in the left upper quadrant, the left flank or at the level of the left shoulder, nausea, vomit, fever, acute anemia (hemorrhage), chronic anemia and thrombocytopenia (disseminated intravascular coagulation). The US study is generally performed in the setting of the general characterization of systemic diseases or of other organs, or in the suspicion of complications of these diseases. In many cases the demonstration of a disease to the spleen is completely incidental (<1% of US abdominal studies). However, the spleen should be evaluated in all patients with chronic liver disease or lymphoma. Selective indication instead may be chronic cryptogenic fever, hematologic or infectious splenomegaly (particularly in the suspicion of complications), splenomegaly of doubtful origin, left upper quadrant and left flank pain (together with study of the other structures such as the kidney).

US is the first-choice technique in the study of the spleen. The exploration should be part of the study of any patient with a suspected disease of the upper abdomen. Often a diagnosis cannot be reached on the basis of the US findings alone and the addition of other imaging modalities is required, especially CT. It is not unusual for US- or CT-guided biopsy to be required. CD is useful for demonstrating perisplenic varices and dilatation of the splenic vein in portal hypertension, for demonstrating patency of the splenic vein or for analyzing blood flow in parenchymal lesions.

Focal splenic lesions are many and varied, with 57% being benign, 36% lymphomatous and 7% metastatic. The majority of focal lesions consist of cysts, pseudocysts (including pancreatic pseudocysts with intrasplenic development), intrasplenic collections (abscesses, hematomas, etc.), inflammatory pseudotumors, lymphangiomas, hamartomas, teratomas, hemangiomas, metastases, sarcomas and lymphomas [120,121].

Splenic **cysts** may be true cysts (25%), and therefore covered by epithelium, which in turn may be congenital (epithelial), parasitic (echinococcosis) or nonparasitic (cystic teratomas, cystic lymphangiomas, cavernous hemangiomas, etc.). False cysts (75%) are instead pseudocysts due to the organization of hematomas, infarctions or abscesses, and so are not covered by epithelium (Fig. 5.162). Identifying these formations is simple: they appear as one or more intraparenchymal cystic masses with homogeneous anechoic appearance and enhanced through-transmission. These well-defined and possibly lobulated or septated structures are in many cases located at the periphery of the organ, possibly with a patently elongated subcapsular appearance.

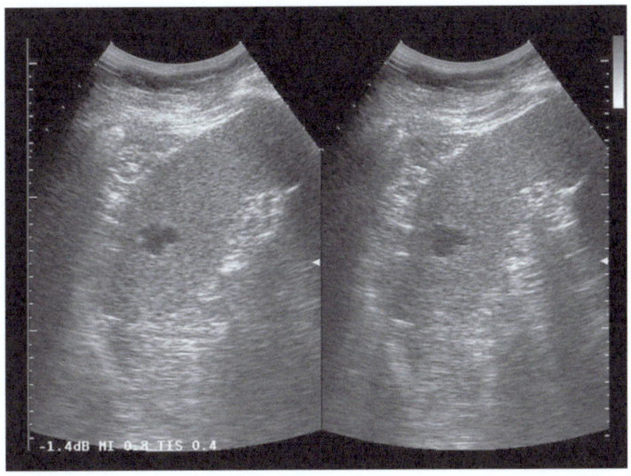

Fig. 5.162 Splenic cyst. Lobulated hypo-anechoic mass in the parenchyma of the spleen

Epidermoid cysts may have a thick wall with irregular internal echoes.

Lymphangiomas, which are predominantly found in pediatric patients, may be solitary but tend to be characterized above all by a honeycomb appearance of the spleen, with multiple cystic areas with heterogeneous size and thin walls. Splenomegaly and the presence of lymphangiomas in other sites may be associated [122] (Figs. 5.163, 5.164).

In **Echinococcus cysts** there may be a mixed solid component, or daughter cysts may be identified internally. The membrane may become detached, with a scalloped appearance while the wall may undergo calcification. In special cases it may be necessary to differentiate between splenic cysts of varying nature and solid focal lesions with a cystic-like appearance such as those seen in lymphoma, abscesses or in some cases of metastasis. In addition, cysts show no vascular signals at CD nor are signs of enhancement seen at CEUS [123] (Fig. 5.165).

Hyperechoic focal lesions of the spleen, with generally well-defined margins and homogeneous

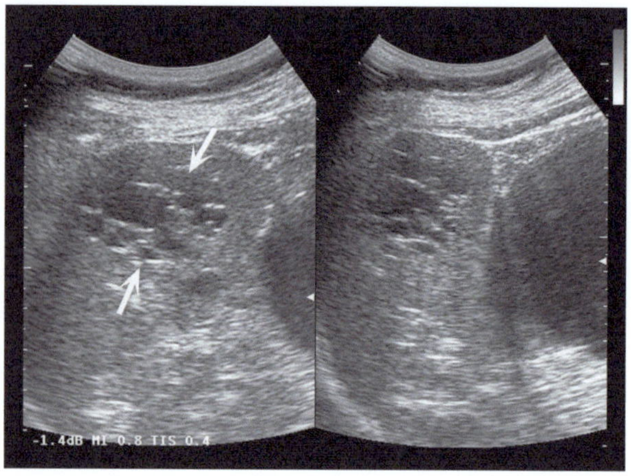

Fig. 5.163 Splenic cystic lymphangioma. Multilocular anechoic mass of the spleen (*arrows*)

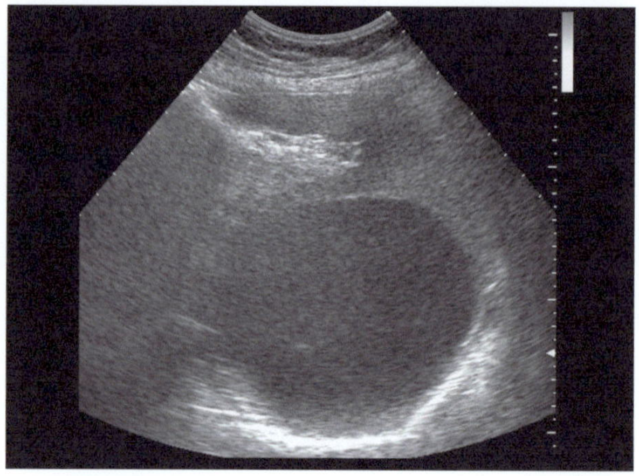

Fig. 5.164 Splenic cystic lymphangioma. Large unilocular and relatively homogeneous cystic mass

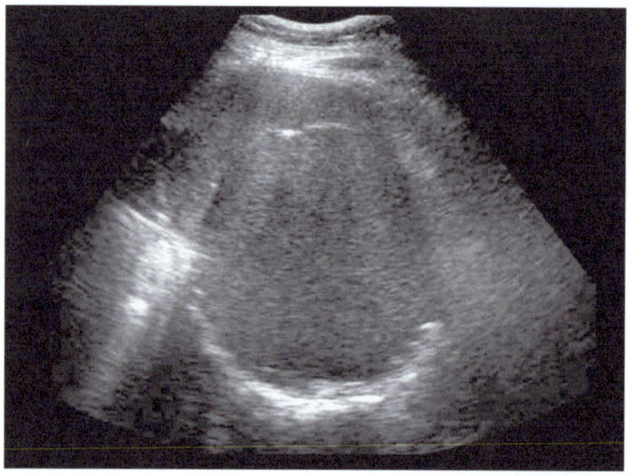

Fig. 5.165 Splenic echinococcosis. Large hypoechoic cystic mass with calcified walls

echotexture and possible posterior acoustic shadowing, include hemangioma, hamartoma (splenoma), abscesses (only rarely, in the case of gas content or resolution), siderotic nodules (Gamma-Gandy bodies, generally secondary to portal hypertension), parenchymal scarring, sarcoidosis, histoplasmosis, (miliary) tuberculosis, thesaurismosis, infarction (chronic phase), extramedullary hematopoiesis, metastasis (rarely), Kaposi sarcoma and calcified lesions. In particular, punctate echogenic foci may be due to sarcoidosis, histoplasmosis, tuberculosis or disseminated infection from *P. carinii* (AIDS) [59,124,125].

Hemangioma is the most common solid focal splenic lesion, being found at postmortem in 14% of individuals. The lesions are often small (<2 cm) and frequently multiple, up to the point of hemangiomatosis. The appearance is generally homogeneous echogenic and substantially avascular at CD [126]. Nonetheless, atypical appearances may be seen: a well-defined anechoic area with enhanced through-transmission, a hypoechoic halo, cystic areas, calcified spots or arterial signals [30,127] (Figs. 5.166–5.168, Video 5.23). There may even be a mixed appearance, i.e. a heterogeneous hypoechoic area with slightly enhanced through-transmission [120,121] (Figs. 5.169, 5.170). In the presence of a homogeneous hyperechoic lesion with no hypoechoic halo the US examination is virtually diagnostic, even in subjects with heterotopic malignancies – in fact only in exceptional circumstances are hyperechoic lesions malignant. Otherwise, work-up with CEUS, CT or MR is required or US follow-up with an interval of a few months. CEUS is able to demonstrate substantial isovascularity in all phases for small hemangiomas and intense, persistent and possibly heterogeneous opacification for large cavernous hemangiomas [123].

Hamartoma is infrequent (0.13% of postmortem studies), is often identified in young subjects and is generally <3 cm. The appearance is solid and often heterogeneous due to the presence of echogenic areas, calcifications and cystic spaces. CD shows moderate vascularity, with multiple vessels distributed radially (Figs. 5.171, 5.172, Video 5.24).

Hypoechoic lesions of the spleen, with or without associated splenomegaly, can be due to non-recent hematomas, infarctions, inflammatory pseudotumors, abscesses, complicated cysts, hemangiomas (rarely) lymphangiomas, Osler nodules, glycogenosis, hemosiderosis (areas of sparing), metastases and lymphomas. Except for particular clinical settings, a patently nodular hypoechoic lesion is generally malignant, especially when it is significant in size [59,125].

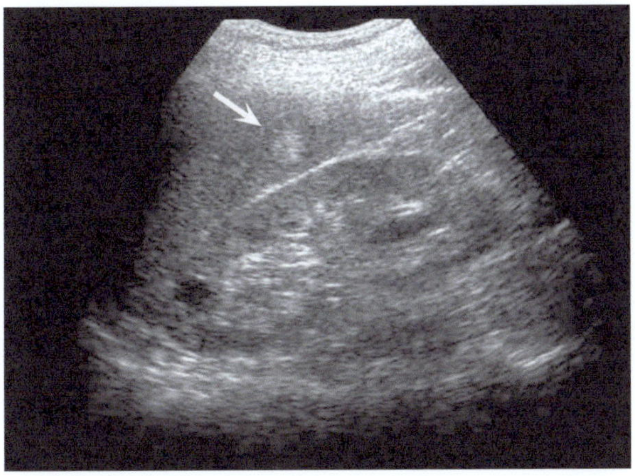

Fig. 5.166 Splenic hemangioma. Hyperechoic mass in the splenic parenchyma (*arrow*)

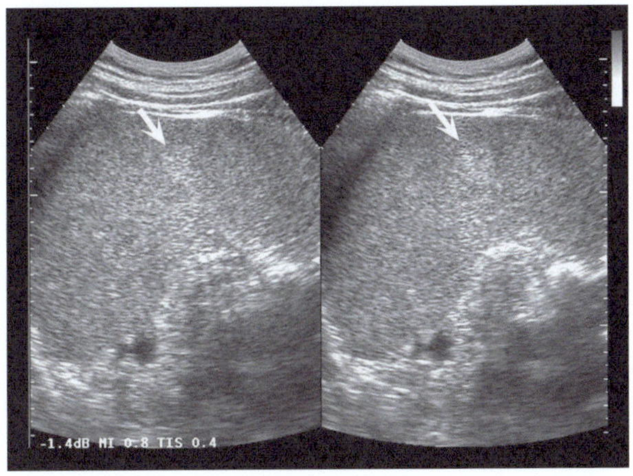

Fig. 5.167 Splenic hemangioma. Mildly hyperechoic mass in the splenic parenchyma (*arrows*)

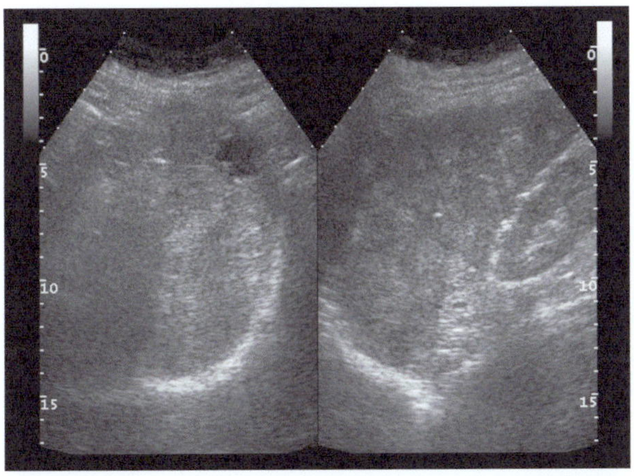

Fig. 5.168 Splenic hemangiomatosis. Spleen disrupted by anechoic cystic spaces and echogenic hemangiomatous patches

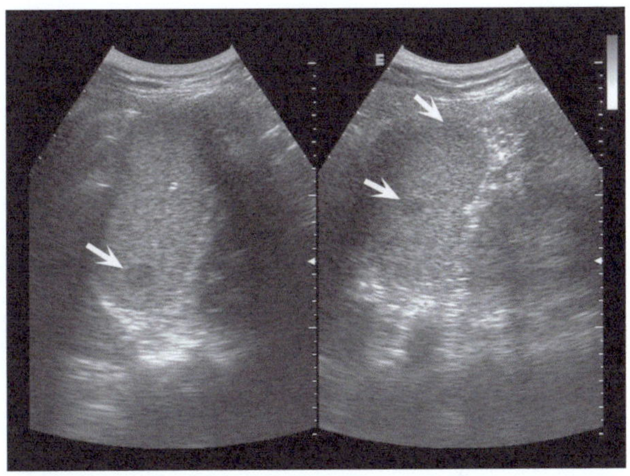

Fig. 5.169 Splenic hemangiomas. Heterogeneous hypo-anechoic masses (*arrows*)

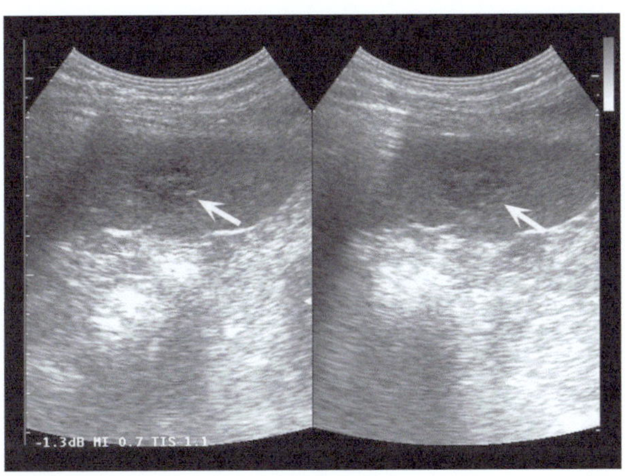

Fig. 5.170 Splenic angioma. Heterogeneous hypo-anechoic mass (*arrows*)

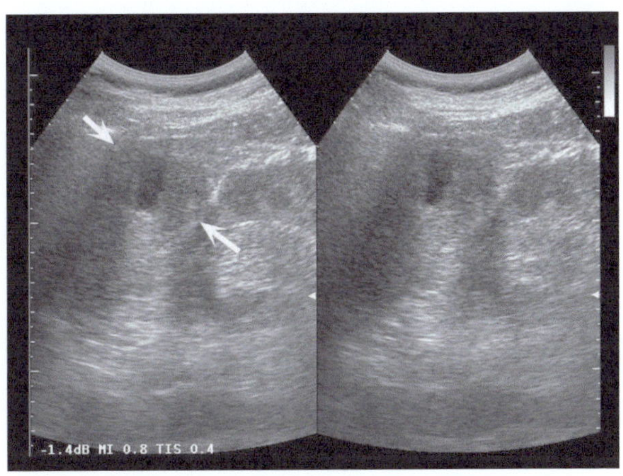

Fig. 5.171 Splenic hamartoma. Hypo-anechoic mass of the spleen (*arrows*)

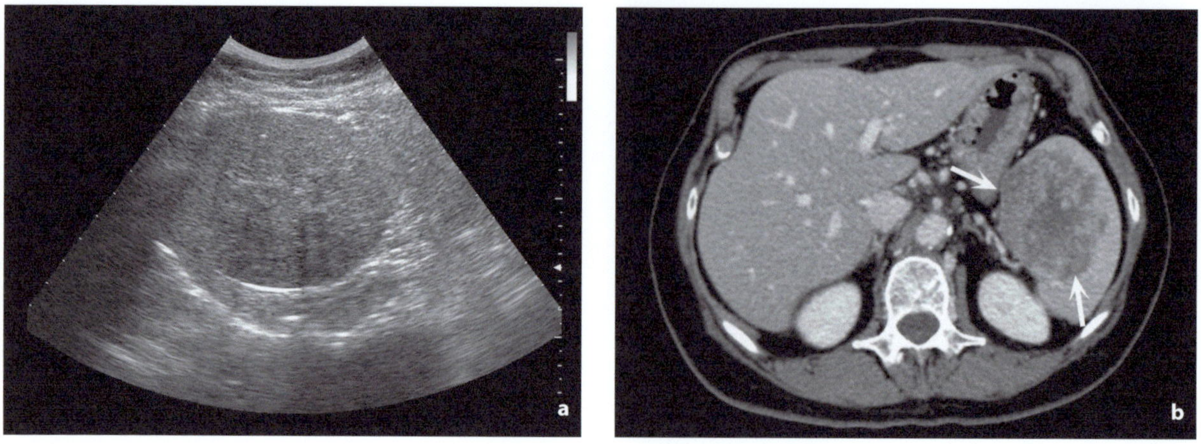

Fig. 5.172a,b Splenic hamartoma. Rounded and relatively homogeneous hypoechoic splenic mass (**a**) which instead in the venous phase axial CT scan displays a heterogeneous appearance, especially in the center of the lesion (**b**, *arrows*)

The spleen is often involved in lymphomatous and leukemic processes, whereas primary forms are rare and consist above all of NHL. The organ is often involved in systemic cases of **Hodgkin's disease** and **non-Hodgkin's lymphoma**. All patients with lymphoma should undergo a study of the spleen for the purpose of disease staging, since involvement of this organ occurs in 30% of patients with lymphoma. US is the technique of first choice, although a CT or PET study is usually required to search for possible combined involvement of the retroperitoneal lymph node stations, as well as to provide a panoramic characterization of the cervical, thoracic, abdominal and pelvic structures [128,129]. In general the presentation is splenomegaly with micro- and macroscopic lymphomatous infiltration. In most cases the spleen is enlarged but with no direct evidence of focal lesions. It should be borne in mind that this does not necessarily indicate direct splenic involvement, since in 1/3 of cases this is simply the expression of congestion or reactive hyperplasia. In other cases, especially in subjects with Hodgkin's disease, the spleen may be of normal size or enlarged, but with the presence of focal lesions. Miliary lesions, however, are not always identifiable with US [73]. There are four patterns of non-diffuse splenic involvement: micronodular (no lesion >3 cm), macronodular (at least one lesion >3 cm), bulky (at least one massive lesion possibly protruding from the profile of the organ) and perisplenic infiltrating (capsular) [59]. The size of the focal lesions seems to correlate with the grade of malignancy of the process: in low-grade lymphomas splenomegaly and small lesions prevail, whereas in high-grade forms there is a predominance of macronodular and massive lesions [128]. Focal lesions, whether single or multiple, are usually heterogeneously hypoechoic in appearance. In some cases the hypoechogenicity is particularly sharp and can mimic cystic disease. Occasionally the foci can even appear echogenic. CD displays limited vascular signals, prevalently perilesional or peripheral intralesional, and provides little additional information of note [129]. In general there is associated lymphadenopathy of the splenic hilar and lumbar lymph nodes [129] (Figs. 5.173–5.181, Video 5.25, 5.26).

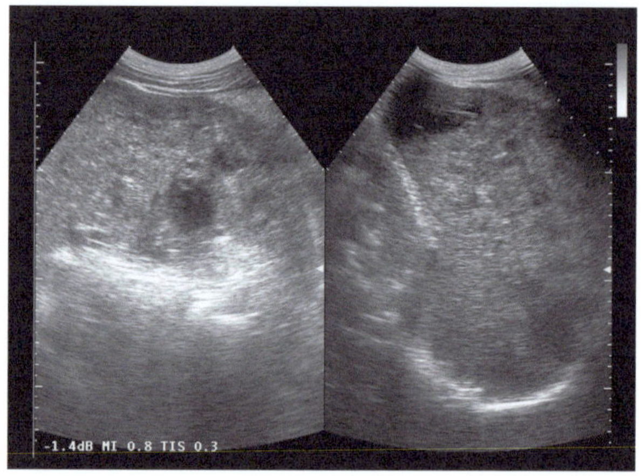

Fig. 5.173 Splenic lesions from acute myeloid leukemia. Enlarged spleen disrupted by multiple hypo-anechoic areas that are heterogeneous in size. Differential diagnosis should especially be made with abscesses

Primary sarcomas and especially angiosarcoma are rare (1–2% of all soft tissue sarcomas) and aggressive tumors associated with early metastases. Occasionally they present with rupture and hemoperitoneum. The spleen may be enlarged and the mass can appear with variable echogenicity, heterogeneous

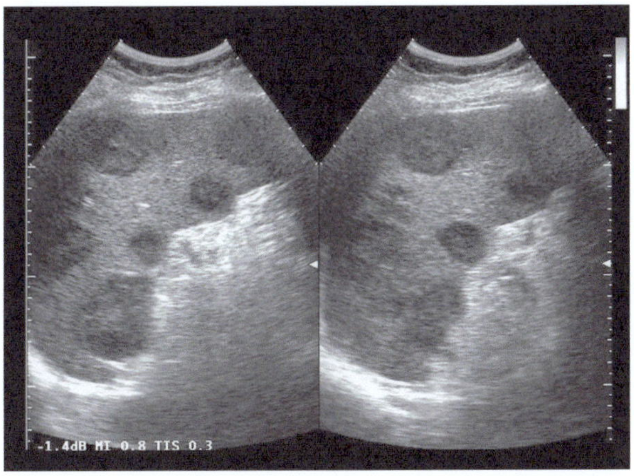

Fig. 5.174 High-grade splenic NHL. Multiple macronodular heterogeneous hypo-anechoic lesions scattered throughout the parenchyma of the spleen

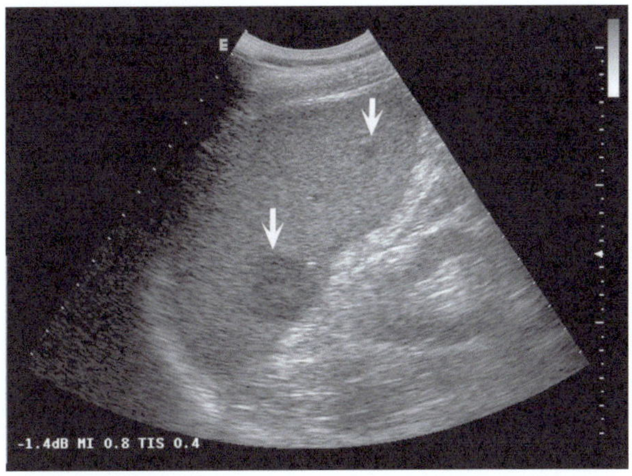

Fig. 5.175 Splenic lymphoma. Two heterogeneous hypoechoic nodules of the spleen (*arrows*)

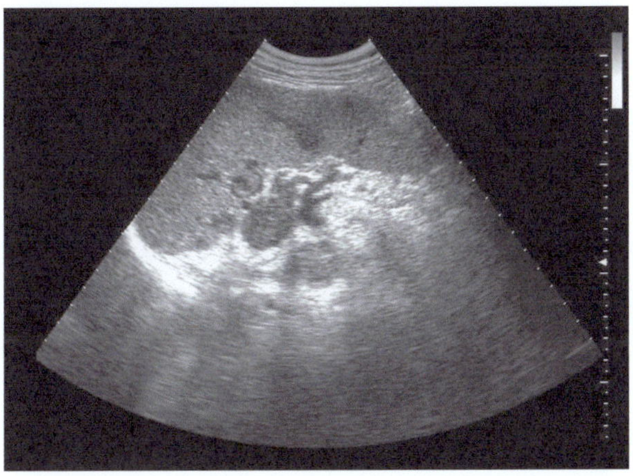

Fig. 5.176 Splenic lymphoma. Hypoechoic nodules of the spleen associated with hilar lymphadenopathies

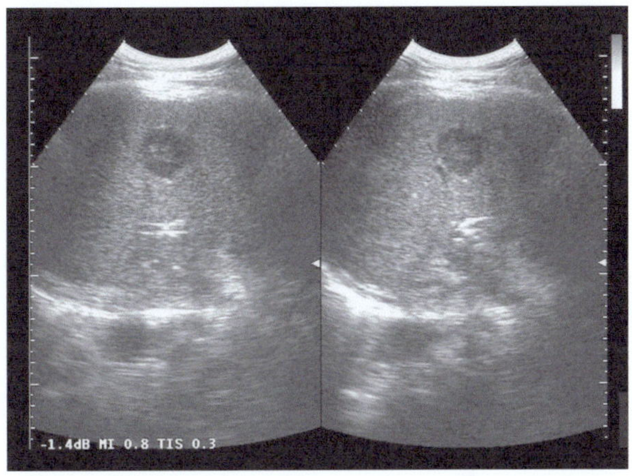

Fig. 5.177 Splenic lymphoma. Solitary heterogeneous hypoechoic nodule of the spleen

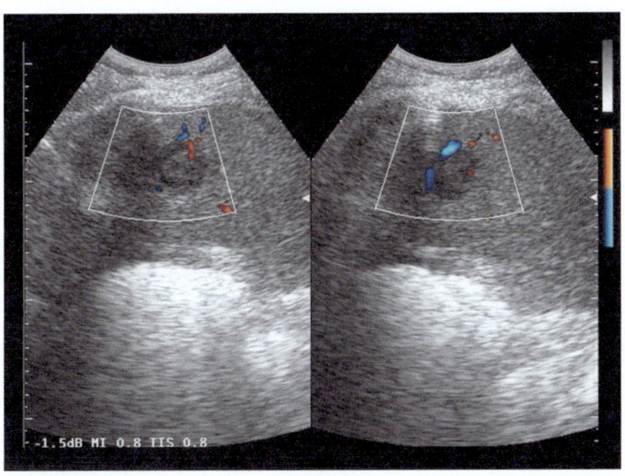

Fig. 5.178 Splenic lymphoma. Heterogeneous hypoechoic nodule of the spleen with some internal vascular signals at directional PD

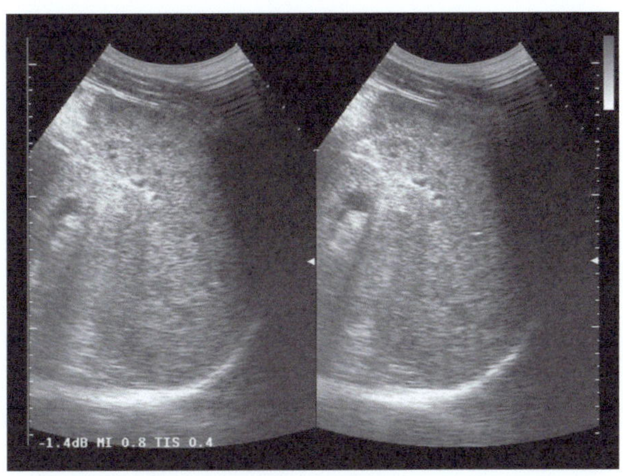

Fig. 5.179 Splenic lymphoma. Diffuse and tenuous miliary lesions of the splenic parenchyma

echotexture and irregular and occasionally jagged margins. Necrotic areas and subcapsular or intraperitoneal hemorrhage are possible [120,121]. Kaposi sarcoma is characterized by multiple hyperechoic areas and overall hemangioma-like appearance.

Inflammatory pseudotumors are characterized by spindle cell proliferation and marked inflammatory reaction. They often appear hypoechoic, well circumscribed and with limited vascular signals.

Despite the significant vascularity of this organ, nonlymphomatous splenic **metastases** are rare (0.3–10% of cancer patients), often late (widespread metastases phase) and usually in the form of micrometastasis not identifiable at US. Contiguous spread is rare and usually only occurs with tumors of the greater curvature of the stomach or the tail of the pancreas. Hematogenous spread is generally due to colon cancer, breast cancer, uterine cancer, ovarian cancer or even melanoma. Rarer sites include the lung and the stomach. Ovarian cancer can reach the surface of the spleen with intraperitoneal spread, and develop superficial implants similar to those of the liver. Superficial lesions are more typical of ovarian cancer at presentation, whereas hematogenous parenchymal lesions are found mainly in cases of recurrence. In most cases single or multiple oval hypoechoic lesions are commonly located in the periphery, although occasionally the appearance is more complex, with internal heterogeneity or with hypoechogenicity more marked at the center than the periphery of the lesion. A target appearance is also possible in lymphomas, although it is more characteristic of metastases (peripheral hypoechoic halo in 20% of cases). In some cases diffuse heterogeneity of the splenic echotexture may be seen

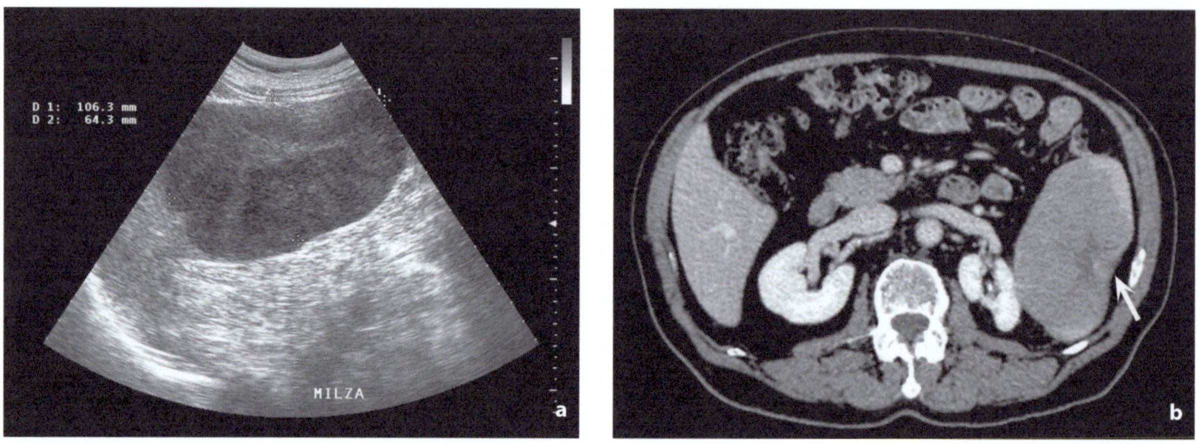

Fig. 5.180a,b Non-Hodgkin's splenic lymphoma, single lesion. Large, relatively homogeneous and rather hypoechoic mass with a central scar-like echogenic image seen widening the inferior half of the organ (**a**). Axial CT scan in the venous phase (**b**) shows an intralesional structure similar to that seen at US (*arrow*)

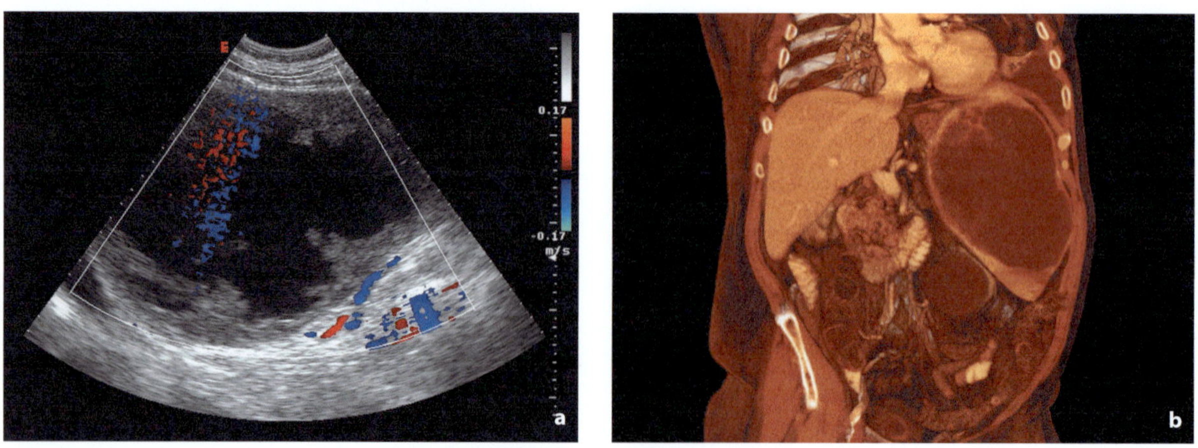

Fig. 5.181a,b High-grade non-Hodgkin's splenic lymphoma, single lesion. Large liquefactive splenic mass without vascular signals at CD (**a**). Corresponding volume rendering CT image (**b**)

in the absence of individual measurable foci. In metastases from ovarian cancer large capsular calcifications and/or cystic-like masses may be observed with thick walls, septations or internal solid components [30]. CD reveals some intranodular vascular signals which are not specific and usually of little help [125]. CEUS shows a hypoechogenicity with internal "microcirculation" which becomes increasingly evident in the venous phase [123] (Figs. 5.182–5.186).

It should be recalled that splenic **infarction**, which is also hypoechoic, may take on a rounded or oval appearance and therefore mimic a tumor. In the early stages in fact, the appearance is nonspecific and often cannot be distinguished with US alone from abscesses, mycotic lesions, metastases and lymphomas. In the acute phase, edema, inflammation and necrosis give rise to a well-circumscribed hypoechoic area which is generally wedge-shaped with irregular margins, although it may take on a more rounded morphology or be relatively echogenic [125]. Occasionally the areas are multiple or tending to confluence. CD is not able to identify flow signals in the diseased area [126]. In doubtful cases, extemporaneous CEUS is recommended, which demonstrates the avascularity, or a US study after an interval of a few days [123]. Although generally identified in a different clinical setting, similar considerations are valid for **abscesses**, which can have a heterogeneous hypoechoic internal structure and not patently fluid or corpuscular, and may show little or no enhanced through-transmission. Fungal and tubercular abscesses and microabscesses, with hypoechoic or echogenic appearance and

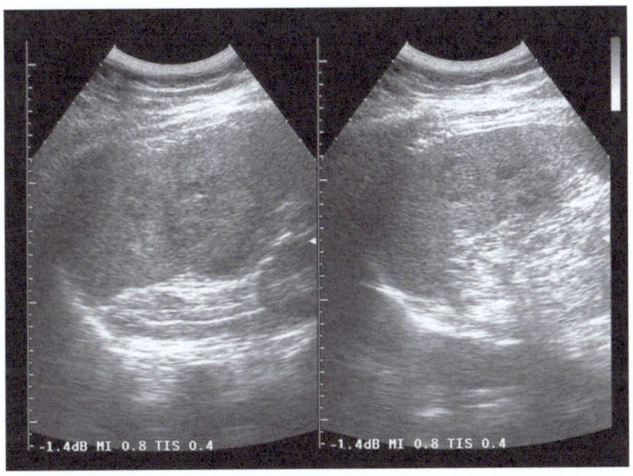

Fig. 5.182 Splenic metastasis from melanoma. Heterogeneous hypo-isoechoic mass with peripheral hypoechoic halo in the spleen

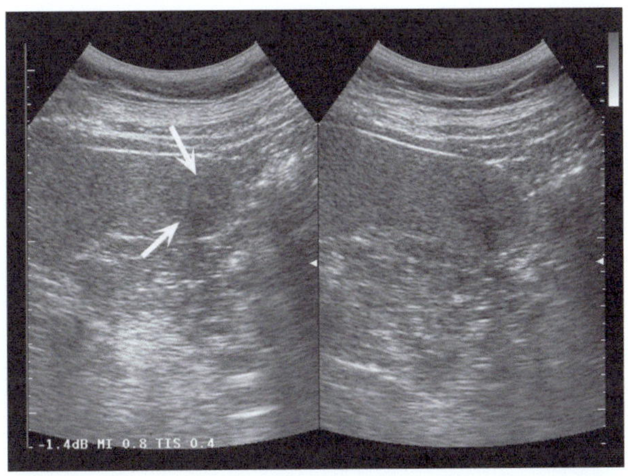

Fig. 5.183 Splenic metastasis from breast cancer. Heterogeneous hypo-anechoic mass in the lower pole of the spleen (*arrows*)

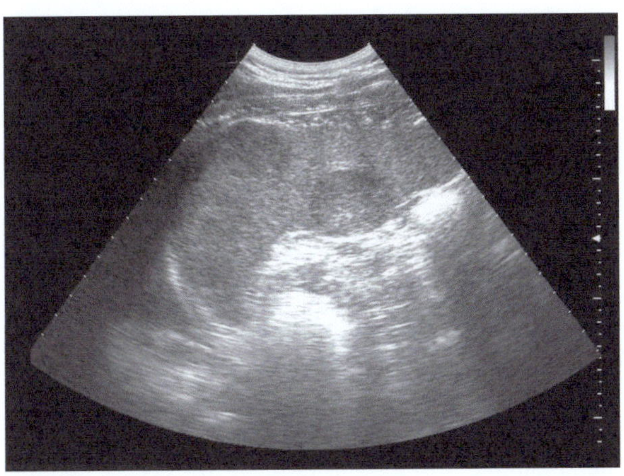

Fig. 5.184 Splenic metastasis from melanoma. Well-defined heterogeneous hypoechoic mass within the spleen seen bulging from the profile of the organ

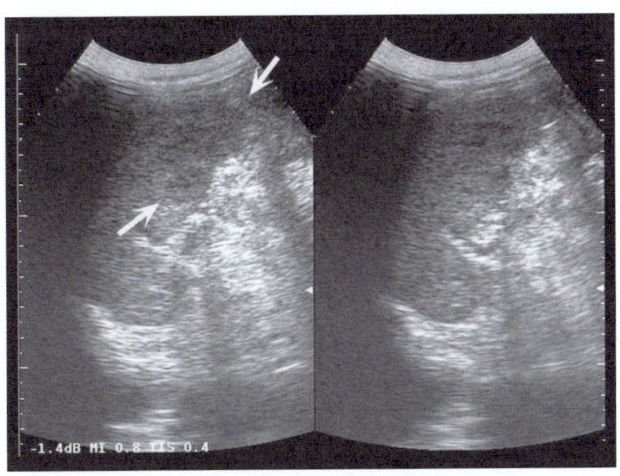

Fig. 5.185 Splenic metastasis from ovarian carcinoma. Heterogeneous hypoechoic area on the anterior portion of the spleen (*arrows*)

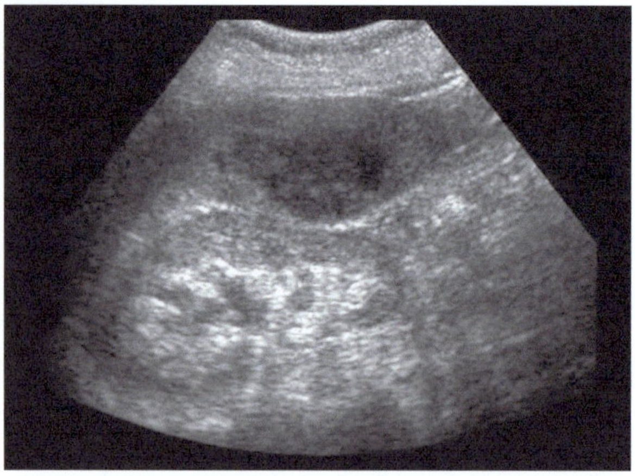

Fig. 5.186 Splenic metastasis from rhinopharyngeal carcinoma. Heterogeneous and clearly hypoechoic lesion deforming the spleen

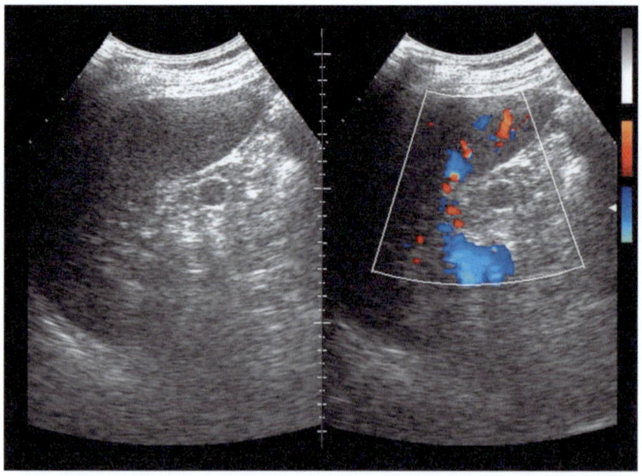

Fig. 5.187 Accessory spleen. Small rounded mass isoechoic to the adjacent splenic parenchyma with no vascular signals at CD

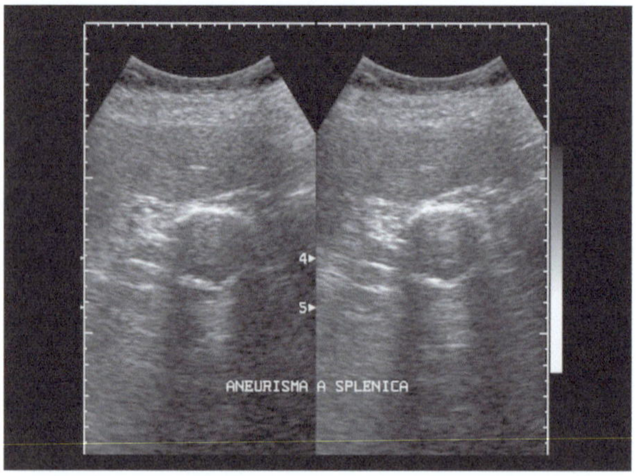

Fig. 5.188 Aneurysm of the splenic artery. Hypo-anechoic mass with marked calcified shell adjacent to the splenic hilum

peripheral hypoechoic halo, can mimic miliary lesions from metastases or especially from lymphoma, since the hematologic, immunodepressed patient is also prone to opportunistic infections [30].

Brief mention should also be made of perisplenic alterations, especially **accessory spleens**. These are present in postmortem findings in 10–30% of individuals and subject to enlargement due to splenomegaly or splenectomy [130]. They generally create no difficulties in differential diagnosis and typically present with limited size (<3 cm), well-defined margins, oval-rounded shape, echotexture similar to the adjacent spleen, and parahilar location (Fig. 5.187). The differential diagnosis includes lymph nodes, left adrenal lesions, lesions of the tail of the pancreas (pseudocysts, tumors), aneurysms of the splenic artery (especially if thrombosed), thrombosis, aneurysm or varicosity of the splenic vein, collapsed jejunal loops and normal left colic flexure [130] (Fig. 5.188).

5.8 Abdominal Lymphadenopathies

Lymphatic drainage of the lower limbs, the pelvic structures and the abdominal organs is guaranteed by the lymph vessels which run parallel to the inferior vena cava and the aorta. The main lymph node stations which make up this system are the lumbar chain (peri-aortic and para-aortic lymph nodes), the lymph nodes adjacent to the celiac trunk, the hepatic hilum, the renal hilum, and the pericaval and mesenteric lymph nodes (Fig. 5.189). The common, internal and external iliac stations drain the entire pelvic area.

Study of these stations is not performed by choice with US, although the technique is able to identify lymph node disease during the course of examinations performed for other indications or on the occasion of the study of disease of the organ associated with adenopathy. US is performed in the routine evaluation of retroperitoneal structures such as the kidneys, the pancreas and the aorta. In these cases, or during any US examination of the abdomen or pelvis, US is able to identify enlarged lymph nodes.

US plays a secondary but not negligible role in the evaluation of abdominal-pelvic lymph nodes. Often the stations, and especially the deep stations, are difficult to access and the accuracy of US in identifying, but above all in ruling out, the presence of adenopathies is limited. Moreover, for US, as with the other imaging modalities, the only discriminating criterion is size.

Under **normal conditions** the lymph nodes are only

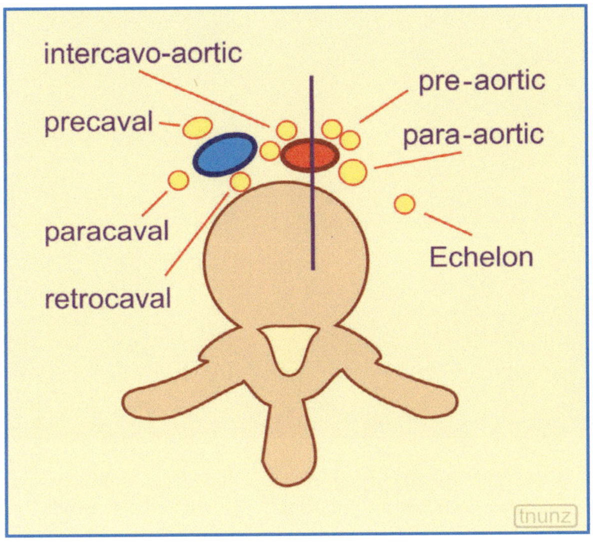

Fig. 5.189 Nomenclature of the retroperitoneal lymph nodes. Terminology of the lumbar lymph nodes in relation to the major retroperitoneal vessels

rarely visible. Their limited size and their echogenicity, which is similar to the retroperitoneal connective tissue, makes their identification challenging [131]. Lymph nodes are considered enlarged when their long-axis diameter exceeds 10 or 15 mm. The presence of a group of nodes of 6–10 mm is already cause for suspicion but this is rarely found with US and is usually the prerogative of CT. Many authors recommend measurement of the short-axis (transverse) diameter of the lymph node or both diameters. Adenopathies may consist of multiple enlarged and independent lymph nodes, clusters of lymph nodes which are still distinguishable from each other, or large clusters of lymph nodes whose shape and volume are difficult to distinguish one from the other.

Except when particularly large, **lymph node enlargements** are generally not sufficient to enable a study of the internal architecture, which appears generically hypoechoic. Unlike superficial adenopathies, neither the echostructure nor the vascular pattern at CD is helpful in the differentiation of enlarged lymph nodes, or in the identification of necrosis or adipose metaplasia of the lymph nodes, which are not generally identifiable at US, at least not as well as at CT. Enlarged lymph nodes may appear hypoechoic or echogenic, with or without posterior acoustic shadowing, often with lobulated margins, rounded or oval, single or confluent. Large lymph node clusters may be identified as heterogeneous, hypoechoic, lobulated masses with possible internal calcifications. The enlarged lymph node may imprint or compress the adjacent vessels, both the inferior vena cava and even the aorta, and may extend from the iliac vessels up to the diaphragmatic hiatus of the aorta and the inferior vena cava. The para-aortic lymph nodes often obliterate the anterior border of the aorta, producing an "ultrasound silhouette" which helps to distinguish a lymphadenopathy from aortic disease. Mesenteric lymphadenopathies may appear with the morphology of a "pseudokidney". The isolated involvement of a lymph node is less common than multiple lymphadenopathies, with enlarged lymph nodes occasionally conglomerated to form a mass proper. Size alone is not a valid diagnostic element for the distinction of a benign from a malignant lymph node, and the hilum of deep lymph nodes is rarely identifiable. Although pathologic lymph nodes are generally characterized by sparse echoes, they can be of medium intensity. Often the metastatic lymph node is more echogenic that the lymphomatous node. In doubtful cases, in both large clusters and small adenopathies, CT- or even US-guided biopsy may be necessary [132].

A presumed **enlarged lymph node** needs to be differentiated from vessels (aorta and its visceral branches, inferior vena cava, portal system, gonadal vein, etc.), vascular anomalies (aneurysms, left inferior vena cava, dilatation of the azygos vein or the gonadal vein, varices from portal hypertension, etc.), dilated uterus, bowel loops, fluid collections, cystic masses, retroperitoneal fibrosis, crura of the diaphragm, psoas muscle and its variants [131]. With the exception of the aorta and the vena cava, all of the other vascular structures are, under normal conditions, of limited size transversally – less than an enlarged lymph node. Intestinal segments such as the duodenum at the level of the head of the pancreas and the initial loops of the jejunum between the splenic hilum, tail of the pancreas and the left retroperitoneum can mimic lymphadenopathies. However, the site, presence of peristalsis and visibility of intraluminal gas generally allow for adequate differentiation. Retroperitoneal venous alterations can also mimic lymph nodes, especially when viewed in the axial plane, e.g. in the case of retroperitoneal varices from portal hypertension. The same can be said for anomalies of the inferior vena cava as in the case of distended and dilated ascending lumbar veins. In all of these cases the study of vascular flow with CD can prove useful. At the level of the hepatic hilum, the inferior margin of the caudate lobe and its papillary process can mimic a lymphadenopathy. The distinction between them is based on continuity with the rest of the hepatic parenchyma [76].

The development of **metastatic lymphadenopathies** is a negative prognostic factor for most malignancies. Most tumors are unable to create a lymphatic network for themselves similar to their vascular neoangiogenetic network and penetrate the lymphatic collectors with direct infiltration or cellular invagination of the lymphatic endothelium, reaching the nearest lymph nodes with the development of metastatic foci beginning from the subcapsular sinus [133]. Testicular and ovarian tumors cause lumbar lymphadenopathies in particular. Testicular tumors, especially, involve the ipsilateral lumbar lymph nodes, whereas isolated involvement of the contralateral lymph nodes is very rare. Metastases arising from the left testicle spread first, in the case of a single lymph node, to the ipsilateral renal hilum immediately caudal to the renal vein, and then extend to the interaortocaval and pre-aortic regions but not contralaterally, whereas those arising from the right testicle tend to spread to the median level (single interaortocaval or right paracaval lymph node), being then able to extend even to the other side, in correspondence with the renal hilum. Pelvic lymph node metastasis from tumors on normally descended testicles are instead rather infrequent and usually subsequent to massive retroperitoneal metastases, with which mesenteric or retrocrural adenopathies can be associated. Ovarian cancers can involve the iliac and inguinal lymph nodes, but tend to be prevalent in the lumbar region. Carcinomas of the right ovary tend to spread to the right paracaval and precaval lymph nodes, from the aortic bifurcation to the level of the ipsilateral renal hilum, whereas carcinomas of the left ovary tend to spread first to the left para-aortic and renal hilar lymph nodes at a level generally higher than on the opposite side. Cancers of the head and body of the uterus, as well as bladder and prostate cancers, tend to spread first to the internal and external iliac lymph nodes before spreading upwards. Stomach cancer involves the perigastric, peripancreatic and celiac lymph nodes and the lymph nodes of the lesser omentum and only in a later phase the lumbar and hepatic hilar nodes (Figs. 5.190–5.194).

Lymphomas can spread to any abdominal and pelvic lymph node station, with a certain prevalence in the lumbar retroperitoneal lymph nodes (25–35% of patients with Hodgkin's disease and 45–55% of those with non-Hodgkin's lymphoma at presentation), the iliac lymph nodes, and in NHL the mesenteric lymph nodes (at times an isolated site of spread from low-grade non-Hodgkin's lymphoma). Spread to the hepatic hilum and splenic hilum is relatively more common in non-Hodgkin's lymphoma [134]. Hodgkin's disease is characterized by small non-confluent lymph nodes with contiguous spread, whereas in NHL the distribution can be more irregular, with bulky masses and frequent extranodal lesions to the abdominal viscera [134]. A characteristic of the lymphomatous forms is in fact the extensive involvement of enlarged, rounded and often lobulated lymph

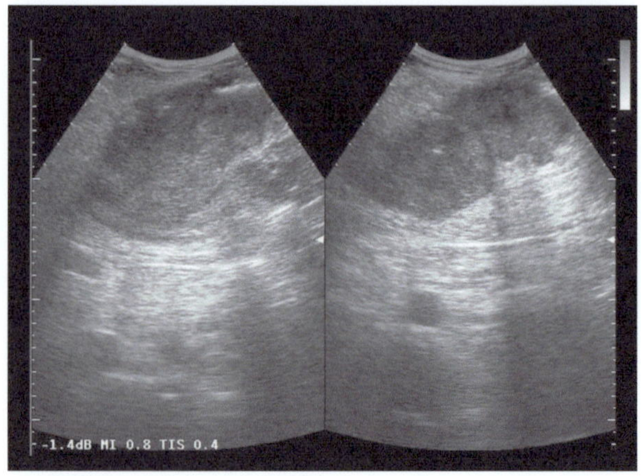

Fig. 5.190 Metastatic lymphadenopathies from colon cancer. Nodal mass between the pancreatic region and the stomach

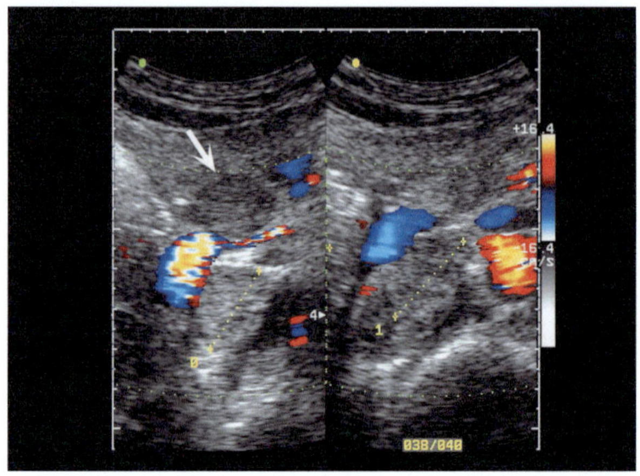

Fig. 5.191 Enlarged metastatic lymph nodes from fibrillar HCC. Relatively homogeneous and echogenic adenopathies located at the interaortocaval and portacaval level (*arrow*)

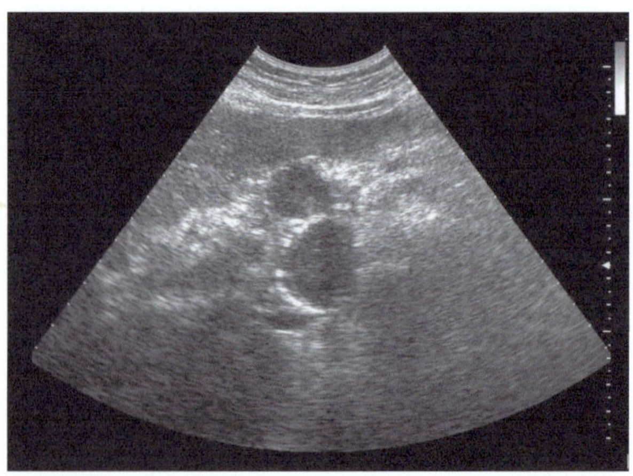

Fig. 5.192 Peripancreatic metastatic lymphadenopathies from stomach cancer. Two markedly hypoechoic lymph nodes in retrogastric location

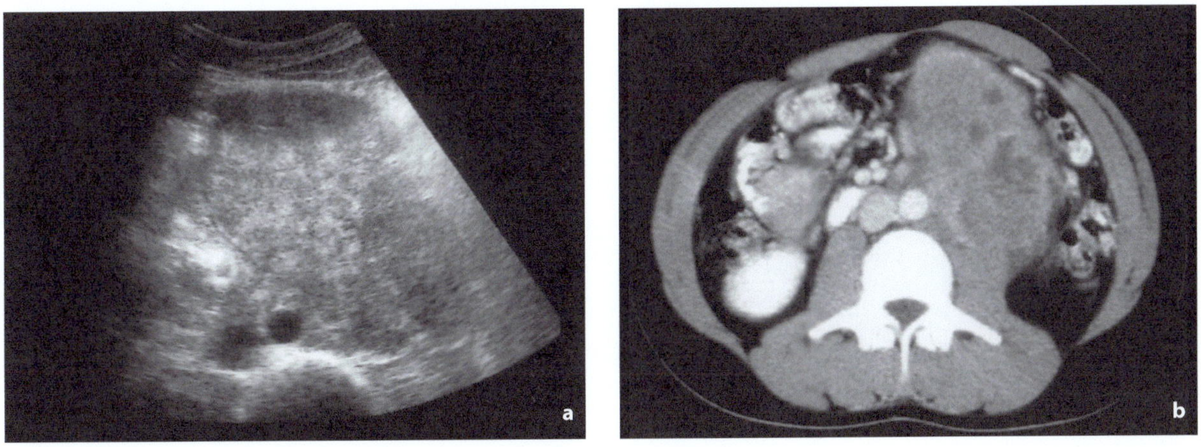

Fig. 5.193a,b Retroperitoneal metastatic lymphadenopathy from seminoma. Large heterogeneous echogenic mass with left para-aortic origin and marked anterior bulging (a). CT correlation (b) confirms the heterogeneous hypo-attenuating mass in left retroperitoneal location

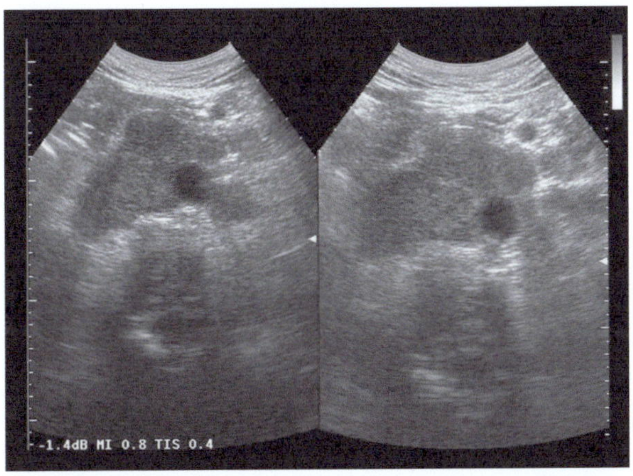

Fig. 5.194 Lumbar lymphadenopathies from colon cancer. Confluent retroperitoneal lymph nodes

nodes with the formation of large clusters [135]. A significant finding for diagnostic purposes is the simultaneous presence of lymphomatous metastases in the kidneys, liver, spleen and adrenal glands. The lymphomatous involvement of the mesenteric lymph nodes which run alongside the mesenteric vessels is characteristic. In these cases a "sandwich" appearance is seen with the lymphadenopathies placed anterior and posterior to the vessels, in front of the aorta and the vena cava. This appearance is identifiable at US and even more so at CD [135,136]. CD is able to demonstrate the relations between the retroperitoneal vessels with their visceral branches and the absence of turbulence in those vessels, as well as to distinguish between peripancreatic lymphadenopathies and a carcinoma of the pancreas, since vascular involvement is only seen in the latter (Figs. 5.195–5.203, Video 5.27).

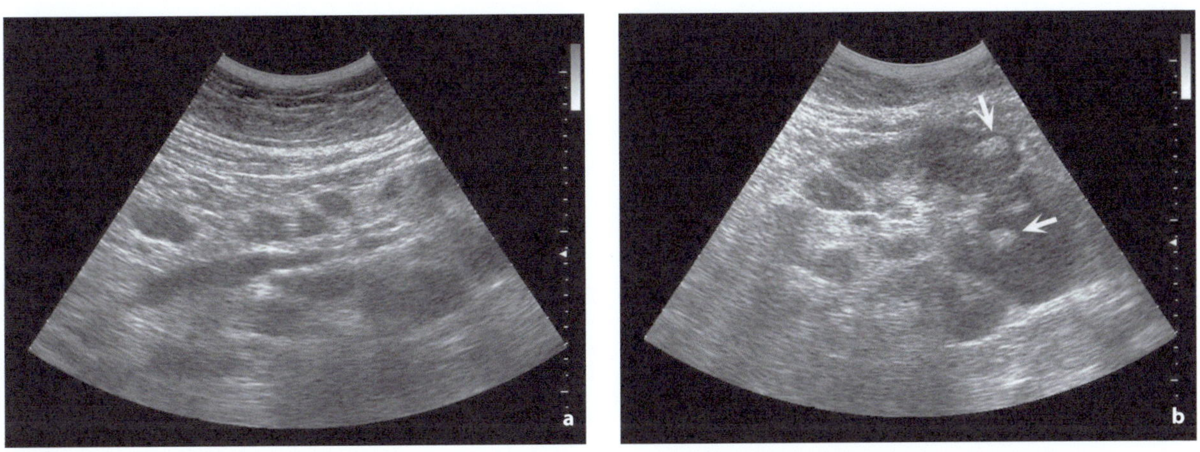

Fig. 5.195a,b Mesenteric lymphadenopathies from chronic lymphatic leukemia. Multiple, non-confluent, hypoechoic lymph nodes distributed ventral and dorsal to the longitudinally sectioned mesenteric vessels (a). The transverse section (b) confirms the enlarged lymph nodes, some of which show internal calcified echogenic foci (*arrows*)

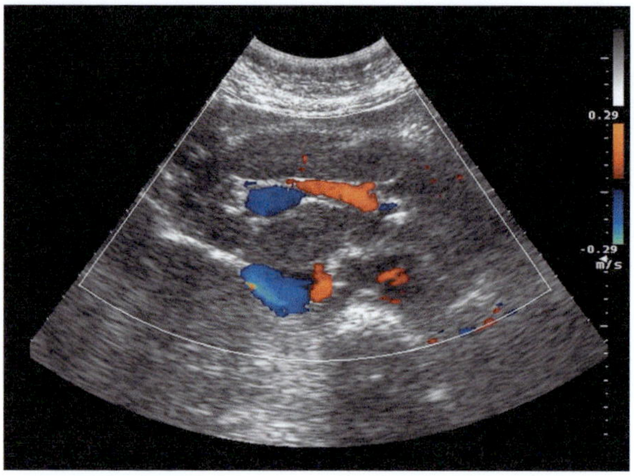

Fig. 5.196 Retroperitoneal and mesenteric lymphoma, "sandwich" sign. CD shows how the enlarged lymph nodes are sandwiched between the retroperitoneal and mesenteric vessels

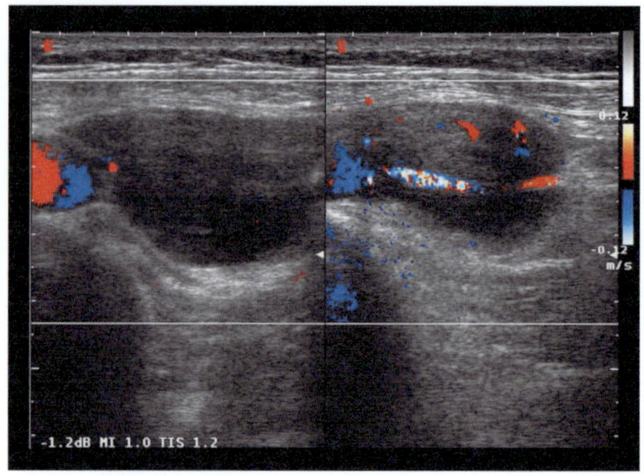

Fig. 5.197 Retroperitoneal lymphoma. In a particularly thin subject, the use of the superficial transducer makes it possible to identify the enlarged left para-aortic hypo-anechoic lymph node which can be seen encircling the inferior mesenteric artery

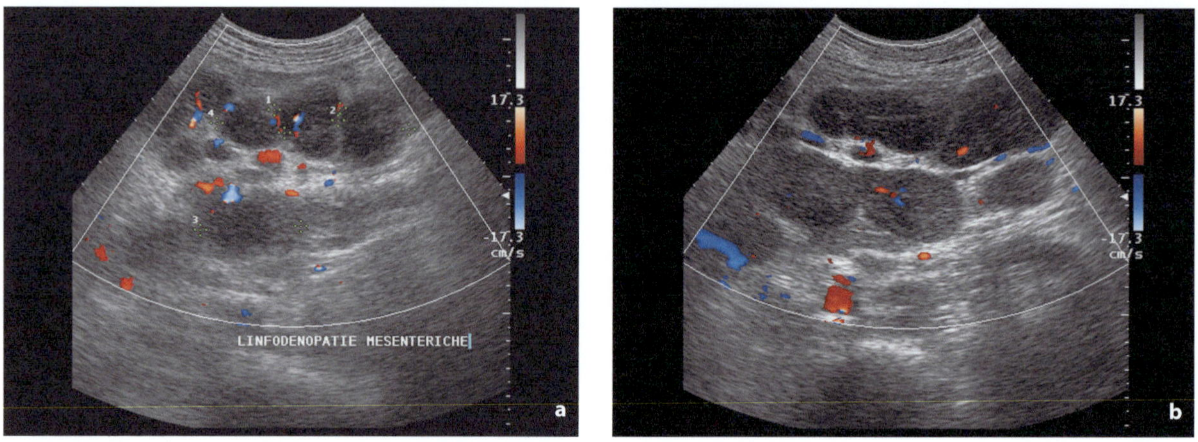

Fig. 5.198a,b Mesenteric lymphoma. Numerous non-confluent enlarged lymph nodes with relatively homogeneous hypoechoic appearance and poor vascular signals at CD located between the mesenteric folds

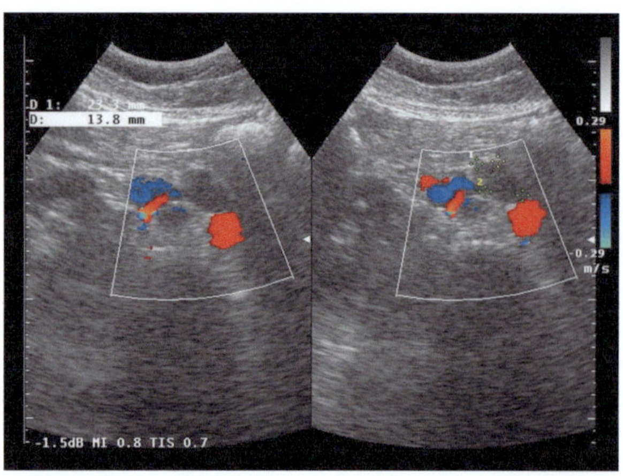

Fig. 5.199 Retroperitoneal lymphoma. Two interaortocaval lymphadenopathies (one *between the calipers*) distinguishable from the vessels at CD

The remaining conditions which could give rise to abdominal adenopathies, in particular mesenteric and retroperitoneal adenopathies, are **Castleman disease** (angiofollicular lymphadenopathy) and the **intestinal malabsorption syndromes** (especially Whipple's disease). A characteristic of the former is the hypervascularity of the lesions seen at CD [137,138] (Fig. 5.204).

Involvement of the **lymph nodes** of the **hepatoduodenal ligament** is a special problem. Around 10% of lymphomatous processes involve the lymph nodes of this ligament, but they are also commonly involved in chronic liver disease. A lymphadenopathy of the lymph nodes of the hepatic hilum is present in chronic liver disease (up to 39% of cases), as well as in liver metastases, gallbladder disease (with or without cholangitis) and occasionally in cases of gastritis and

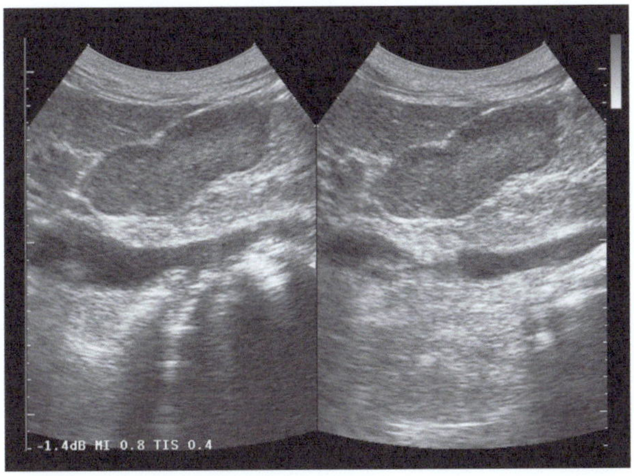

Fig. 5.200 Hodgkin's lymphoma, abdominal lymphadenopathies. Large circumscribed cluster of lymph nodes with relatively homogeneous hypoechoic appearance can be identified below the liver

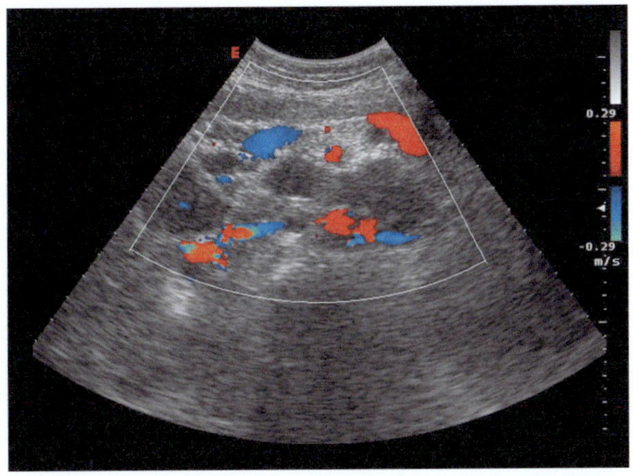

Fig. 5.201 Retroperitoneal lymphoma. CD is able to distinguish between the lumbar vessels and the hypoechoic lymphadenopathies

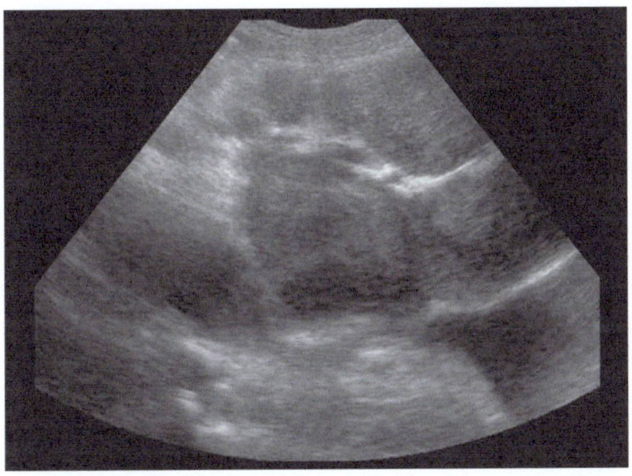

Fig. 5.202 Mesenteric lymphoma. Large hypoechoic lymphadenopathies of the mesenteric root

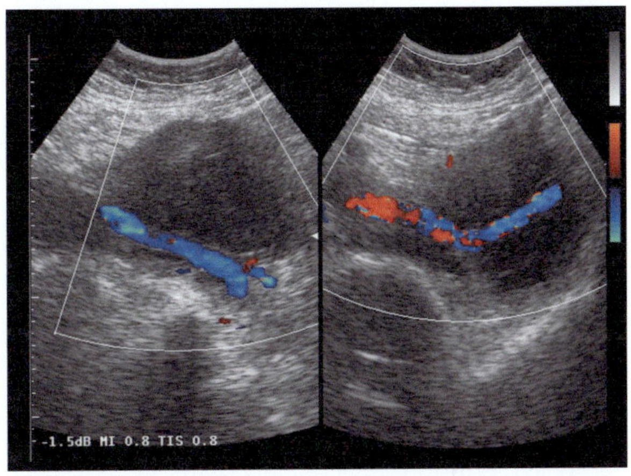

Fig. 5.203 Iliac lymphoma. Large hypoechoic adenopathies in external iliac location are seen encircling the vessels at that level

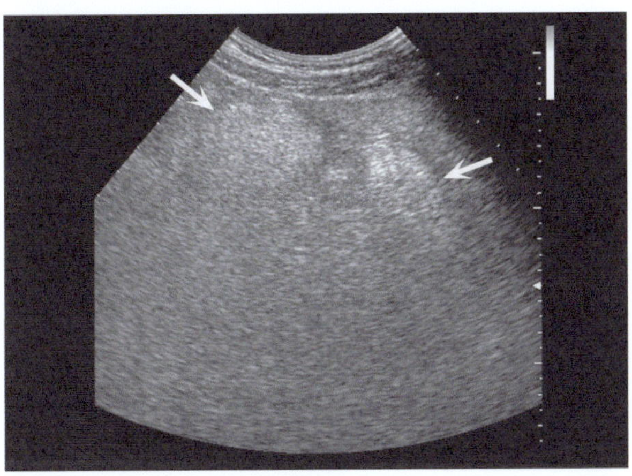

Fig. 5.204 Adipose lymphadenopathies from Whipple's disease. Massive adipose infiltration of enlarged mesenteric lymph nodes, which are identifiable in their profile only anteriorly (*arrows*)

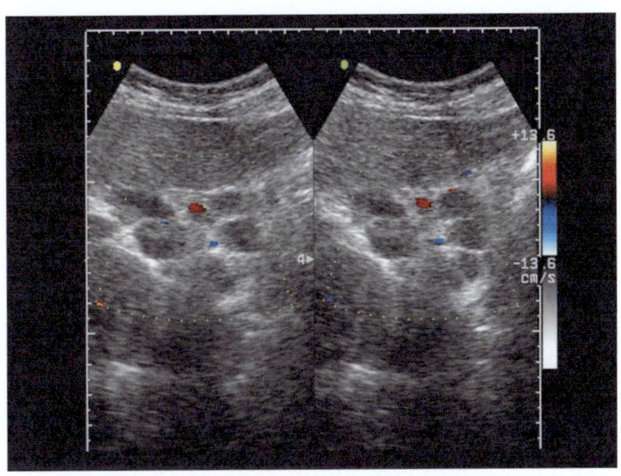

Fig. 5.205 Lymphadenopathies of the lesser omentum from stomach cancer. Multiple non-confluent small lymph nodes between the hepatic hilum and the region of the head of the pancreas

pancreatitis [137,139,140] (Fig. 5.205). With regard to chronic liver disease, enlargement of the hilar lymph nodes is seen particularly in HCV+ subjects or with biliary cirrhosis and constitute on the one hand a sign the process is active, and on the other a prognostic element, since it is found especially in the more severe forms of disease [140]. Even in carriers of HCC it has been seen in the majority of cases that enlarged lymph nodes of the hepatic hilum and the lesser omentum are an expression of the underlying disease and not a neoplastic complication.

5.9 Peritoneal Carcinomatosis

Tumors may spread to the peritoneum directly along the ligaments, mesentery and omenta (cancer of the stomach, colon, pancreas, ovary, etc.) or via cellular dissemination in the peritoneal fluid (intraperitoneal seeding, particularly in the sloping recesses, typical but not exclusive of ovarian cancer), or with lymphatic (e.g. mesenteric lymphoma) or hematogenous spread (embolism, particularly from extra-abdominal tumors, with the development of moderately sized masses in the peritoneum and/or retroperitoneum). In some cases spontaneous rupture of the tumor (e.g. HCC) or instrumental procedures (surgery, biopsy, etc.) are responsible for the seeding of tumor cells in the peritoneal cavity [141]. Pleural effusion is often associated, especially right-sided (e.g. Meigs' syndrome of ovarian tumors). Like other diagnostic imaging modalites and even more so, US tends to underestimate the presence of **peritoneal carcinosis**. In most cases the presence of peritoneal effusion in a patient with an advanced abdominal tumor is clearly indicative of diffuse involvement of the serosa. However, the direct demonstration of peritoneal involvement is often difficult, and is particularly complex in the absence of associated effusion. Nonetheless, a thorough exploration of the various abdominal-pelvic peritoneal regions is often able to identify peritoneal involvement in patients with an adequate suspicion. To this end an appropriate technique is essential, one which involves the use of higher-frequency transducers for the identification of omental invasion, anterior hepatic capsular lesions (especially of the left hepatic lobe) and nodules in the anterior wall of the peritoneum (Figs. 5.206–5.216).

The **"initial" forms** of carcinosis, which are often more extensive than estimated by US, consist of small nodules of plaques on the surface of the bowel loops and the abdominal parenchymas (especially the liver) and on the peritoneal profile underlying the anterior abdominal wall. Peritoneal implants appear as hypoechoic nodulations and are especially identifiable when surrounded by peritoneal effusion. In the

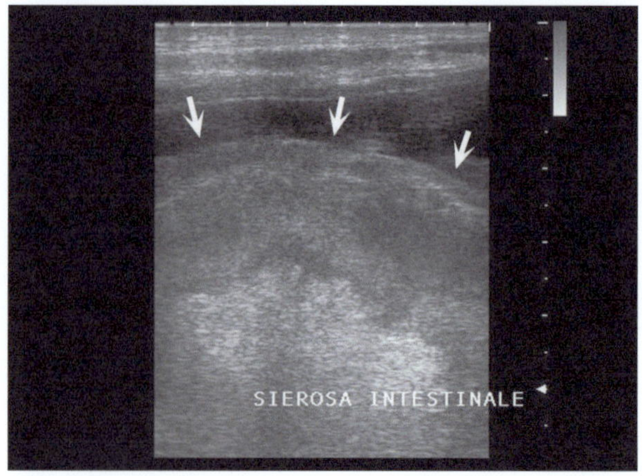

Fig. 5.206 Peritoneal carcinosis from ovarian cancer, thickening of the intestinal serosa. Hypoechoic bands (*arrows*) diffusely thicken the serosa and the bowel loops. Peritoneal effusion is associated

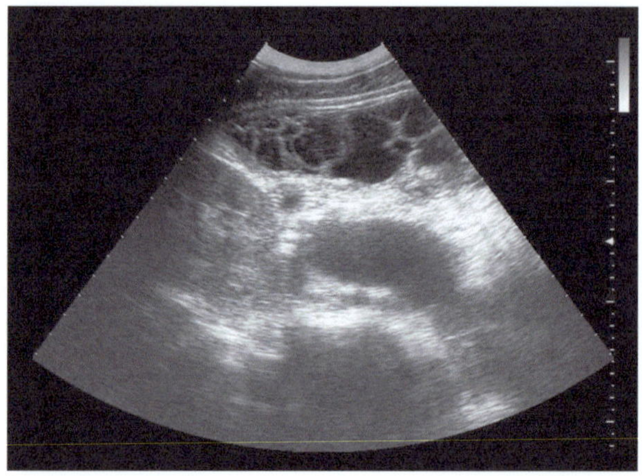

Fig. 5.207 Peritoneal carcinosis from ovarian cancer. Diffuse septated loculations

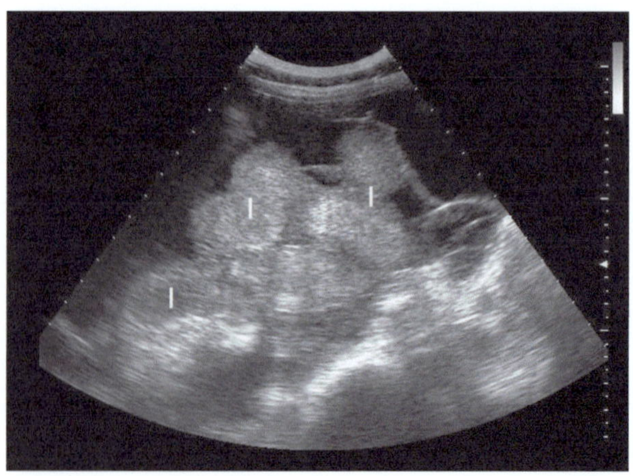

Fig. 5.208 Peritoneal carcinosis from ovarian cancer. Effusion with internal sedimentation circumscribing the bowel loops which are adhering to each other due to blocked diffusion. *I*, intestine

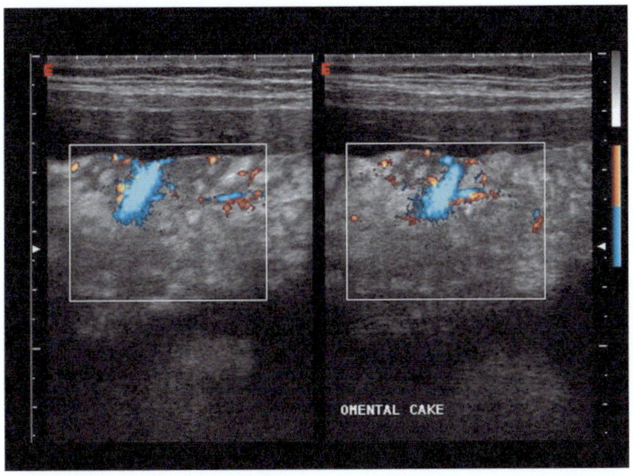

Fig. 5.209 Peritoneal carcinosis from uterine cancer, invasion of the greater omentum. Marked heterogeneous echogenic thickening of the omentum with moderate vascular signals at directional PD

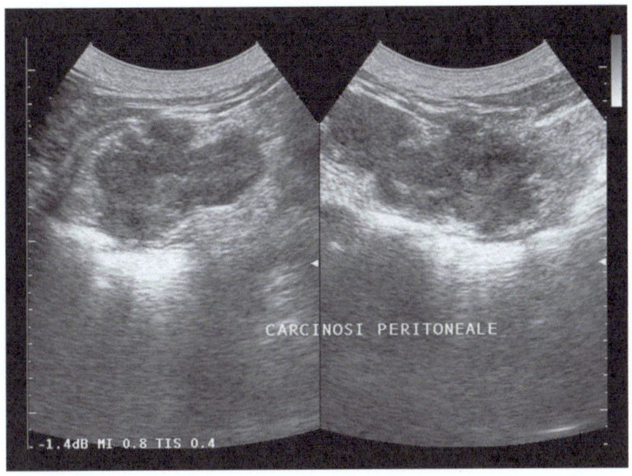

Fig. 5.210 Peritoneal metastasis from melanoma. Lobulated heterogeneous hypoechoic nodule in a right paracolic location

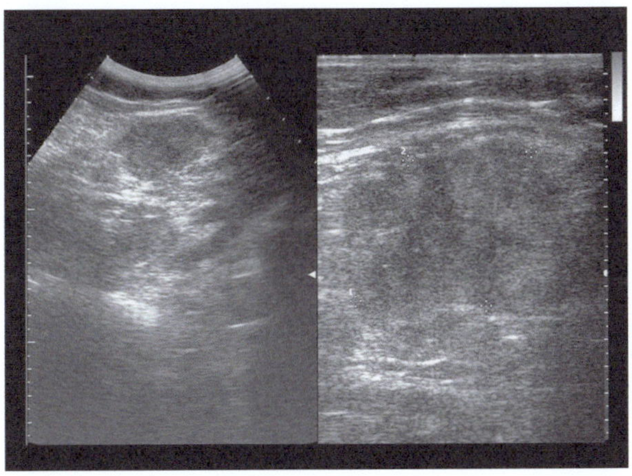

Fig. 5.211 Peritoneal metastasis from ovarian cancer. Lobulated heterogeneous hypoechoic nodule located in the right iliac fossa (*left*). The use of the superficial transducer makes possible a much more accurate definition of the echostructure of the lesion (*right*)

presence of ascites even lesions of few millimeters in size may be identified, but in the absence of this carcinosis may only be visualized in the macronodular and mass forms [30,142,143]. Evaluation of the arrangement of the **peritoneal effusion** itself can be helpful. A significant quantity in some sites and simultaneous absence in others may indicate "blocked spread", e.g. between the mesenteric folds with conglomeration of the bowel loops, and therefore indirectly suggest carcinosis. In benign ascites the loops instead float freely together with their respective mesenteric layers, with an overall "anemone" appearance [59]. Another highly suspicious sign is a corpuscular appearance of the effusion with some echoes floating in the anechoic fluid, the visualization of loculations or the presence of irregular septations [30]. The **peritoneal ligaments** distended by the fluid, such as the falciform ligament, may appear thickened or be the site of solid polypoid implants. The external surface of the loops becomes thickened and rigid. The greater omentum infiltrated by carcinosis appears as a broad heterogeneous echogenic plate (**omental cake**) and can be identified anteriorly between the abdominal wall and the bowel loops [143,144]. The mesenteric nodular infiltrations are particularly difficult to identify at US, especially when deep [141]. Hypoechoic deposits may be seen on the liver, especially on the anterior profile of the left lobe and the lateral profile of the right lobe, and less frequently on the spleen. These deposits tend to thicken the capsule, causing retraction (**scalloping**) of the organ's profile at that site. Therefore a focal undulation of the parenchymal surface should be considered suspicious. Patently cystic images with possible internal echogenic debris or calcified deposits in the peritoneum or on the parenchymal surfaces may be seen especially in metastases from ovarian cancer. In general, superficial liver metastases with no frank appearance of a capsular implant but nonetheless located peripherally with irregularity of the hepatic surface, may suggest a coexisting carcinosis, and this is regardless of whether the peritoneal colonization may have caused the hepatic lesion or vice versa. It should be borne in mind that these appearances all refer to carcinosis of a certain entity, in cases where the clinical suspicion often already exists. These findings may be particularly useful in the distinction

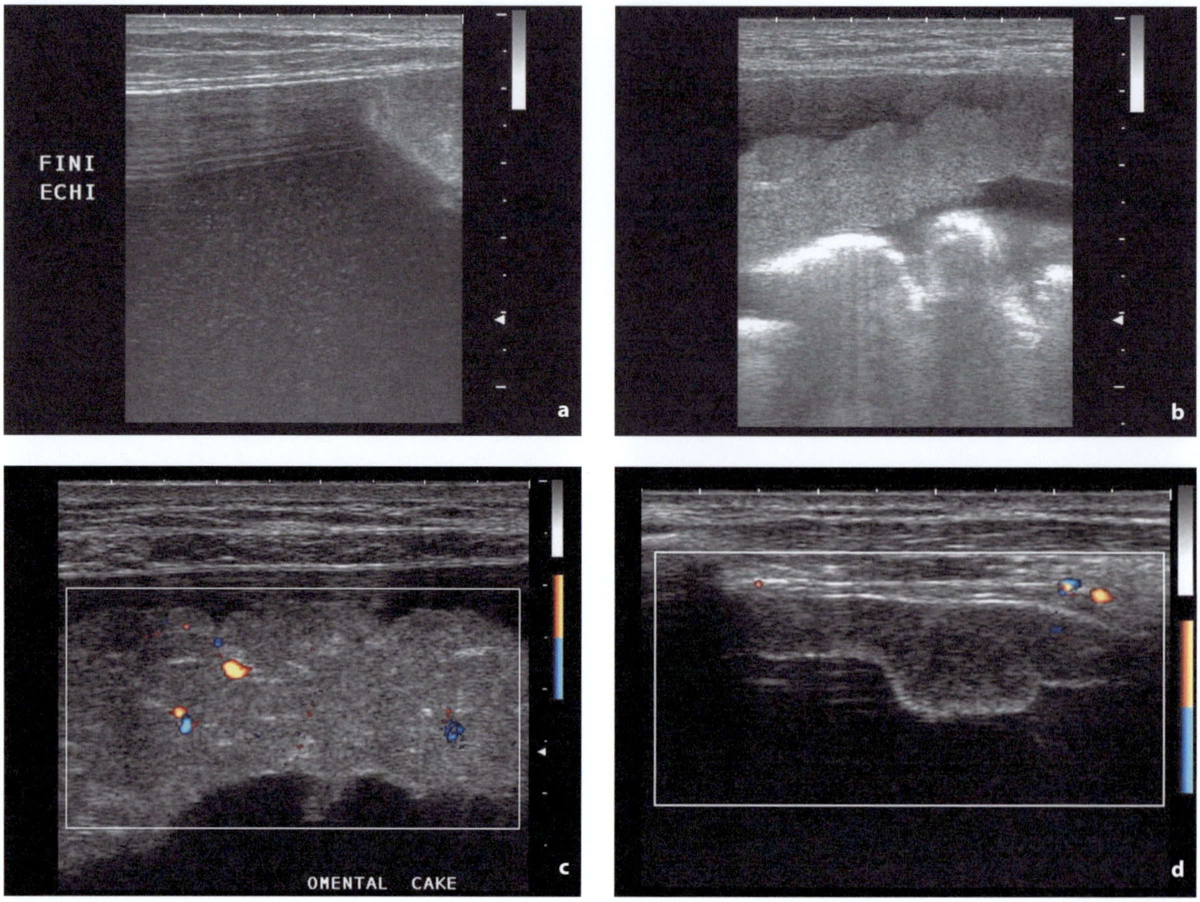

Fig. 5.212a-d Peritoneal carcinosis from ovarian cancer. Multiple signs of peritoneal involvement: finely corpuscular peritoneal effusion (**a**), marked heterogeneous hypoechoic thickening of the greater omentum (**b**) with vascular signals at directional PD (**c**), solid vascularized mural lesion (**d**)

between malignant and **benign ascites**. The finding of peritoneal effusion, especially in patients with no clear history of cancer, may be the expression of other conditions, such as chronic liver disease, congestive heart failure or renal failure. Therefore, the finding of direct signs of carcinosis enables correct characterization of the effusion [142]. Additional elements may be blocked spread of the fluid, failure to identify a state of portal hypertension or thin appearance of the gallbladder walls. In benign ascites, in fact, the gallbladder walls appear diffusely thickened due to edema, and occasionally even stratified. It should also be recalled that if the patient has a coexisting hypoalbuminemia, the gallbladder wall may appear thickened even in malignant ascites [145].

A particular form is **pseudomyxoma peritonei**, which is due to the rupture of a cystadenoma or mucinous cystadenocarcinoma of the ovary, or occasionally of the appendages. In these cases the peritoneal cavity fills with dense mucoid material and at US large fluid-filled loculations, possibly with calcified walls, scalloping of the hepatic profile and displacement of the bowel loops may be seen [146].

The **differential diagnosis** of carcinosis should take into consideration the different forms of thickening, heterogeneity or nodularity of the mesenteric-peritoneal structures, which may be produced in a generally diffuse manner as a consequence of congestion (portal hypertension), ischemia or inflammation (primary inflammation, inflammation of the appendages, diverticulitis, tubo-ovarian inflammation, etc.) (Figs. 5.217, 5.218).

US can be also be useful to guide aspiration of the peritoneal fluid for diagnostic purposes and palliative drainage of the liquid itself when diffuse, or the more extensive and symptomatic fluid sacs when locular. In

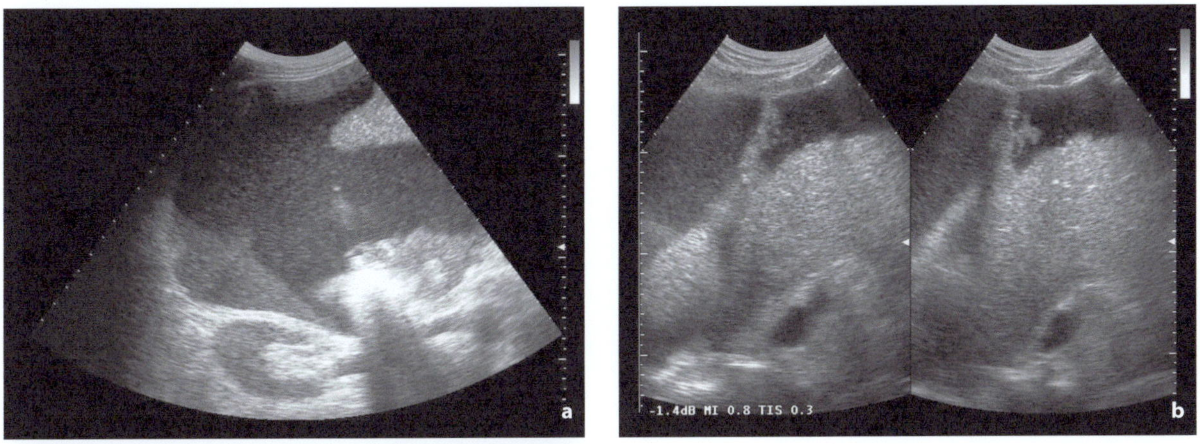

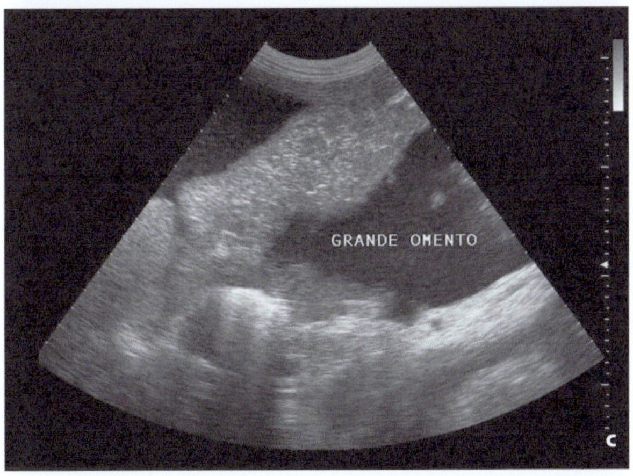

Fig. 5.213a-c Peritoneal carcinosis from colon cancer. Multiple signs of peritoneal involvement: markedly corpuscular peritoneal effusion, thicker in the dependent portions (**a**), solid polypoid lesions at the level of the falciform ligament (**b**), heterogeneous hypoechoic thickening of the greater omentum (**c**)

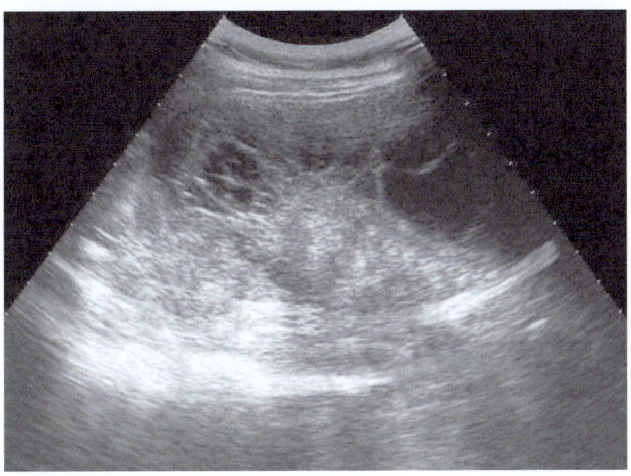

Fig. 5.214 Peritoneal carcinosis of unknown origin. Complex mass with solid deep echogenic components and multiple septations and loculations anteriorly

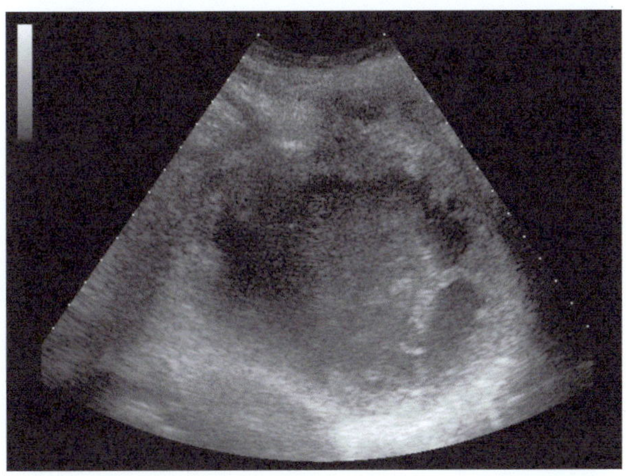

Fig. 5.215 Peritoneal carcinosis from ovarian cancer. Complex mass with numerous heterogeneous fluid-filled components

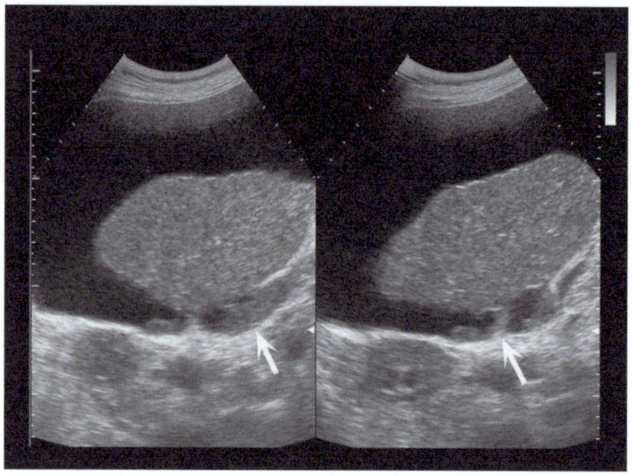

Fig. 5.216 Peritoneal carcinosis from ovarian cancer. Solid perihepatic peritoneal lesions (*arrows*). Liver appears retracted and pseudocirrhotic due to diffuse metastatic involvement

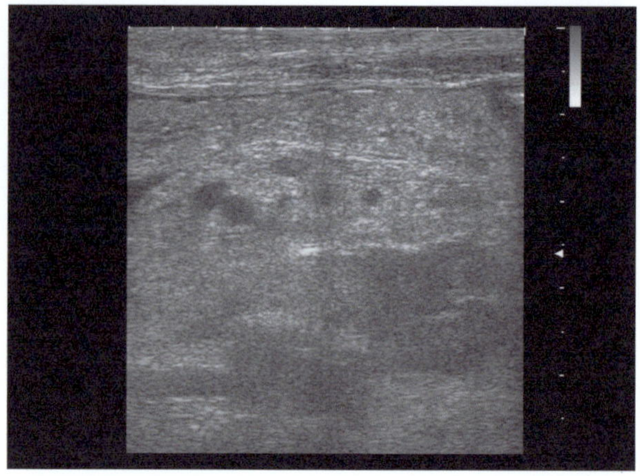

Fig. 5.217 Omental congestion mimicking carcinosis in a patient with HCC and portal thrombosis. Hyperechoic edematous appearance of the omentum with internal hypoechoic areas indicative of dilated vessels

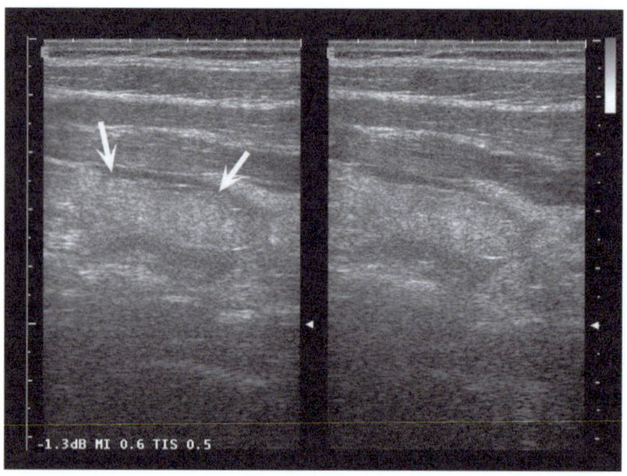

Fig. 5.218 Segmental infarction of the greater omentum mimicking carcinosis in a patient with a history of renal cell carcinoma. Hypoechoic thickening of the greater omentum with thin hypoechoic border (*arrows*)

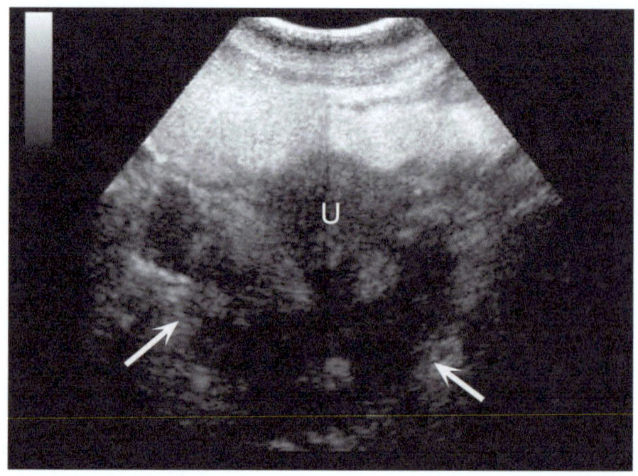

Fig. 5.219 Intraperitoneal injection of US contrast medium, which identifies "blocked diffusion" in a patient with pancreatic carcinoma. At the time of therapeutic paracentesis SonoVue is injected into the cavity which enhances the anterior pelvic spaces but is unable to reach the posterior spaces (*arrows*). *U*, uterus

addition, a study after the introduction of contrast medium into the peritoneal cavity may prove useful (Fig. 5.219). Identification of the peritoneal spaces where the contrast medium is unable to spread due to the "blocked" spread induced by carcinosis can in fact be important in centers where intraperitoneal chemotherapy is performed. It may, for example, influence the placement of intraperitoneal ports or prompt their repositioning [147].

5.10 Gastrointestinal Tract Tumors

US is without doubt not the technique of choice in the study of a suspected tumor of the gastrointestinal tract, since other modalities such as radiographic and endoscopic techniques are much more suited to the task. Nonetheless, it is not uncommon for a tumor of the alimentary tract to be identified in a subject examined with abdominal US for nonspecific symptoms, weight loss and anemia, or in an individual examined for a different indication. Even in the patient with known gastrointestinal tumor and examined with US for other reasons such as the search for liver metastases, the opportunity should be taken to explore the primary tumor, since signs of spread within the surrounding peritoneal cavity or in the lymph nodes of the stations adjacent to the lesion, and useful for treatment planning, can be identified.

With the abdominal transducer the classic appearance of tumors of the alimentary tract is the "pseudokidney", with the hypoechoic invaded intestinal wall comparable to the renal cortex and the echogenic mucosa-lumen complex comparable to the fat of the renal sinus [148] (Fig. 5.220). With use of the superficial transducer and the technique of graded compression, the lesion can be analyzed in much greater detail. The normal stratification of the digestive wall is disrupted, unlike benign mural thickening where, with the exception of advanced transmural forms of Crohn's disease, the stratification is retained or even accentuated as a consequence of preferential inflammatory involvement of one or another layer (Figs. 5.221, 5.222). The luminal surface appears irregular, with possible ulcerations that appear as loss of wall substance into which the hyperechogenicity of the luminal gas penetrates [30]. Endoscopic transducers, especially for the upper digestive tract, and transrectal transducers, for rectal tumors, are used in evaluation of the extramucosal component of the wall lesions, for the identification of lymphadenopathies and the study of the surrounding organs (Fig. 5.223, 5.224).

Carcinoma of the stomach may be located at the cardias (25% of cases) and accessible to US only in very thin subjects, at the level of the body (25%) and in the antrum (50%), which is the most accessible site to US. The lesion presents as a thickening of the gastric wall (>5 mm), being circular or asymmetric in shape with discontinuity of the normal stratification of the organ. The echogenic content of the stomach indirectly displays the luminal stenosis and displacement. The tract involved appears hypoperistaltic and little compressible with possible calcifications. Lymphadenopathies are often observed adjacent to the lesion, anterior to the gastric antrum, in the lesser omentum and with peripancreatic location (Figs. 5.225–5.228).

In **carcinoma of the duodenum** (0.3% of all malignant gastrointestinal tumors) US can be useful for the detection of the carcinoma (sensitivity 87%) as well as identification of a possible portal or caval invasion (tumors of the 2nd and 3rd part of the duodenum), a biliary obstruction (tumors of the 2nd part), lymphadenopathies, peritoneal effusion and liver metastases [149]. US is able to identify ill-defined

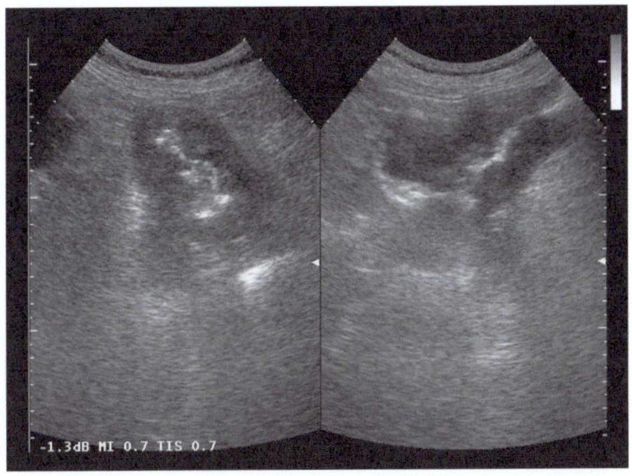

Fig. 5.220 Carcinoma of the left colic flexure, image of "pseudokidney". Marked focal wall thickening of the left colic angle with internal hyperechogenicity corresponding to luminal gas

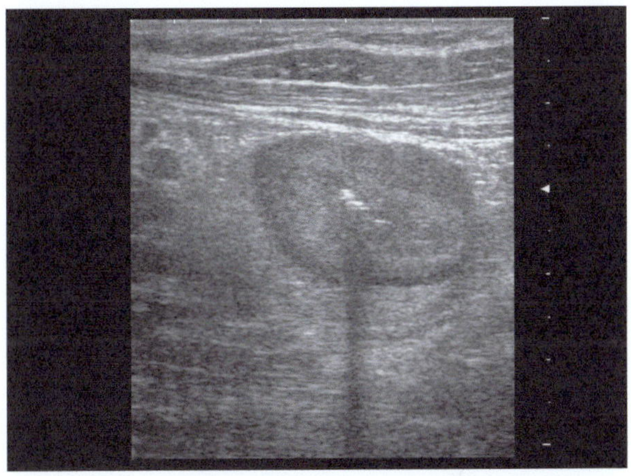

Fig. 5.221 Acute colitis. Diffuse circumferential thickening of the colon wall with conserved mural stratification

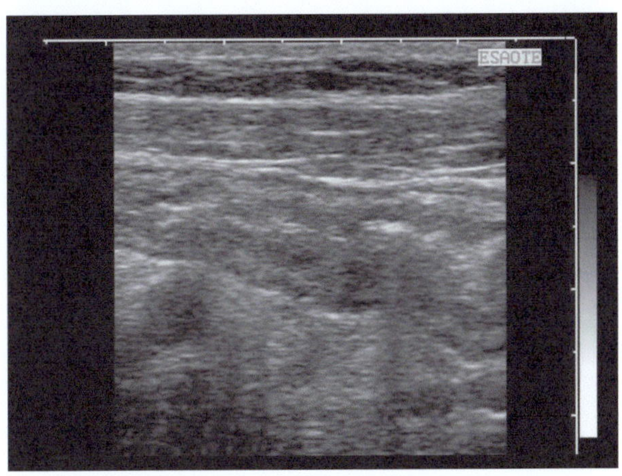

Fig. 5.222 Crohn's disease. Mild thickening of the final ileal bowel loop, particularly involving the hyperechoic submucosa, with mural stratification substantially conserved

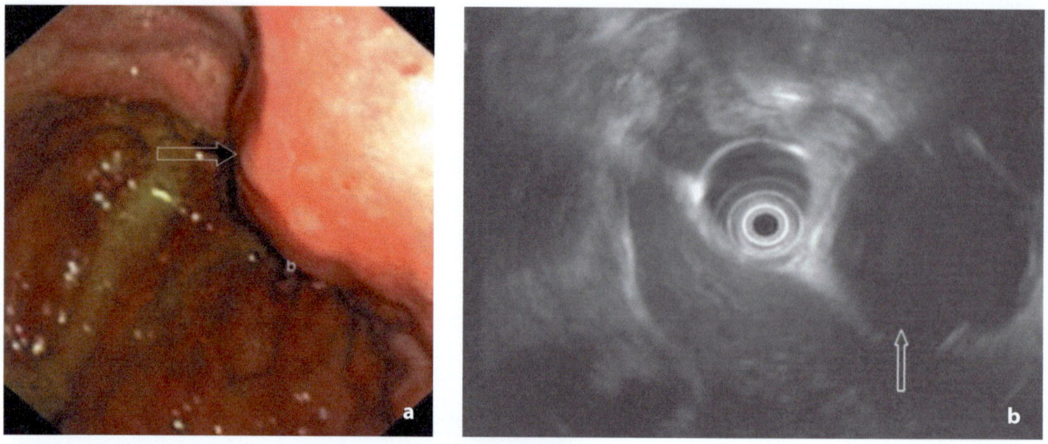

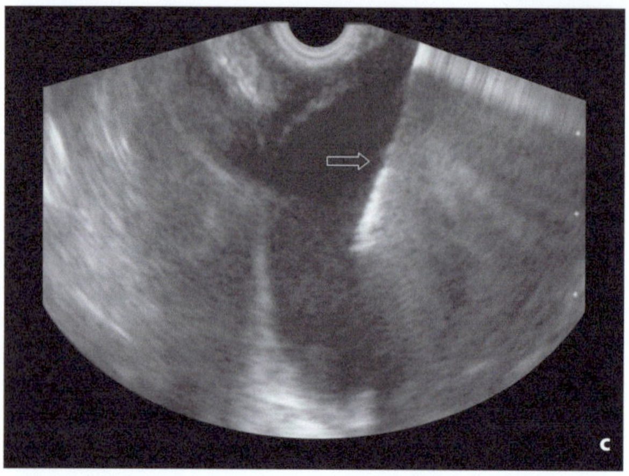

Fig. 5.223a-c Pancreatic mass causing bulging on the gastric lumen. Endoscopy: extrinsic compression of the posterior wall of the gastric antrum (**a**). Radial scan EUS (**b**) with 7.5 MHz transducer: oval hypo-anechoic area (*arrow*) of the body of the pancreas in relation to the pancreatic duct. Linear scan EUS (**c**): Transgastric FNAC of the lesion (22 G needle, *arrow*). Courtersy P. Marone, Italy

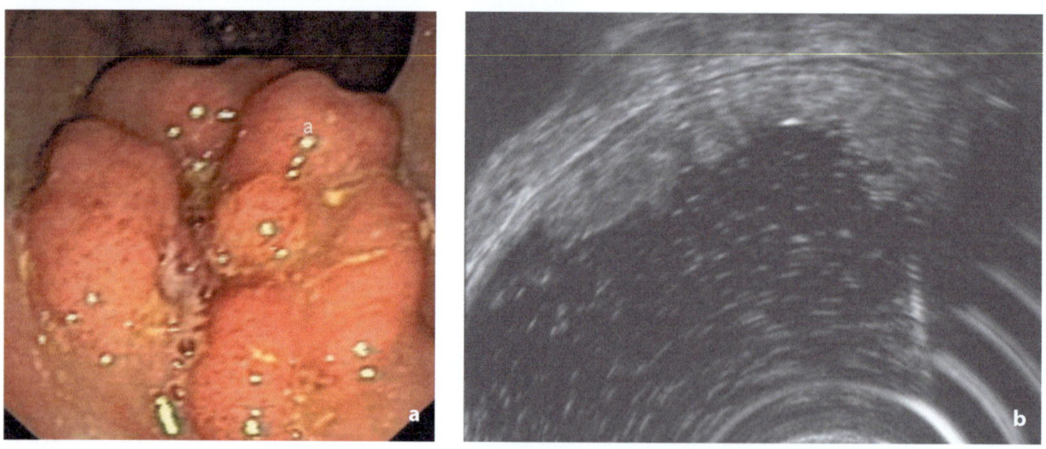

Fig. 5.224a,b Villous adenoma of the rectum with carcinomatous foci. Endoscopy (**a**): polypoid invasion of the rectum. Radial scan EUS (**b**) with multifrequency (5–20 MHz) transducer: sessile area with irregular shape and margins, mixed echogenicity, involvement of the mucosa and submucosa and integrity of the hypoechoic layer indicating the muscular propria. Courtesy P. Marone, Italy

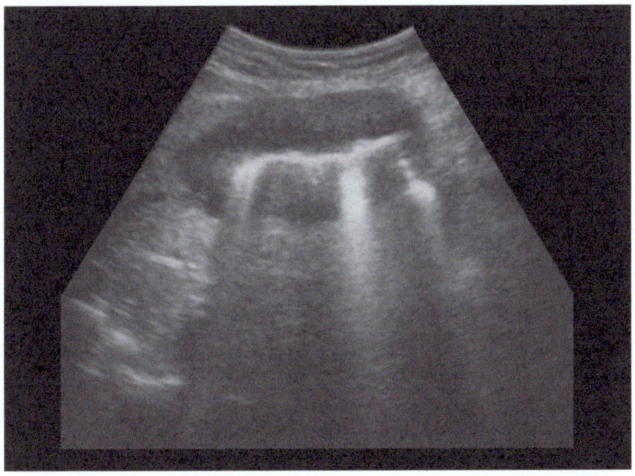

Fig. 5.225 Carcinoma of the gastric antrum. Marked diffuse hypoechoic thickening of the gastric antrum wall, with fixity of the luminal gas content

heterogeneous hypoechoic masses. Deep lesions may be difficult to identify, but in these cases even the US suspicion is important, as it prompts diagnostic work-up such as suggesting extension of the endoscopic examination to include the entire duodenum.

Adenocarcinoma of the **small bowel** is rare, with prevalence in the jejunum. The characteristic appearance is "cockade-like", with thickened walls (>3 mm), luminal stenosis, hypoperistalsis, poor compressibility and possible dilatation of the proximal bowel loops or mesenteric adenopathies. Since the stomach is well identifiable topographically and the colon can generally be followed for all or most of its length, the result is that any image of a "digestive tract tumor" not ascribable to these two portions is related to the small bowel.

Carcinoid is predominantly found in the appendix and the distal ileum (80% of cases). It appears as an

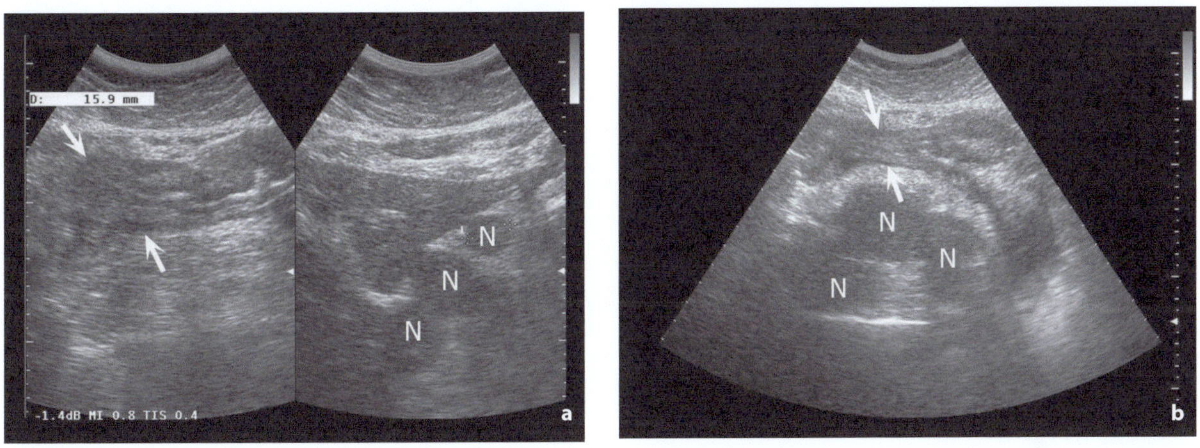

Fig. 5.226a,b Carcinoma of the gastric antrum with lymph node metastases. Thickening of the stomach wall at the level of the antrum (*arrows*) associated with multiple enlarged lymph nodes of the lesser omentum and peripancreatic chain. *N*, lymph nodes

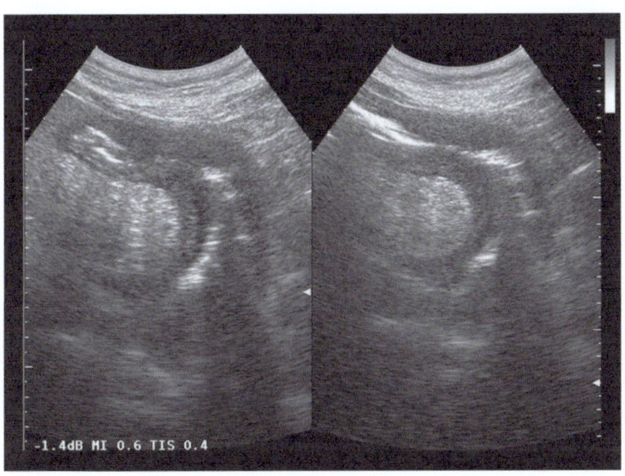

Fig. 5.227 Scirrhous gastric carcinoma. Marked and diffuse hypoechoic wall thickening of the gastric body and antrum

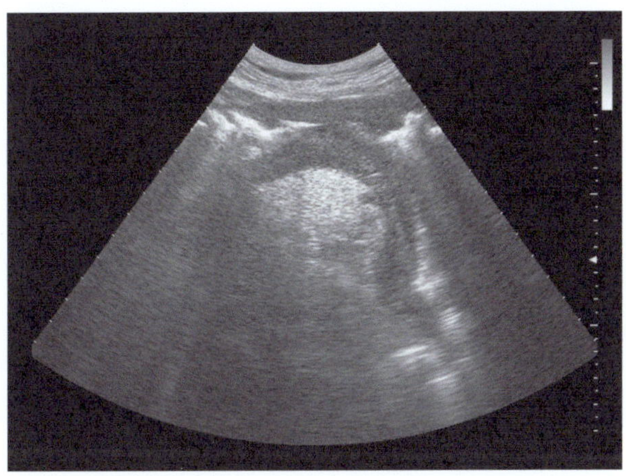

Fig. 5.228 Stomach cancer. Notable irregular thickening and loss of the normal mural stratification, at the level of the antrum, especially evident on the posterior wall

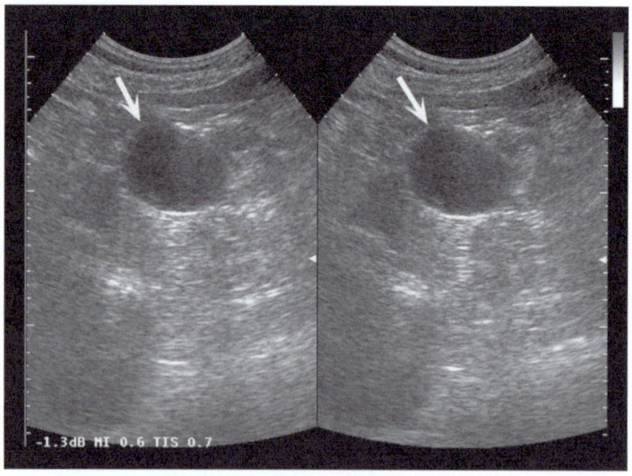

Fig. 5.229 Gastric GIST. Hypoechoic nodulation with relatively homogeneous echotexture and well-defined margins in relation to the posterior wall of the gastric antrum (*arrows*)

intraluminal hypoechoic lesion smaller in size than carcinoma, with associated invasion of the intestinal wall and metastases, especially to the liver (95% of carcinoids >2 cm) [150].

Gastrointestinal stromal tumors are prevalently found in the stomach and small bowel and appear as moderately sized heterogeneous hypoechoic masses with possible internal cavitation or frank pseudocystic appearance. The often exophytic growth of GISTs creates difficulties for differential diagnosis with other abdominal-pelvic masses, hence the need to identify its inseparability from the digestive structures. Perilesional lymphadenopathies are rare, whereas liver metastases are common (Figs. 5.229–5.232).

The alimentary tract is the most common site of primary extranodal metastasis from **lymphomas** (5–10% of adults) [134]. The stomach is most frequently involved in both primary and secondary

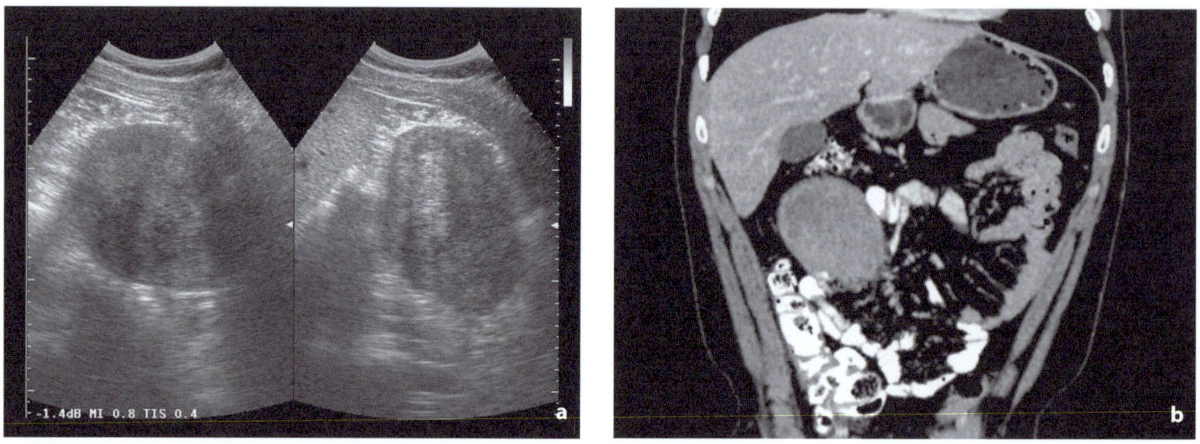

Fig. 5.230a,b Jejunal GIST. Solid, well-defined heterogeneous hypoechoic mass in subhepatic location (**a**). Coronal CT reconstruction better defines the spatial relations of the mass (**b**)

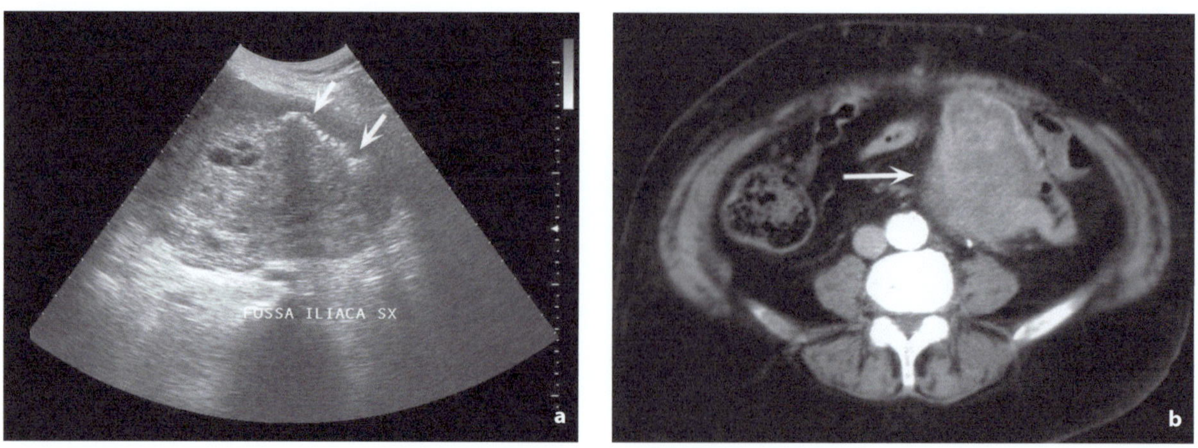

Fig. 5.231a,b Sigmoid colon GIST. Heterogeneous hypoechoic mass with necrotic-liquefactive areas (**a**), appearing eccentric with respect to the sigmoid lumen (*arrows*). CT scan (**b**) confirms the relation of the mass with the sigmoid colon (*arrow*)

forms (51% of cases), followed by the small bowel (33%) and the colon-rectum (16%). A distinction needs to be made between MALTomas, which are prevalent in the stomach, and T-cell intestinal lymphomas, which are rarer, occasionally associated with celiac disease and usually found in the ileum. The appearance is of single or multiple submucosal nodulations or masses which may degenerate with necrosis and ulceration and possibly cause thickening of the intestinal wall and/or the corresponding mesentery. In other cases the thickened wall is associated with an "aneurysmal" dilatation of the loop, a finding which is also possible in melanoma [136]. Adjacent lymphadenopathies are frequent, especially perigastric and mesenteric (Fig. 5.232).

Carcinoma of the **colon** is found in the sigmoid colon in 25% of cases, the descending colon in 5%, the transverse colon in 15% and the ascending colon/cecum in 25%. Lesions located in the left colic flexure or the rectosigmoid junction may be difficult to identify with US, whereas lesions in the ascending and sigmoid colon are relatively easy to study. Lesions located in the rectum (20%) cannot be accessed with the transabdominal approach, but only with a transrectal transducer [150]. In particular, lesions of the posterior colic wall are difficult to identify, even with adequate compression. One option for overcoming these difficulties is distension of the colic lumen with the retrograde introduction of water and possible drug-induced hypotony. This notably improves the ultrasound transmission and enables better definition of wall lesions. US shows a short segment with irregular, asymmetrically thickened, hypoechoic wall (>4 mm) with disruption of the mural stratification, luminal stenosis, fixity of the finding, poor compressibility and possible adjacent adenopathies (10% of cases) (Figs. 5.233–5.236). The pericolic fat may be mildly heterogeneous, but the absence of significant alterations is a useful element for differentiation with inflammatory processes.

Hematogenous **intestinal metastases** are predominantly found in the small bowel, especially on the antimesenteric side, and usually appear as areas of segmental thickening of the intestinal wall, with loss of normal mural stratification and peristaltic activity at the site of the lesion (Fig. 5.237). They are generally identified in a rather advanced stage, when they have become symptomatic or cause complications such as

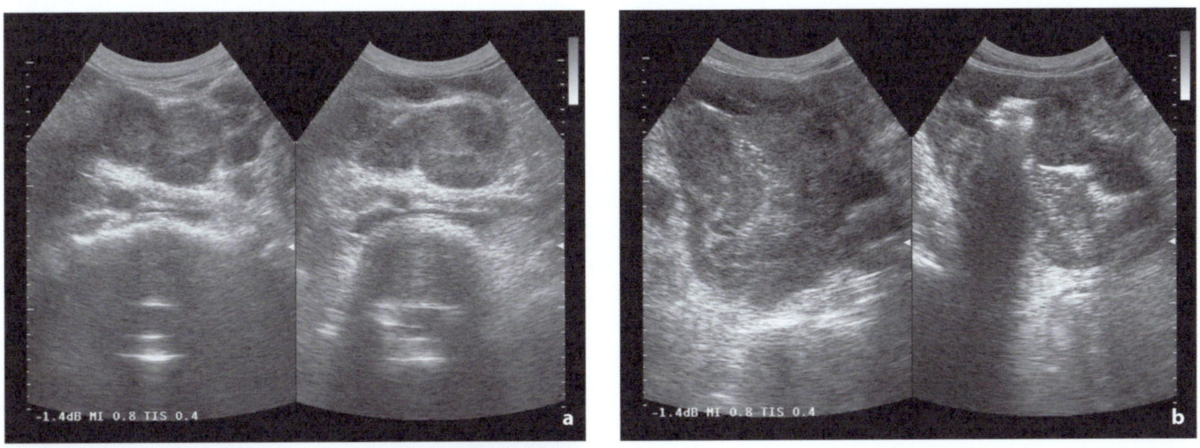

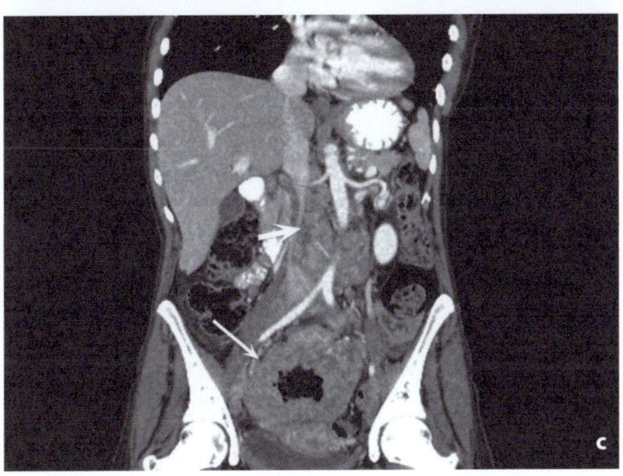

Fig. 5.232a-c Intestinal and mesenteric lymphoma. Multiple enlarged mesenteric lymph nodes (**a**) associated with dilatation of an ileal loop with diffusely thickened walls (**b**). Coronal CT reconstruction confirms both the mesenteric and retroperitoneal adenopathies (*short arrow*) and the "aneurysmal" dilatation of the ileal loop (**c**, *long arrow*)

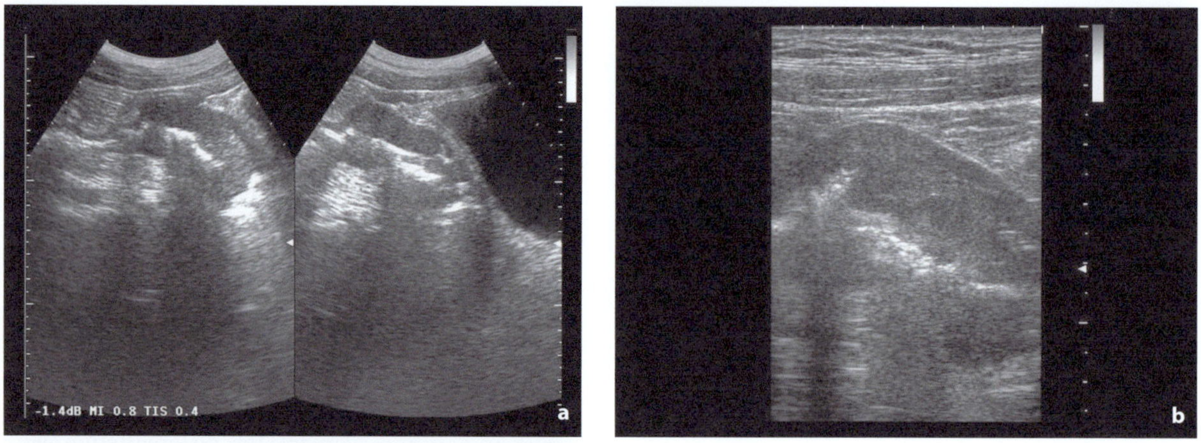

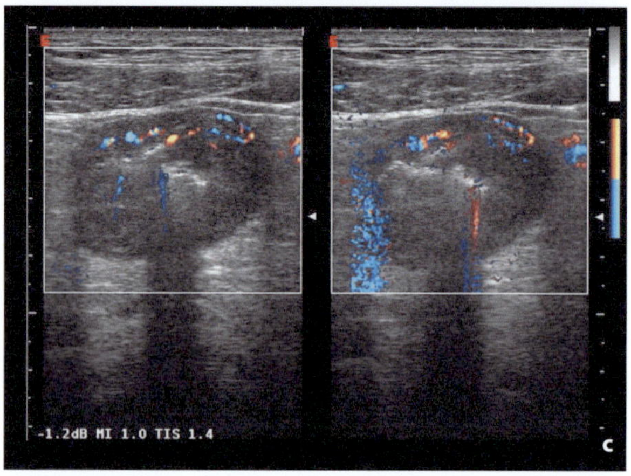

Fig. 5.233a-c Carcinoma of the sigmoid colon. The abdominal transducer is used to visualize a marked hypoechoic thickening of the sigmoid colon at the supravesical level (**a**). The use of a high-frequency transducer enables better definition of the asymmetric thickening and the absence of stratification of the colon wall (**b**). Moderate vascular signals can be distinguished at directional PD (**c**)

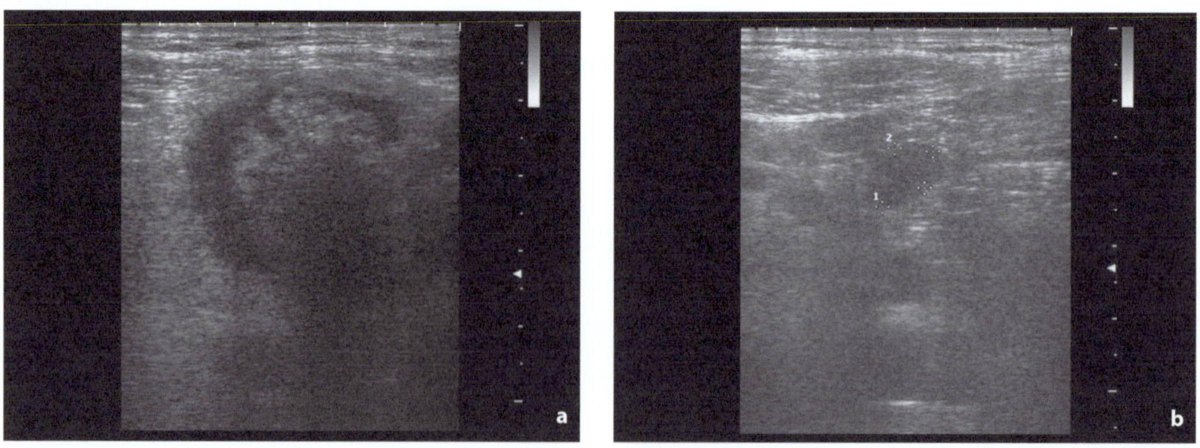

Fig. 2.234a,b Carcinoma of the sigmoid colon. The superficial transducer is able to accurately visualize the asymmetric and heterogeneous thickening of the sigmoid wall (**a**) and also reveals a paracolic lymphadenopathy (**b**, *between the calipers*)

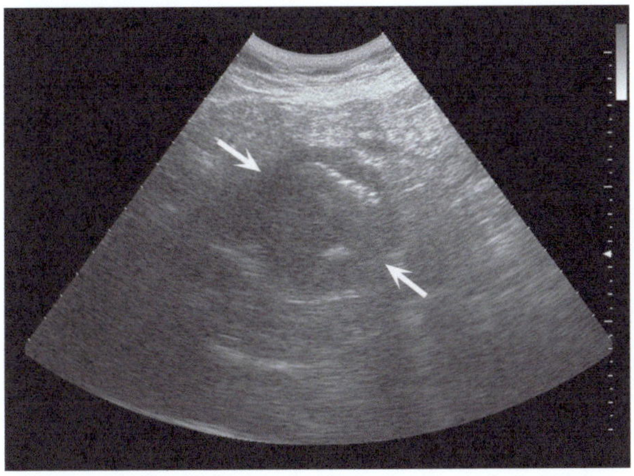

Fig. 5.235 Carcinoma of the ascending colon. Focal asymmetric hypoechoic wall thickening of the deep colic wall (*arrows*)

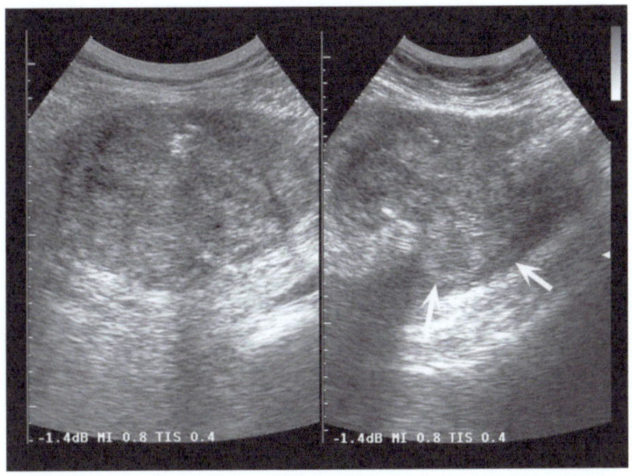

Fig. 5.236 Carcinoma of the cecum invading the psoas muscle. Marked heterogeneous thickening of the cecum with evident protrusion (*arrows*) in the setting of the psoas muscle, which appears hypoechoic to the mass

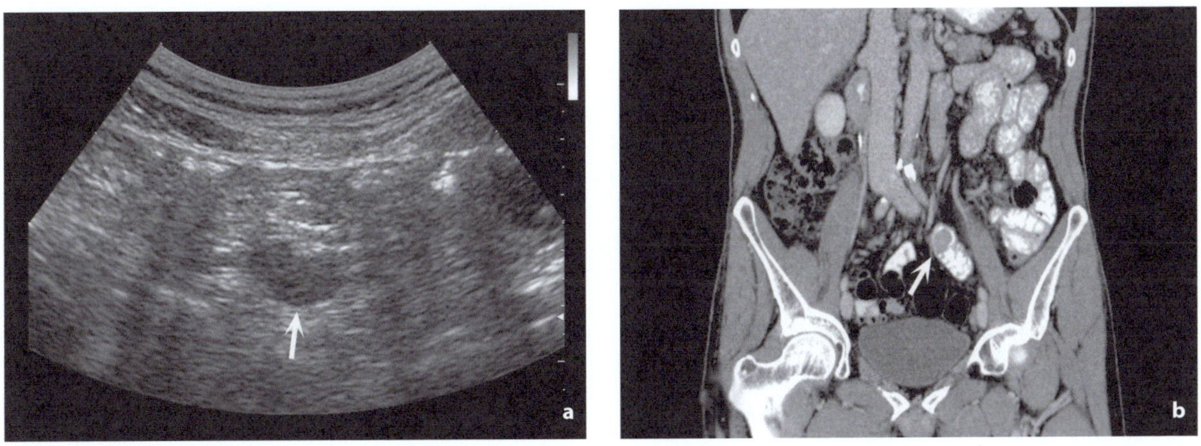

Fig. 5.237a,b Intestinal metastases from melanoma. Hypoechoic nodule in the lumen of an ileal loop (**a**, *arrow*). Correlation with coronal CT reconstruction (**b**, *arrow*)

perforation, obstruction and especially intussusception [151] (Video 5.28).

In the event a tumor causes **intestinal obstruction**, the proximal bowel loops appear dilated such that by following these the site of the obstruction can be reached. Obstruction of the small bowel is diagnosed in cases of bowel loops with a diameter >3 cm and with a length >10 cm. These bowel loops tend to display initial hyperperistalsis, with intense movements of the liquid luminal content. At a later stage the contents become increasingly dense and corpuscular and the peristalsis rather ineffective, with a characteristic pendulum-like movement (antegrade and retrograde) of the luminal material. The distal digestive tract, including the entire colon if the obstruction involves the small bowel, appears collapsed. The level of the obstruction can be defined by the topography of the dilated loops (upper left quadrant for the jejunal loops and lower quadrants for the ileal loops) and the characteristics of the intestinal folds (well represented in the jejunum and increasingly thinned in the ileum). The thickening of the intestinal folds and the presence of effusion between the loops can indicate a "decompensated" or patently complicated obstruction, with vascular suffering of the loops involved. Moreover, in the case of tumors the peritoneal effusion may be an expression of peritoneal spread [152].

References

1. DiSantis DJ et al (2000) Imaging evaluation of the palpable abdominal mass. American College of Radiology. ACR Appropriateness Criteria. Radiology 215(Suppl):201-202
2. Barker CS et al (1990) Ultrasound of the palpable abdominal mass. Clin Radiol 41:98-99
3. Haddad MC et al (2001) The gamut of abdominal and pelvic cystic masses in children. Eur Radiol 11:148-166
4. Khong PL et al (2003) Ultrasonography of intra-abdominal cystic lesions in the newborn. Clin Radiol 58:449-454
5. Wootton-Gorges SL et al (2005) Giant cystic abdominal masses in children. Pediatr Radiol 35:1277-1288
6. Spevak MR et al (2002) Ultrasonography of the adolescent female pelvis. Ultrasound Q 18:275-288
7. Sammour RN et al (2005) Decidualization of ovarian endometriosis during pregnancy mimicking malignancy. J Ultrasound Med 24:1289-1294
8. Chiang G et al (2004) Imaging of adnexal masses in pregnancy. J Ultrasound Med 23:805-819
9. Lucey BC et al (2007) Spontaneous hemoperitoneum: a bloody mess. Emerg Radiol 14:65-75
10. Yunoki et al (1999) Intraperitoneal seeding of ruptured hepatocellular carcinoma: case report. Abdom Imaging 24:398-400
11. Casillas VJ et al (2000) Imaging of nontraumatic hemorrhagic hepatic lesions. Radiographics 20:367-378
12. Chen ZY et al (2002) Etiology and management of hemorrhage in spontaneous liver rupture: a report of 70 cases. World J Gastroenterol 8:1063-1066
13. Hertzberg BS et al (1999) Ovarian cyst rupture causing hemoperitoneum: imaging findings and potential for misdiagnosis. Abdom Imaging 24:304-308
14. Hora M et al (2004) Rupture of papillary renal cell carcinoma. Scand J Urol Nephrol 38:481-484
15. Yip KH et al (1998) Spontaneous rupture of renal tumours: the role of imaging in diagnosis and management. Br J Radiol 71:146-154
16. Yamakado K et al (2002) Renal angiomyolipoma: relationship between tumor size, aneurysm formation, and rupture. Radiology 225:78-82
17. Belloir A et al (1983) Ultrasonographic study of retroperitoneal and abdominopelvic hematomas. J Radiol 64:621-625
18. Lotterman S (2008) Massive hemoperitoneum resulting from spontaneous rupture of uterine leiomyoma. Am J Emerg Med 26:974
19. Ishida H et al (1998) Sonographic and color Doppler findings of rupture of liver tumors. Abdom Imaging 23:587-591
20. Mortele KJ et al (2003) Spontaneous intraperitoneal hemorrhage: imaging features. Radiol Clin North Am 41:1183-1201
21. Jeffrey RB et al (1982) Echogenic clot: a useful sign of pelvic hemoperitoneum. Radiology 145:139-141
22. Mahlke R et al (1995) Acute abdominal pain in chronic pancreatitis: hemorrhage from a pseudoaneurysm? Z Gastroenterol 33:404-407
23. Catalano O et al (2005) Real-time, contrast-enhanced sonography: a new tool for detecting active bleeding. J Trauma 59:933-939
24. Catalano O et al (2006) Active abdominal bleeding: contrast-enhanced sonography. Abdom Imaging 31:9-16
25. Auslender R et al (2002) Coiling of the ovarian vessels: a color Doppler sign for adnexal torsion without strangulation. Ultrasound Obstet Gynecol 20:96-97
26. Scoutt LM et al (2007) Imaging of adnexal torsion. Ultrasound Clin North Am 2:311-325
27. Vijayaraghavan SB (2004) Sonographic whirlpool sign in ovarian torsion. J Ultrasound Med 23:1643-1649
28. Albayram F et al (2001) Ovarian and adnexal torsion. Spectrum of sonographic findings with pathologic correlation. J Ultrasound Med 20:1083-1089
29. Choi J (2006) Imaging of hepatic metastases. Cancer Contr 13:6-12
30. Jeffrey RB et al (1995) Sonography of the abdomen. Raven Press, New York
31. Kopljar M et al (2004) Nature of Doppler perfusion index changes in patients with colorectal cancer liver metastases. J Ultrasound Med 23:1295-1300
32. Leen E et al (1993) Early detection of occult colorectal metastases using duplex colour Doppler sonography. Br J Surg 80:1249-1251
33. Öktar SO et al (2006) Doppler sonographic evaluation of hemodynamic changes in colorectal liver metastases relative to liver size. J Ultrasound Med 25:575-582
34. Leen E et al (1996) Prognostic power of Doppler perfusion index in colorectal cancer. Correlation with survival. Ann Surg 223:199-203
35. Leen E et al (2000) Potential role of Doppler perfusion index in selection of patients with colorectal cancer for adjuvant chemotherapy. Lancet 355:34-37
36. Gultekin S et al (2006) The role of late-phase pulse inversion harmonic imaging in the detection of occult hepatic metastases. J Ultrasound Med 25:1139-1145
37. Oldenburg A et al (2005) Detection of hepatic metastases with low MI real time contrast enhanced sonography and SonoVue. Ultraschall Med 26:277-284
38. Blomley MJ et al (1998) Liver vascular transit time analyzed with dynamic hepatic venography with bolus injections of a US contrast agent: early experience in seven patients with metastases. Radiology 209:862-866
39. Clayton RAE et al (2003) Incidence of benign pathology in patients undergoing hepatic resection for suspected malignancy. Surgeon 1:32-38
40. Tchelepi H et al (2004) Ultrasound of the focal liver masses. Ultrasound Q 20:155-169
41. Jones EC et al (1992) The frequency and significance of small hepatic lesions (less than or equal to 15 mm) detected by CT. AJR Am J Roentgenol 158:535-539
42. Schwartz LH et al (1999) Prevalence and importance of small hepatic lesions found at CT in patients with cancer. Radiology 210:71-74
43. Brick SH et al (1987) The mistaken or indeterminate CT diagnosis of hepatic metastases: the value of sonography. AJR Am J Roentgenol 148:723-726
44. Eberhardt SC et al (2003) Utility of sonography for small hepatic lesions found on computed tomography in patients with cancer. J Ultrasound Med 22:335-343
45. Middleton WD et al (1997) Small (1.5 cm or less) liver metastases: US-guided biopsy. Radiology 205:729-732
46. Yu SCH et al (2001) US-guided percutaneous biopsy of small (1-cm) hepatic lesions. Radiology 218:195-199
47. Robinson PJA (2004) The liver. In: Husband JE et al (eds) Imaging in oncology, II Edition. Taylor & Francis, London, 1059-1084
48. Della Vigna P et al (2007) Contrast-enhanced ultrasonog-

raphy in the follow-up of patients with hepatic metastases from breast carcinoma. Radiol Med 112:47-55
49. Wernecke K et al (1992) The distinction between benign and malignant tumors on sonography: value of hypoechoic halo. AJR Am J Roentgenol 159:1005-1009
50. Cosgrove DO (2001) Malignant liver disease. In: Meire H et al (eds) Abdominal and general ultrasound, II Edition. Churchill Livingstone, London, 209-233
51. Nino-Murcia et al (1992) Color Doppler characterization of focal hepatic lesions. AJR Am J Roentgenol 159:1195-1197
52. Tanaka S et al (1990) Color-Doppler imaging of liver tumors. AJR Am J Roentgenol 154:509-514
53. Catalano O et al (2005) Real-time harmonic contrast material-specific US of focal liver lesions. Radiographics 25:333-349
54. Lassau N et al (2006) Gastrointestinal stromal tumors treated with Imatinib: monitoring response with contrast-enhanced sonography. AJR Am J Roentgenol 187:1267-1273
55. De Giorgi U et al (2005) Effect of angiosonography to monitor response during Imatinib treatment in patients with metastatic gastrointestinal stromal tumors. Clin Cancer Res 11:6171-6176
56. Delorme S et al (2006) Contrast-enhanced ultrasound for examining tumor biology. Cancer Imaging 6:148-152
57. Krix M (2005) Quantification of enhancement in contrast ultrasound: a tool for monitoring of therapies in liver metastases. Eur Radiol 15(Suppl 5):104-108
58. Piscaglia F et al (2003) Liver metastases from rectal carcinoma: disease progression during chemotherapy despite loss of arterial-phase hypervascularity on real-time contrast-enhanced harmonic sonography at low acoustic energy. J Clin Ultrasound 31:387-391
59. Schmidt G (2006) Differential diagnosis in ultrasound imaging. Georg Thieme Verlag, Stuttgart
60. Moody AR et al (1993) Atypical hepatic hemangioma: a suggestive sonographic morphology. Radiology 188:413-417
61. Wachsberg RH et al (1999) Duplex Doppler sonography of small (<3 cm diameter) liver tumours: intralesional arterial flow does not exclude cavernous hemangioma. Clin Radiol 54:103-106
62. Kim KA et al (2006) Unusual mesenchymal liver tumors in adults: radiologic-pathologic correlation. AJR Am J Roentgenol 187:W481-W489
63. Smith SL et al (2001) Cystic mesenchymal hamartoma mimicking hepatic hydatid disease. Clin Radiol 56:599-601
64. Markhardt BK et al (2006) Sonographic features of biliary hamartomas with histopathologic correlation. J Ultrasound Med 25:1631-1633
65. Uggowitzer M et al (1997) Power Doppler imaging and evaluation of the resistive index in focal nodular hyperplasia of the liver. Abdom Imaging 22:268-273
66. Lizardi-Cervera J et al (2006) Focal nodular hyperplasia and hepatic adenoma: a review. Ann Hepatol 5:206-211
67. Hung C-H et al (2001) Sonographic features of hepatic adenomas with pathologic correlation. Abdom Imaging 26:500-506
68. Clounet M et al (1999) Imaging features of nodular regenerative hyperplasia of the liver mimicking hepatic metastases. Abdom Imaging 24:258-261
69. Aytaç S et al (1999) Focal intrahepatic extramedullary hematopoiesis: color Doppler US and CT findings. Abdom Imaging 24:366-368
70. Yoo et al (2003) Focal eosinophilic infiltration in the liver: radiologic findings and clinical course. Abdom Imging 28:326-332
71. Catalano O et al (2004) Low mechanical index contrast-enhanced sonographic findings of pyogenic hepatic abscesses. AJR Am J Roentgenol 182:447-450
72. Castroagudín JF et al (2007) Sonographic features of liver involvement by lymphoma. J Ultrasound Med 26:791-796
73. Siniluoto T et al (1991) Ultrasonography of spleen and liver in staging Hodgkin's disease. Eur J Radiol 13:181-186
74. Konno K et al (2001) Liver tumors in fatty liver: difficulty in ultrasonographic interpretation. Abdom Imaging 26:487-491
75. Catalano O et al (2007) Transient hepatic echogenicity difference on contrast-enhanced ultrasonography. Sonographic sign and pitfall. J Ultrasound Med 26:337-345
76. Johnson DB et al (2000) Hepatic sonography. In: Shirkhoda A (ed) Variants and pitfalls in body imaging. Lippincott Williams & Wilkins, Philadelphia, 233-246
77. Bruix J et al (2005) Management of hepatocellular carcinoma. Hepatology 42:1208-1236
78. Kanematsu M et al (1999) Small hepatic nodules in cirrhosis: ultrasonographic, CT, and MR imaging findings. Abdom Imaging 24:47-55
79. Bruix J et al (2001) Clinical management of hepatocellular carcinoma. Conclusions of the Barcelona-2000 EASL conference. European Association for the Study of the Liver. J Hepatol 35:4214-30
80. Kim MJ et al (2003) Correlation between the echogenicity of dysplastic nodules and their histopathologically determined fat content. J Ultrasound Med 22:237-334
81. Bennett GL et al (2002) Sonographic detection of hepatocellular carcinoma and dysplastic nodules in cirrhosis: correlation of pretransplantation sonography and liver explant pathology in 200 patients. AJR Am J Roentgenol 179:75-80
82. Colombo M (2005) Natural history of hepatocellular carcinoma. Cancer Imaging 5:85-88
83. Caturelli E et al (2001) Hemangioma-like lesions in patients with chronic liver disease: differential diagnosis. Radiology 220:337-342
84. Ghittoni G et al (2004) Hyperechoic focal liver lesions in patients with hepatic cirrhosis. Giorn It Ecogr 7:209-214
85. Liu WC et al (2003) Poor sensitivity of sonography in detection of hepatocellular carcinoma in advanced liver cirrhosis: accuracy of pretransplantation sonography in 118 patients. Eur Radiol 13:1693-1698
86. Maruyama H et al (2000) Enhanced color flow images in small hepatocellular carcinoma. Abdom Imaging 25:164-171
87. Kubota K et al (2000) Evaluation of the intratumoral vasculature of hepatocellular carcinoma by power Doppler sonography: advantages and disadvantages versus conventional color Doppler sonography. Abdom Imaging 25:172-178
88. Catalano O et al (2004) Hepatocellular carcinoma: spectrum of contrast-enhanced gray-scale harmonic sonography findings. Abdom Imaging 29:341-347
89. Llovet JM et al (2001) Increased risk of tumour seeding after percutaneous radiofrequency ablation of a single hepatocellular carcinoma. Hepatology 33:1336-1337
90. Gandolfi L et al (2003) The role of ultrasound in biliary and pancreatic disease. Eur J Ultrasound 16:141-159
91. Komatsuda T et al (2000) Gallbladder carcinoma: color Doppler sonography. Abdom Imaging 25:194-197
92. Azuma T et al (2001) Differential diagnosis of polypoid lesions of the gallbladder by endoscopic ultrasonography. Am J Surg 181:65-70

93. Xu H-X et al (2003) Comparison of three- and two-dimensional sonography in diagnosis of gallbladder diseases. J Ultrasound Med 22:181-191
94. Weiner SN et al (1984) Sonography and computed tomography in the diagnosis of carcinoma of the gallbladder. AJR Am J Roentgenol 142:735-739
95. Wittekind CH et al (2005) TNM atlas. Springer-Verlag Berlin
96. Bressler EL et al (1987) Sonographic parallel channel sign: a reappraisal. Radiology 151:343-346
97. Wing VW et al (1985) Sonographic differentiation of enlarged hepatic arteries from dilated intrahepatic bile ducts. AJR Am J Roentgenol 145:57-61
98. Darweesh RMA et al (1988) Fatty-meal sonography for evaluating patients with suspected partial common duct obstruction. AJR Am J Roentgenol 151:63-68
99. Jeffrey RB (2004) Pancreatic malignancy. In: Husband JE et al (eds) Imaging in oncology, II Edition. Taylor & Francis, London, 325-341
100. Angeli E et al (1997) Color-Doppler imaging in the assessment of vascular involvement by pancreatic carcinoma. AJR Am J Roentgenol 168:193-197
101. Midwinter MJ et al (1999) Correlation between spiral computed tomography, endoscopic ultrasonography and findings at operation in pancreatic and ampullary tumors. Br J Surg 86:189-193
102. Calculli L et al (2002) The usefulness of spiral computed tomography and colour-Doppler ultrasonography to predict portal-mesenteric trunk involvement in pancreatic cancer. Radiol Med 104:307-315
103. Scialpi M et al (2005) Pancreatic carcinoma versus chronic focal pancreatitis: contrast-enhanced power Doppler ultrasonography findings. Abdom Imaging 30:222-227
104. Saftoiu A et al (2006) Power Doppler endoscopic ultrasonography for the differential diagnosis between pancreatic cancer and pseudotumoral chronic pancreatitis. J Ultrasound Med 25:363-372
105. Ozawa Y et al (2002) Contrast-enhanced sonography of small pancreatic mass lesions. J Ultrasound Med 21:983-991
106. Chang KJ et al (1997) The clinical utility of ultrasound-guided fine-needle aspiration in the diagnosis and staging of pancreatic carcinoma. Gastrointest Endosc 45:387-393
107. Solmi L et al (1992) Comparison between echo-guided fine-needle aspiration cytology and microhistology in diagnosing pancreatic masses. Surg Endosc 6:222-224
108. Francis IR (2003) Cystic pancreatic neoplasms. Cancer Imaging 3:111-116
109. D'Onofrio M et al (2007) Comparison of contrast-enhanced sonography and MRI in displaying anatomic features of cystic pancreatic masses. AJR Am J Roentgenol 189:1435-1442
110. Demos TC et al (2002) Cystic lesions of the pancreas. AJR Am J Roentgenol 179:1375-1386
111. Prasad SR et al (2003) Intraductal papillary mucinous tumors of the pancreas. Abdom imaging 28:357-365
112. Procacci C et al (1996) Intraductal mucin-producing tumors of the pancreas: imaging findings. Radiology 198:249-257
113. Buetow PC et al (1997) Islet cell tumors of the pancreas: clinical, radiologic and pathologic correlation in diagnosis and localization. Radiographics 17:453-472
114. D'Onofrio M et al (2003) Contrast-enhanced ultrasonographic detection of small pancreatic insulinoma. J Ultrasound Med 22:413-417
115. Ueno N et al (1996) Utility of endoscopic ultrasonography with color Doppler function for the diagnosis of islet cell tumor. Am J Gastroenterol 91:772-776
116. Anderson MA et al (2000) Endoscopic ultrasound is highly accurate and directs management in patients with neuroendocrine tumors of the pancreas. Am J Gastroenterol 95:2271-2277
117. Galiber AK et al (1988) Localization of pancreatic insulinoma: comparison of pre- and intraoperative US with CT and angiography. Radiology 166:405-408
118. Merkle EM et al (2000) Imaging findings in pancreatic lymphoma. AJR Am J Roentgenol 174:671-675
119. Sato M et al (2001) Pancreatic metastasis: sonographic findings. Abdom Imaging 26:72-75
120. Görg C et al (1991) Splenic lesions: sonographic patterns, follow-up, differential diagnosis. Eur J Radiol 13:59-66
121. Görg C et al (1991) Sonography of focal lesions of the spleen. AJR Am J Roentgenol 156:949-953
122. Komatsuda T et al (1999) Splenic lymphangioma: US and CT diagnosis and clinical manifestations. Abdom Imaging 24:414-417
123. Catalano O et al (2006) Contrast-enhanced sonography of the spleen. Semin Ultrasound CT and MRI 27:426-433
124. Bhatt S et al (2006) Gamma-Gandy bodies. Sonographic features with histopathologic correlation. J Ultrasound Med 25:1625-1629
125. Robertson F et al (2001) Radiology of the spleen. Eur Radiol 11:80-95
126. Görg C et al (1994) Color Doppler imaging of focal splenic masses. Eur J Radiol 18:214-219
127. Duddy MJ et al (1989) Cystic hemangioma of the spleen: findings on ultrasound and computed tomography. Br J Radiol 62:180-182
128. Görg C et al (1997) Malignant splenic lymphoma: sonographic patterns, diagnosis and follow-up. Clin Radiol 52: 535-540
129. Shirkhoda A et al (1990) Lymphoma of the solid abdominal viscera. Radiol Clin North Am 28:785-799
130. Görg C (2001) The spleen. In: Meire H et al (eds) Abdominal and general ultrasound, II Edition. Churchill Livingstone, London, 379-445
131. Smeets AJ et al (1990) Evaluation of abdominal lymph nodes by ultrasound. J Ultrasound Med 9:325-331
132. Fisher AJ et al (1997) Small lymph nodes of the abdomen, pelvis and retroperitoneum: usefulness of sonographically guided biopsy. Radiology 205:185-190
133. Carrington BM (2004) Lymph node metastases. In: Husband JE et al (eds) Imaging in oncology, II Edition. Taylor & Francis, London, 999-1022
134. Reznek RH et al (2004) Lymphoma. In: Husband JE et al (eds) Imaging in oncology, II Edition. Taylor & Francis, London, 817-874
135. Wojnar J et al (1992) Sonography in the diagnosis and therapy monitoring of lymphomas. Neoplasma 39:261-266
136. Bragg DG et al (2002) Hodgkin's disease, lymphomas, and the lymphoproliferative disorders. In: Bragg DG et al (eds) Oncologic imaging. WB Saunders Company, Philadelphia, 629-645
137. Gimondo P et al (1996) Abdominal lymphadenopathy in

benign diseases: sonographic detection and clinical significance. J Ultrasound Med 15:353-359
138. Konno K et al (1998) Color Doppler findings in Castleman's disease of the mesentery. J Clin Ultrasound 26:474-478
139. Cassani F et al (1990) Prevalence and significance of abdominal lymphadenopathy in patients with chronic liver disease: an ultrasound study. J Clin Gastroenterol 12:42-46
140. Soresi M et al (2003) Ultrasound detection of abdominal lymph nodes in chronic liver diseases. A retrospective analysis. Clin Radiol 58:372-377
141. Healy JC et al (2004) Peritoneal metastases. In: Husband JE et al (eds) Imaging in oncology, II Edition. Taylor & Francis, London, 1125-1138
142. Görg C et al (1991) Malignant ascites: sonographic signs of peritoneal carcinomatosis. Eur J Cancer 27:720-723
143. Yeh HC (1979) Ultrasonography of peritoneal tumors. Radiology 133:419-424
144. Derchi LE et al (1987) Normal anatomy and pathologic changes of the small bowel mesentery: US appearance. Radiology 164:649-652
145. Huang Y-S (1989) Utility of sonographic gallbladder wall patterns in differentiating malignant from cirrhotic ascites. J Clin Ultrasound 17:187-192
146. Lersch C et al (2001) Gray-scale sonographic findings in a patient with pseudomyxoma peritonei. J Clin Ultrasound 29:186-191
147. Puls R et al (2003) Intraperitoneal distribution of ultrasound contrast medium imaged with B-mode ultrasound and colour-stimulated acoustic emission imaging. Eur Radiol 13:695-699
148. Bluth EI et al (1979) Ultrasonic evaluation of the stomach, small bowel, and colon. Radiology 133:677-680
149. Ishida H et al (2001) Duodenal carcinoma: sonographic findings. Abdom Imaging 26:469-473
150. Kala Z et al (2007) A shift in the diagnostic of the small intestine tumors. Eur J Radiol 62:160-165
151. Ledermann HP et al (2001) Diagnosis of symptomatic intestinal metastases using transabdominal sonography and sonographically guided puncture. AJR Am J Roentgenol 176:155-158
152. Di Mizio R et al (1995) Uncompensated small bowel obstruction in adults. Ultrasonographic findings of free fluid between loops and its prognostic value. Radiol Med 89:787-791

The Urogenital Tract 6

6.1 Adrenal Masses

US evaluation of the **adrenal glands** requires that particular attention be paid to the scan technique, possibly involving a painstaking study to find the best approach to the organs. This is particularly true in the assessment of subjects who are obese and/or have intestinal gas. US is unable to explore all of the adrenal gland, nor in all cases, especially on the left, it is always able to visualize or at least rule out significant enlargement of the glands. In cases initially studied with US and persistent suspicion of hyperplasia despite a negative US finding, work-up with CT or MR is advisable. US can also be used as an alternative to CT in the percutaneous biopsy of adrenal masses (after pharmacologic prophylaxis in the suspicion of pheochromocytoma) and also in PEI of adenomas.

The **right adrenal gland** can be better examined than its counterpart. Excellent visualization can be achieved with the subject in the right anterior oblique position or prone, and by exploiting the liver as an acoustic window. In thinner subjects the evaluation can be performed with an anterior, transversal approach with the patient supine. The upper renal pole and the inferior vena cava constitute useful anatomic landmarks. The **left adrenal gland** is more difficult to study due to the presence of intragastric gas, the narrower splenic acoustic window and the limited availability of anatomic landmarks. The gland may be visualized with the patient in the left anterior oblique position or prone using the spleen as an acoustic window and with scans from the midaxillary line to the anterior axillary line. In thin subjects the visualization of the left adrenal gland may be achieved with the patient supine after having distended the stomach with water. The primary anatomic landmark is provided by the upper pole of the kidney, and secondarily by the tail of the pancreas [1].

The adrenal glands can be studied with imaging modalities when they are responsible for an **endocrine disorder** leading to primary or secondary hypersecretion of their hormones or a hypofunction caused by enzyme deficit or other conditions which lead to a reduction in hormone production. Cushing's syndrome, with the suppression of ACTH due to a hypersecretion of cortisol, can be caused by a adrenal adenoma or more rarely by a bilateral hyperplasia or a carcinoma (20–30% of cases of adrenal Cushing's syndrome in adults). Conn's syndrome is characterized by a hypersecretion of aldosterone and may result from an adenoma (generally <2 cm) or a bilateral hyperplasia and only exceptionally (2% of cases) from a carcinoma. The hypersecretion of catecholamine is present in pheochromocytoma, which can be bilateral in 10% of cases. In all of these forms the diagnostic hypothesis is based on clinical and laboratory findings, and the imaging evaluation is done with CT/MR.

Lesions of the adrenal glands **without endocrine function** include nonfunctioning adenomas and carcinomas, myelolipomas, cysts and rare forms (ganglioneuroma, lymphoma, hematoma, granulomatosis). In addition, these glands are a rather common site of hematogenous metastases and their evaluation is a part of the staging and follow-up of a number of tumors, particularly of the lung. With the increasingly widespread diffusion of tomographic imaging modalities, the incidental finding of adrenal masses in asymptomatic cancer and non-cancer patients has become a less than rare event. When a lesion <4–5 cm is identified in a patient with no history of extraadrenal tumor, a complete evaluation of the adrenal hormone profile needs to be done. Hyperfunctioning lesions are treated, whereas non-hyperfunctioning lesions are subject to follow-up for the subsequent 18 months (with US if accessible) and if the size stabilizes they are labeled as nonfunctioning adenomas and no longer monitored. Lesions >4–5 cm are generally indicated for surgical treatment, unless the appearance is patently adipose. In fact biopsy has limited accuracy (54–86%), in excluding a primary carcinoma, the probability of which is 6% for adrenal lesions between 4 cm and 6 cm, but 25% for masses >6 cm. The patient with a synchronous or prior extra-adrenal tumor is a more complicated case. The incidental finding of an adrenal mass not associated with an endocrine disorder has a likelihood of 32–72% of being metastatic and therefore should be evaluated with a targeted CT or PET study. In the event these examinations are suspicious or equivocal, biopsy may be done, whereas the non-suspicious forms are indicated for monitoring with US or CT [2,3].

US can provide a good visualization of **adrenal masses** and has a relative possibility of characterizing them. The positive predictive value is without doubt greater than the negative predictive value and if in doubt, other imaging and/or nuclear medicine modalities should always be used. Only a thorough technique is able to visualize the adrenal glands with a sufficiently high degree of reproducibility and safety, while bearing in mind that in the adult US is not the technique of choice, a role which is played primarily by CT (or alternatively MR) [4]. However, US is the first technique used in the suspicion of a disease of the upper abdomen, and it should also be borne in mind that adrenal disease may be present even in the absence of specific symptoms. For example, a metastasis may be found during a US evaluation of liver metastases, or a primary adrenal tumor may be discovered during an abdominal or renal examination done for another indication. In the presence of the clinical suspicion of a adrenal endocrine disorder, the diagnosis should first be confirmed with specific hormone assays and then the disease should be investigated with imaging, rather than directly proceeding with diagnostic work-up. A similar consideration is valid for patients with arterial hypertension in whom excluding a secondary nature of the condition is desirable.

Cystic lesions of the adrenal glands are rather infrequent, generally asymptomatic and of limited intrinsic diagnostic interest. Over half of the cases are congenital (lymphangioma) or degenerative (pseudocysts). Alternatively, cystic lesions can originate from hemorrhage in an adenoma or another necrotic adrenal tumor such as pheochromocytoma or neuroblastoma [5,6]. It is not unusual for metastases to undergo cystic degeneration. The lesions present a typical cystic appearance: rounded/oval mass, anechoic with thin and well-defined walls and enhanced through-transmission. The cysts may display an internal anechoic or finely corpuscular content, with thin or thick walls and the possible presence of wall calcifications (ranging from isolated calcifications to a circumferential calcified rim) or even thin internal septations [5]. However, the distinction between a large adrenal cyst and an exophytic cyst of the upper renal pole can often be challenging. In cases of cysts formed from neoplastic degeneration, a solid component is often present or at least an irregularity in the walls. All cases where the appearance is not that of a simple cyst should be investigated further or undergo percutaneous aspiration, otherwise no additional diagnostic work-up or monitoring over time is required.

An adrenal **hyperplasia** may be asymptomatic or manifest with signs of glandular insufficiency, such as Cushing's syndrome, adrenogenital syndrome or Conn's syndrome. Cushing's syndrome and Cushing's disease are characterized by a diffuse enlargement of the adrenal glands bilaterally, but with the integrity of the glandular structure and morphology maintained. The appearance is of well-defined hypoechoic masses. Diffuse adrenal enlargement occurs in tuberculosis, histoplasmosis and other infectious diseases. In these cases the glands appear diffusely and symmetrically enlarged, with rounded contours and often with increased echogenicity. Most cases of hyperaldosteronism (Conn's syndrome) are characterized by bilateral adrenal hyperplasia, often accompanied by subcentimeter hyperplastic nodules which cannot always be identified with US (Fig. 6.1).

An **adenoma** with a diameter <2.5 cm is found at postmortem in 2–9% of individuals and is generally nonfunctioning. The frequency in clinical practice is much lower. In general, the finding of an adrenal adenoma is completely incidental, during a US study done for other reasons. Around half of the patients who present symptoms of hyperaldosteronism have an adenoma which is usually unilateral and small in size

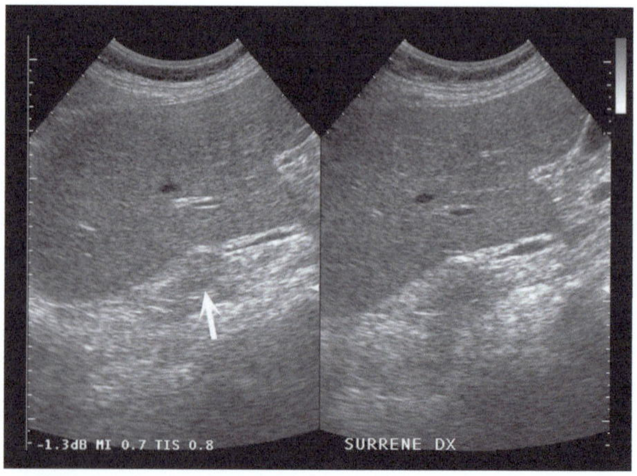

Fig. 6.1 Adrenal hyperplasia. Vaguely nodular and minimal thickening of the right adrenal gland (*arrow*)

(2–2.5 cm). Around half of these cases are due to bilateral hyperplasia. The appearance is of a well-defined hypoechoic mass. When the solitary adenoma is small, it can be difficult if not impossible to differentiate from a hyperplastic nodule. In general hyperplastic nodules are multiple, whereas a functioning adenoma is associated with atrophy of the contralateral adrenal gland (Fig. 6.2).

Adrenal **carcinoma** is a tumor with a high grade of malignancy and poor prognosis, in part because in 70% of cases it is diagnosed in stage III/IV. It is rare (0.05–0.2% of all malignancies), occasionally familial and has a peak incidence between the 4th and 7th decade of life, although it also occurs in early childhood. Functioning tumors (59%) are more common among women, whereas nonfunctioning tumors (41%) are more frequently found in men [7]. The size of the tumors varies considerably, from 3 to 22 cm in diameter, and are often rather large at presentation, especially if nonfunctioning. The distinction between adenoma and carcinoma is challenging and may even be difficult histologically. In 50% of cases adrenal carcinoma is hyperfunctioning and tends to be large. It can calcify and undergo cystic degeneration. It appears as a heterogeneous mass with hypoechoic necrotic components of variable size and amorphous calcifications. The appearance of small carcinomas (2–6 cm) is of a homogeneous mass with moderate echogenicity, whereas larger masses tend to have an anechoic central focus due to necrosis or hemorrhage. Calcifications are present in 19% of cases. The tumor tends to invade the adrenal and renal veins to then reach the inferior vena cava, and then the right atrium. This venous invasion occurs in 10% of cases and can be studied with CD. Sites of frequent metastasization and which are accessible to US include the liver, lymph nodes, retroperitoneum and peritoneal cavity.

Myelolipoma is a non-rare benign tumor containing blood vessels, adipose tissue and cellular elements of the bone marrow in variable proportions. The lesion is generally unilateral and may be microscopic or even reach 30 cm. Myelolipomas are generally asymptomatic, but the onset of hemorrhage in the setting of tumor can cause flank pain. The prevalently adipose forms are easier to characterize and appear as echogenic or prevalently echogenic masses in the adrenal space. A greater presence of myelomatous tissue can produce an appearance of hypo-anechoic areas within the lesion, with hemorrhagic phenomena causing the formation of hypo-anechoic foci. Calcified nuclei may create punctate echogenic images, but often these calcifications are too small to be identified with US. A small myelolipoma may be concealed by the perirenal fat, while an accumulation of this fat or an exophytic angiomyolipoma of the upper renal pole can mimic an adrenal myelolipoma [8] (Fig. 6.3, Video 6.1).

Pheochromocytoma arises from the adrenal medulla in 90% of cases and from extra-adrenal structures (paravertebral sympathetic ganglia or bladder wall) in the remaining 10%. This rare, slow-growing tumor shows a predilection for adults (4th–6th decade of life) although it may also occur in childhood. It may be a part of MEN: in this case the tumor is present from infancy, is often multicentric and generally has a low grade of malignancy. The secretion of catecholamine (adrenalin and noradrenalin) by this tumor causes tachycardia, headache and arterial hypertension and can be demonstrated with urinalysis. Pheochromocytoma is malignant in 5–13% of cases, especially if located in an extra-adrenal site. The

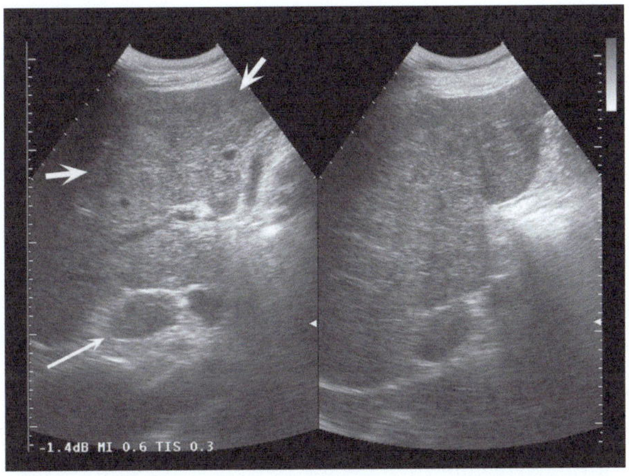

Fig. 6.2 Adrenal adenoma in patient with liver metastasis from pulmonary carcinoma. Hypoechoic mass of the right adrenal gland (*long arrow*) associated with hypoechoic hepatic invasion (*short arrows*)

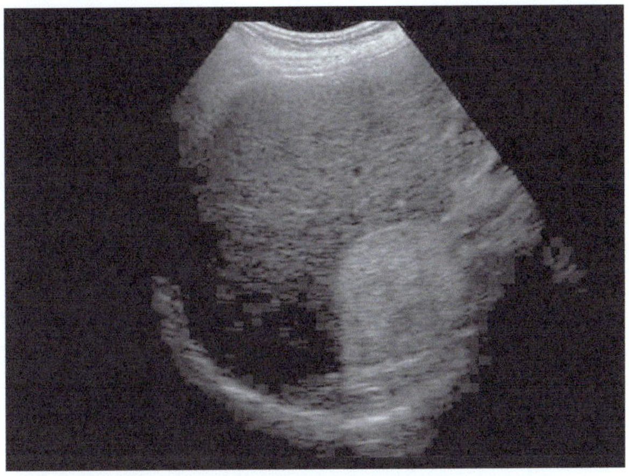

Fig. 6.3 Adrenal myelolipoma. Relatively well-defined and homogeneous hyperechoic mass of the right adrenal gland

invasion of adjacent tissue is not an indication of malignancy, whereas the development of lymphadenopathies and (liver) metastasis is. In 10% of cases, especially in children, pheochromocytoma is multicentric and in 5% of cases bilateral. The US study has a high degree of sensitivity, with a presentation not dissimilar from that of carcinoma. The tumor tends to be large (mean 5–6 cm) with a generally homogeneous hypoechoic appearance and relatively well-defined margins. Hemorrhage or necrosis cause the formation at the center of the mass of a hypo-anechoic area or bestow upon the lesion a "complex" appearance. Pheochromocytoma can be wholly cystic and present fluid-fluid levels or give rise to calcifications [7].

Neuroblastoma is the most common childhood extracranial solid tumor, with a peak incidence in the first five years of life and occasionally appearing as functionally active [9,10]. Although it may be located anywhere along the chains of the sympathetic network – from the neck to the pelvis – it tends to show a predilection for the abdomen (2/3 of cases) and especially the adrenal glands (50–75% of cases). Some cases are diagnosed in the prenatal period, thanks to US identification of the mass in the adrenal space. For the purposes of diagnosis more weight should be given to the age of the subject than the US appearance of the lesion, since this may vary considerably although there is a tendency towards hyperechogenicity [11]. The mass may be prevalently adrenal or paravertebral and display a heterogeneous echotexture due to the presence of hypo-anechoic necrotic-hemorrhagic areas, cystic-like spaces and calcified echogenic foci [10]. Particularly significant is the presence of calcifications in the neoplasm, which appear as hyperechoic nuclei possibly accompanied by posterior acoustic shadowing. The most typical cases in fact present as heterogeneous mass with medium-to-large calcified inclusions [9,11]. CD demonstrates moderate vascularity with peripheral, central or diffuse distribution. Important criteria for staging include the spread or not of disease beyond the median line, lymph node involvement, local extension (adjacent organs, vessels, lumbar muscles, vertebral canal, etc.) and liver metastasization. The differential diagnosis includes nephroblastoma, another high-frequency pediatric neoplasm. The rare cystic variant which is particularly found in neonates needs to be differentiated from other adrenal and peri-adrenal cystic masses. The larger forms which markedly compress the liver also need to be distinguished from hepatic masses, particularly hepatoblastoma [9]. In the presence of a mass with the abovementioned characteristic, a thoraco-abdominal CT and bone scintigraphy are indicated.

Adrenal **metastases** are very common, being the fourth most frequent site of tumor spread after the lung, liver and bone. Lung cancer is the most common primary (30–40% of cases in metastasis), followed by the less frequent cancers of the stomach, breast, kidney and pancreas, or also melanoma. It should, however, be borne in mind that some ACTH-secreting tumors can cause a non-metastatic adrenal hyperplasia. In addition, in 50% of cases the metastatic involvement is bilateral such that a mass in both adrenal glands in no way constitutes a differential criterion with respect to hyperplasia and adenoma. The metastases manifest in the form of masses with a maximum mean diameter of 3.5 cm, partly because those that are <2 cm are difficult to identify at US. The appearance of the metastases is not absolutely specific – the echogenicity can vary, although in most cases hypoechogenicity prevails. The lesions are generally rounded or oval in shape and limited in size. The larger masses generally present heterogeneous areas of necrosis or hemorrhage and occasionally have a cystic-like appearance, especially in the center of the lesion. Calcifications are rare. When associated with metastases in other sites, e.g. in the liver, no further diagnostic work-up is required. If the enlargement of the gland is instead isolated and unilateral, the presence of a nonfunctioning adenoma should first be ruled out: the notable size (90–95% of lesions >3 cm are malignant) and/or heterogeneous echotexture are suggestive of metastasis, although US and CD are often insufficient, and additional studies with CT or MR, FNAC or short-term follow-up are required [12] (Figs. 6.4–6.10).

Primary adrenal **lymphoma** is rare, whereas secondary adrenal involvement is common and generally bilateral. Non Hodgkin's lymphomas are generally responsible for the involvement, which can be diffuse, giving rise to hyperplasia, or be characterized by a mass. Retroperitoneal lymphadenopathies or involvement of other abdominal organs are often present. The generally hypoechoic appearance is nonspecific, although it may also appear anechoic and mimic a cystic mass. Lymphomatous masses may even present as echogenic. In this case the appearance of one adrenal gland is different from the contralateral gland (Fig. 6.11).

The diaphragmatic pillars can be the cause of **interpretation errors**, as they can be mistaken for the adrenal gland [13]. A similar consideration holds on the right with the inferior vena cava, which in transverse images can mimic an enlarged adrenal gland. In addition a nodular adrenal gland may be poorly distinguishable from the internal hepatic profile and therefore may pass unrecognized, while an exophytic hepatic lesion can mimic an adrenal lesion. In addition to simple hyperplasia or small nodular masses, false negatives of US for adrenal nodulations may be due to the presence of more significant adrenal enlargements

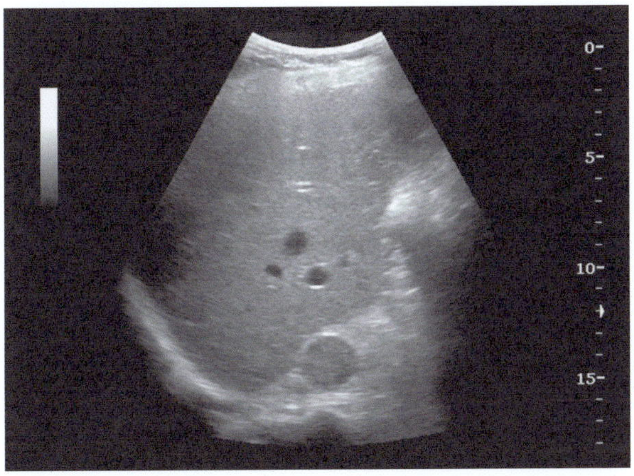

Fig. 6.4 Adrenal metastasis from pulmonary adenocarcinoma. Small rounded nodule with relatively homogeneous echotexture and well-defined margins of the right adrenal gland

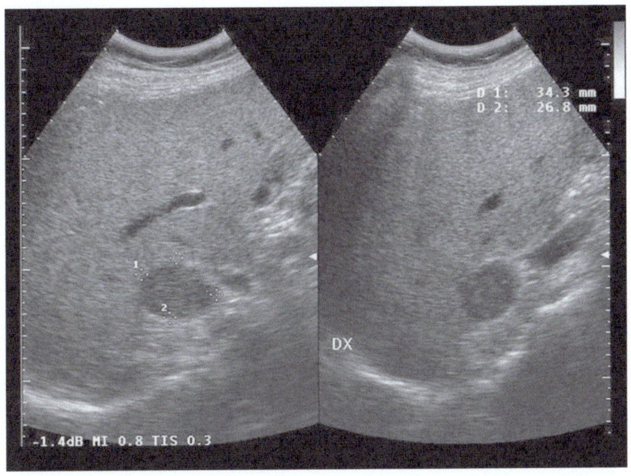

Fig. 6.5 Adrenal metastasis from melanoma. Clearly hypoechoic nodule of the left adrenal gland

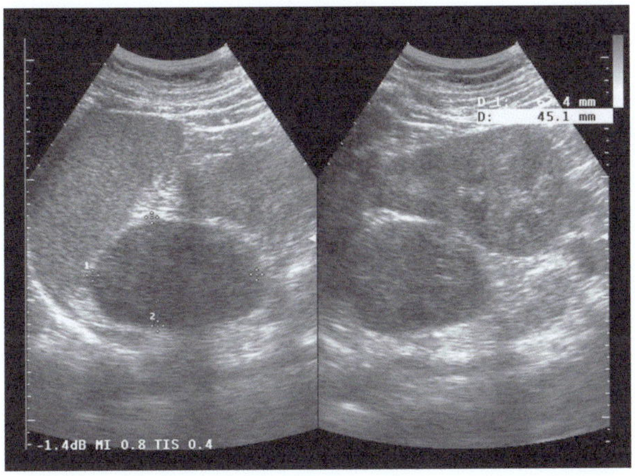

Fig. 6.6 Adrenal metastasis from melanoma. Clearly hypoechoic nodule of the left adrenal gland

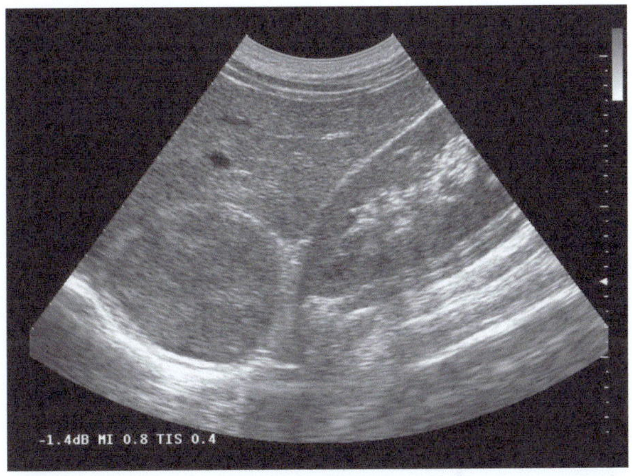

Fig. 6.7 Adrenal metastasis from melanoma. Well-defined heterogeneous hypoechoic mass of the right adrenal gland

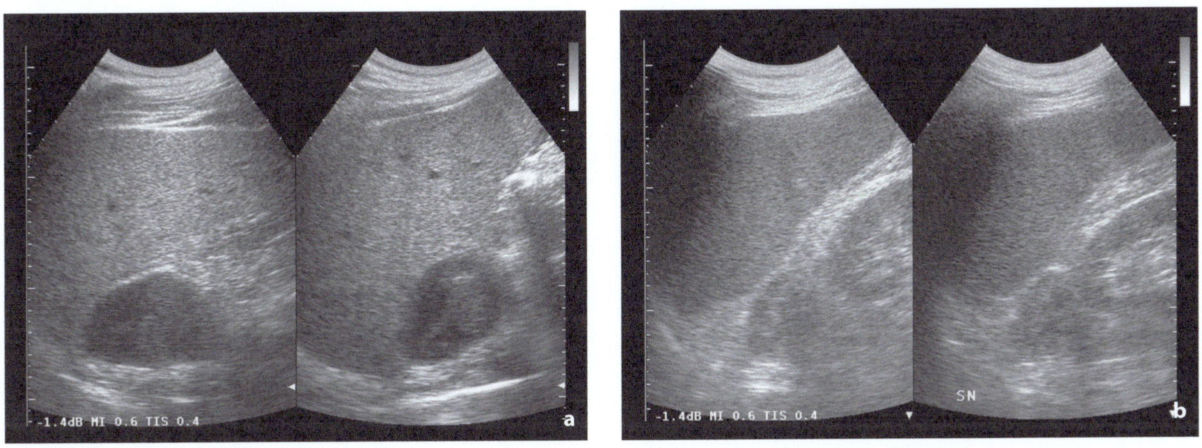

Fig. 6.8a,b Bilateral adrenal metastasis. Large mass of the adrenal glands, with well-defined margins and hypoechoic appearance on the right (a) and on the left (b)

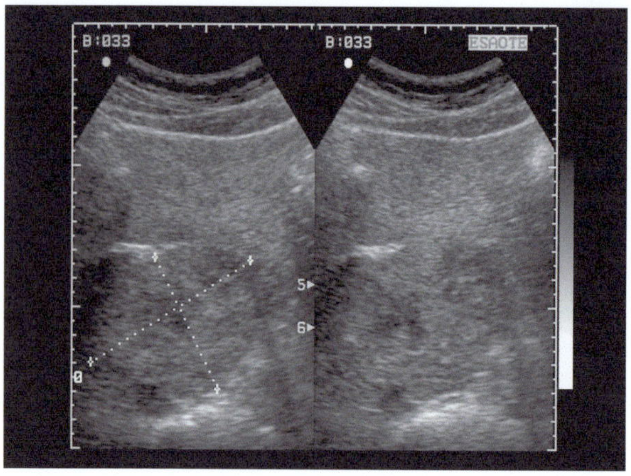

Fig. 6.9 Adrenal metastasis from pulmonary microcytoma. Heterogeneous hypoechoic mass of the right adrenal gland

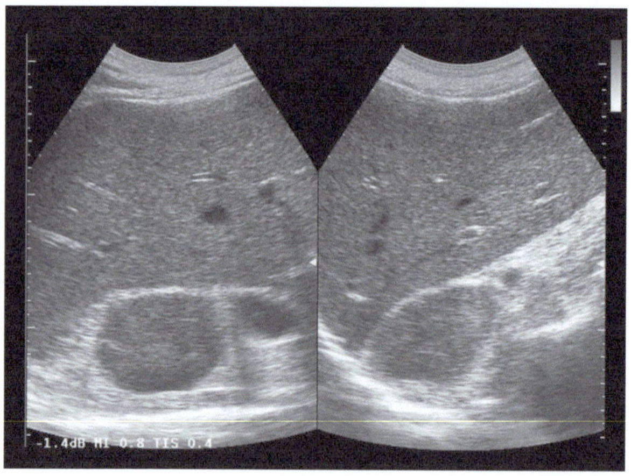

Fig. 6.11 Adrenal lymphoma. Relatively well-defined and homogeneous hypoechoic nodule of the right adrenal gland

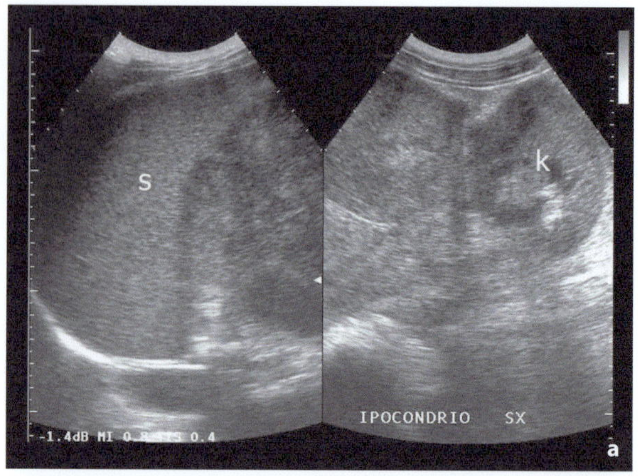

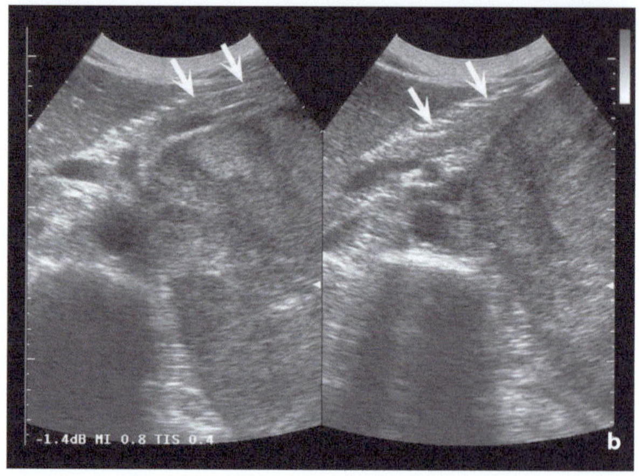

Fig. 6.10a,b Adrenal metastasis from melanoma. Large heterogeneous hypoechoic mass extending from the left adrenal gland can be seen in contact with the spleen (*s*) and the left kidney (*k*) as well as markedly displacing the pancreas and the splenic vein (*arrows*). The latter finding demonstrates the retroperitoneal origin of the lesion

which, due to their echogenicity, are difficult to differentiate from the surrounding retroperitoneal adipose tissue. With regard to larger adrenal masses US often has difficulty in defining the organ of origin, such that from this point of view CT and MR are more panoramic and accurate [14].

6.2 Small Renal Tumors

A **small renal tumor** is defined as an expansive lesion of the kidney with a diameter <3 cm. This size creates particular difficulties for their identification and characterization which are generally absent in larger tumors. First of all there is the need to be certain that there effectively is an expansive lesion in the site where US demonstrates a morphostructural anomaly, by differentiating it from other events such as pseudotumors. Secondly, there is the need to characterize the lesion by making the fundamental distinction between carcinoma and other typologies and in particular angiomyolipoma, which is the most common alternative.

The "**mimickers" of renal tumors** include first and foremost the hyperechoic pseudonodules which simulate a small echogenic carcinoma or a small angiomyolipoma. Congenital (junctional) or acquired (e.g. after enucleation of cysts or nodules) cortical defects, occupied by echogenic retroperitoneal fat, can be characterized because the former are in communication with the echogenic renal hilum, whereas the latter are correlated with a history of prior surgery. Occasionally even adipose components of the renal sinus protrude locally into the deep cortex, thus also mimicking an echogenic nodule [15,16]. Hematomas and arteriovenous fistulas can mimic solid hypoechoic lesions. There are other anatomic variants which can have the appearance of a pseudotumor. A lobar dysmorphism appears as a deep and well-defined nodulation isoechoic to the cortex, and may be associated with a hypertrophic hypoechoic pyramid, thus mimicking an endophytic lesion. However, CD shows segmental and interlobar branches which originate external to the "lesion" and run to its sides up to the corticomedullary junction and possibly with the arcuate arteries within the dysmorphic area. Persistent fetal lobulations and dromedary hump kidney manifest as irregularities in the renal contour, which can simulate an isoechoic focal lesion bulging from the renal cortex, especially on the left midrenal external contour. However, CD is useful in this case too, demonstrating vascular structures in the suspicious area similar to those of adjacent areas [16]. CD with contrast medium may prove useful in the characterization of suspected pseudomasses [17]. Lastly, the CEUS study may prove useful in ruling out a focal lesion by demonstrating the constant isoechogenicity (isovascularity) of the presumed focal lesion with respect to the surrounding parenchyma (Figs. 6.12, 6.13).

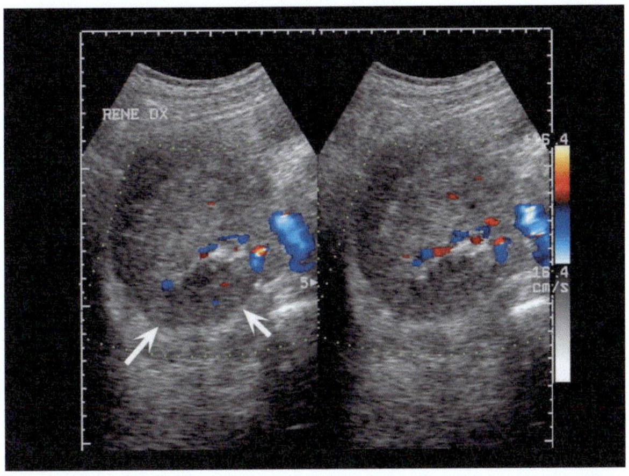

Fig. 6.12 Focal nephritis. Heterogeneous hypoechoic focus appearing hypovascular at CD (*arrows*)

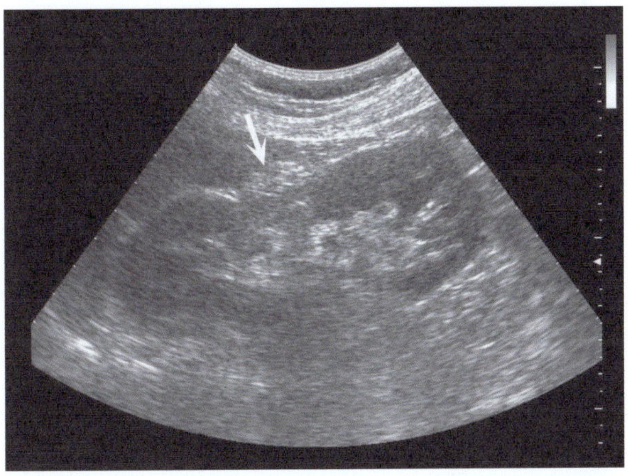

Fig. 6.13 Outcome of enucleation due to benign renal lesions, pseudotumor. Localized alteration of the profile and echogenicity of the parenchyma (*arrow*) creates a false image of an expansive lesion

The possibility of **identifying** renal lesions with US is largely dependent on the physical characteristics of the patient and the size of the lesion, with the technique proving particularly effective with lesions >2 cm. Small renal tumors are generally round in shape with an associated focal bulging of the renal contour in the case of exophytic growth or deformation of the fat of the renal sinus with endophytic growth. The limits of US detection are linked to isoechoic, polar and exophytic lesions, especially when the kidneys are located deep or concealed by colic gas. Moreover, there is the risk of confusing a solid hypoechoic lesion with an anechoic cystic lesion and vice versa. The sensitivity of US, however, does not appear to be exceptional. A US preoperative study performed on a group of patients with a cancer risk (von Hippel–Lindau syndrome or hereditary renal papillary carcinoma) identified 0% of lesions 0–5 mm, 21% of lesions 5–10 mm, 28% of lesions 10–15 mm, 58% of lesions 15–20 mm, 79% of lesions 20–25 mm and 100% of lesions 35–30 mm. Detection was therefore markedly influenced by lesion size and not by parameters such as left or right side, polar site or otherwise, solid or cystic nature, superficial or deep location, whereas specificity, which was not dependent on size, was 82% (only considering lesions 10–35 mm) [18]. In general, US is less effective than CT and MR in both identification and characterization of renal tumors <3 cm. Currently the use of tissue harmonic imaging and CD can improve identification, but a thorough and patient exploration is required in these cases, which includes all of the parts of both kidneys and also takes into consideration the possibility of exophytic and isoechoic forms. The possibilities of CEUS in identifying and characterizing these small lesions still need to be verified on large patient populations, although the injection of contrast medium is probably useful in select cases when faced with specific doubts (e.g. pseudotumors) [19]. US-guided percutaneous biopsy is little used for these lesions. Both FNAC and **core biopsy** have been shown often to be ineffective for an adequate differential diagnosis of these lesions, which are frequently heterogeneous and therefore can easily create sampling problems. In particular there can be difficulties in distinguishing oncocytomas and carcinomas, and some angiomyolipomas can be considered malignant. The indication for percutaneous biopsy may instead be given in the suspicion of lymphoma or renal metastasis. When the lesion remains indeterminate despite accurate imaging, follow-up over time may be a rational option while bearing in mind that most small renal cell carcinomas identified incidentally grow particularly slowly, especially if well circumscribed (to the point of suggesting in the particularly elderly subject or with an elevated surgical risk a wait-and-see approach in place of surgery) [20,21].

Renal cell carcinoma (RCC) accounts for 68–87% of solid small renal tumors [21]. It is generally solitary and found in the thickness of the parenchyma or protruding towards the renal sinus or more often towards the outside. The echogenicity tends to be variable, with 61–77% of lesions <3 cm (especially if papillary) being hyperechoic, whereas the larger forms tend to be iso-hypoechoic with more-or-less heterogeneous echotexture [21,22]. Occasionally an adjacent cyst is present – the "sentinel" cyst [23]. Structural homogeneity may be suggestive of oncocytoma, although some 35% of carcinomas also have a homogeneous appearance. The presence of a perilesional hypoechoic rim, which indicates the presence of a pseudocapsule, and multiple intralesional microcysts are rather specific findings for RCC but unfortunately rather infrequent (sensitivity of 8–84% and 12–31%, respectively). Carcinomas present moderate and especially peripheral vascularity with elevated flow velocity. Internal low-resistance sinusoidal vessels are detected with little systolic-diastolic modulation. The vascular peripheral rim may make the identification of otherwise unrecognizable isoechoic nodules possible. Five vascular patterns of focal renal lesions have been identified: 0, no signal; 1, some intralesional signals; 2, penetrating vessels; 3, peripheral nodular vascularity; 4, mixed penetrating and peripheral vascularity. Carcinomas tend to be characterized only by patterns 3 and 4, whereas some 80% of angiomyolipomas have been shown to have patterns 0–2 [24]. Nonetheless, the vascularity of RCC can appear greater than the adjacent healthy parenchyma but also less, in which case an isoechoic nodule can stand out as a defect in the parenchymal vascular map [16]. The CD findings are insufficient, and while it is true that the presence of hypervascularity should always raise suspicion, it is also true that these findings need to be integrated with the US morphologic findings (Figs. 6.14–6.20, Video 6.2).

Renal **angiomyolipoma** is a hamartomatous tumor consisting of variable quantities of thick-walled newly formed vessels, smooth muscle cells and mature adipose tissue. The tumor is predominant in women >40 years of age. Around 80% of patients with tuberous sclerosis, being generally middle-aged women, have renal angiomyolipomas, often multiple (synchronous or metachronous) and bilateral. In contrast, less than 40% of patients with an incidental finding of angiomyolipoma are subsequently diagnosed with tuberous sclerosis. In typical cases, the small angiomyolipoma manifests as a hyperechoic mass (similar to if not greater than the fat of the renal sinus and with no direct correlation with the effective adipose content in the nodule) with homogeneous echotexture, well-defined margins and possible post-

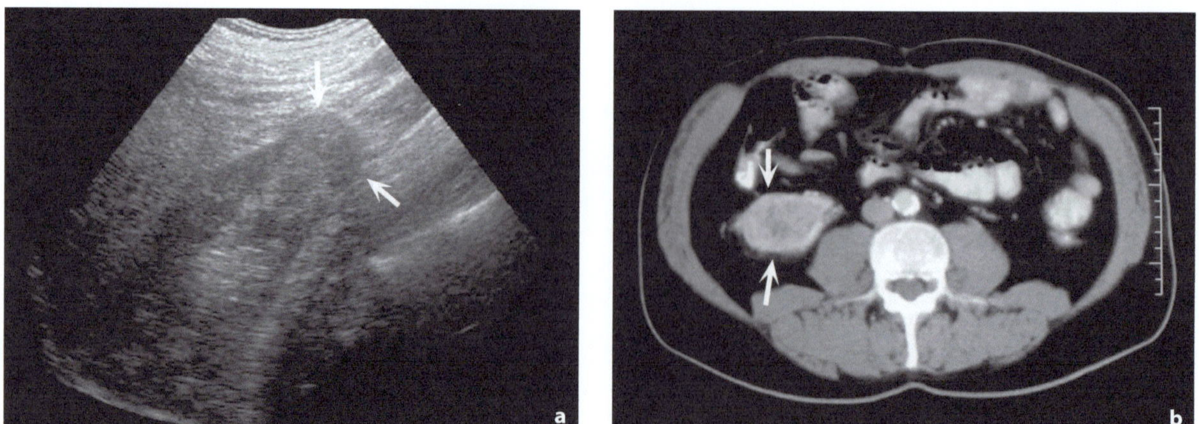

Fig. 6.14a,b Renal cell carcinoma. Mildly hyperechoic deformation of the right lower renal pole (**a**, *arrows*). CT scan confirms the renal nodule (**b**, *arrows*)

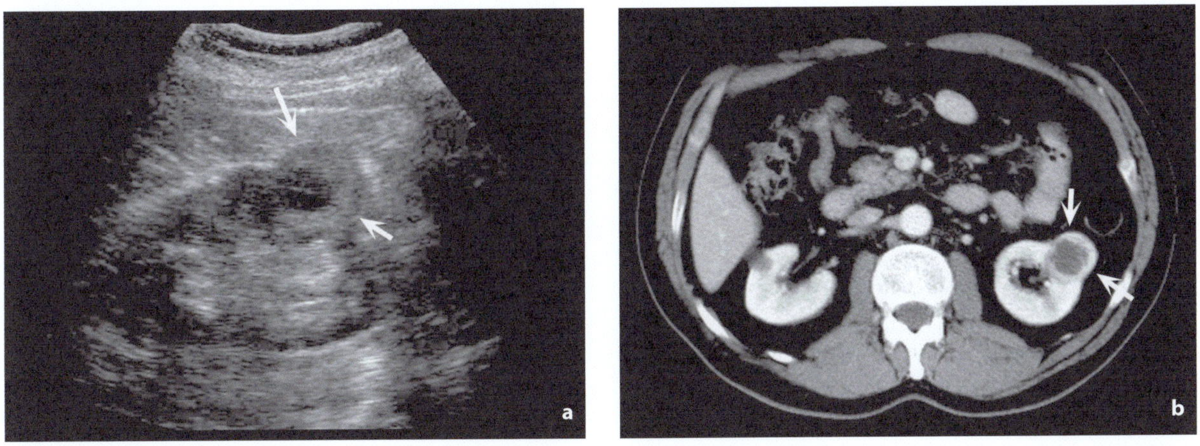

Fig. 6.15a,b Renal cell carcinoma, alveolar type. Exophytic echogenic mass (**a**, *arrows*) with internal eccentric hypo-anechoic area. CT scan in total nephrographic phase shows excellent morphologic correlation (**b**, *arrows*)

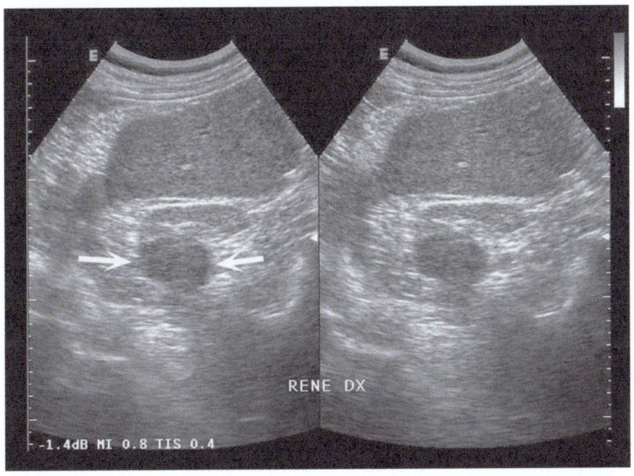

Fig. 6.16 Renal cell carcinoma. Hypoechoic nodule deforming the renal contour (*arrows*)

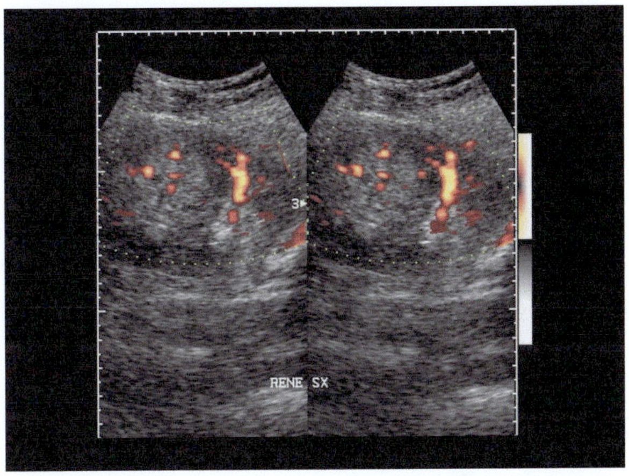

Fig. 6.17 Renal cell carcinoma. Hyperechoic nodule with central color signals at PD

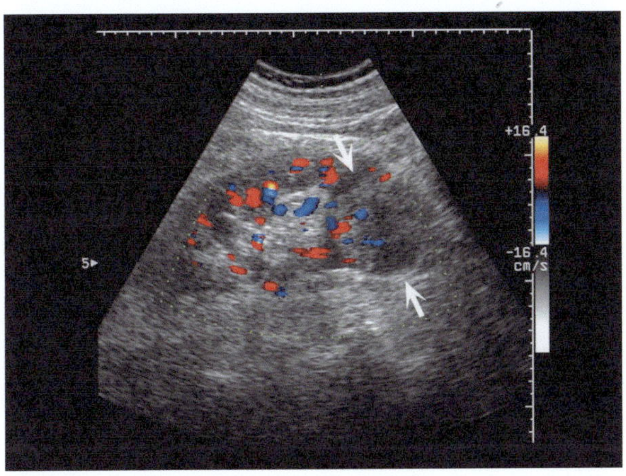

Fig. 6.18 Renal cell carcinoma. Heterogeneous and mildly hypoechoic nodule with some vascular signals at CD (*arrows*)

erior acoustic shadowing (21–40% of cases) and few internal vascular signals or some penetrating vessels at CD [16]. The appearance can, however, be isoechoic to the parenchyma (29% of cases) or even hypoechoic (6%) and heterogeneous internal portions may be present, but microcystic images or perilesional hypoechoic pseudocapsular halo are generally not seen (Figs. 6.21–6.24). The probability that the typical presentation of a small "brilliant" mass with posterior acoustic shadowing is a carcinoma is very low. Nonetheless performing a direct CT scan to identify adipose attenuation or US follow-up over time may be advisable. In the less typical forms, e.g. with hyperechogenicity lower than the renal sinus, US monitoring is less rational because carcinoma also grows very slowly and therefore, considering also the fluctuations in measurements, the finding of no growth or

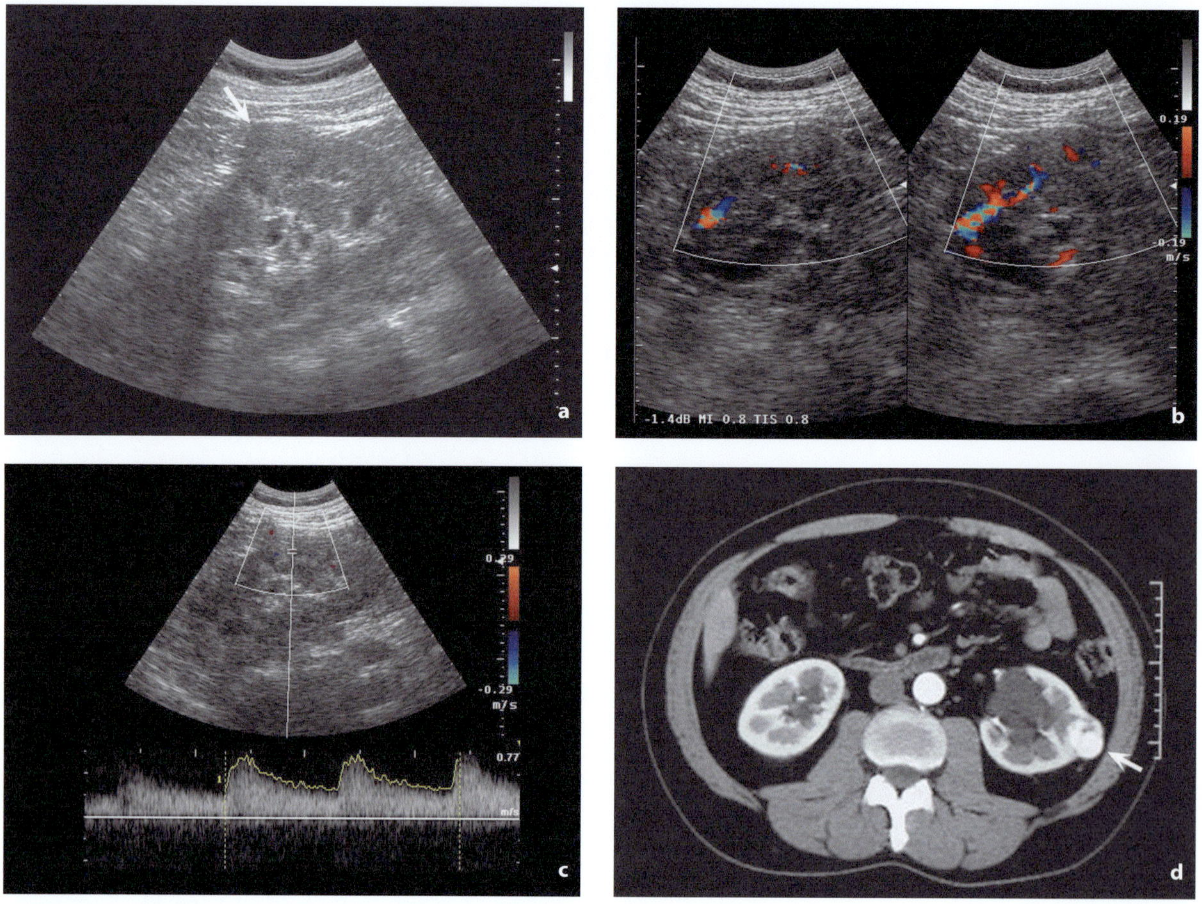

Fig. 6.19a-d Renal cell carcinoma. Mildly hypoechoic nodule forming a bulge in the renal contour (**a**, *arrow*). Nodule shows some central vascular signals at CD (**b**), and low-resistance flow at spectral analysis (**c**). CT scan in the cortical phase shows the intense vascularity of the lesion (**d**, *arrow*)

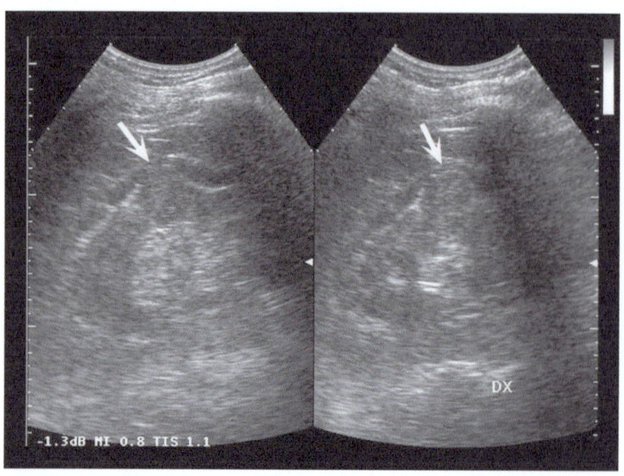

Fig. 6.20 Renal cell carcinoma. Substantially isoechoic nodule seen widening the parenchyma and forming a bulge in the renal contour (*arrows*)

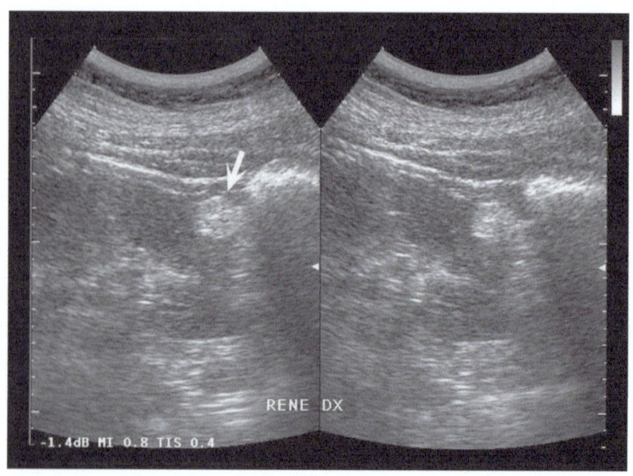

Fig. 6.21 Renal angiomyolipoma. Homogeneous and clearly hyperechoic nodule in the renal parenchyma (*arrow*)

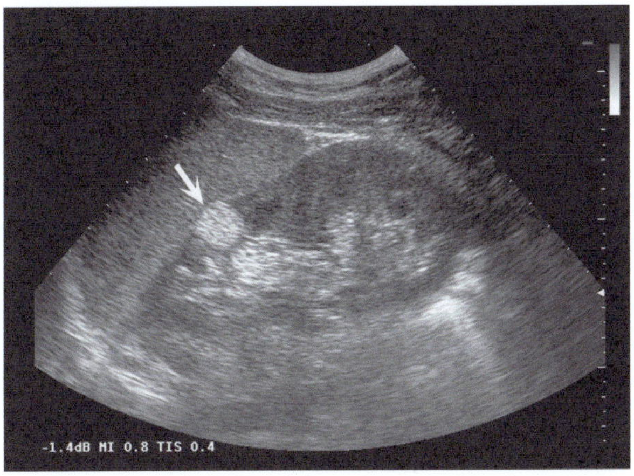

Fig. 6.22 Renal angiomyolipoma. Homogeneous and clearly hyperechoic nodule in the parenchyma of the left kidney (*arrow*)

limited growth cannot rule out carcinoma unless the diameters have stabilized after a number of years. A more advisable approach in less typical cases, therefore, is diagnostic work-up with CT or MR. The ability of CEUS to differentiate these lesions still needs to be confirmed with large patient populations, although it is clear that angiomyolipomas with a significant vascular component can be difficult to distinguish from carcinomas. CD with contrast medium has proved ineffective in this task [17,25]. Once the diagnosis of angiomyolipoma has been confirmed with one test or another, lesions >4–5 cm tend to be treated surgically, especially due to the risk of spontaneous bleeding, whereas smaller lesions undergo monitoring, even though periodic follow-up at least of lesions <2 cm does not appear to have a sufficiently robust rationale. Follow-up can of course be an opportunity for defini-

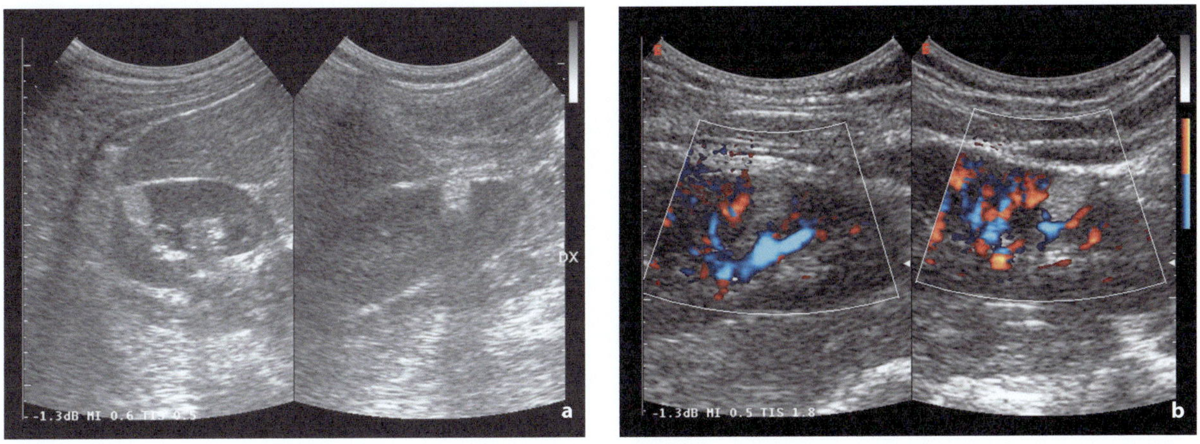

Fig. 6.23a,b Renal angiomyolipoma. Small intraparenchymal nodule with homogeneous hyperechoic appearance, well-defined margins and slight acoustic shadowing (**a**). No color signals can be identified at directional PD (**b**)

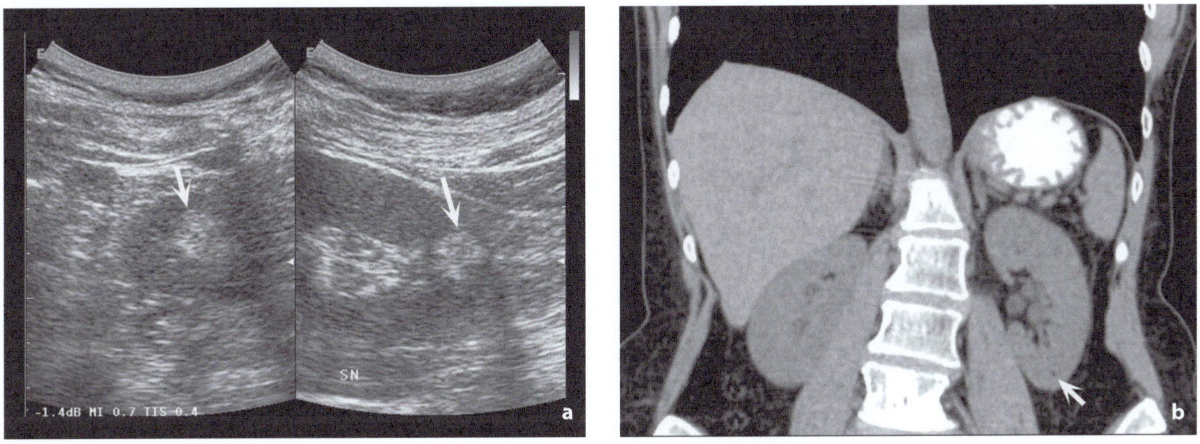

Fig. 6.24a,b Renal angiomyolipoma. Mildly echogenic nodule within the renal parenchyma (**a**, *arrows*). Coronal CT reconstruction shows small nucleus of adipose hypoattenuation (**b**, *arrow*) whereas the rest of the nodule is not recognizable as such

tively ruling out a small echogenic carcinoma, but it should be recalled that small renal cell carcinomas identified incidentally can have very slow growth [20], and that even angiomyolipomas can increase in size over time, albeit slowly, especially when multiple and regardless of the amount their adipose component [26].

Adenoma is not recognized by all pathologists as a distinct pathologic entity. At any rate the appearance is similar to a small RCC, with a particular tendency towards homogeneity [23].

Oncocytoma (8–27% of small renal tumors) is a proximal collecting duct adenoma composed of large cells with granular eosinophilic cytoplasm. Generally benign and solitary with a hypo- or isoechoic appearance to the parenchyma, as stated above it may display typically homogeneous echotexture. However, the differentiation from carcinoma cannot usually be made with US [16,21].

Renal **metastases** are rather infrequent and usually found in an advanced phase of metastasization (especially melanoma or carcinomas of the breast, lung, colon, female reproductive system or the contralateral kidney, possibly already operated on). In the patient with an advanced primary extrarenal tumor, a new renal lesion is more likely to be secondary than primary. They may be single or multiple, occasionally bilateral and are often found in the parenchyma thickness or more often towards the periphery. It is not uncommon that the effective site of metastasization in, for example, melanoma is the perirenal fat, with later extension to the underlying parenchyma. The appearance is generally more-or-less circumscribed, heterogeneous hypoechoic with some vascular signals at CD and with bulging of the renal contour at the site of the lesion. In some cases an enlargement and deformity of the kidney may be seen without the appearance of a definite focal lesions but with diffuse heterogeneity [2,22] (Figs. 6.25–6.30, Video 6.3).

6.3 Renal Masses

Renal masses can be classified in masses with expansive growth and masses with invasive growth. The former include most renal cell carcinomas (RCCs), angiomyolipomas and oncocytomas as well as most metastases and lymphomas. Invasive lesions include transitional cell carcinomas, rare RCCs, a minority of metastases and lymphomas, and some infrequent primary carcinomas (medullary carcinoma and collecting duct carcinoma).

RCCs in the adult account for 80–90% of cases of clear-cell adenocarcinoma (conventional RCC accounts for 75% of all renal neoplasm in surgical series). Papillary cystadenocarcinoma (10–15%) and

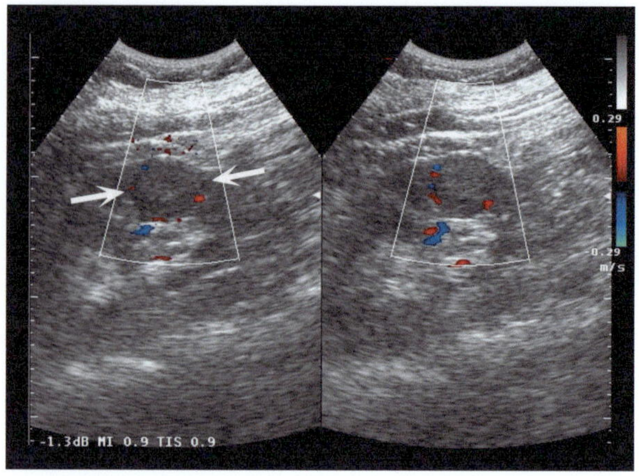

Fig. 6.25 Renal metastasis from bronchial carcinoid. Moderately hypoechoic nodule (*arrows*) seen displacing the renal vessels at CD

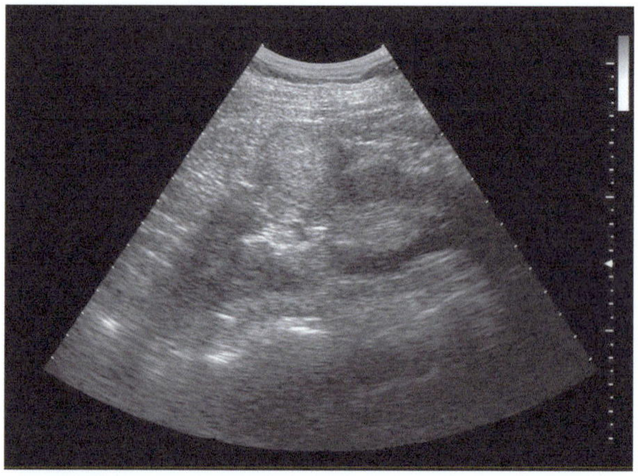

Fig. 6.26 Renal metastasis from lung cancer. Patently exophytic, heterogeneous hyperechoic nodule

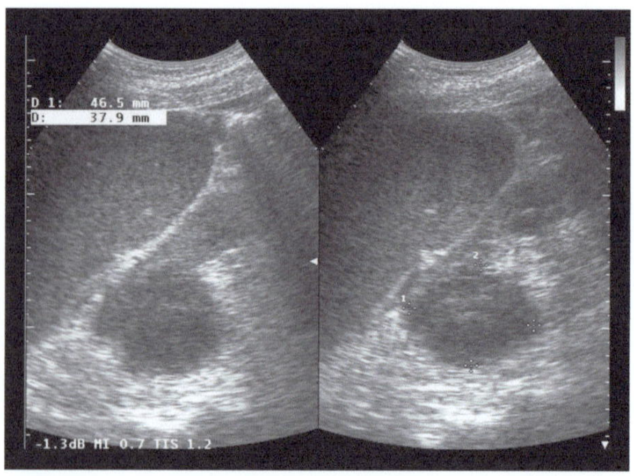

Fig. 6.27 Renal metastasis from anaplastic carcinoma of the thyroid. Heterogeneous hypoechoic nodule with ill-defined margins, located in the left upper renal pole

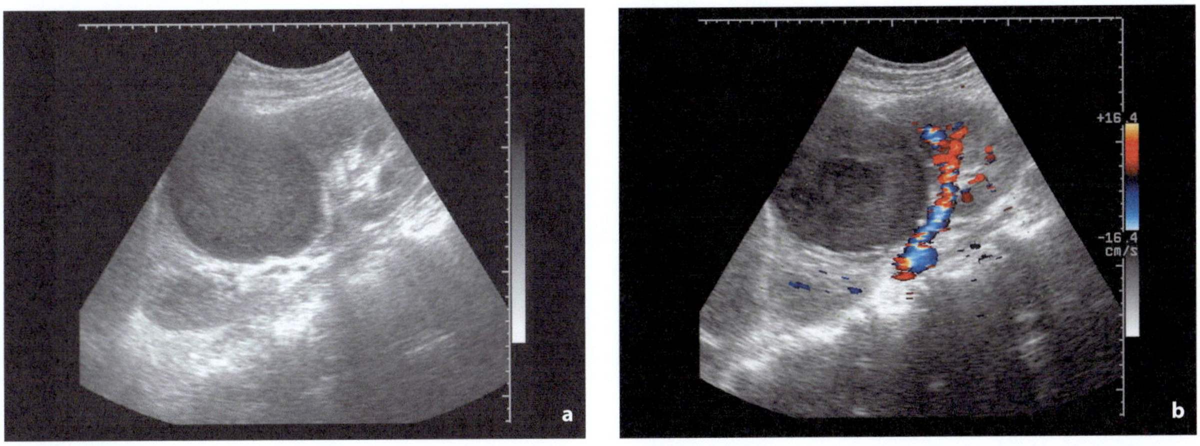

Fig. 6.28a,b Renal metastasis from melanoma. Hypoechoic lesion with anechoic center (**a**) and hypovascular appearance at CD (**b**)

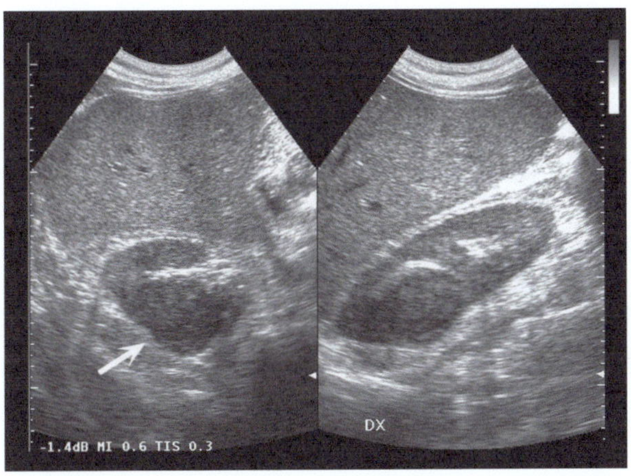

Fig. 6.29 Renal metastasis from lung cancer. Heterogeneous hypoechoic nodulation (*arrow*) which imprints both the renal sinus and the external contour of the organ

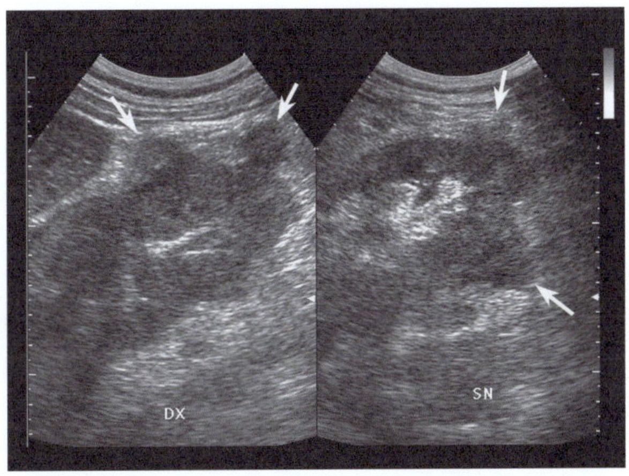

Fig. 6.30 Perirenal metastasis from pulmonary carcinoma. Several hypoechoic nodulations of the renal contour can be distinguished bilaterally (*arrows*)

transitional cell carcinoma (5–7%, from the calices and the pelvis) are rarer [27]. RCC is predominant in males (M/F 2:1), with a peak incidence in the 5th–7th decade of life. Risk factors include von Hippel–Lindau syndrome (36% of patients), dialysis-correlated cystic disease (incidence 3–6 times higher than the general population), possibly polycystic kidney syndrome and to a lesser extent conditions such as obesity, smoking and exposure to certain chemicals [22]. The increasing incidence in recent years is for the most part only apparent, being due to increasing life expectancy and the elevated diffusion of imaging examinations, with incidental findings in 70–83% of cases [16,27,28]. Incidentally identified renal tumors are on average smaller and have a lower stage and grade and greater disease-free survival than symptomatic lesions [16,21,29]. In one study on renal lesions <7 cm, it was seen that 16% of benign lesions were operated on for suspected malignancy. "Benign" nephrectomies were particularly frequent among women, whereas there was no probabilistic correlation with lesion size [30].

The **extension** of RCC is the main prognostic factor and is without doubt much more important than the size of the mass alone. In TNM, T1 is <7 cm, whereas T2 is >7 cm and T3a is characterized by extrarenal spread into the retroperitoneal fat (an element which cannot be readily identified with US) (Figs. 6.31, 6.32). Stage T3b is characterized by invasion of the renal vein and/or the inferior vena cava. Most urologists refer to the Robson classification: stage I, tumor confined to the capsule; stage II, spread to the perirenal fat but confined to the perirenal fascia; stage III, renal

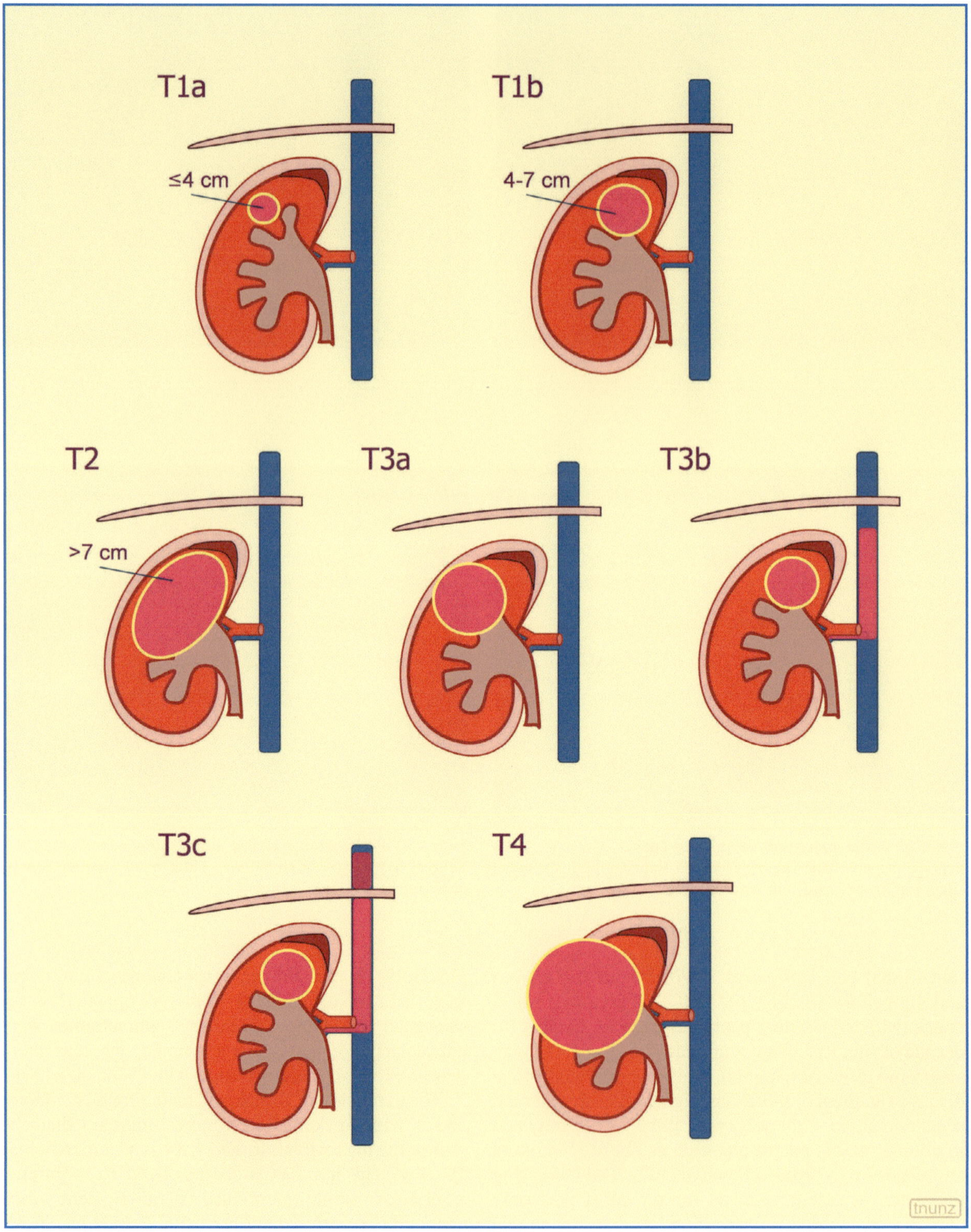

Fig. 6.31 Staging of renal tumors. *T1a*, tumor ≤4 cm confined to the kidney; *T1b*, tumor 4–7 cm confined to the kidney; *T2*, tumor >7 cm confined to the kidney; *T3a*, tumor of any size extends to the adrenal gland or perirenal tissue but not beyond the perirenal fascia; *T3b*, tumor of any size invades the renal vein or the inferior vena cava below diaphragm; *T3c*, tumor of any size invades the inferior vena cava above diaphragm; *T4*, tumor of any size extends beyond perirenal fascia. Modified from [31]

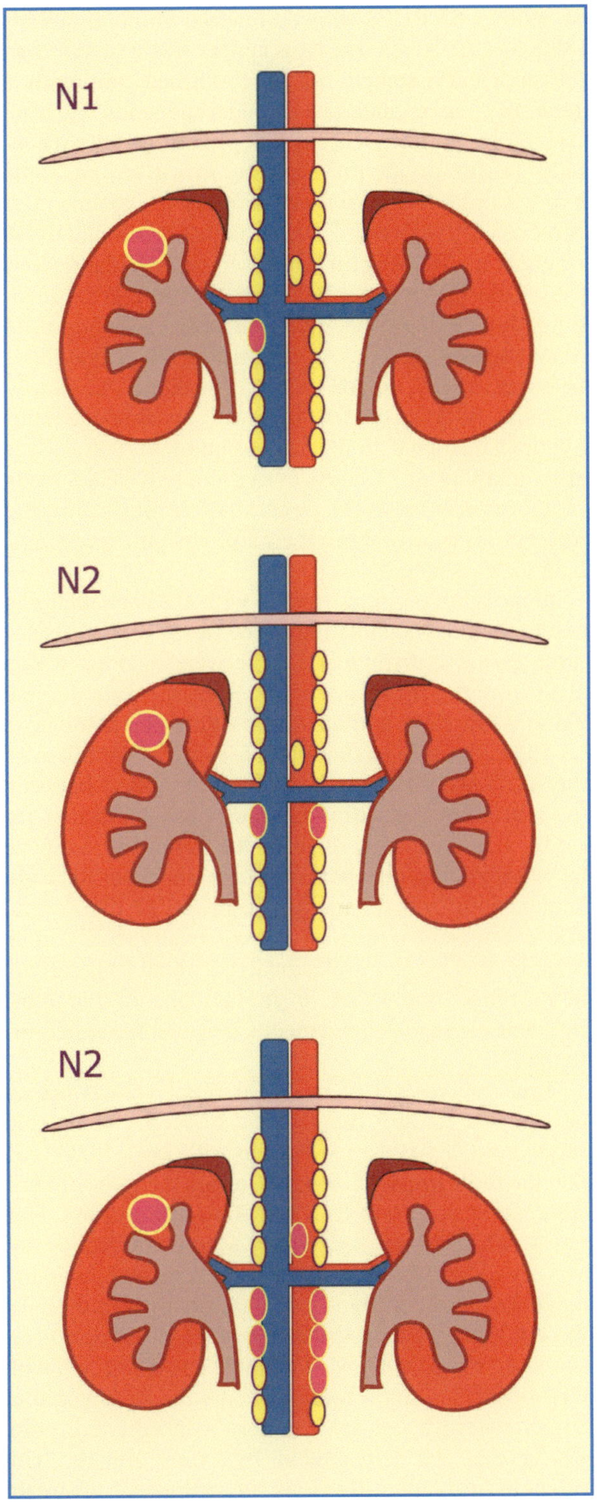

Fig. 6.32 N parameter for renal tumors. Regional lymph nodes include renal hilar, para-aortic, preaortic, interaortocaval, para-caval, retrocaval and retroaortic. *N1* refers to metastasis to a single regional lymph node, whether ipsi- or contralateral, and *N2* metastasis to more than one lymph node, whether ipsi- or contralateral. Modified from [31]

vein, inferior vena cava and/or regional lymph node involvement; stage IV, invasion of adjacent organs and/or metastasis [32] (Fig. 6.33).

Patients with a normal contralateral kidney in morphologic and functional terms generally undergo radical nephrectomy, even though attempts are increasingly being made to adopt **nephron-sparing** surgery (partial nephrectomy or enucleation with sparing of the adrenal gland), which is especially indicated in monofocal small (<4 cm) tumors in an early stage (stage I Robson or stage T1/2 TNM) and adequately accessible. Clearly, surgery of this kind requires particularly accurate staging. From this point of view, US is unable to distinguish between Robson stage I and stage II (T1/2 and T3a), because it is generally unable to identify the perirenal fascia. However, CEUS has recently demonstrated the possibility of identifying the tumor pseudocapsule as a rim of **contrast enhancement** which increases in echogenicity towards the late phases (21% of carcinomas in baseline scans vs. 81% with contrast medium) [33].

The **appearance** of RCC is generally an iso-hypoechoic mass with heterogeneity due to necrotic phenomena, especially central, with possible cystic areas and/or scattered calcifications. Masses with echogenicity equal to or greater than that of the fat of the renal sinus are rarer, especially for masses >3 cm [27]. The calcifications (8–18% of cases) can be peripheral or more often central, diffuse or punctate [22]. The margins are often irregular and ill-defined. The size of the mass can vary, possibly reaching several tens of centimeters at diagnosis, and in general the probability of malignancy of a renal mass is correlated with its size, with a threshold at 4 cm [34], even though one study showed that the incidence of benign lesions among patients who underwent nephrectomy for suspected tumor did not depend on lesion size [30]. The invasive forms of RCC may show signs of obliteration of the renal sinus fat, dilatation of the calices associated with invasion of the pelvis, and heterogeneity of the perirenal adipose tissue. In some cases (5–15%) the appearance is uni- or more often multilocular cystic, with thick and irregular walls and internal septations, mural nodularity and thick septal or mural calcifications, elements which enable differentiation from benign cysts [22]. CD usually shows moderate and especially peripheral vascularity of RCC with high-flow vessels and possible arteriovenous fistulas, although slow flows or spectra with little systolic-diastolic modulation and low RI are also possible. In reality, little difference has been found in terms of RI between benign and malignant lesions. In a large retrospective study on 299 operated renal lesions, 92% of those with vascular signals – regardless of the pattern – turned out to be malignant (RCC). Prospectively, 83%

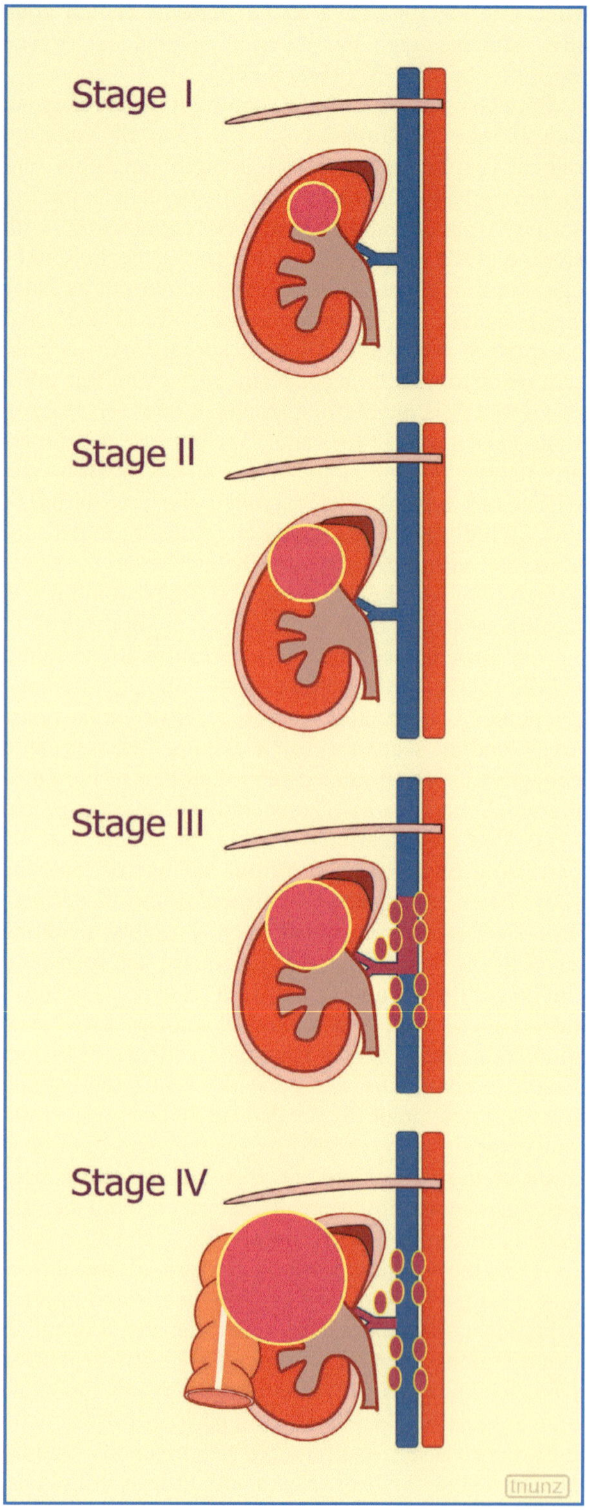

Fig. 6.33 Robson staging of renal cell carcinoma. *Stage I*, confined to renal capsule; *stage II*, tumor with invasion of perirenal fat; *stage III*, tumor also extends to renal vein and inferior vena cava and/or regional lymph nodes; *stage IV*, tumor also extends beyond perirenal fascia with invasion of adjacent organs or structures

of another 65 RCCs showed internal vascular signals [35]. At CEUS, renal masses appear less vascular than the adjacent parenchyma, well-defined and with a generally accentuated and heterogeneous internal "microcirculation". CEUS has proven to be particularly useful in identifying low flows within some hypovascular lesions with an efficacy greater than CD and even CT (risk of mistaken diagnosis of small cyst), whereas its utility is limited for hypervascular lesions [36]. Late-phase hyperenhancement has a 96% sensitivity but a 77% specificity in characterizing solid renal masses <5 cm. An additional RCC feature is heterogeneous enhancement, whereas angiomyolipoma is usually characterized by homogeneous hypoenhancement in the arterial and late phases. It is also clear that a CD study, even more so a CEUS study of these masses, is in general of limited practical interest, especially when their size is significant (Figs. 6.34–6.39, Video 6.4–6.6).

Identifying perirenal spread with US is challenging due to the nonvisualization of the fascia. In the case of large masses, distinguishing between lesions which arise from the right upper renal pole, the right adrenal gland or the deep surface of the right hepatic lobe can be difficult, more so than with CT or MR. In this case the study should search for a cleavage plane between the mass and the various organs (also important for ruling out invasion), identify the echogenic adipose layer separating retroperitoneal masses from the right hepatic lobe and recognize the origin of the arterial afferent vessels to the mass. Occasionally RCC can be complicated by an intralesional, perirenal or pararenal hemorrhage: the lesion is in fact one of the most frequent causes of spontaneous peri/pararenal hemorrhage [37].

The involvement of the main **renal vein** is not an uncommon finding (up to 30% of RCCs in the old series but 0% in cases of lesions <2.5 cm). RCC is in fact the most frequent tumor to invade the inferior vena cava (up to 5–10% of RCCs in non-recent series). This event, which is not necessarily a contraindication for surgery although it does modify the approach, is found more frequently in right-sided tumors than in those of the left kidney due to the different length of the corresponding renal vein [23]. Thrombi can be detected with CD, which reveals a more-or-less echogenic vascular defect within a normal, or more often dilated, vein, which may be surrounded by color signals with possible slowing of flow immediately upstream (Fig. 6.40). The presence of intrathrombotic vascular signals definitively indicates the at least partial neoplastic nature of the thrombus, but this finding is very difficult to identify [16]. The sensitivity of US for caval invasion is only 54% (but 100% with CD). Nonetheless the identification of the most important

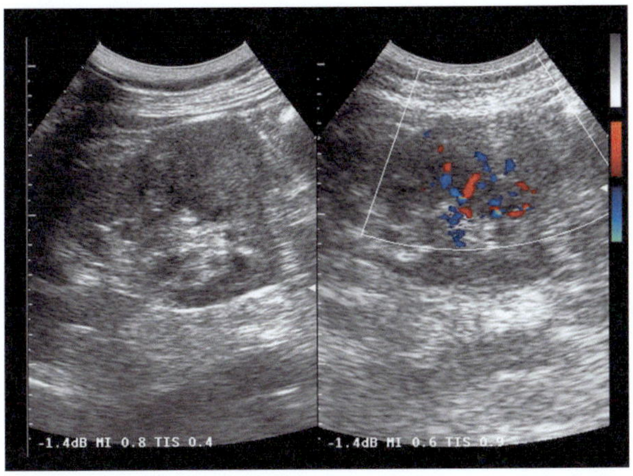

Fig. 6.34 Renal cell carcinoma. Heterogeneous hypo-isoechoic lesion with hypervascular appearance at CD especially in the deep portion

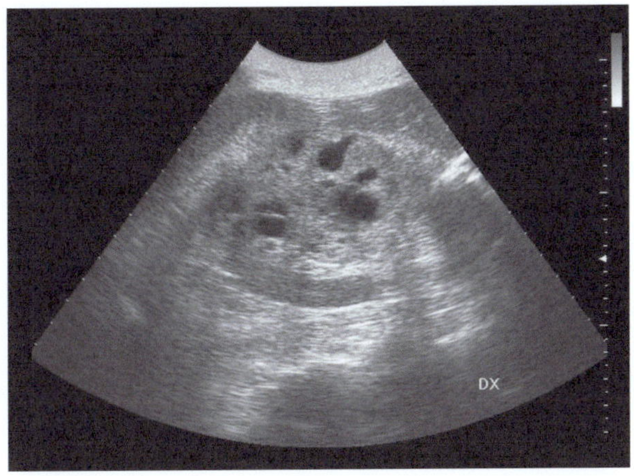

Fig. 6.35 Renal cell carcinoma. Echogenic mass with multiple cystic areas

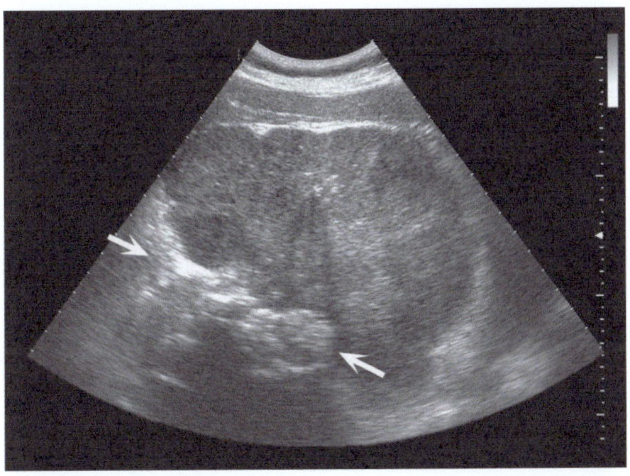

Fig. 6.36 Renal cell carcinoma. Large heterogeneous hypoechoic mass with extensive calcified components resulting from prior embolization (*arrows*)

forms, i.e. those extending to the retrohepatic tract of the vein, occurs frequently, and the limit of cranial extension should always be indicated in the report [38,39]. Thorough evaluation of the contralateral kidney is crucial, not only for an assessment of its overall morphofunctional state, but also because bilateral lesions and contralateral metastasization are not rare events (1–2%). Other possible sites of metastasization which are accessible to US and which should be evaluated include the liver and the ipsilateral (6% of cases of RCC) and contralateral adrenal glands. Hematogenous liver metastases have a variable appearance. Moreover, this organ can also be subject to invasion by direct extension. Lumbar lymphadenopathies are indubitably better identified with CT and MR, as is invasion of the posterior muscles. When they are visible at US, they appear heterogeneously hypoechoic,

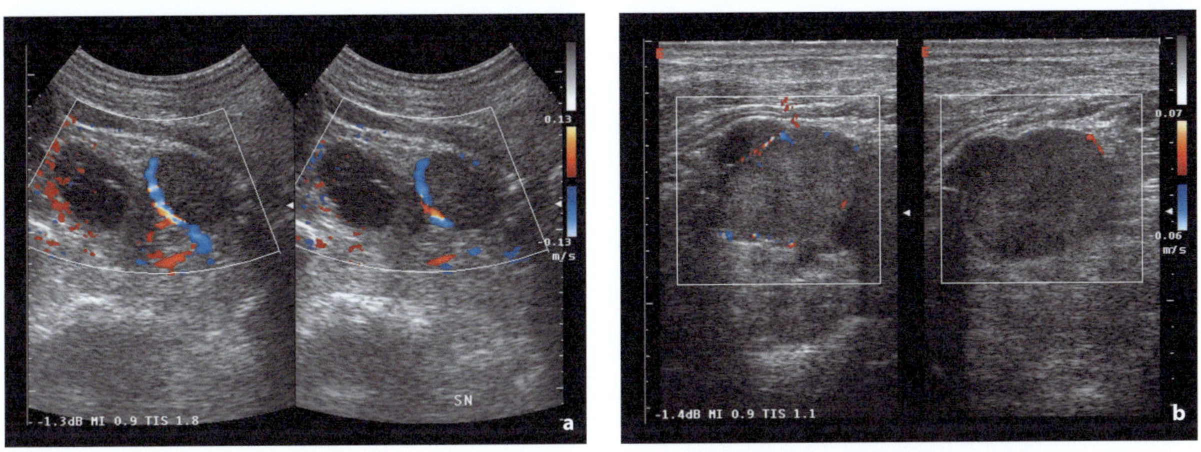

Fig. 6.37a,b Renal cell carcinoma in patient undergoing dialysis. In a subject with renal atrophy and multiple simple cortical cysts a hypoechoic nodule (**a**) can be seen which displaces the adjacent vessels at CD. The use of the superficial transducer makes possible the visualization of signals of intralesional flow at CD (**b**), thus enabling differentiation from a complicated cyst

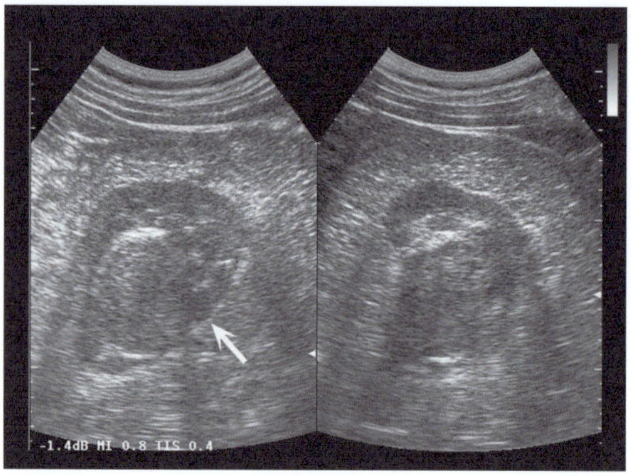

Fig. 6.38 Renal cell carcinoma in renal sinus. Solid mass appearing substantially isoechoic to the adjacent renal parenchyma (*arrow*) with endophytic development and marked obliteration of the renal sinus

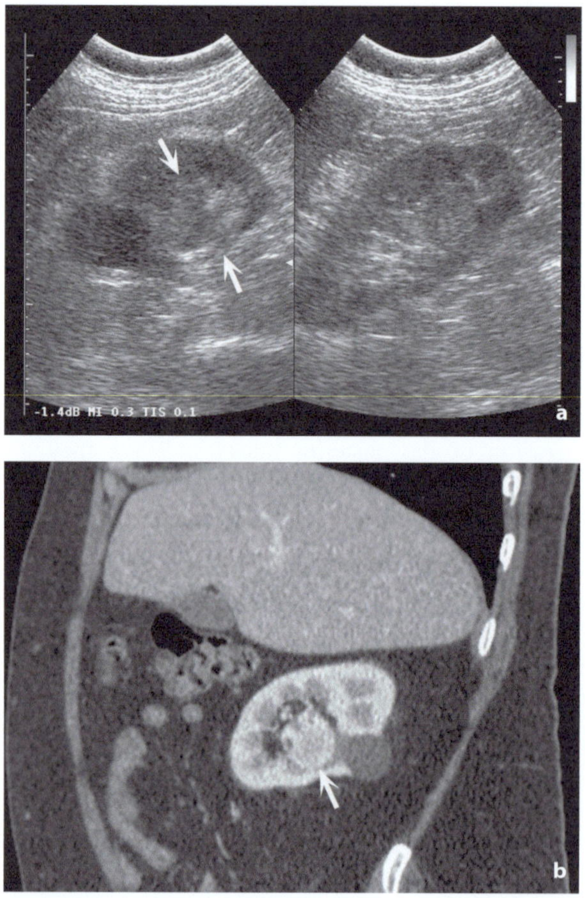

Fig. 6.39a,b Renal cell carcinoma in renal sinus. Mildly hypoechoic mass with poorly defined margins located in the echogenic sinus (**a**, *arrows*). Sagittal CT reconstruction in the cortical phase shows hypervascular endophytic lesion (**b**, *arrow*)

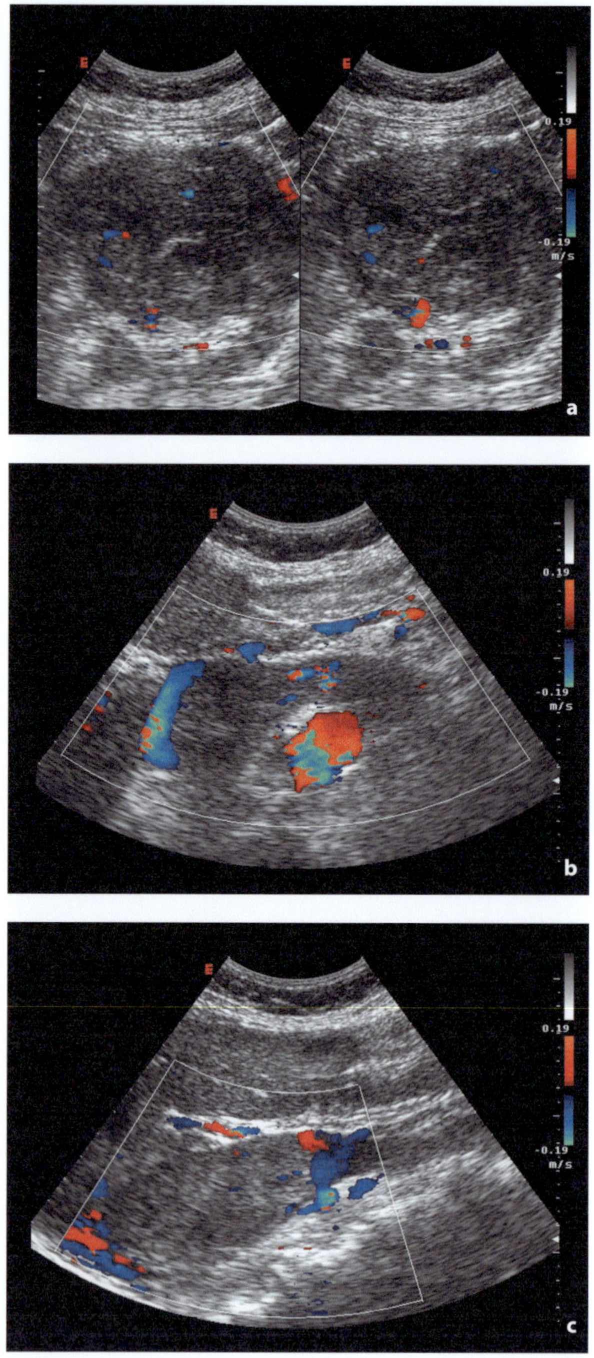

Fig. 6.40a-c Renal cell carcinoma with venous invasion. Hypoechoic renal mass (**a**) extending in the renal vein seen in transverse scan (**b**) and in the inferior vena cava (**c**) shown longitudinally. The small flow signals in the thrombus are arterial and indicate the malignant nature of the lesion

and are typically located on the lumbar side corresponding to the pathologic side of the kidney, or in an interaortocaval location. Overall, the accuracy of US in the staging of RCC is 50–70%, but except in cases of evident inoperability further staging is performed with MR and especially CT [23].

Oncocytoma (5% of renal tumors) prevails in men, with a peak incidence in the 5th–6th decades of life [23,27]. It may grow to a significant size and appear homogeneous or display a hypo- or hyperechoic central scar with a stellate appearance, or even necrosis or calcifications. CD may occasionally identify the "wheel" pattern, with a radial distribution of the vessels [16,22] (Fig. 6.41).

Large **angiomyolipomas** tend to have a heterogeneous internal structure and poorly defined margins with possible vascular signals at CD. These characteristics in many cases render the lesions difficult to distinguish from carcinomas. Calcifications are not usually encountered. The real size of forms which bulge from the renal contour or which are frankly exophytic is difficult to define because they tend to be lost in the echogenicity of the perirenal fat. In addition the frankly extrarenal forms need to be differentiated from sarcomas and especially from retroperitoneal liposarcomas, a distinction which can be challenging with US. CD can show single or multiple intralesional pseudoaneurysms which appear as small anechoic areas with vascular signals at CD or with enhancement at CEUS. In the event of hemorrhage, marked heterogeneity of the angiomyolipoma may be seen, together with the presence of perirenal fluid collections (Fig. 6.42, Video 6.7).

Multilocular cystic nephroma is an uncommon benign tumor with a prevalence in male children and female adults. It appears as a mass with a thick capsule and multiple fluid-filled internal loculations separated by septations with the possible presence of calcifications. Its location within the renal sinus and the relatively regular distribution of the septations are suggestive of the diagnosis, although a US differential diagnosis with multilocular cystic RCC is challenging [23] (Fig. 6.43).

Transitional cell (urothelial) **carcinoma** of the renal calices and pelvis (7% of renal tumors, 4–5 times less frequent than parenchymal carcinoma) can mimic a parenchymal tumor, especially when it reaches a conspicuous size and invades the adjacent renal tissue. In these cases, distinguishing between a parenchymal and urothelial origin is often not possible. The tumors are often multiple and bilateral and can especially be identified when associated with dilatation of the pelvis and/or calices, whereas this may be difficult to identify if the lesions are small [22]. Transitional cell carcinoma appears as a hypoechoic defect in the lumen of the possibly dilated pelvicaliceal system, with a sessile or pedunculated base, possible calcifications (differential diagnosis with calculi) and some vascular signals at CD, especially with moderately sized lesions. Alternatively, a hypoechoic nodulation may be identified within the echogenic fat of the renal sinus without pelvicaliceal dilatation. In this sense it should be recalled that the fat of the renal sinus can occasionally appear partly hypoechoic. However, this hypoechogenicity appears central, symmetrical and poorly defined, with posterior acoustic shadowing and normal vessels running through the area. In contrast, the hypoechogenicity induced by the urothelial tumor

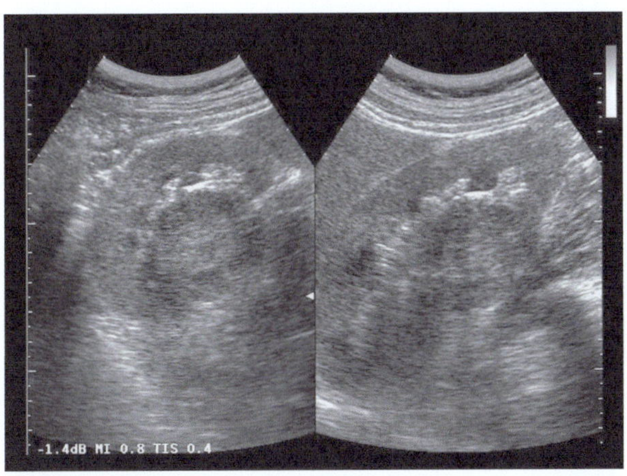

Fig. 6.41 Renal oncocytoma. Heterogeneous mass appearing more echogenic centrally protruding from the renal parenchyma

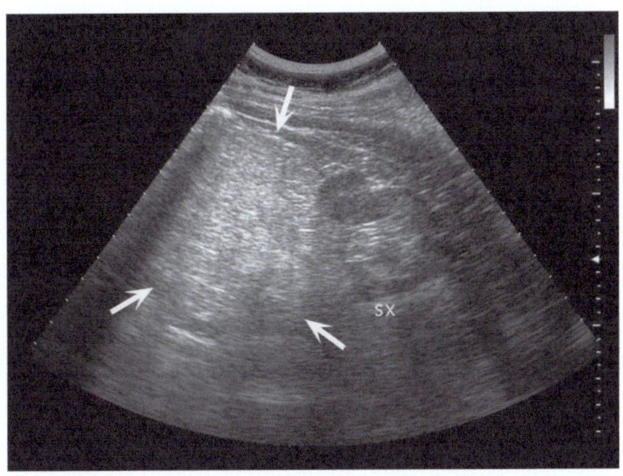

Fig. 6.42 Exophytic renal angiomyolipoma. Large, relatively homogeneous hyperechoic mass with ill-defined margins (*arrows*) in the differential diagnosis with retroperitoneal liposarcoma

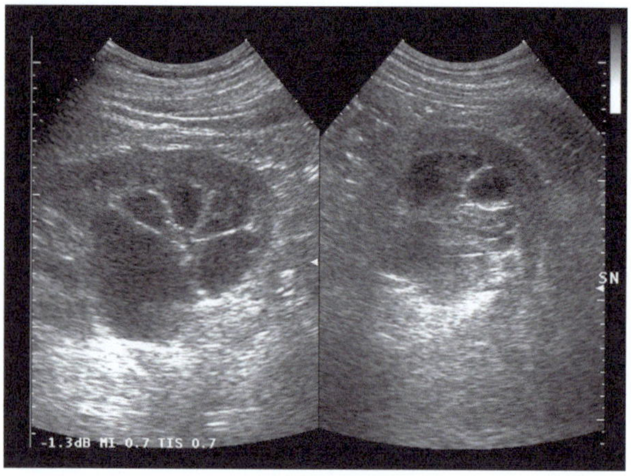

Fig. 6.43 Multinodular cystic nephroma. Multilocular cystic mass of the kidney

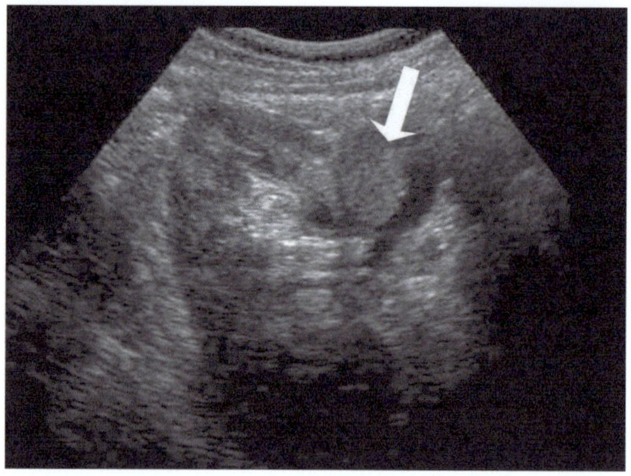

Fig. 6.44 Transitional cell carcinoma of the renal pelvis. Echogenic sessile lesion (*arrow*) protruding into the lumen of the dilated renal pelvis

appears more eccentric and circumscribed, without posterior acoustic shadowing and with more irregular vascularity [40]. Lastly, there are also forms with diffuse invasion of the renal parenchyma, which appears widened and disrupted [23] (Figs. 6.44–6.46).

Nephroblastoma (Wilms's tumor) is the most common childhood primary renal tumor (6% of pediatric tumors), with a slight predilection for females and a peak incidence at 3–4 years of age (only 20% of cases present >5 years). Nephroblastoma is bilateral in 5% of cases and presents as an intrarenal mass which distorts the architecture of the organ but which often initially displays an echogenic pseudocapsule. The echostructure appears solid with hypo-anechoic areas due to necrosis and/or hemorrhage and echogenic foci of calcifications or fat. Occasionally prevalently cystic and multiseptated forms may be seen, which are not terribly dissimilar from multilocular cystic nephroma, in which, however, the cysts are never located within the septations themselves [41]. As it grows, the lesion first tends towards exophytic development and then to extrarenal spread, with a pattern similar to the intravascular spread of RCC, i.e. into the renal vein and the inferior vena cava [42] (Fig. 6.47).

Primary renal **lymphomas** are rare, since the kidney does not possess lymphoid tissue, whereas secondary lesions linked to Hodgkin's and especially non-Hodgkin's lymphoma are not uncommon (5–6% of subjects at presentation, 33–41% at postmortem) [2]. The US appearance is variable: solitary lesion (10–20% of cases at postmortem but 50% of cases detected at imaging), multiple lesions (30–60% or diffuse parenchymal invasion (20%), with bilateral lesions being common [43]. Monofocal forms can be indistinguishable from carcinoma. The lesions tend to be limited in size with a relatively homogeneous

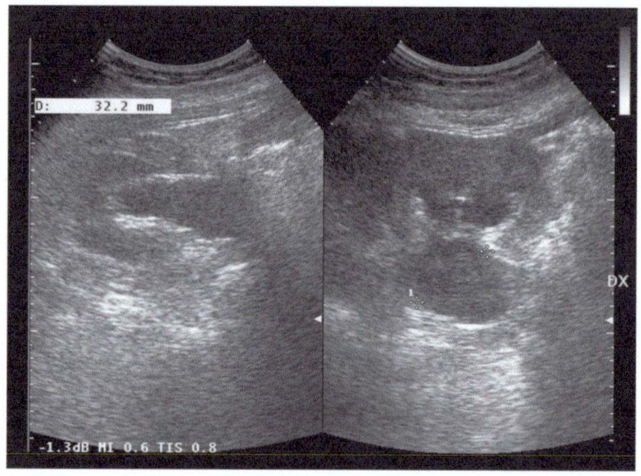

Fig. 6.45 Urothelial tumor of the renal pelvis. Moderate pelvicaliceal dilatation with mildly echogenic tissue within the renal pelvis (*between the calipers*)

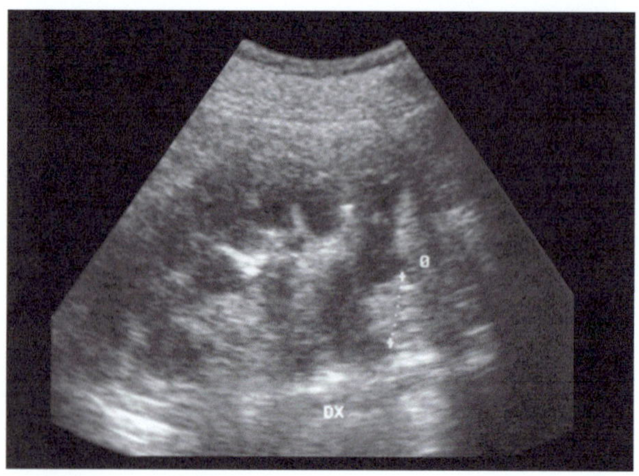

Fig. 6.46 Urothelial tumor of the renal pelvis. Pelvic dilatation with internal echogenic mass (*between the calipers*)

hypoechoic appearance, although they may appear anechoic or associated with moderately enhanced through-transmission and as such mimic a cyst [22]. CD generally shows a poorly vascular lesion. In the diffuse forms a hypoechoic or hyperechoic disruption of the renal parenchyma may be seen without definite signs of focal lesions. In many cases subcapsular or perirenal nodulations are associated and indicative of direct extension of the lesion. Moreover, around half of the patients present retroperitoneal adenopathies. The "halo" produced by perirenal infiltrate needs to be distinguished from conditions such as perirenal metastasis with desmoplastic reaction, retroperitoneal fibrosis with unusual perirenal location, perirenal urinomas and inflammation from acute pancreatitis. Both when it is thin or much more marked, however, the appearance of the perirenal lymphomatous lesion creates a sort of "floating" of the intrinsically normal kidney with the perirenal hypoechoic image distributed in a relatively uniform manner around the organ [44] (Figs. 6.48–6.51, Video 6.8).

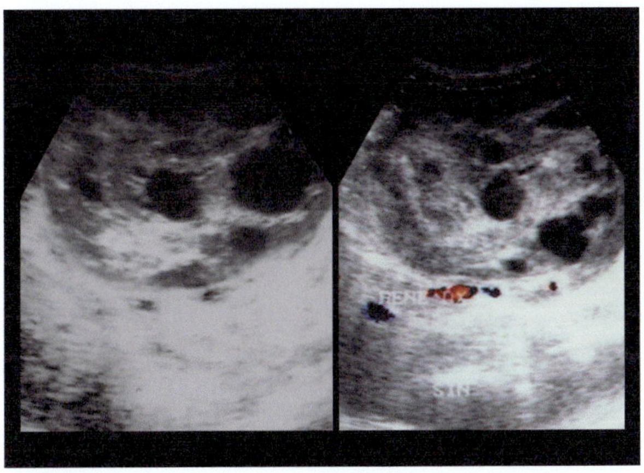

Fig. 6.47 Nephroblastoma. Echogenic mass with internal cystic-like components and poor vascular signals at CD

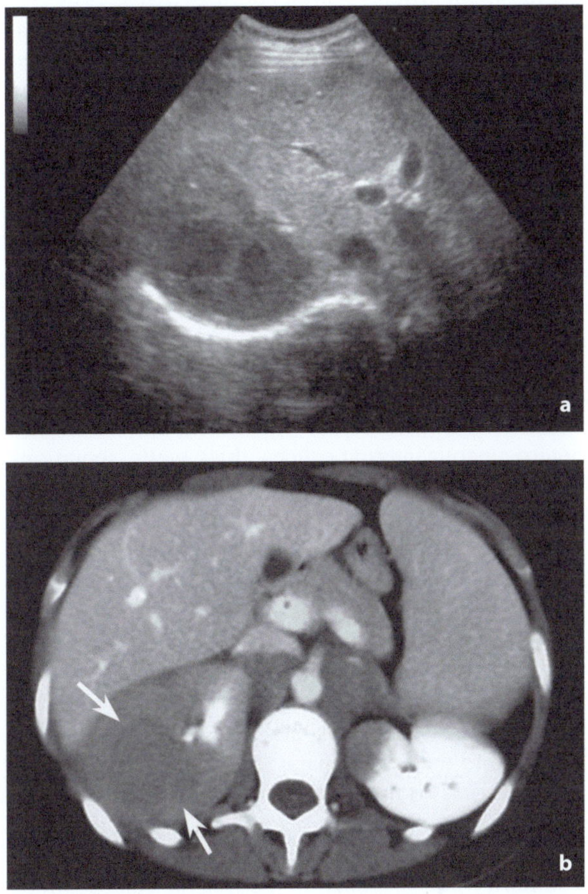

Fig. 6.48a,b Renal lymphoma. Total hypo-anechoic disruption of the right kidney (**a**). Axial CT scan (**b**) confirms the hypo-attenuating renal disruption (*arrows*) and visualizes some retroperitoneal lymphadenopathies

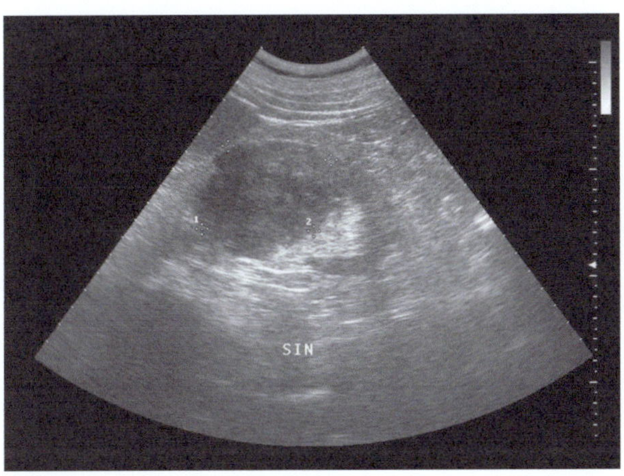

Fig. 6.49 Renal lymphoma. Heterogeneous hypoechoic mass in the upper pole of the kidney

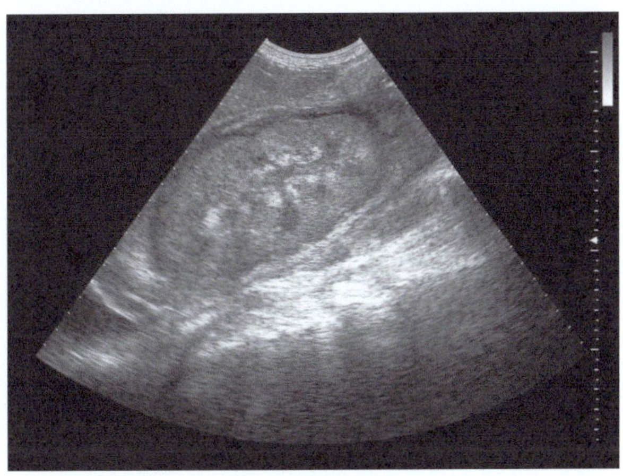

Fig. 6.50 Perirenal lymphoma. Thin hypo-anechoic tissue diffusely distributed around the kidney

6.4 Atypical Renal Cysts

Renal masses with a complex cystic appearance are a common incidental finding during US, CT or MR examinations done for other reasons. The lesions may be simple cortical cysts, complicated cysts (septated, infected, hemorrhagic, calcified), parapelvic cysts, multilocular cystic nephromas, unilocular or multilocular cystic or necrotic RCC, adult polycystic kidney, multicystic kidney, caliceal diverticula, dilated calices (including tumor-filled calix from neoplastic pelvic obstruction), pus-filled calix, blood-filled calix, liquefied parenchymal hematomas, abscesses, hydatidosis or aneurysms [23]. In most cases (95%) they are simple cysts with no malignant potential which are commonly found in middle-aged and elderly subjects. Occasionally, however, these cysts have a complex structure with a potential neoplastic degeneration – heterogeneous internal echoes, thick walls, septations, calcifications and mural nodularity [22]. Internal echoes may be due to infected or hemorrhagic content, while septations – possibly the expression of the progressive coalescence of adjacent cysts – are especially suspicious if thick (>1 mm), irregular and incomplete (i.e. not attached to the wall of the cyst). Calcifications can be small or large, linear or rounded, located in the wall or the septations. They are particularly suspicious if thick and irregular. Nodularities adhering to the septations or the walls are also highly suspicious. The probability of malignancy therefore depends on morphologic features such as number and thickness of the internal septations, presence of mural nodularity and presence of peripheral calcifications. These elements are at the basis of the CT classification of atypical cysts proposed by Bosniak [45].

The US study of atypical renal cysts is not always easy, since the technique is unable to detect the presence of lesion vascularity, which is an element of considerable suspicion. However, even CT has some limitations in the study of these lesions: due to the volume averaging effect, CT can have difficulty detecting thin septations or mild heterogeneity. It is not uncommon for a cyst with a "simple" appearance at CT to display a complicated structure at US, even though these are forms with thin septations and no calcifications or nodules so therefore benign [46] (Figs. 6.52–6.54, Video 6.9). Occasionally it may be difficult to demonstrate the macrovascularity even with CT or MR. In addition, in many cases monitoring over time is required such that it would be useful to have an imaging technique with the same reliability as CT but less invasive in terms of exposure to radiation and intravenous contrast media.

Several authors [47] have used PD with contrast medium to detect the vascular signal in the septations

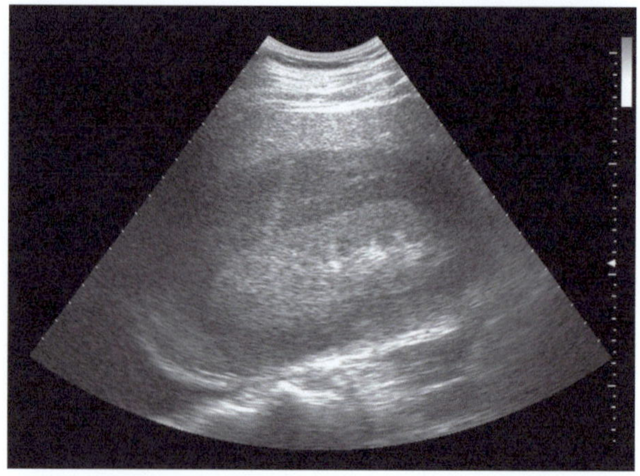

Fig. 6.51 Perirenal non-Hodgkin's lymphoma. Thick heterogeneous hypoechoic tissue completely surrounding the right kidney, intrinsically within the norm

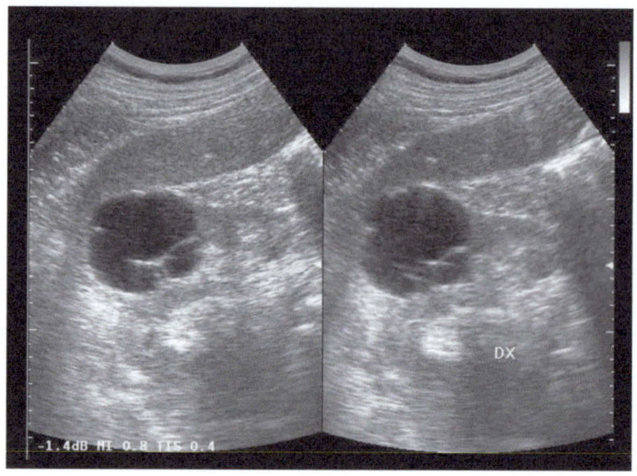

Fig. 6.52 Atypical cortical cyst, classifiable as Bosniak grade II. Cystic mass within the right renal cortex with some thin internal septations

and mural nodules, but this only enables an evaluation of the macrovascularity (Fig. 6.55). Others have suggested that since CEUS is able to study the microcirculation it could be used to this end. With this in mind they have adapted the Bosniak classification to CEUS study [46]: type I, simple cysts, no contrast enhancement; type II, few thin septations or small quantities of mural calcifications, possible contrast enhancement; type III, multiple thin septations or some thick septations or small mural nodulations, possible contrast enhancement; type IV, numerous thick septations, large mural nodule or multiple mural nodularities, possible contrast enhancement. In cystic RCCs there is a progressive contrast enhancement of the lesion wall in the arterial phase, with progressive

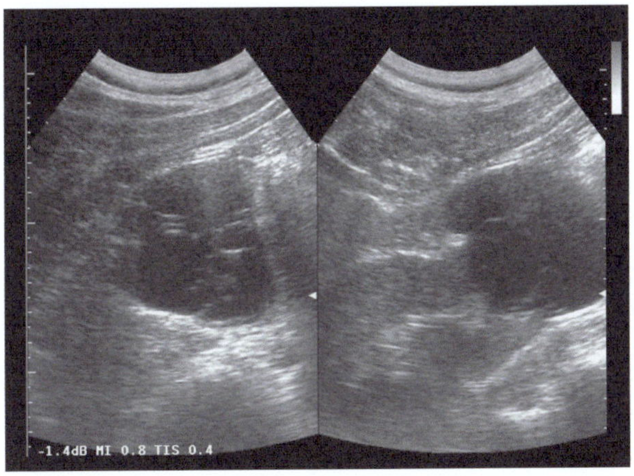

Fig. 6.53 Atypical cortical cyst, classifiable as Bosniak grade II. Cystic mass within the right renal cortex with multiple thin internal septations

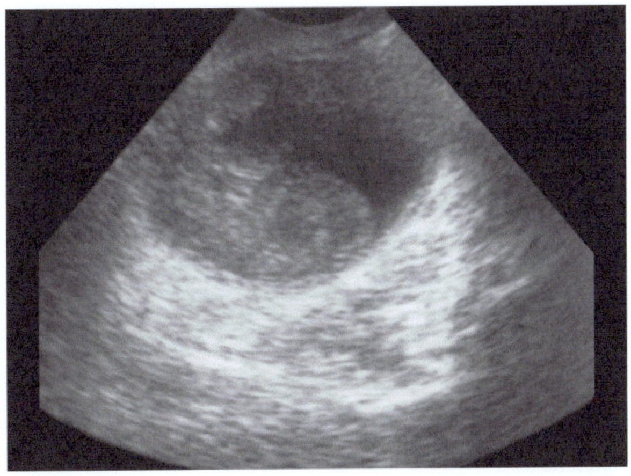

Fig. 6.54 Cystic renal cell carcinoma classifiable as Bosniak grade IV. Cystic mass shows a large mural nodule with heterogeneous hypoechoic appearance

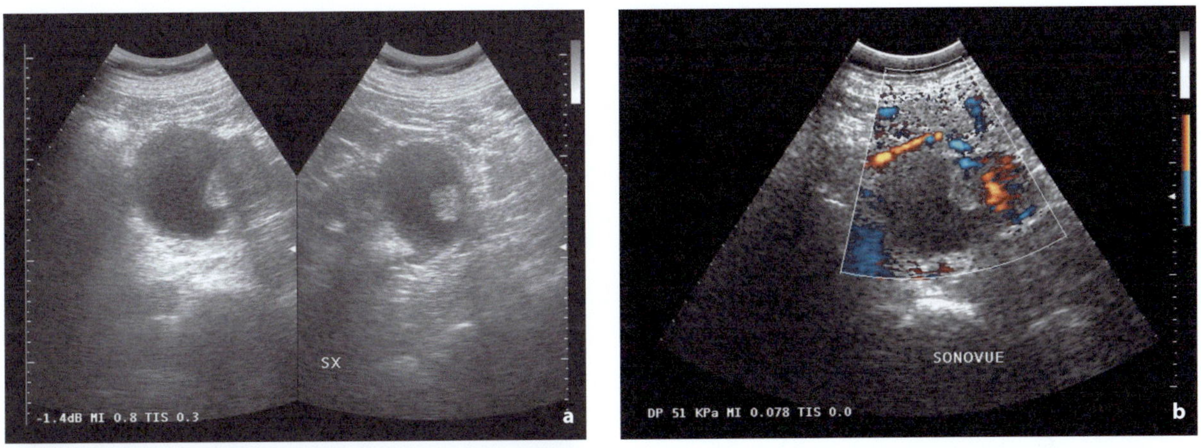

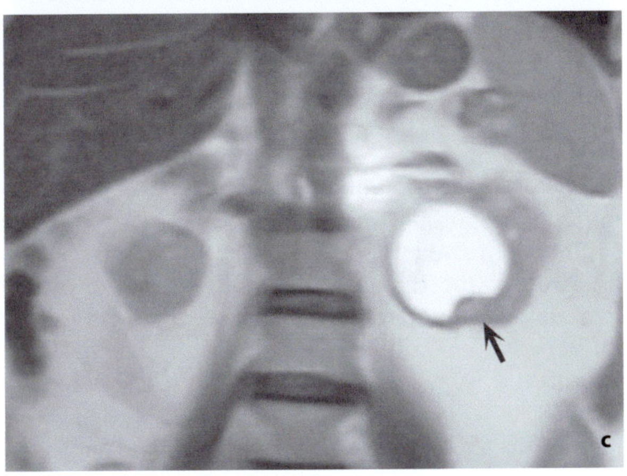

Fig. 6.55a-c Atypical renal cyst. Solid nodule within cystic renal mass (**a**) with no flow signals at directional PD after injection of contrast medium (**b**). Coronal MR correlation (**c**, *arrow*)

wash-out in the late phase. Even the enhancement of septations or mural nodularities is not absolutely indicative of malignancy, since this may be observed in inflammatory forms. It is nonetheless a fundamental finding for orienting the patient towards surgery [25,48] (Fig. 6.56). Since it is comparable to CT in terms of diagnostic accuracy if not superior (in lesions adequately accessible to the study), CEUS could be proposed as a more suitable imaging modality for the monitoring of these lesions [19,48,49].

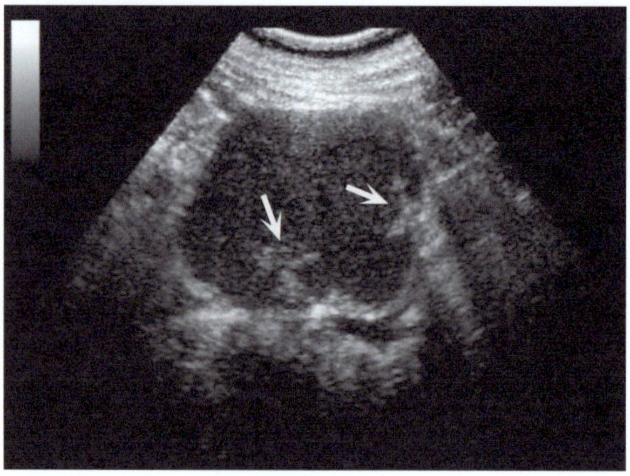

Fig. 6.56 Atypical renal cyst. CEUS study shows enhancement of solid intracystic nodules (*arrows*)

6.5 Ovarian Masses

"Ovarian masses" are a frequent and significant problem. An estimated 5–10% of women undergo surgical procedures at some time during their life for an adnexal mass. In addition, at least 80% of adnexal masses are benign, especially in reproductive-age women (87% of resected masses) and less so in postmenopausal subjects (65%) [50].

The incidence of **ovarian cancer** is increasing. The malignancy currently accounts for 4% of tumors in women and it is the second most common tumor of the female reproductive system and has the highest mortality. Both the incidence of the lesions and the probability of malignancy increases with age, with a range between 40 and 70 years of age and a mean age at diagnosis of 61 years, therefore in postmenopausal age. Some 85% of cases involve women >45 years. The risk factors include nulliparity, late primiparity, infertility, family history (hereditary forms account for as many as 5% of cases, with the possible malignancy developing in premenopausal age) and personal history of colon, breast or uterine cancer. Oral contraceptive use and breast-feeding seem to offer a measure of protection. Given the nonspecific and late symptoms, the majority of cases are identified in a late phase and therefore often associated with a poor prognosis. Lesions identified in stage I – possibly as incidental findings – instead have a five-year survival rate >90% [49,50].

Epithelial tumors account for 60–75% of ovarian neoplasms and 85–95% of malignant lesions and include the following forms: serous (52% of epithelial tumors), mucinous (16%), nondifferentiated (6%), endometrioid (19%, associated in 20–33% of cases of endometrial hyperplasia or carcinoma), clear cell (7%) and Brenner [51,52]. The tumors can be classified as benign, borderline (presence of internal papillary projections but absence of stromal invasion, possible peritoneal metastasization) and malignant. The serous forms (30% of ovarian tumors) are borderline in 15% of cases and malignant in 25%, the mucinous forms (20–25% of ovarian tumors) are borderline in 10% of cases and malignant in 20%, whereas endometrioid forms are generally malignant.

CA-125 is a cancer antigen whose serum levels rise (>35 IU/mL) in 80–85% of cases of ovarian cases, although without a clear correlation between lesion size and levels measured. Many ovarian tumors, however, can give normal CA-125 levels, especially in the initial phase and above all in mucinous types.

Together with CA-125, US is a first-level diagnostic examination in the study of adnexal masses, given its availability, noninvasiveness and high negative predictive value. When the transvaginal approach is used with high-resolution transducers and CD it is the most accurate. The suprapubic approach also plays an important role, in that as well as providing a more panoramic view it is also the approach which often identifies, usually incidentally, an initial ovarian lesion. TVUS is nonetheless more sensitive and more specific and provides additional information in 70% of cases. MR is better able to characterize lesions [53] and is a possible second-level diagnostic modality, while laparoscopy, staging laparotomy and second-look surgery have important roles to play [52]. According to the **FIGO staging** criteria in fact, the role of laparotomy is fundamental: stage I, limited to the ovary; stage II, limited to the pelvis with surgical demonstration of malignant implants; stage III, limited to the abdomen with surgical demonstration of malignant implants; stage IV, with hematogenous or extra-abdominal spread.

The determination of adequate **suspicion of malignancy** is important. Indeed, only 13–21% of women surgically treated for a suspected carcinoma effectively have the diagnosis of malignancy confirmed [52]. In addition, the degree of suspected malignancy influences the surgical approach. A laparoscopic approach is suggested for masses with a moderately suspicious US appearance and no additional risk factors (ascites, diameter >10 cm, bilateral presentation, RI <0.6, CA-125 >35 IU/mL), whereas laparotomy is indicated in the presence of one of these factors [54]. A simple, unilocular and homogeneous cystic mass <5 cm identified in an asymptomatic subject can be simply monitored with US, since it is most likely benign. The **morphologic characteristics** suggestive of malignancy are (in addition to any findings of peritoneal or parenchymal colonization) significant size (>5 cm and even more so if >9–10 cm), bilateral presentation (20% of benign tumors but up to 50% of malignant tumors, especially if serous or endometrioid), solid components without clear adipose appearance (low or moderate echogenicity, without marked hyperreflectivity with acoustic shadowing), thick (>2–3 mm) and irregular walls, mural nodularity (papillary projections emerging from the internal surface of the cystic wall, highly suspicious), hypervascularity and peritoneal effusion (but only if notable) (Figs. 6.57–6.60). The greater or lesser echogenicity of the intracystic fluid does not seem to be a differentiating criterion. Various multiparameter scoring systems have been proposed (Fig. 6.61), which have led to a sensitivity of TVUS for the diagnosis of malignancy of 82–100% with a specificity, however, ranging from 56% to 95% due to the overlap between benign and malignant forms [52,55,56]. A qualitative CD study should always be performed, with both the transabdominal and transvaginal approach, to show the presence of vascularity in the solid components, mural nodularities and papillary projections of the malignant lesions [56,57] (Figs. 6.62–6.66). This has proven particularly useful for example in the differentiation of ovarian carcinomas from other pelvic masses with a complex appearance [58]. CD is able to help identify solid vascular areas and distinguish the various components. This enables an analysis of vascular patterns, thus demonstrating both subjectively and quantitatively the greater vascularity of the malignant lesions with respect to the benign lesions [59].

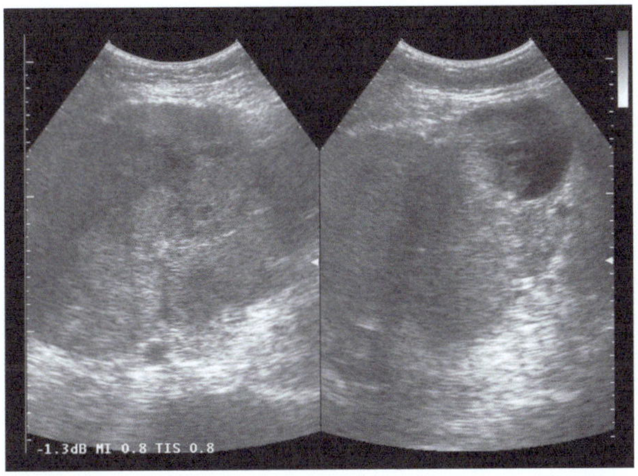

Fig. 6.57 Endometrioid carcinoma of the ovary. Prevalently solid large pelvic mass with heterogeneous hypoechoic appearance

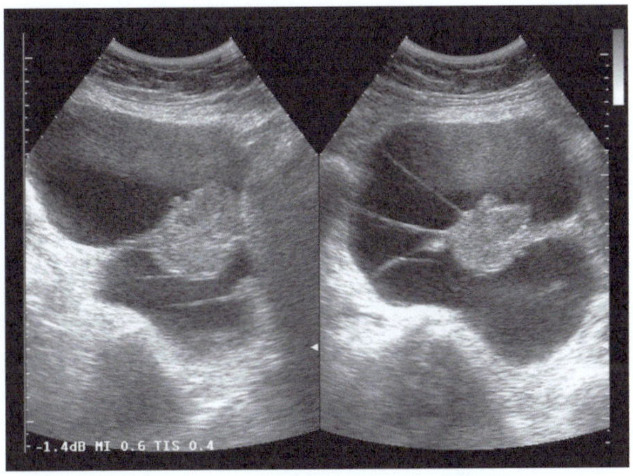

Fig. 6.58 Mucinous cystadenocarcinoma of the ovary. Complex, prevalently cystic mass with solid central component from which multiple septations with variable thickness irradiate

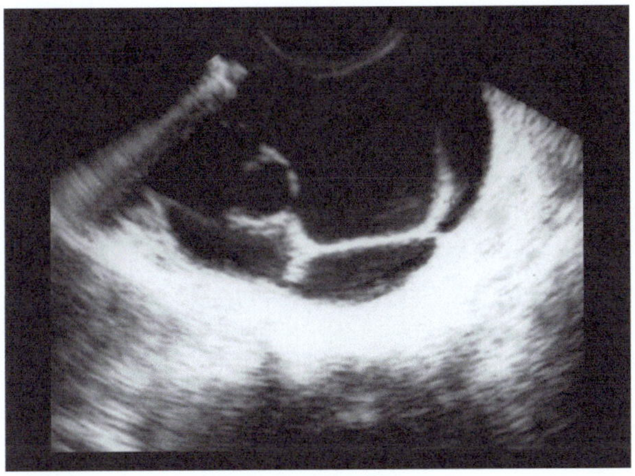

Fig. 6.59 Serous cystadenocarcinoma of the ovary. Adnexal mass with thick and irregular internal septations

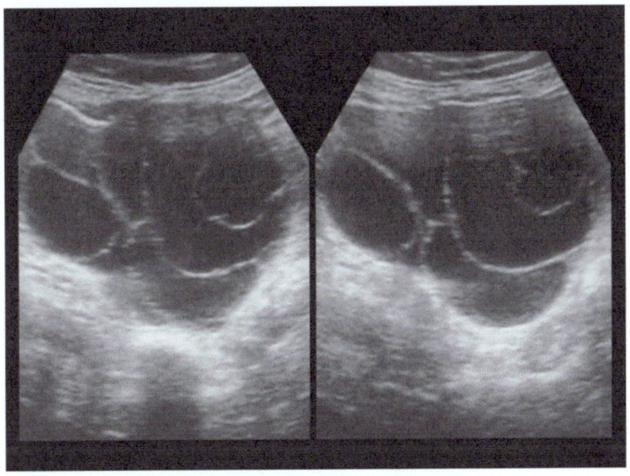

Fig. 6.60 Serous cystadenocarcinoma of the ovary. Ovarian mass with multiple thin internal septations

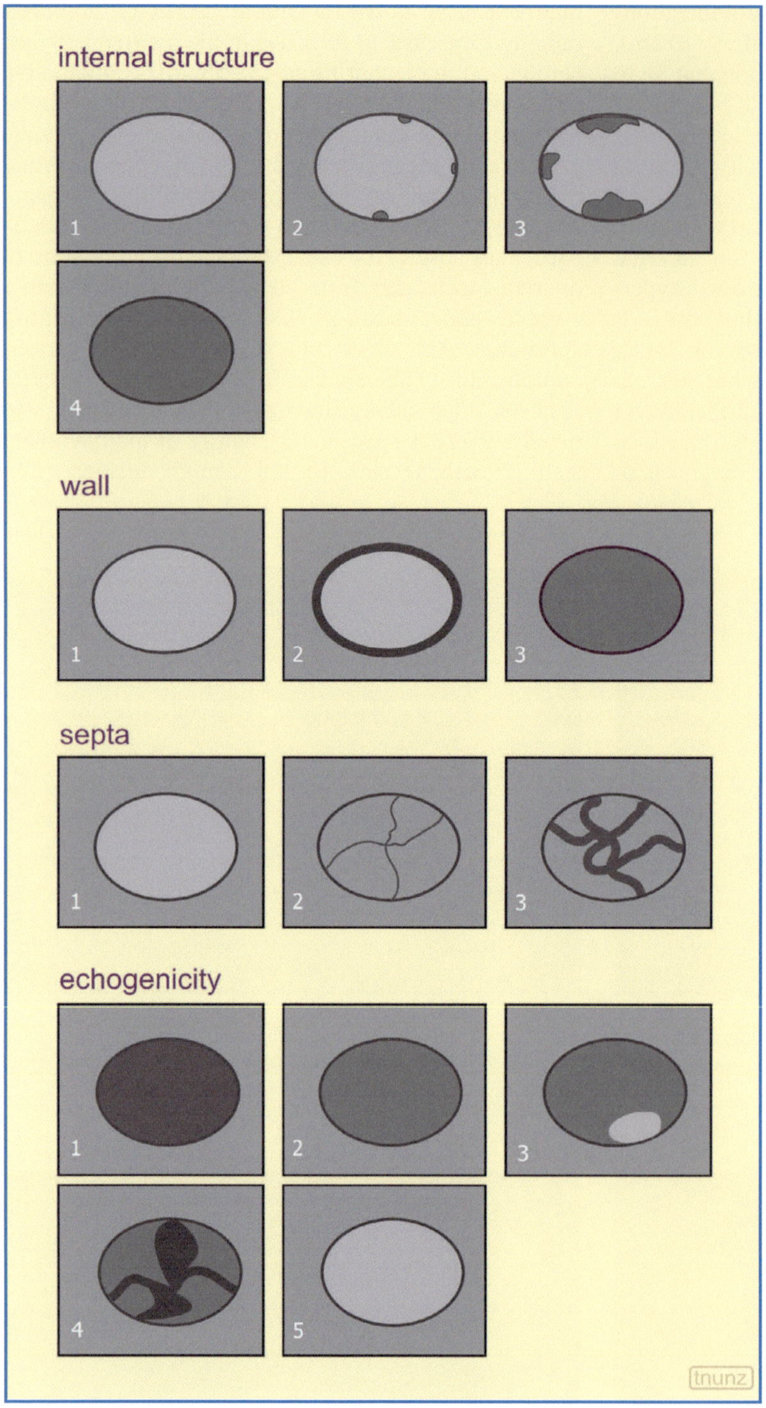

Fig. 6.61 Morphostructural scoring of ovarian masses. According to Sassone et al. [55], there are *1* to *4* typologies for internal structure, *1* to *3* for the wall, *1* to *3* for septations and *1* to *5* for echogenicity

Whereas in benign lesions the formation of vessels occurs mainly in the periphery, malignant lesions display neoangiogenesis which generally originates from the center and is detected in the septations, the papillary projections and the solid components. Nonetheless hypervascular benign forms and malignant forms with no vascular signals are also found [50,51] (Fig. 6.67). CD has proven useful in the differentiation between malignant ovarian tumors and other pelvic masses with complex appearance and is without doubt more specific than US alone and especially than CA-125 plasma levels alone [58]. A more complex

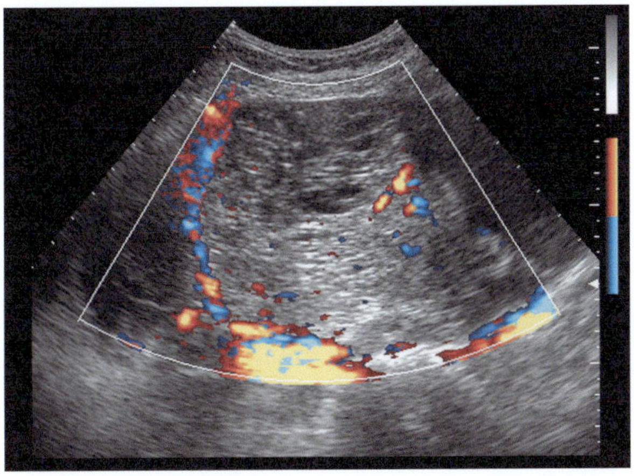

Fig. 6.62 Serous cystadenocarcinoma of the ovary. Complex mass with prevalently solid-microcystic areas characterized by some color signals at directional PD and corpuscular macrocystic areas with color signals in the large septations

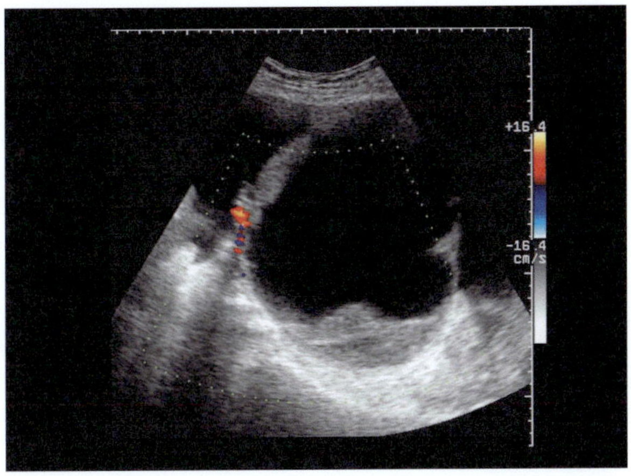

Fig. 6.63 Mucinous cystadenocarcinoma of the ovary. Prevalently cystic mass with peripheral solid components and thick septations showing flow signals at CD

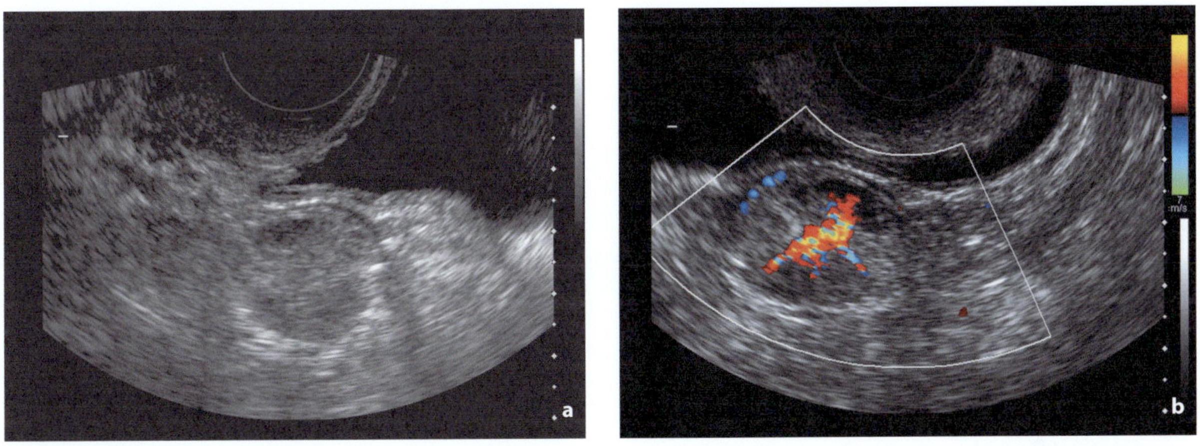

Fig. 6.64a,b Ovarian cancer. Heterogeneous hypoechoic mass is seen widening the ovary (a) and displays moderate and prevalently central vascularity at CD (b)

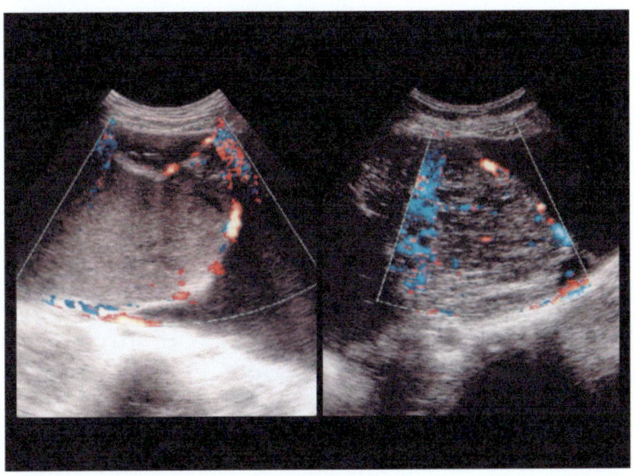

Fig. 6.65 Mucinous cystadenocarcinoma of the ovary. Heterogeneous multilocular cystic mass with flow signals within the thick septations at directional PD

case regards the spectral parameters, which in the past were given considerable weight but the role of which in the diagnosis of malignancy has been re-evaluated in recent years [52]. Spectral Doppler is complex and time consuming since it requires the sampling of flow in various vascular poles. In these vessels without smooth musculature, with poor flow resistance and high incidence of arteriovenous fistulas, the technique shows a significant diastolic component of the spectrum, with consequent poor systolic-diastolic modulation (Fig. 6.68). As a result systolic velocity values are suspicious if >16 cm/s, RI values are suspicious if <0.4–0.8 (most authors however settle on <0.4–0.45) and PI values are suspicious if <1 [52,56,57,60,61] (Fig. 6.69). The sensitivity of the Doppler technique in different series ranges from 50% to 100%, and the

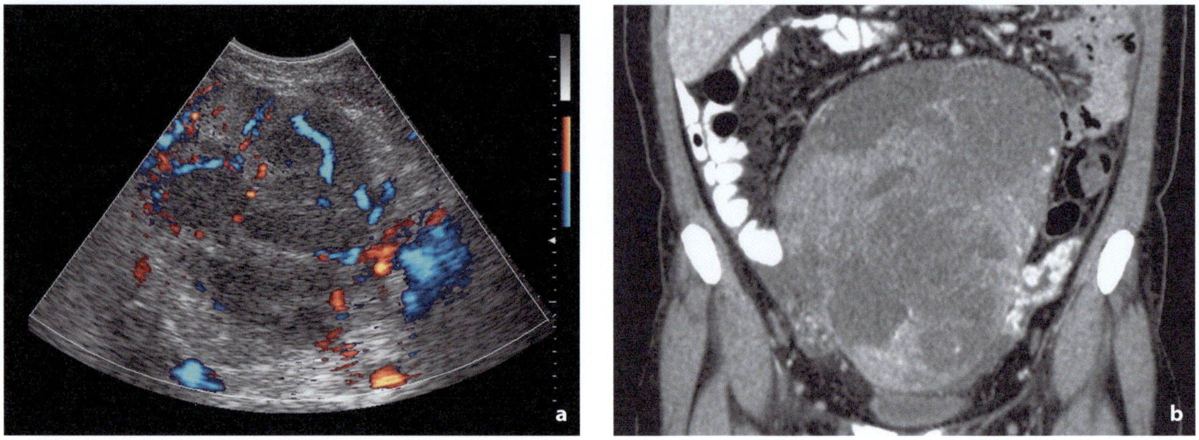

Fig. 6.66a,b Ovarian cancer. Large median pelvic mass with heterogeneous hypoechoic appearance and marked and particularly peripheral vascularity at directional PD (**a**). Coronal CT correlation shows internal texture very similar to the US image (**b**)

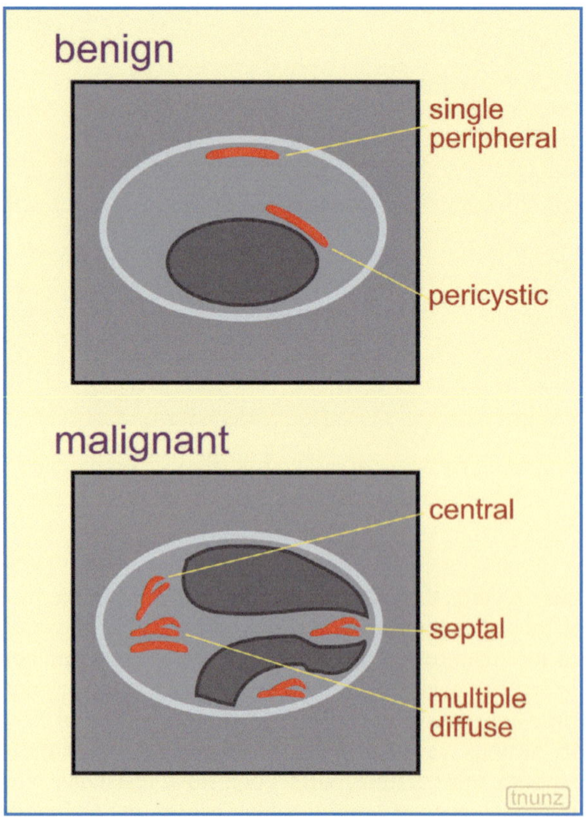

Fig. 6.67 Possible CD distribution patterns of ovarian masses. In the benign forms peripheral and pericystic flows predominate, whereas in malignant lesions central, septal and diffuse flows are more commonly found

specificity from 46% to 100%, in part because there are interfering factors such as the hormonal state of the patient (the findings in postmenopausal women are without doubt more reliable than in premenopausal women, in whom a measurement between the 3rd and 11th day of the menstrual cycle is recommended) and there are benign conditions, such as endometriosis and pelvic inflammatory disease, which can have an acoustic impedance of the "malignant" type. It should also be borne in mind that an adnexal mass can show rather different Doppler spectra in different vascular poles. In this case a mean of the various samplings should not be calculated as would be done in different circumstances, rather the trace which gives the lowest RI and PI values should be used for the suspicion of malignancy. Lastly, with regard to the peak systolic velocity, elevated values have been correlated with malignant forms, and a cut-off value has even been used as an independent parameter in the prognosis of epithelial ovarian tumors [60]. All things considered, the US evaluation needs to integrate the gray-scale morphologic data with the CD findings and possibly those provided by spectral Doppler, to obtain accurate results (sensitivity and specificity of 90%). In a large multicenter study on pelvic masses identified with TVUS and CD and considered to be of extrauterine relevance, 8% were unclassifiable in terms of suspicion of malignancy. These indeterminate lesions were for the most part, as is understandable, borderline ovarian tumors although there were also cases of parametrial myomas, papillary cystadeno(fibro)mas and struma ovarii [62]. The current experiences with contrast media are also limited. It would, however, appear that malignant tumors are characterized by a greater peak enhancement, a slower wash-out and a wider area below the enhancement curve, whereas the time to peak for the most part seems to overlap between benign and malignant lesions. CEUS with

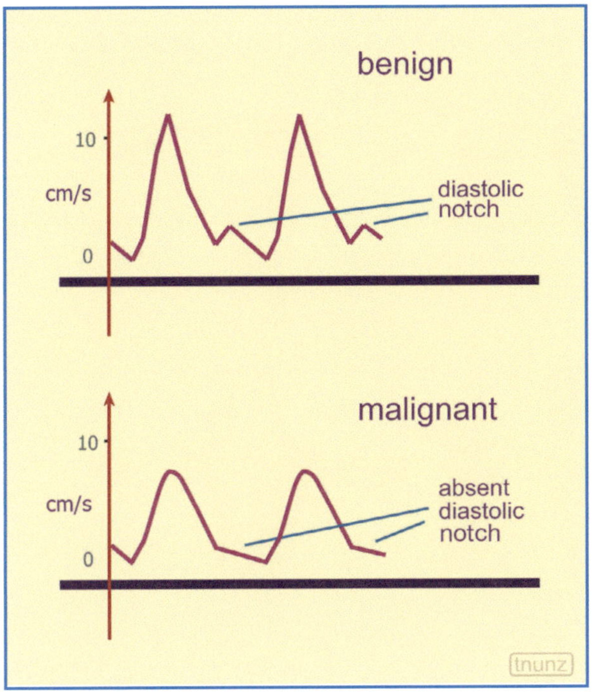

Fig. 6.68 Typical spectral profiles of adnexal masses. In the benign forms the systolic-diastolic difference is greater and a diastolic notch is present, whereas in malignant lesions the modulation is lower and the diastolic notch is absent

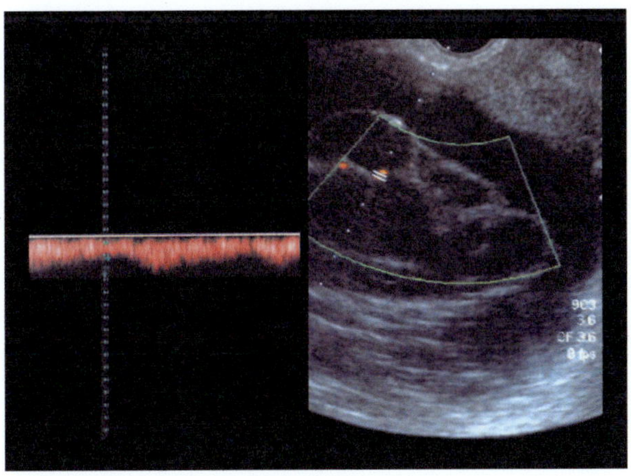

Fig. 6.69 Cystadenocarcinoma of the ovary. Finely and irregularly septated mass. Spectral Doppler of a septal arterial vessel shows a low-resistance spectrum

transvaginal transducer therefore appears to increase reliability in benign-malignant distinction with the identification of intralesional microvascularity [57,63,64].

The **spread pattern** of ovarian carcinoma first of all is by direct extension to the uterine tube, the broad ligaments, the uterus and the contralateral ovary (50% of carcinomas are in fact bilateral, but half of these are the result of spread from the ovary to the opposite side). The advanced phase sees the invasion of the bladder, the rectosigmoid, ileal loops and the pelvic walls (Fig. 6.70). Peritoneal spread, which is still within the T parameter, can be identified at the level of the greater omentum, the hepatic capsule, the right hemidiaphragm, the intestinal serous surface and the rectouterine pouch. The regional lymph nodes include the hypogastric, common iliac, external iliac, lateral sacral, para-aortic and inguinal nodes. Hematogenous metastases are identified in only 1% of cases at presentation but they are frequent in the advanced phases or in disease recurrence – the organs which can be explored are the liver, kidney, adrenal gland, urinary bladder and spleen. Last of all, US with the transabdominal approach, but most of all the transvaginal and transrectal approaches, can be useful in the diagnosis of pelvic recurrence of ovarian cancer (vaginal dome, bladder wall, etc.), with an accuracy of 90%.

With specific regard to other expansive ovarian masses, the most frequent in both pre- and postmenopausal women is without doubt the functional cyst (**follicular cysts** arising from non-ruptured or non-reabsorbed follicles, **corpus luteum cysts** arising from bleeding within a corpus luteum) associated with menstrual irregularities but with no malignant potential. The masses are generally <3 cm (although >10 cm is possible), unilocular with thin, smooth walls and enhanced through-transmission [52]. In the presence of this appearance, no particular additional work-up is generally required, although there is a slight overlap with benign tumors such as serous cystadenoma. With lesions <5 cm (<6 cm in postmenopausal women), a US examination is done after one or two menstrual cycles to identify whether there has been spontaneous regression of the finding, which is rather common if the size of the functional cyst is limited and if the woman is of reproductive age. Often combined hormone therapy is performed to facilitate reabsorption of the cysts, although the real effectiveness of and need for this approach is debatable [65]. Cysts with a simple appearance but with a size greater than the above-mentioned threshold values are probably not functional and are often due to serous cystadenomas, which if persistent can be removed with laparoscopy. The situation however is different when internal bleeding has rendered the content of the cystic mass heterogeneous, with a lacy reticular pattern of echoes (but without septations or solid components). In this case CD is of little help, although it can identify vascular signals, and an additional study is indicated for adequate characterization. **Corpus luteum cysts**

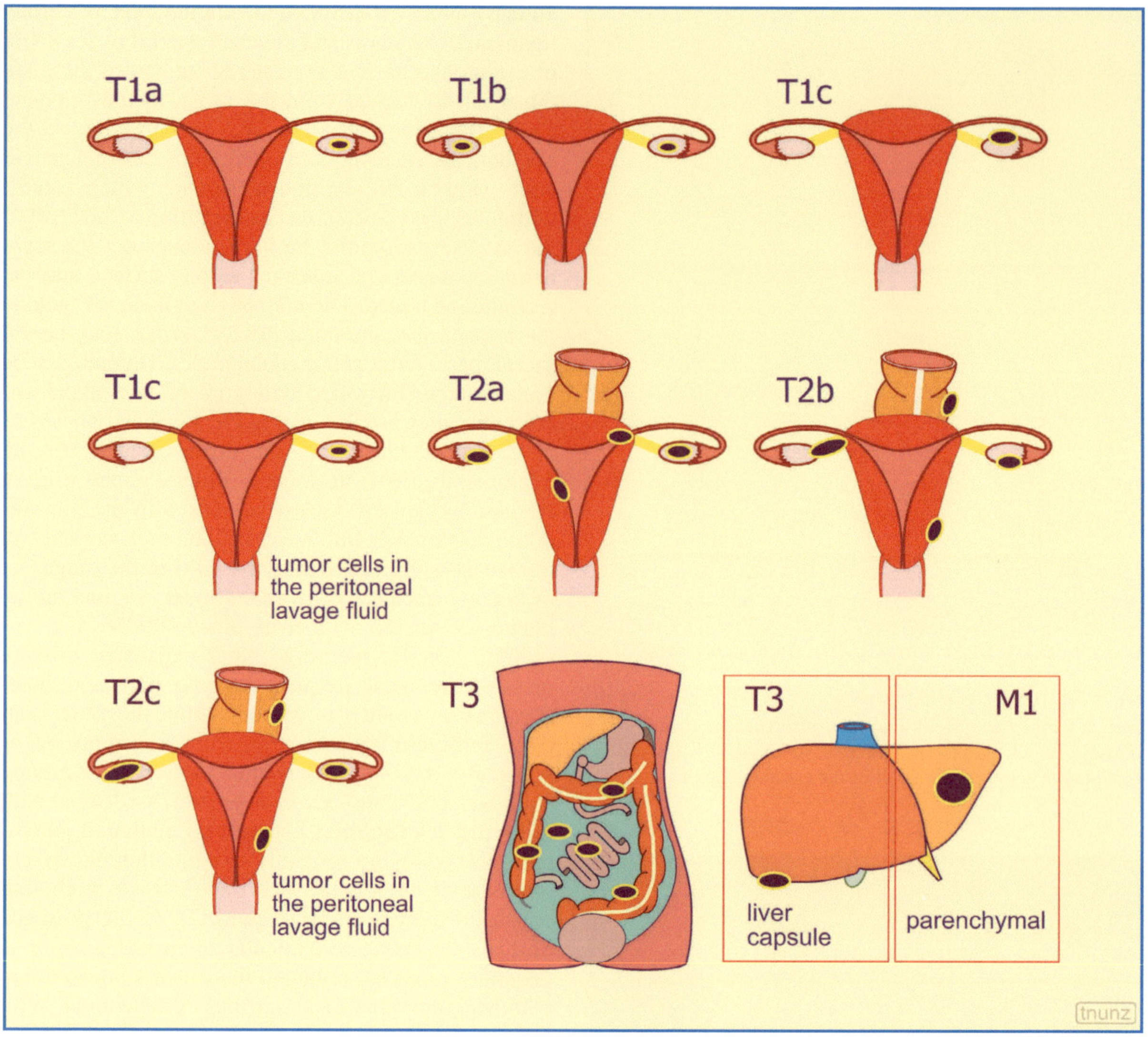

Fig. 6.70 Staging of ovarian cancer. *T1a*, tumor confined to one ovary; *T1b*, tumor is confined to both ovaries; *T1c*, tumor confined to one or both ovaries but with capsular rupture and/or tumor cells in peritoneal lavage fluid; *T2a*, extension to the uterus and/or uterine tube but without tumor cells in peritoneal washings; *T2b*, extension to other pelvic structures but without tumor cells in peritoneal washings; *T2c*, pelvic extension with tumor cells in peritoneal washings; *T3*, extrapelvic metastases, including those at the level of the hepatic capsule. Modified from [31]

can have a varied appearance and not unusually can mimic a carcinoma. They are a relatively frequent occurrence, both as an incidental finding and as a source of pelvic pain and palpable mass, and are typically revealed in the postovulatory phase [66]. Their size is generally 3–3.5 cm, although they can reach 8 cm, and the wall appears thin (2–3 mm), sharp and smooth. The finding of enhanced through-transmission is indicative of their cystic nature. The internal structure is very variable, in relation to the age of the cyst and therefore the evolution of the effused blood: strands of fibrin (echogenic reticulated strands, generally thin and regular), retracted coagulations (pseudosolid and generally homogeneous echogenic components adhering to the cystic wall with a crescent or triangular shape), and fluid-fluid or fluid-debris levels [65,66]. The different morphologic appearances of the clots and the septations can of course mimic a cystic tumor, although the absence of color signals at transvaginal CD constitutes a sufficiently specific sign. In doubtful cases, however, the most rational approach appears to be short-term US follow-up, with demonstration of even partial involution of the lesion (generally no longer recognizable after 6–8 weeks) [65]. Occasionally, however, the cyst may present an annular appearance, with a peripheral echogenic ring and hypoechoic center, which can mimic a uterine tube pregnancy, especially in cases of rupture of the hemorrhagic cysts which produces effusion in the rectouterine pouch [66] (Fig. 6.71–6.73).

Ovarian **endometrioma** (or endometriosis chocolate cyst, 80% of cases of pelvic endometriosis) is predominant in premenopausal women and appears as an adnexal cystic mass with diffuse low-level internal echoes. The size is generally limited, and multiple loculations and/or echogenic cholesterol wall foci may be present, but generally there are no signs suggestive of malignancy such as mural nodulations or thick and irregular septations [52,67]. Internal fluid-fluid or fluid-debris levels are possible (Fig. 6.74).

Mature **cystic teratomas** are generally asymptomatic. They account for 15–54% of ovarian tumors and are bilateral in 10–13% of cases. They typically appear with echogenic dermoid areas (or broad hyperechoic areas), internal fluid-lipid levels (less echogenic fluid in dependent portions and more echogenic fat above), "tip of the iceberg" sign (masking of the deep components due to hyperechoic superficial components) and calcifications. Occasionally multiple intraluminal floating echogenic "balls" 5–40 mm in size may be distinguished [68] (Figs. 6.75, 6.76,

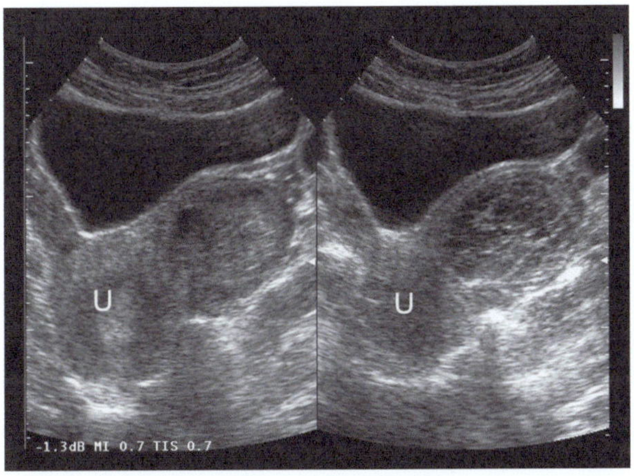

Fig. 6.71 Corpus luteum cyst. Well-defined left adnexal mass with heterogeneous and lacy pattern of fibrinous bands. *U*, uterus (with thickened endometrium)

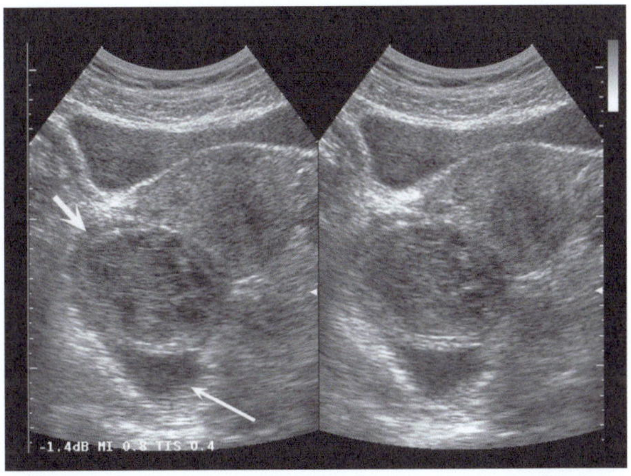

Fig. 6.72 Corpus luteum cyst. Heterogeneous hypoechoic mass of the right ovary (*short arrow*) associated with peritoneal effusion (*long arrow*)

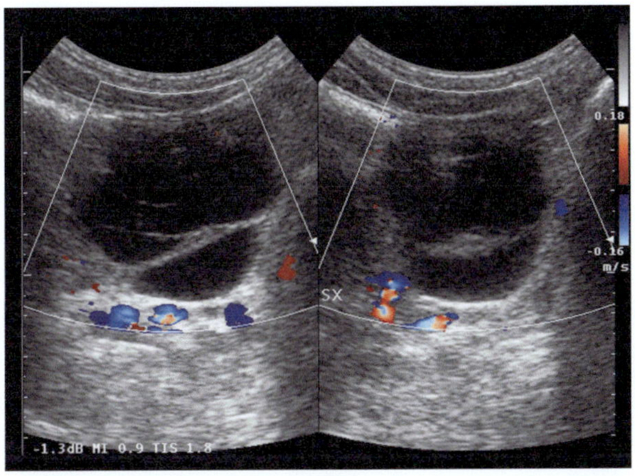

Fig. 6.73 Corpus luteum cyst. Cystic mass with internal septs and inhomogeneous content but without flow signals

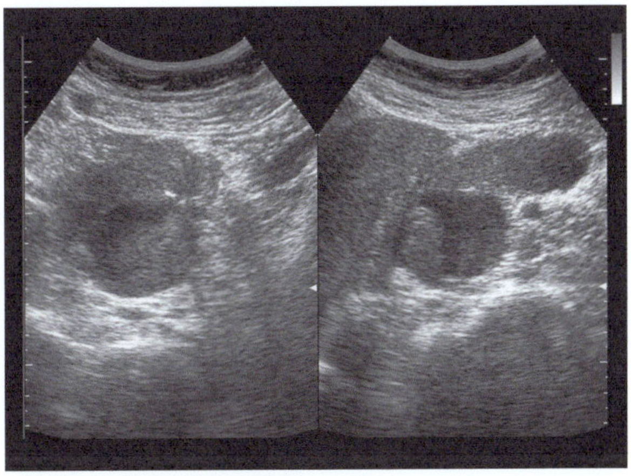

Fig. 6.74 Endometriosis. Cystic mass with partially fluid heterogeneous content

Video 6.10). CD shows substantial avascularity, except for some vascular signs. The overall appearance, with a marked "tip of the iceberg" sign, could in theory mimic a rectosigmoid distended with fecal material [50]. The only other adnexal lesion to contain fat is the rare and malignant immature teratoma, which appears as a prevalently solid mass with small echogenic adipose foci and large calcifications [52].

Serous cystadenoma appears as a clear fluid-filled cystic mass with homogeneous anechoic appearance and some thin internal septations and occasionally some small mural nodulations. **Serous cystadenocarcinoma** tends to have a more complex appearance, with thick walls, multiple thick and irregular septations and solid intralesional polypoid components adhering to the walls or the septations themselves [50].

Mucinous cystadenoma and **cystadenocarcinoma** appear not terribly dissimilar from the corresponding serous lesions, although with a tendency to greater echogenicity of the intracystic fluid content, occasionally with fluid-debris levels and on average more internal septations [50]. A characteristic of the benign mucinous forms is the presence of different degrees of echogenicity between the various intralesional fluid-filled loculations, which is the evident expression of a mucinous production with different chemical composition [69]. In the event of rupture, multiple fluid-filled peritoneal loculations may be observed.

Fibrous tumors (4% of ovarian tumors, 2% of those malignant) – in the various forms of fibromas, thecomas, fibrous thecomas and fibrothecomas – are usually identified incidentally in middle-aged women.

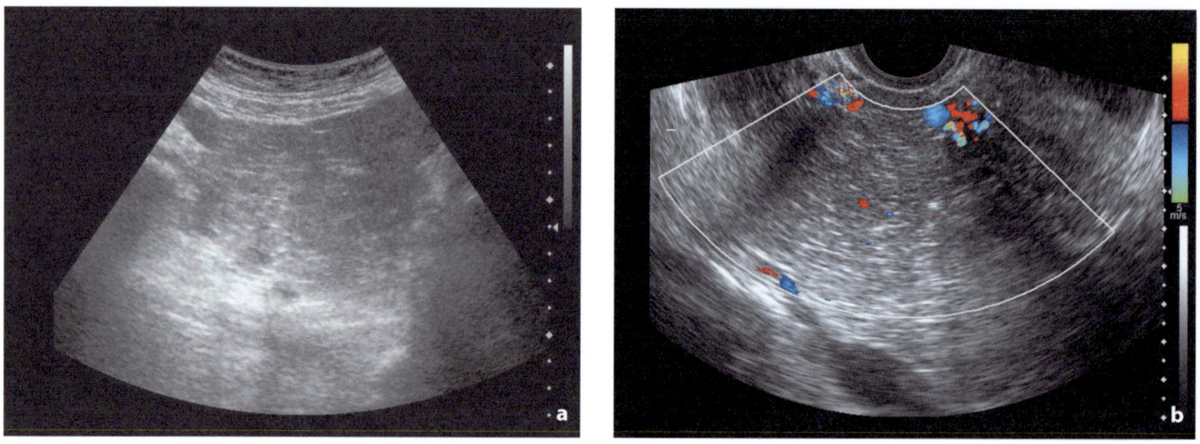

Fig. 6.75a,b Teratoma of the ovary. Poorly defined, mildly heterogeneous echogenic mass (**a**) almost without vascular signals at CD (**b**)

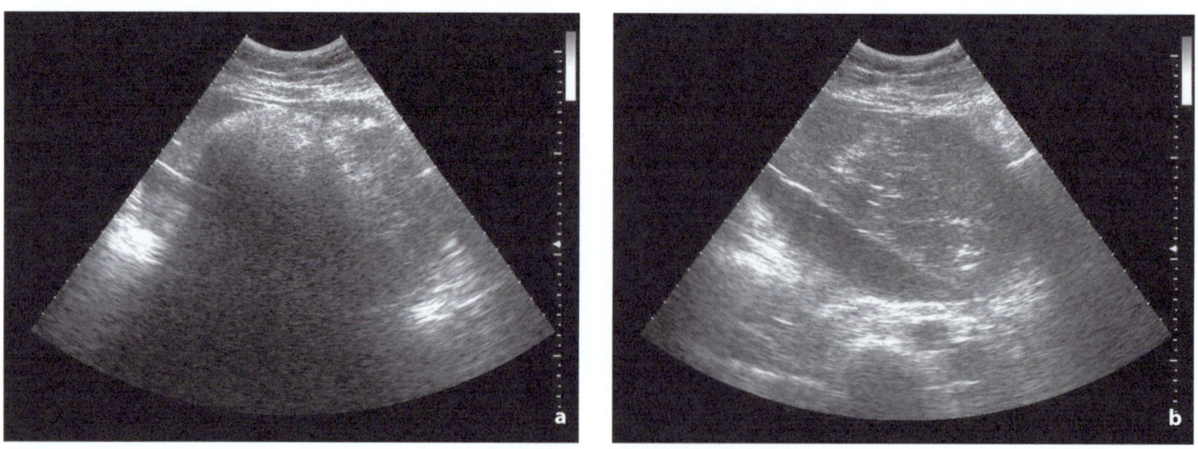

Fig. 6.76a,b Dermoid cyst of the ovary. Complex mass with hyperechoic patches and marked posterior acoustic shadowing (**a**, "tip of the iceberg" sign) as well as hyperechoic adipose areas and hypo-anechoic fluid areas (**b**)

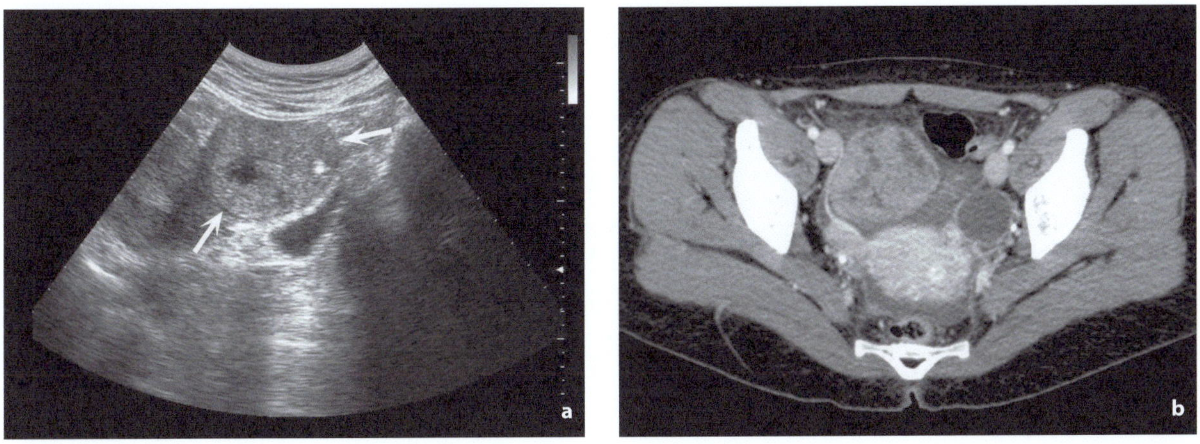

Fig. 6.77a,b Ovarian fibroma. Well-defined echogenic mass (*arrows*) with substantially homogeneous echotexture except for the presence of a calcification and an eccentric liquefactive area (**a**). CT scan (**b**) confirms the right solid adnexal mass. Left adnexal follicular cyst and slight fluid layer in the rectouterine pouch can also be distinguished

They appear as masses with variable echogenicity, generally hypoechoic but possibly hyperechoic with enhanced through-transmission. The solid appearance can mimic a malignant lesion, in part because associated peritoneal and even pleural effusion are not rare events. In the sclerosing forms the appearance is more complex, with rounded cystic components located centrally, and hypervascularity especially with peripheral and central distribution. RI and PI generally have low mean values (0.39 and 0.47, respectively) [70]. CD can be useful in the differentiation from pedunculated subserous uterine myomas by showing the presence of poor, irregularly distributed and slow intralesional flows in the fibrous tumor, whereas myomas tend to be hypervascular. In general, although most of these tumors are benign, the tendency is to surgically remove all solid or prevalently solid ovarian masses, regardless of the age of the patient [65] (Fig. 6.77).

Germ cell tumors (5–15% of malignant ovarian tumors) are for the most part made up of dysgerminomas, which are most frequent in adolescents and young women. An increase in serum AFP and HCG may be associated. The tumors are generally solid, and are bilateral in 80% of cases.

Metastases account for 5–10% of malignant ovarian tumors and often originate from the stomach (30–40% of cases), colon (10–15%), pancreas, breast, endometrium and even the contralateral ovary. Functioning ovaries are at greater risk than those of postmenopausal women [51]. Metastases are difficult to differentiate from primary tumors, as they share many morphostructural and vascular features. Bilateral presentation is common (80%), but as stated above this is not rare in the primary forms. A metastatic lesion may be suspected in the presence of a prevalently or exclusively solid (non-adipose) lesion, but the morphostructural similarities are notable [71] (Figs. 6.78–6.81). With regard to vascularity, metastases show RI and PI values significantly lower than carcinoma, whereas the systolic and diastolic velocities are similar [72].

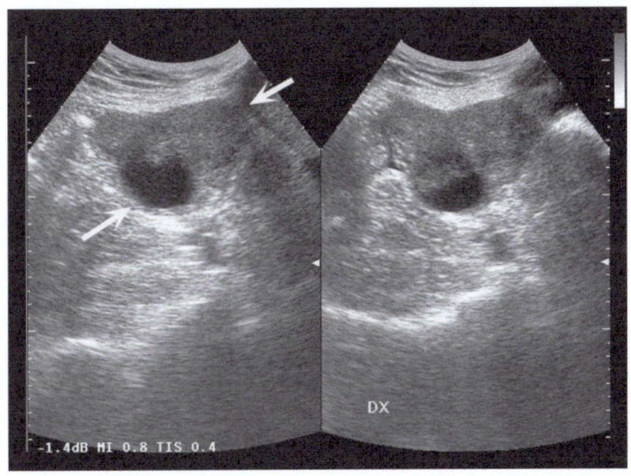

Fig. 6.78 Ovarian metastasis from colon cancer. Right adnexal mass (*arrows*) characterized by hypoechoic solid portions and anechoic cystic portions

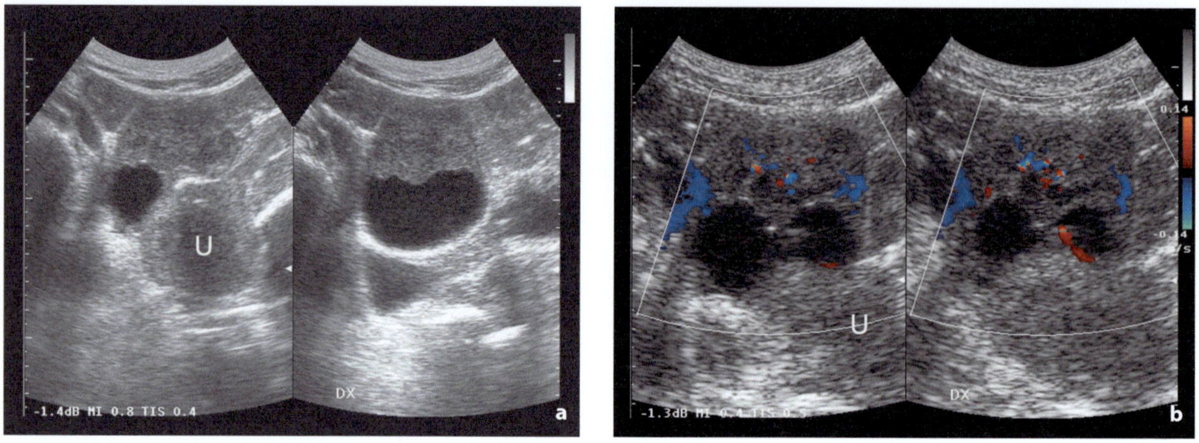

Fig. 6.79a,b Ovarian metastasis from breast cancer. Complex mass of the right ovary, with cystic components and solid nodules (**a**) and moderate vascular signals at CD (**b**). *U*, uterus

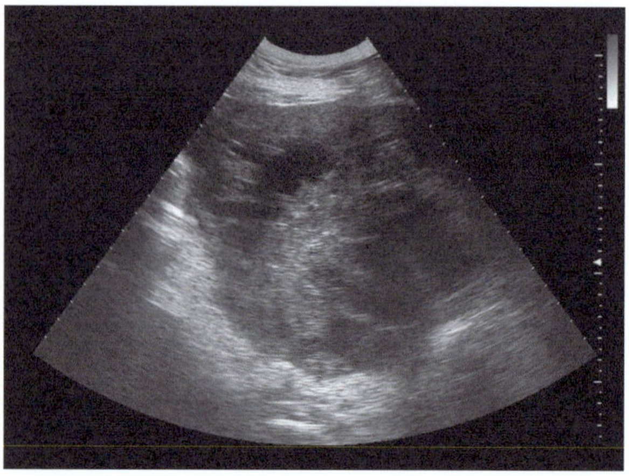

Fig. 6.80 Ovarian metastasis from rectal cancer. Large complex pelvic mass with hypo-anechoic components

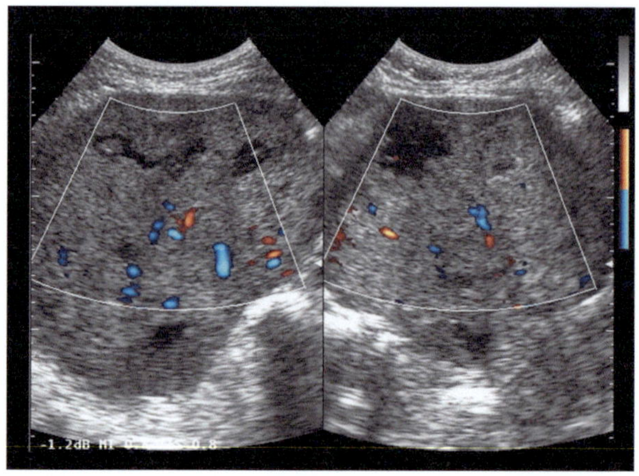

Fig. 6.81 Ovarian metastasis from breast cancer. Large echogenic mass with several hypo-anechoic liquefactive areas and moderate vascularity at directional PD

6.6 Endometrial Thickening

Carcinoma of the uterine body (endometrium) is the most common malignancy of the female reproductive system and the 4th most common malignancy in women, with a rising incidence in industrialized countries. It arises de novo or from a hyperplasia caused by unopposed estrogens [73]. The peak presentation is between 55 and 65 years of age, with 80–88% of cases in postmenopause and <5 % of cases occurring below 40 years of age [74–76]. Adenocarcinoma accounts for 90% of cases (ranging from grade 1, well differentiated to grade 3, anaplastic). Risk factors include early menarche, late menopause, nulliparity, obesity, diabetes, hypertension, hormone therapy with tamoxifen (7.5% relative risk), prolonged hormone replacement therapy (without progestin), polycystic ovary syndrome, hereditary nonpolyposis colon cancer syndrome (40–60% lifetime risk) and estrogen-secreting neoplasms (e.g. granulosa-cell tumor of the ovary) [73,74]. An alteration in the menstrual cycle occurs in premenopausal women, which may vary from amenorrhea to menometrorrhagia. Metrorrhagia or spotting is the most common and earliest symptom of carcinoma in postmenopausal women, and should always prompt diagnostic investigation (>75% of cases are therefore identified when still in stage I, with a five-year survival rate of 76%). Pain is usually a late symptom. In addition, in 80–95% of cases postmenopausal metrorrhagia has benign causes, including endometrial atrophy (the most common etiology, with ulcerations of the atrophied endometrial surface), estrogen therapy (without associated progesterone), endometrial hyperplasia, atrophic vaginitis and cervical or endometrial polyps [74,77,78]. The aim of TVUS in these cases is to select patients for endometrial biopsy, study the endometrium in the search for polyps or submucosal myomas and identify any myometrial invasion by the endometrial carcinoma [50]. Postmenopausal women operated on for breast cancer who are positive for the estrogen receptor are placed on adjuvant hormone therapy with tamoxifen for five years. It has become a consolidated practice, although the utility is still to be confirmed, to have these patients undergo periodic US follow-up to evaluate the endometrium. Indeed the endometrium tends to increase in thickness, especially at the center of the uterine body, and often displays small anechoic areas indicative of hyperplastic phenomena, polypoid changes and cystic degeneration of the endometrium and myometrium [79].

TNM staging of endometrial cancer is shown in Figures 6.82 and 6.83. The 1988 **FIGO classification** includes the following stages: I, limited to the uterine body excluding the isthmus (IA limited to the endometrium, IB invading <50% of the myometrium, IC invading >50% of the myometrium); II, involving the body and cervix (IIA confined to the endometrium, IIB invading the cervical stroma); III, extending beyond the uterus but not beyond the pelvis (IIIA invading the peritoneum of the uterus, the adnexa, positive peritoneal cytology, IIIB vaginal metastases, IIIC, metastases to the pelvis or pelvic and/or lumbar lymph nodes); IV, extending beyond the pelvis or invading the mucosa of the rectum or the bladder (IVA invasion of the bladder, rectum, sigmoid colon and small bowel, IVB distant metastases including intra-abdominal and/or inguinal lymph nodes). In terms of tumor grading a distinction is made between well-differentiated, moderately differentiated and poorly differentiated forms.

Gynecologic examination and TVUS are the initial elements for characterizing postmenopausal metrorrhagia. However, the final diagnosis, based on the initial findings provided by US or alternatively by hysterosonography, is generally reached with the second-level diagnostic technique of hysteroscopy and/or biopsy. MR also has a fundamental role to play, especially in staging, which should not be performed solely with TVUS. US study of the endometrial cavity and entire uterus can benefit from the use of the Doppler techniques, tissue harmonic imaging, 3D imaging and EFOV, which may also be performed with the transvaginal approach [80]. In some cases the addition of **hysterosonography** may be useful, performed with TVUS after distension of the endometrial cavity with liquid (single-use injector with inflatable balloon) (Fig. 6.84). This technique can be useful in the event of a poorly defined endometrium or a thickened endometrium, being able to distinguish in the latter case between true thickenings and false positives of TVUS [76].

At TVUS, the **endometrial thickness** is measured at the level of the hyperechoic central line produced by the mirror image of the uterine cavity. In the sagittal scan at the widest point, the two facing endometrial layers are added (from one endometrial-myometrial junction to the other) without considering the sub-endometrial hypoechoic layer (halo) (corresponding to the internal third of the myometrium, which appears compact and moderately vascular). Any fluid in the open cavitary lumen should be subtracted from the overall endometrial thickness when the latter is measured [79] (Fig. 6.85). The accumulation of intracavitary fluid is not a rare finding in menopause, especially in women undergoing hormone replacement therapy, and its actual pathologic significance is debatable. At any rate further work-up is recommended if the fluid layer is >3 mm thick and/or echogenic [81] (Fig. 6.86). The intra- and interobserver reliability of the measurement of endometrial thickness is more than sufficient for effective clinical use [82]. In premenopausal women the endometrium is <4 mm in the menstrual phase, 4–8 mm in the proliferative phase and 7–14 mm in the secretive phase, when it also becomes more echogenic [79] (Fig. 6.87). In postmenopausal women the endometrium atrophies due to the lack of epithelial stimulation and appears as a thin strip <4 mm and generally around 2 mm with a progressive thinning over the years and a substantial difference between the first five years after menopause and later years. Continuous hormone replacement therapy, with estrogen or combined (low-dose estrogen and progesterone), increases the thickness on average by 1–1.5 mm; sequential therapy by 3 mm [78]. If the measured thickness is <4 mm, the postmenopausal menorrhagia is put down to endometrial atrophy and no further diagnostic work-up is needed. In addition, measurement of the endometrial thickness cannot be considered an absolute criterion since a thickened endometrium can be found for example in women with no problems of metrorrhagia. In these cases, therefore, the decision to perform a biopsy should be based on clinical findings and family history, as well as the US and CD findings [50,82].

Stage I **endometrial carcinoma** presents as a focal thickening of the endometrial lining, which becomes more echogenic and heterogeneous. The endometrial thickness in postmenopausal women is considered pathologic if >5 mm (>7 mm in women undergoing hormone replacement therapy and >10 mm in those undergoing treatment with tamoxifen). The

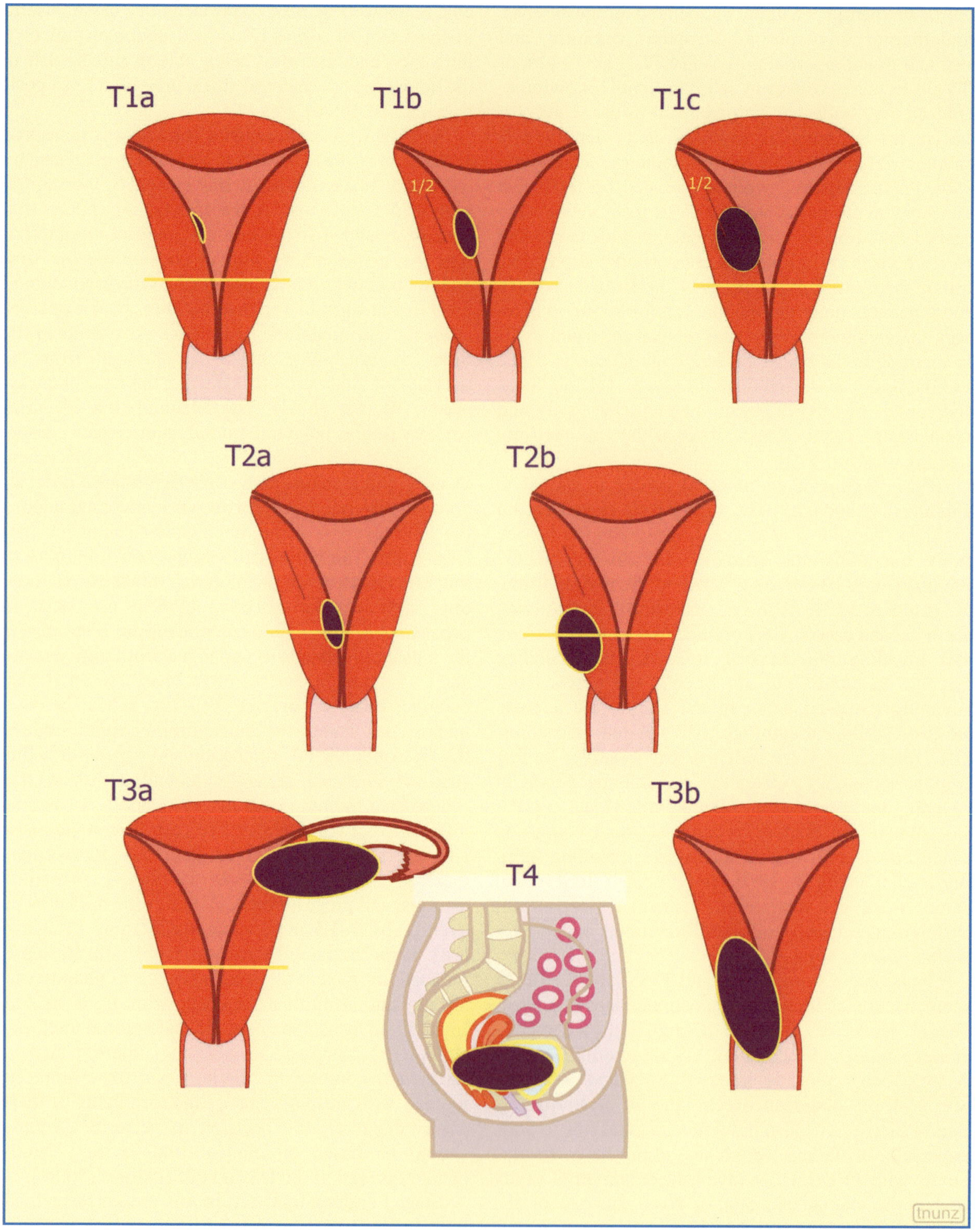

Fig. 6.82 Staging of endometrial cancer. *T1a*, tumor limited to the endometrium; *T1b*, invasion of <50% of the myometrium; *T1c*, invasion of >50% of the myometrium; *T2a*, invasion of glandular cells in the endocervical canal; *T2b*, invasion of the stromal layer of the cervix; *T3a*, spread to the serosa and/or the adnexae; *T3b*, spread to the vagina; *T4*, spread to the bladder or intestinal mucosa. Modified from [31]

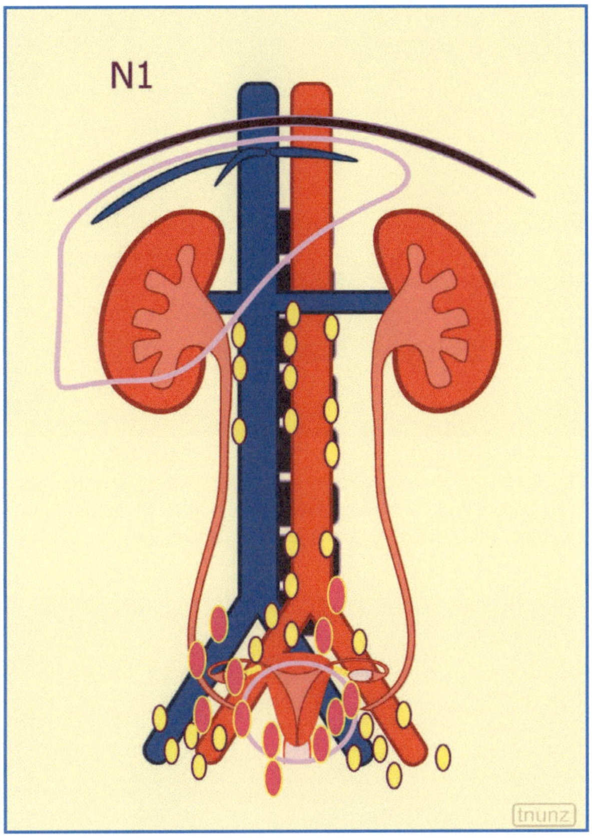

Fig. 6.83 N parameter for endometrial cancer. Regional lymph nodes include the pelvic lymph nodes (hypogastric, common iliac, external iliac, lateral sacral, parametrial, presacral, lateral sacral) and para-aortic lymph nodes (including paracaval and interaortocaval). *N1* includes metastasis to one or more of these stations. Modified from [31]

demonstration of a normal thickness virtually rules out carcinoma (indication for biopsy only in cases of repeated bleeding), whereas a postmenopausal thickness >10.5 mm has a sensitivity of 88% and a specificity of 61% in the diagnosis of malignancy [74,77]. In women with polycystic ovary syndrome, the endometrium appears thickened and occasionally with heterogeneous microcystic areas as a result of hyperplasia induced by a chronic state of anovulation [83]. Even after menopause there are other causes of endometrial thickening: endometrial hyperplasia, cystic atrophy, polyps, synechia and adjuvant treatment for breast cancer. In these conditions there is a certain degree of similarity in the imaging characteristics, although cystic areas may suggest a polyp, homogeneous thickening a hyperplasia and marked, hyperechoic and heterogeneous thickening a malignancy [50] (Figs. 6.88, 6.89).

Saline infusion hysterosonography is used by some authors in cases of endometrial thickening, to identify the imaging characteristics of different causes of bleeding. In this case, if the endometrium is not really thickened (single wall <2 mm), the diagnostic protocol is concluded, whereas in the presence of focal or polypoid thickenings hysteroscopy-guided biopsy is indicated and with diffuse thickening either conventional biopsy or a dilatation and curettage procedure is performed [50]. The risk of disseminating malignant cells is approximately 7% [73].

CD study is performed with longitudinal scans and is aimed at identifying the most vascular areas, where the spectral analysis should be performed [77]. Histologically, the development of an endometrial

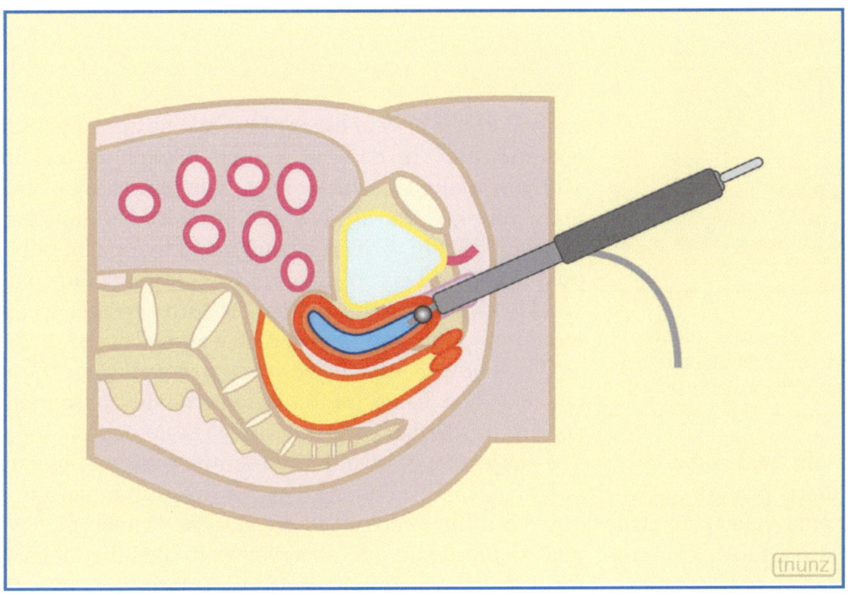

Fig. 6.84 Hysterosonography. Liquid distension of the uterine cavity for TVUS

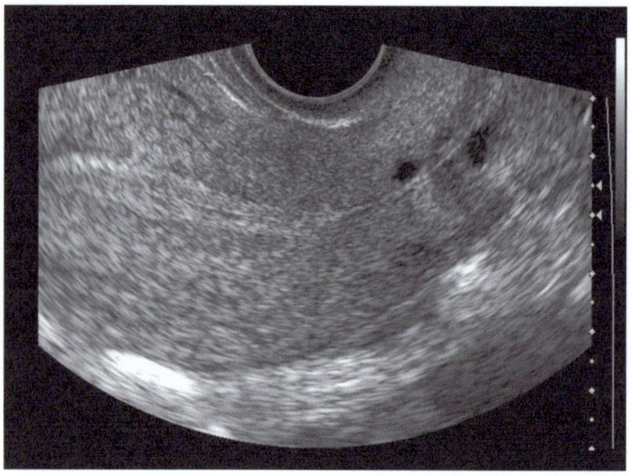

Fig. 6.85 Endometrial anatomy. Endometrium in reproductive-age woman, visualized as a relatively homogeneous band

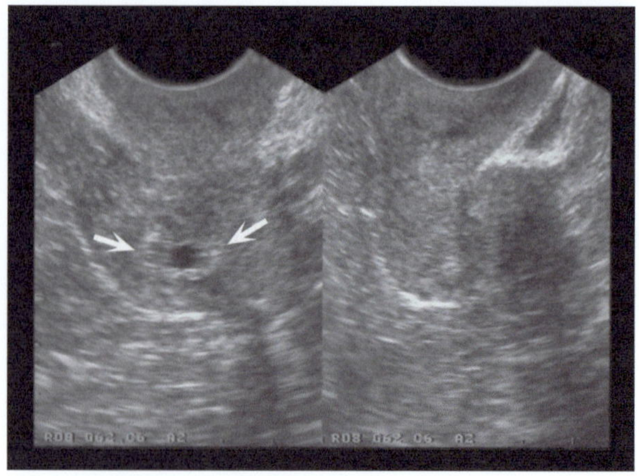

Fig. 6.86 Benign endometrial thickening. Increase in the post-menopausal endometrial thickness (*arrows*), with minimal intracavitary fluid collection at the level of the fundus

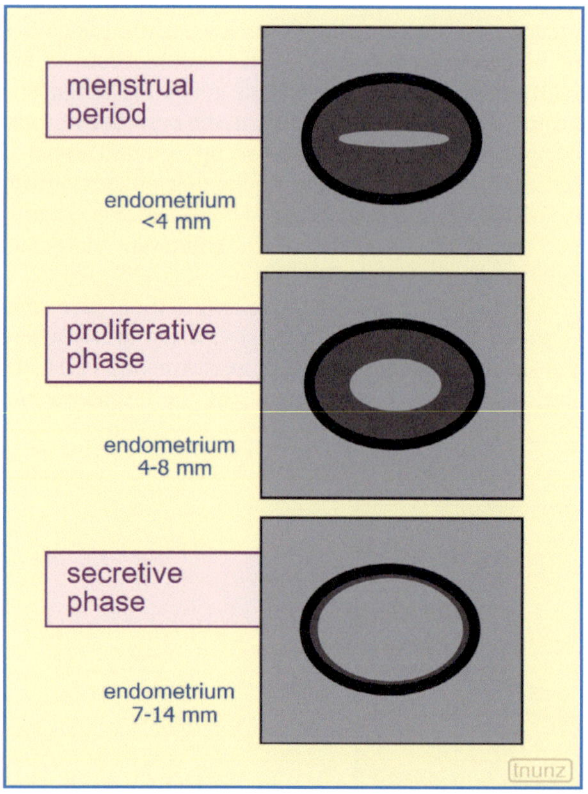

Fig. 6.87 Physiologic variations of the endometrial thickness. Differences in endometrial thickness in reproductive-age females in relation to the different phases of the menstrual cycle

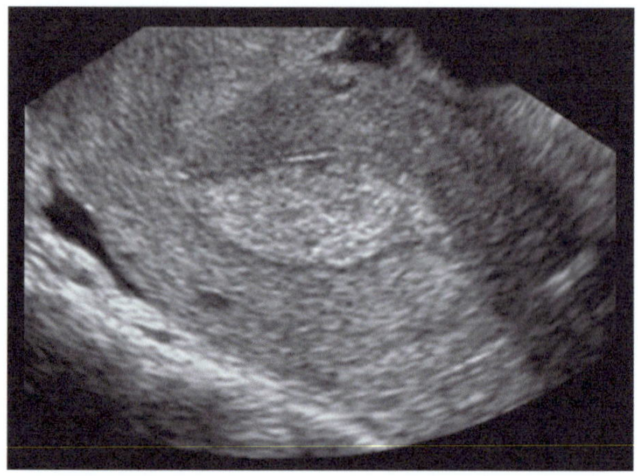

Fig. 6.88 Endometrial atrophy. Homogeneous thickening of the postmenopausal endometrium. Effusion is identifiable

malignancy is correlated with thin and randomly distributed vessels (without muscularis propria), often grouped together in hypervascular areas and associated with numerous arteriovenous microfistulas. Current systems are able to detect vascular signals at transvaginal PD in 77% of cases of normal postmenopausal endometrium, in 85% of benign thickening and in 100% of malignant thickenings, whereas study of the main uterine arteries has not produced significant results [77] (Fig. 6.90). In benign and malignant polypoid lesions, CD is able to detect signals of peduncular vessels, which in the malignant form are generally more numerous and ramified as well as being associated with lower-impedance spectral waveforms. These elements may be useful for deciding on the appropriate approach, whether polypectomy or hysterectomy [84]. The subjective or quantitative demonstration of hypervascularity in the endometrium or in the endometrium-myometrium interface is suggestive of malignancy, with an intra- and interobserver reproducibility at least for expert sonographers [85]. Tumor vessels are

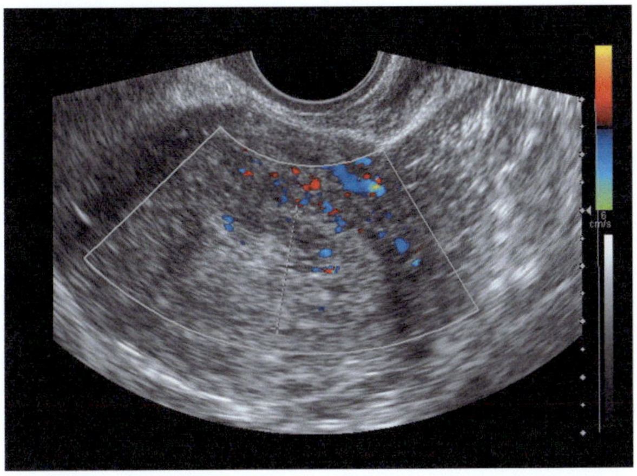

Fig. 6.89 Endometrial hyperplasia. Marked heterogeneous echogenic thickening of the endometrium which also displays some internal anechoic areas. No significant internal flow signals are detected. Regular appearance of the endometrial-myometrial interface

characterized by rather high flow (V_{max} suspicious if >18 cm/s) and low resistance (RI 0.34–0.6, suspicious if <0.5, PI suspicious if <1). The diagnostic efficacy of spectral measurements is nonetheless controversial, and some studies report a substantial overlap of the vascularity between benign and malignant thickening of the endometrium, in particular with RI and PI values not terribly dissimilar (considering also normal values for age and parity) [77,79,86]. In some studies, however, the degree of vascularity is correlated with the probability of malignancy, regardless of the degree of endometrial thickness. The vascularity is greater with lower RI in the more advanced stages of disease and correlates with the grade, degree of myometrial invasion, probability of lymph node involvement and prognosis [77,87].

In locally advanced forms, the US diagnosis of endometrial neoplasm clearly becomes easier, with evidence of uterine enlargement, marked and heterogeneous endometrial thickening, distension of the uterine cavity with fluid, echogenic and/or papillary material, discontinuity of the periendometrial hypoechoic halo and invasion of the myometrium (Fig. 6.91).

Myometrial invasion is the single most important prognostic factor and is predictive of the risk of lymph node metastasis (3% of cases of superficial myometrial invasion and 40% of those with deep invasion) [88]. At US the internal myometrium surrounds the endometrial hyperechogenicity and has a low echogenicity, lower than that of the more external myometrium. The absence of a normal subendometrial hypoechoic halo, especially a focal thinning, as well as

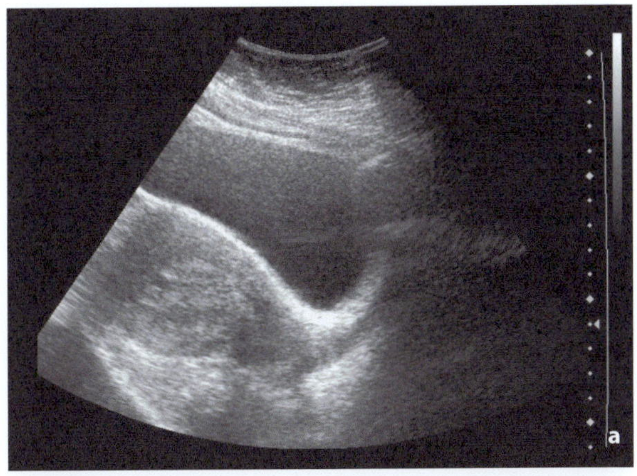

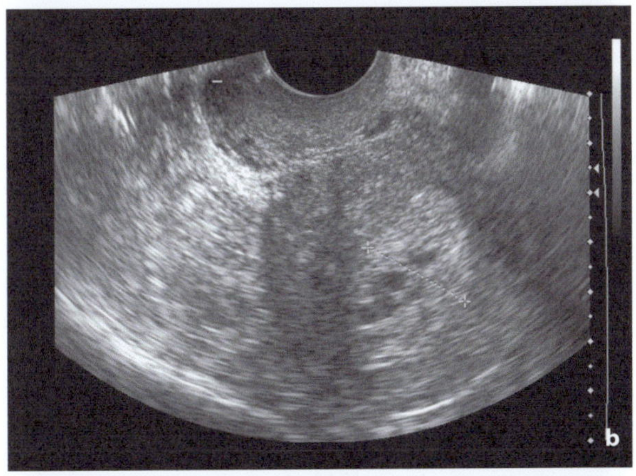

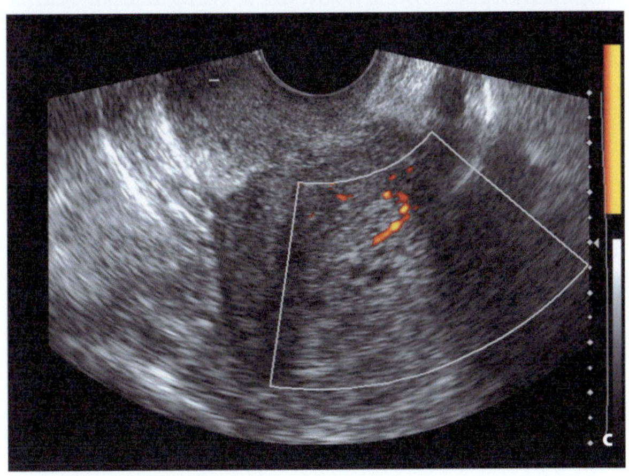

Fig. 6.90a-c Endometrial cancer. Diffuse heterogeneous thickening of the endometrium visualized with the suprapubic (a) and transvaginal (b) approach. Presence of arterial signals at PD (c)

irregularity of the endometrium-myometrium junction may be suggestive of invasion of the latter. Complete obliteration of the hypoechoic myometrial layer suggests deep wall infiltration (>50% of the myometrium). Malignant endometrial lesions with a significant polypoid component can appear to thin the

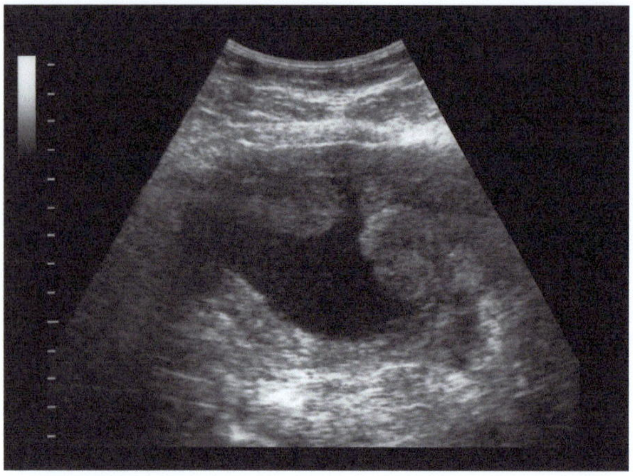

Fig. 6.91 Endometrial cancer. Marked irregular thickening of the uterine wall with the cavity distended by fluid

myometrium at that level, possibly due to compression, and therefore cause an overstaging of the deep spread of the disease. The same can be said for myometrial atrophy or the presence of myomas, hematometra or pyometra. False negatives can instead arise from superficial tumor spread or endometrial microinvasion [74]. TVUS has demonstrated an overall accuracy of 73–99% in the diagnosis of myometrial invasion [50,73.89], whereas hysterosonography has shown a sensitivity of 88% and a specificity of 100% [76]. In a comparative series, TVUS showed an accuracy of 76% and 86% in the detection of superficial and deep myometrial invasion, respectively, while saline infusion US had an accuracy of 72% and 96%, respectively [90]. Involvement of the cervix, which is an indication for adjuvant radiation therapy, can be suspected in the presence of heterogeneity of the normal echogenic stroma of the cervix and is identified with an accuracy of 93–96% [50,91]. Lastly, extrauterine spread, by both direct extension and lymphatic spread, is poorly defined by US and requires the contribution of MR [92].

6.7 Bladder Wall Lesions

A **circumscribed thickening** of the **bladder wall**, whether real or presumed, can be the result of very few conditions outside of carcinoma. These include mesenchymal tumors (hemangioma, plasmocytoma, neurofibroma, solitary fibrous tumor, lipoma, leiomyoma, paraganglioma, sarcoma and lymphoma), blood clots, wall hypertrophy, wall edema (e.g. indwelling catheter), prostatic adenoma and surgical outcomes [93,94].

Bladder cancer is the most common neoplasm of the excretory tract (70% of cases), with an increasing incidence. Onset is after 40 years in 97% of cases and the risk increases with age (peak between 60 and 70 years). The M/F ratio is 3–4:1 [94,95]. Risk factors include exposure to dyestuffs (e.g. aniline), therapy with some drugs (e.g. cyclophosphamide and phenacetin), exposure to radiation, smoking and schistosomiasis. There are two main types, a **papillary form** (80% of cases) with a broad or thin base but with a regular profile protruding into the bladder lumen, and an invasive **sessile form** with no peduncle (20%). Carcinoma of the bladder is histologically urothelial (transitional cell) in 90–95% of cases, squamous in 5–10% of cases, adenocarcinomatous in 2% of cases and mixed in 10% [96]. Painless gross hematuria is the first symptom in over 80% of cases [94].

The preferred **site** of transitional cell carcinomas is the lateral walls and posterior surface. Tumors located on the bladder dome account for 6–9% of cases, the lateral walls 38–63%, the posterior wall 9–11%, the trigone 15–27%, the neck 2–6% and the anterior wall 2–8%. This distribution is somewhat comforting for the sonographer, since the anterior wall and the bladder neck are the two portions that are most difficult to access.

Multifocal lesions account for 15–30% of cases and have a significant tendency to recur, with recurrent lesions each time being of a higher-grade malignancy than the previous. Recurrences are particularly common in the invasive, multifocal and large forms. Occasionally a lesion does not recur within the bladder but at the level of the upper urinary tract.

The **stage** of the disease (Fig. 6.92) influences treatment. The **superficial forms** (Tis, Ta and T1), without invasion of the muscularis propria, have a tendency to recur and in 10–20% of cases progress towards advanced lesions. The preferred treatment option is cystoscopy with transurethral resection, which is also the clinical system for their differentiation with higher stages. The **advanced forms** (T2, T3 and T4a) with invasion of the muscle layer or beyond have a less favorable prognosis and are more difficult to define at cystoscopy (errors in 25–50% of cases). These tumors are generally treated with cystectomy and lymphadenectomy. Some T4a tumors, in addition to those that have spread to the pelvic or abdominal wall (T4b) or are associated with metastases, are treated with neoadjuvant chemotherapy or palliative radiation therapy [96,97].

US is the technique of first choice in evaluation of the subject with painless gross hematuria or microhematuria, the two classic presentations of this tumor. In some cases the tumor is also identified incidentally. In special cases a transrectal or transvaginal approach may be used, which can be particularly useful for

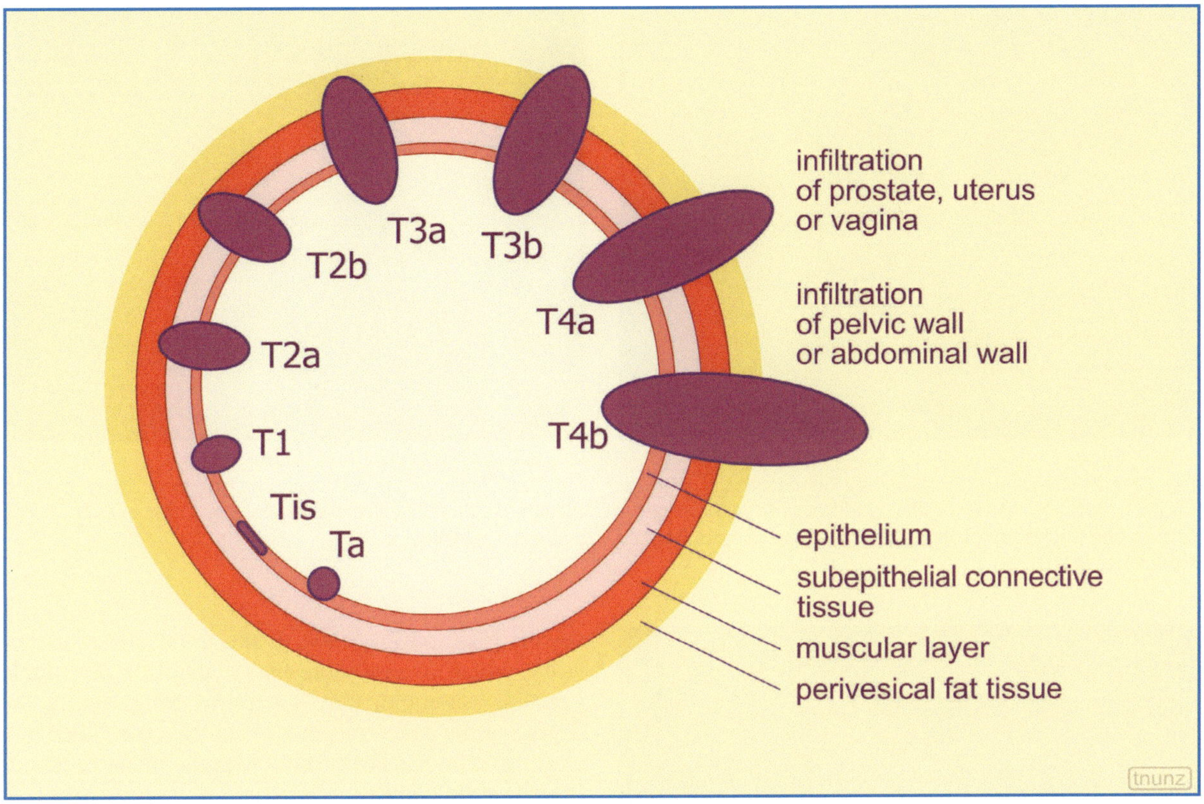

Fig. 6.92 Staging of bladder cancer. *Tis*, flat tumor, in situ; *Ta*, noninvasive papillary carcinoma; *T1*, invasion of the subepithelial connective tissue; *T2a*, invasion of <50% of the muscle layer; *T2b*, invasion of >50% of the muscle layer; *T3a*, microscopic invasion of the perivesical tissue; *T3b*, macroscopic invasion of the perivesical tissue; *T4a*, invasion of the prostate or uterus or vagina; *T4b*, invasion of the pelvic wall or abdominal wall. Modified from [31]

study of the trigone (differential diagnosis with vaginal and prostatic tumors) or the bladder neck (the voiding phase is also useful), or a transluminal approach, with endourethral transducers which are especially effective for staging. Transabdominal US has a sensitivity of 80%–90% for bladder lesions >5 mm but only 33% for lesions <5 mm [94] (Fig. 6.93).

In a recent series with state of the art equipment, US proved 91% sensitive and 79% specific in evaluating focal abnormalities of the bladder wall in patients referred to cystoscopy [98]. The difficulty in detection is largely related to cases of insufficient distension of the bladder, flat lesions or lesions located on the bladder dome (possibly concealed by intestinal gas) or on the anterior wall (possible "compression" in the initial centimeters of the ultrasound beam and/or masking in the common reverberation artifacts from urine). Multiplanar and 3D reconstruction images (so-called virtual cystoscopy) can improve the US display of bladder tumors, and correlate well with conventional cystoscopy [99]. **Transurethral US** has demonstrated a variable accuracy from 62% to 92%, with difficulty particularly in the more invasive forms [96.97].

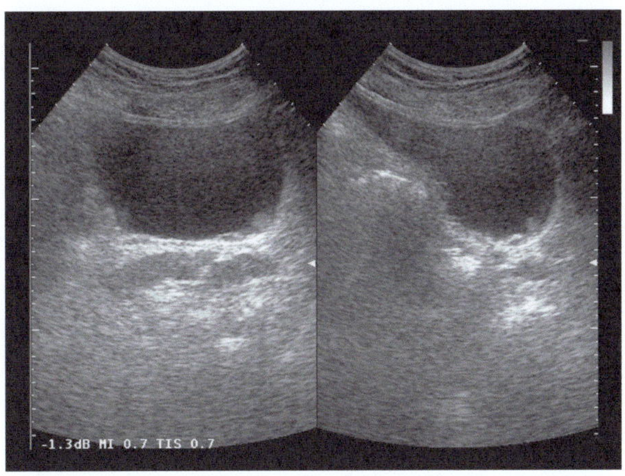

Fig. 6.93 Vesical papilloma. Small lesion protruding into the bladder lumen

The US study should evaluate the site, number and size of lesions (measuring both the height and the width at the base), the characteristics of the attachment (thin or wide), the appearance of the underlying

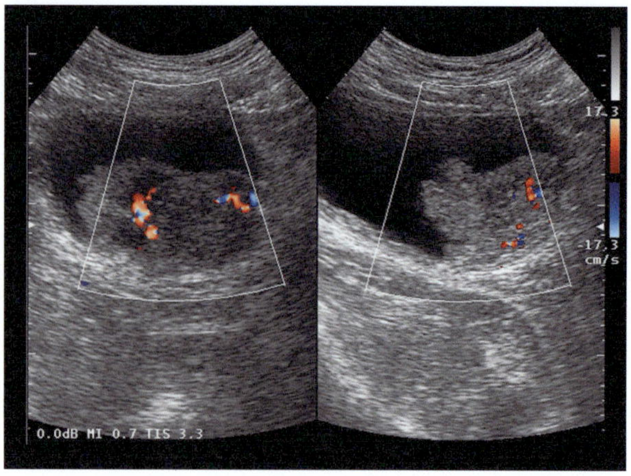

Fig. 6.94 Transitional cell carcinoma of the urinary bladder. Large hypoechoic mass of the bladder wall with irregular surface and thickening of the bladder wall at the base. Marked vascularity at CD

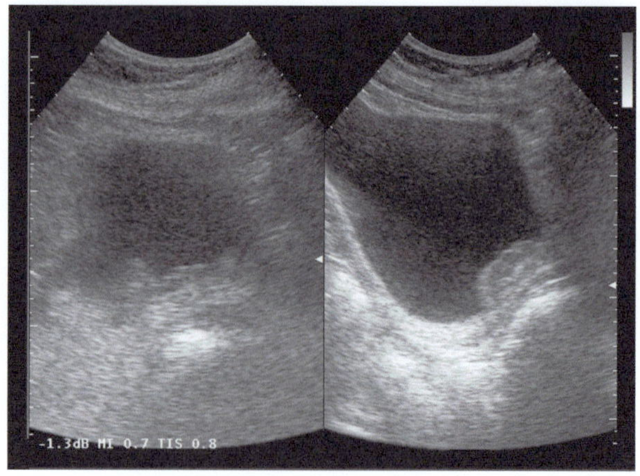

Fig. 6.95 Transitional cell carcinoma of the urinary bladder. Plaque-like thin but extensive hypoechoic lesion of the posterior and inferior bladder wall

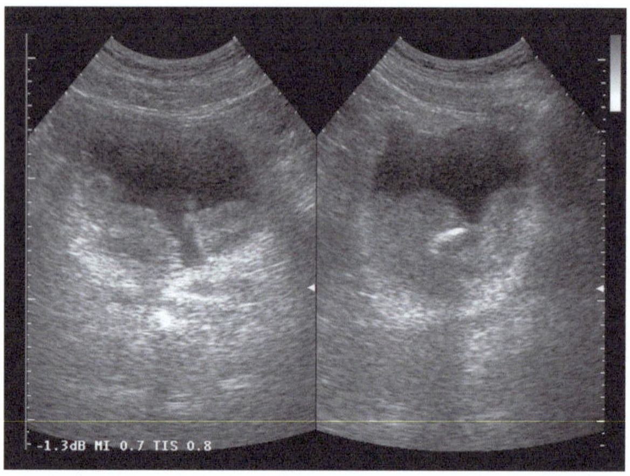

Fig. 6.96 Transitional cell carcinoma of the urinary bladder. Multifocal lesion with a broad base and large internal calcification

bladder wall and the perivesical fat, and the state of the ureters and the kidneys. Papillary lesions appear as echogenic masses protruding into the bladder lumen, with a generally irregular surface, absence of posterior acoustic shadowing and heterogeneous internal echotexture (Figs. 6.94–6.96). The echogenicity is greater than that of urine and usually moderately lower than that of the bladder wall. These characteristics often make it possible to distinguish between superficial forms with an integral parietal layer and deep forms with an interrupted parietal layer. In the presence of markedly calcified lesions, evaluating the underlying bladder wall may prove challenging. In other cases only small intralesional calcifications may be identified: these may give rise to the twinkling artifact at CD, which should not be confused with vascular signals (Fig. 6.97). Study of the intralesional vascularity, which generally presents in the form of a single vascular peduncle, may be useful for defining the degree of the cancerous process since a certain degree of correlation has been found with the invasiveness of the lesion (in contrast to RI).

Superficial lesions do not produce changes to the underlying **bladder wall**, which instead appears locally interrupted and heterogeneous in invasive lesions. In addition, invasive tumors show a wider contact length (41.5 mm threshold) and a lower tumor height-to-length ratio (0.605 threshold) than superficial tumors [100]. Moreover, the distinction between forms that invade the superficial portion of the detrusor (T2a) and forms that are also invading the deep portion (T2b) cannot be made with certainty. Over time, especially in cases of invasion of the entire thickness, the wall becomes thick and rigid. **Extravesical spread** can be difficult to visualize, although hypoechoic bands or even protrusions into the hyperechoic perivesical fat may be identified, especially at the level of the lateral walls. Invasion of the seminal vesicles may be suspected in the event of loss of the angle between the bladder and the vesicle. Invasion of the uterus, vagina and rectum are more difficult to identify. In general, however, transabdominal US tends to overstage superficial lesions and understage deep lesions. Edema, intravesical clots and intralesional calcifications may all cause tumor overstaging [94].

Trigonal lesions tend to obstruct the ureteral orifice, causing hydronephrosis and, over the long term, atrophy of the renal parenchyma. The CD study of ureteral jet can detect a deviation in the jet itself or its partial (low and subcontinous flow) or total obliteration.

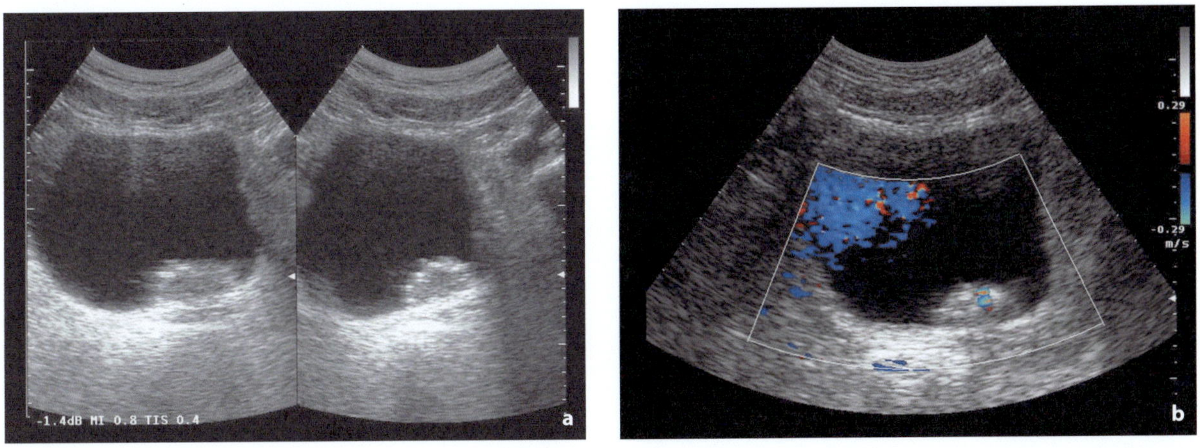

Fig. 6.97a,b Transitional cell carcinoma of the urinary bladder. Hypoechoic sessile lesion with hyperechoic surface located on the left portion of the posterior bladder wall (**a**). CD shows a twinkling artifact generated by an intralesional calcification which should not be confused with a flow signal (**b**)

Bladder carcinomas are generally slow growing and are especially characterized by local invasion. The **lymph nodes** classified as regional are those in the lesser pelvis, i.e. those below a plane passing through the bifurcation of the common iliac arteries. Lymph node metastases, the identification of which is a significant prognostic indicator, are mainly at the level of the external iliac lymph nodes of the medial group (obturator) and the middle group, which are difficult to identify with US, as are those subsequent to the common iliac and lumbar lymph nodes. US is able to identify only larger pelvic lymphadenopathies. The technique can be useful for liver **metastases**, which are the most common together with lung and bone metastases, although like these they are a relatively late manifestation. The search for and quantification of a possible hydronephrosis, whether uni- or bilateral, should be constantly performed [96,97].

Differential diagnosis consists of a relatively limited number of conditions. Reverberation artifacts immediately posterior to the anterior bladder wall can mimic (or even conceal) a mural protrusion, although adjusting the gray gain should be able to dispel any doubt. The various forms of chronic cystitis, if the wall thickening is particularly irregular and distributed in an asymmetrical manner on the bladder wall, can mimic plaque-like lesions [98] (Fig. 6.98). Bladder stones change position with a shift in patient posture, present no vascular signals at CD, and are echogenic and possibly accompanied by posterior acoustic shadowing (they can mimic a calcified tumor). Even blood clots are generally mobile and separable from the bladder wall, as well as being without flow at CD. It should be borne in mind that bladder cancer can present with massive hematuria and therefore be associated with clots, which may lead to an overestimation of the size of the lesion (Fig. 6.99). Ureterocele typically is located in the trigone and has an anechoic center, although a tumor may arise from the mucosa of an ureterocele (Figs. 6.100, 6.101). If the bladder is not sufficiently distended, normal or pathologic perivesical structures (uterus, prostatic adenomyomas, gynecologic masses, etc.), can mimic an intraluminal lesion. If the bladder is collapsed, a cystic pelvic mass can mimic the bladder and any solid components of the mass can, in turn, mimic bladder lesions [101]. **Nonepithelial bladder cancers** (<10% of cases) are of intramural origin and have a different US appearance, with a thickened wall, echogenicity generally

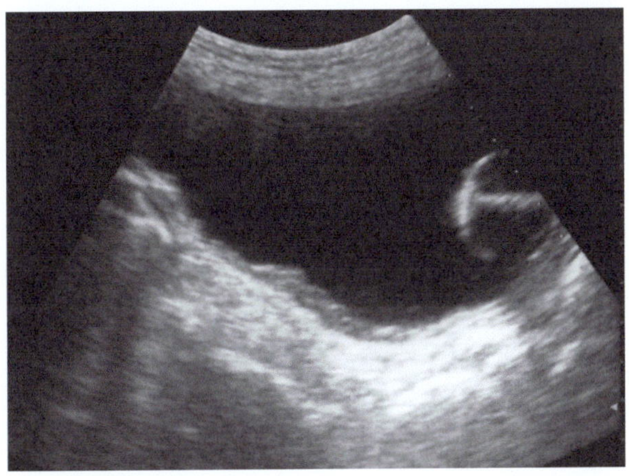

Fig. 6.98 Catheter-induced chronic cystitis. Diffuse thickening of the bladder wall in a subject with indwelling catheter (balloon of the Foley catheter is visible) appears more marked on the posterior wall prompting differential diagnosis with a productive urothelial lesion

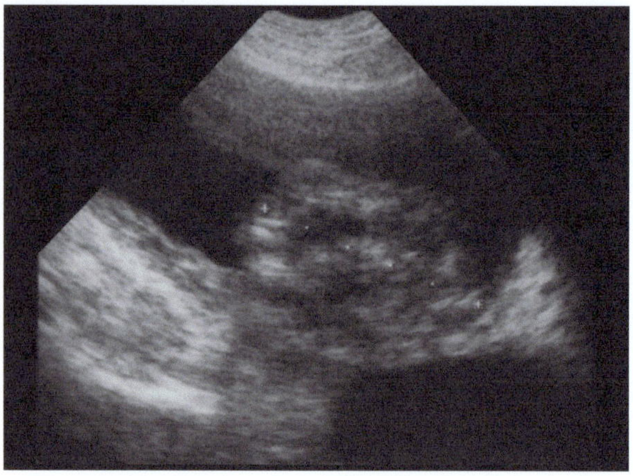

Fig. 6.99 Bladder clot. Large heterogeneous echogenic blood clot (*between the calipers*) in the bladder lumen mimicking an intraluminal polypoid mass

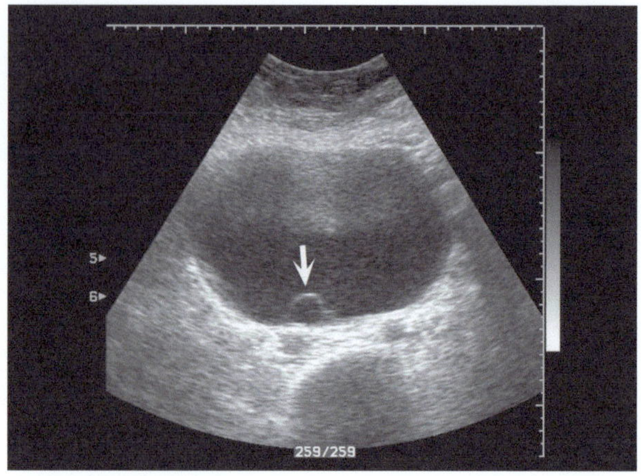

Fig. 6.100 Ureterocele. Small anechoic mass (*arrow*) with well-defined margins located at the right ureteral outlet

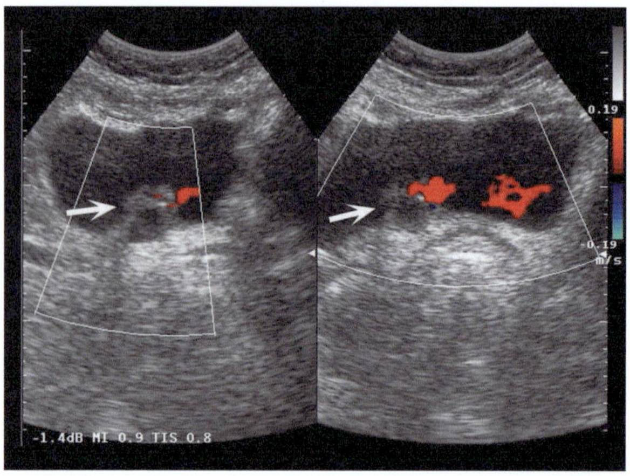

Fig. 6.101 Papilloma on ureterocele. Anechoic mass (*arrows*) projecting into the bladder lumen from the right ureteral outlet with a thick and irregular appearance of the external surface. CD identifies the ureteral jet bilaterally

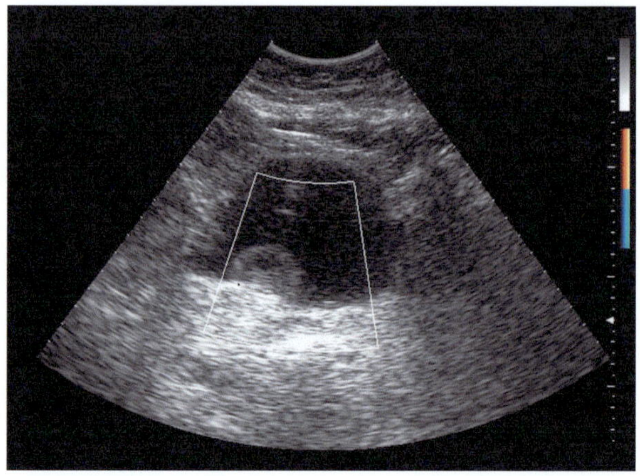

Fig. 6.102 Lymphoma of the urinary bladder. Sessile hypoechoic mass with initial internal liquefaction and no vascular signal at directional PD can be distinguished protruding into the bladder lumen

greater than the rest of the wall, a secondary interruption of the echogenic mucous line and an obtuse angle with the surface of the mucosa itself (Figs. 6.102, 6.103).

Follow-up should be tailored to the individual subject and is based on alternation between cystoscopy and the combination suprapubic US + urinary cytology in an initial phase and then on the use of US and cytology alone in a later phase, with cystoscopy performed in all suspicious cases (Figs. 6.104, 6.105). Cystoscopy is more sensitive but also more costly, more invasive and poorly tolerated by patients. Moreover, the technique does not enable monitoring of the upper urinary tract. Even the combined approach TRUS + suprapubic US may be a reasonable alternative to cystoscopy, as well as being less costly [95].

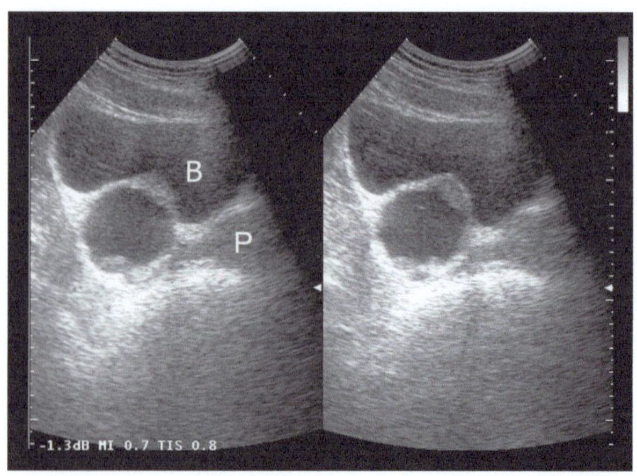

Fig. 6.103 Bladder wall metastasis from melanoma. Prevalently cystic complex mass with solid nodulations imprinting the bladder lumen. *B*, bladder; *P*, prostate

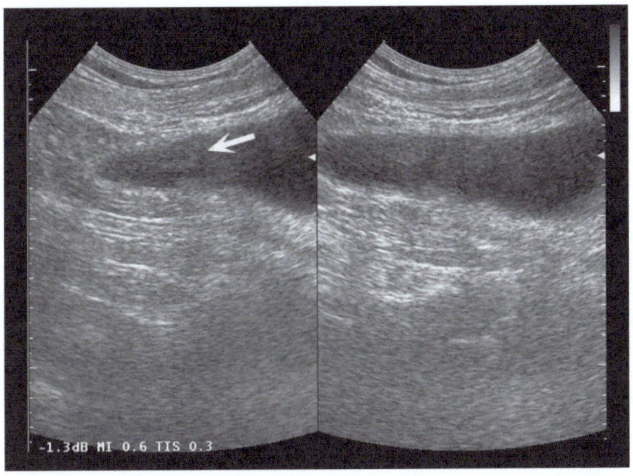

Fig. 6.104 Papilloma of the urinary bladder. In a patient with prior resection of the bladder due to transitional cell carcinoma and presenting with gross hematuria, a small polypoid lesion (*arrow*) on the residual anterior bladder wall can be distinguished, almost concealed among the reverberation artifacts which are common at this level

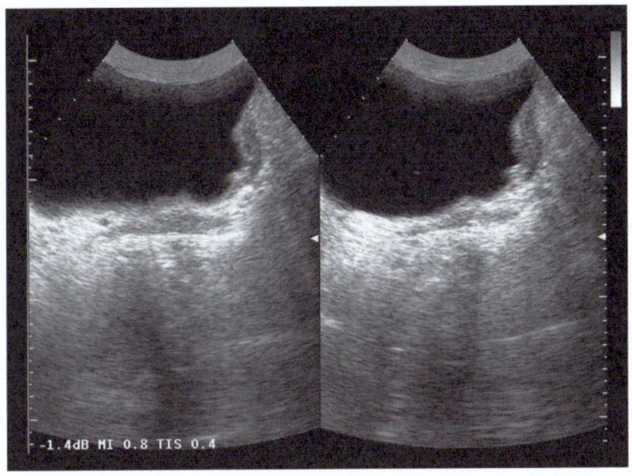

Fig. 6.105 Transitional cell carcinoma of the urinary bladder, recurrence. At the site of bladder resection new slight but extensive wall thickening can be seen, which is more evident than for simple scarring, and absent in previous examinations

6.8 Prostate Nodules

Prostatic adenocarcinoma (95% of prostate cancers) is a tumor that is prevalent in older males (80% of cases diagnosed >65 years) which is common in the clinically manifest form and even more so in the silent microscopic form (present in 30% of individuals >50 years). Risk factors include advanced age, ethnicity (African-Americans) and family history [102]. The tumor arises in the central zone of the gland in 10% of cases, in the transition zone (site of benign prostatic hyperplasia and therefore hyperrepresented in the elderly) in around 20% and in the peripheral zone in some 70% of cases (with equal distribution between the anterior and the posterior portions) [103] (Fig. 6.106). Tumor grading is based on the Gleason score, which ranges from grade 1, well differentiated, to grade 5, poorly differentiated. The system sums the scores of the two most common types of cancer cell patterns seen at low-power microscopy. The score may therefore range from 2 (the least aggressive) to 10 (the most aggressive) [104].

Prostate specific antigen (PSA) is largely used in the screening, diagnosis and formulation of the prognosis of prostate cancer. Several scientific societies recommend an annual PSA assay after 50 years of age.

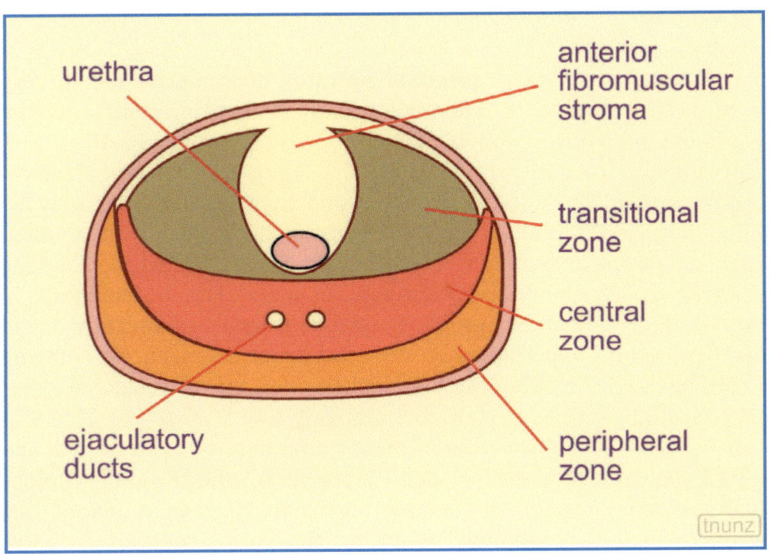

Fig. 6.106 Zonal anatomy of the prostate. Anatomic subdivision of the prostate gland into zones

PSA is found to be increased in 16–86% of subjects with benign hyperplasia and in 60–70% of those with carcinoma, as well as in cases of prostatitis or recent TRUS, prostate biopsy, cystoscopy or bladder catheterization. The normal values of serum PSA are <4 ng/mL and tend to vary with the size of the gland and with age [103]. An additional diagnostic indicator is the ratio between free PSA (i.e. not bound to a protein) and total PSA – the value of this ratio decreases in the presence of a carcinoma. It is also important to define the rate of increase in the PSA value over time, which is diagnostically significant if >0.4–0.75 ng/mL/year.

The US study of the prostate with the suprapubic approach is only able to provide an evaluation of the size and a general study of the structure of the gland. Additional information regarding the structure of the gland can be obtained with the transperineal approach. The only modality capable of studying prostatic nodules is TRUS, performed with high-frequency (6–9 MHz) intraluminal transducers in sagittal and transverse or coronal planes. The technique is able to identify the less echogenic central zone and the more echogenic peripheral zone.

The initial **tumor nodule** in general appears hypoechoic, although not all cancerous lesions are hypoechoic and not all hypoechoic lesions are cancerous. The suspicion of malignancy of the hypoechoic lesion increases with the size, digital rectal examination (DRE) findings and PSA value (Fig. 6.107). Small prostatic carcinomas are hypoechoic in 60–75% of cases and isoechoic in 12–40%. In contrast, the hyperechoic forms or hypoechoic with echogenic foci are rare (<5%). In addition, there seems to be no correlation between echogenicity and prognosis [95,103]. Well-differentiated nodules arising in the peripheral portion can appear isoechoic to the surrounding tissue, just as initial lesions developing in the central zone often do. These nodules therefore can only be recognized as a bulge in the prostatic profile or a distortion of the periprostatic fat. A TRUS finding of multiple nodules is not unusual. It should be borne in mind that nodules and pseudonodules can be the result of benign processes that should be included in the **differential diagnosis**: adenomyoma, chronic granulomatous inflammation, malakoplakia, parenchymal atrophy, acinar dilatation, "dirty" cysts, infarcted areas, scarring, fibrosis (prior transurethral prostatic resection), tubercular infection, acute infection, primary lymphoma, peripheral muscle tissue and dilated peripheral vessels (CD value!) (Fig. 6.108). The probability of malignancy of a hypoechoic lesion increases with its diameter, palpability and the PSA value. Adenomyoma presents as two tendentially hypoechoic nodulations lateral to the urethra or as a mass which

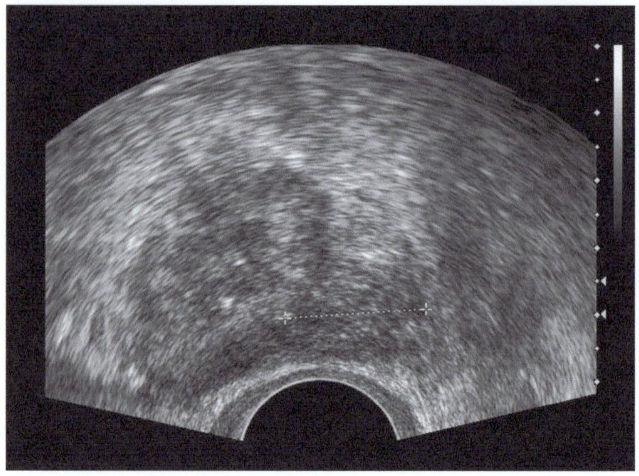

Fig. 6.107 Prostate cancer. Peripheral nodule with heterogeneous hypoechoic appearance (*between the calipers*)

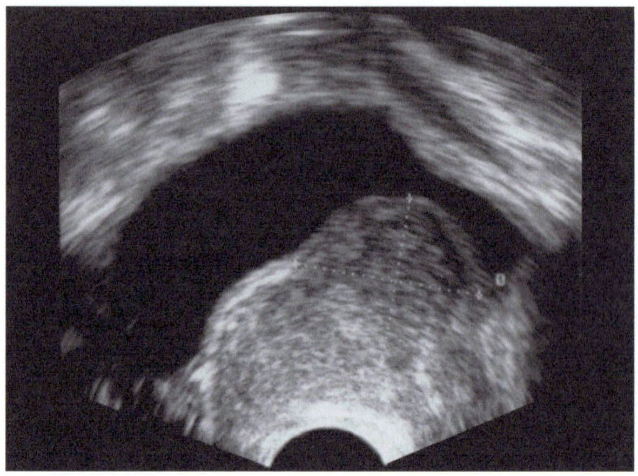

Fig. 6.108 Adenomyoma of the prostate. Large heterogeneous hypoechoic nodule protruding from the prostatic surface towards the bladder lumen

tends to protrude upwards and imprint the urinary bladder. The main characteristic of prostatitis is large calcifications, which should be topographically correlated with any DRE finding of firmness. Heterogeneous hypoechoic and hyperechoic areas may be found, which are difficult to distinguish from an invasive tumor. Lastly, there is also the problem of the glandular background. In many cases the carcinoma in fact develops in a gland with coarse echotexture due to hyperplastic or inflammatory phenomena, thus making its identification challenging. All of these considerations explain the relatively low accuracy of TRUS in the detection of these initial tumors. With growth and progressive dedifferentiation, the lesion becomes easier to identify and may take on a plaque-like morphology. Even in these cases, however, invasive growth can lead to diffuse disruption of the glandular echostructure, thus reducing the possibility of detecting definite lesions.

Even with the transrectal approach, therefore, US has limited sensitivity and specificity for the detection of carcinoma of the prostate, with around 30% of tumors being unidentifiable and only 21–56% of hypoechoic nodules proving to effectively be malignant. Spectral Doppler does not seem to be much help, since the values of systolic velocity and RI are similar in benign and malignant lesions. The hyperemia of the hypo-isoechoic lesions, possibly also studied with the injection of intravenous contrast medium, correlates with the Gleason score but does not appear to significantly increase the accuracy of the technique (increase of only 7%), because although most carcinomas are hypervascular, there are also isovascular and hypovascular forms. Some authors have also investigated the spectral waveforms of prostate feeding arteries (capsular arteries): PI was found to be significantly lower in patients with malignant nodules (mean 1.49) than in those with benign lesions (mean 1.71), while RI was lower, although not significantly, in patients with malignant nodules (mean 0.78) than in those with benign lesions (mean 0.82) [105]. The impact of elastography and transrectal CEUS, while promising, needs to be verified in large studies [103,106,107] (Figs. 6.109, 6.110). CD and CEUS can nonetheless help in the identification of isoechoic forms in some cases, even identifying the relative vascular peduncles. In addition, the degree of Doppler vascularity seems to correlate with the Gleason score and with the stage of the disease and therefore with prognosis [103,107,108]. Moreover, CD with contrast medium and CEUS can be used for biopsy guidance. With respect to gray-scale US guidance, CD is able to obtain an increase in biopsy accuracy estimated at 10%. Of course this is in reference to the more aggressive tumors, which as stated above tend to be hypervascular [107,108].

The sensitivity of TRUS can be increased by combining it with the PSA value: 1 g of normal or hyperplastic tissue produces around 0.3 ng/mL, whereas each gram of cancerous tissue produces as much as 3.5 ng/mL. Clearly there is a correlation between the prostate volume measured with TRUS and the probability of malignancy based on the serum PSA levels. While recognizing that the PSA value can be influenced as stated above by a recent urologic examination, a recent TRUS and especially a recent biopsy, several useful categories can be distinguished for diagnostic and therapeutic management. If PSA is <3–4 ng/mL, the probability of malignancy is very low, although there are very well-differentiated and very poorly differentiated tumors accompanied by normal PSA values. In this case if DRE is normal there is no need to perform TRUS, whereas TRUS may be useful if the DRE findings are anomalous. If PSA is between 3–4 and 10 ng/mL, then calculation of the **PSA density** (PSAD) is important, i.e. the ratio between serum PSA and the prostate volume measured at TRUS. If the PSAD is >0.10–0.15, then biopsy guided by the DRE or TRUS findings is required, or multiple biopsies if both DRE and TRUS are of little help (0.14 is the threshold which gives the maximum sensitivity with a moderate specificity). Lastly, if the PSA is >10 ng/mL, the probability of a neoplasm is high and multiple biopsies should be performed even in the case of negative findings at DRE and TRUS [109,110].

In most cases TRUS is sufficient for local characterization. **Biopsy** generally follows, possibly US-guided, which can be systematic (sextant, with at least three cores from the periphery of both lobes) and/or

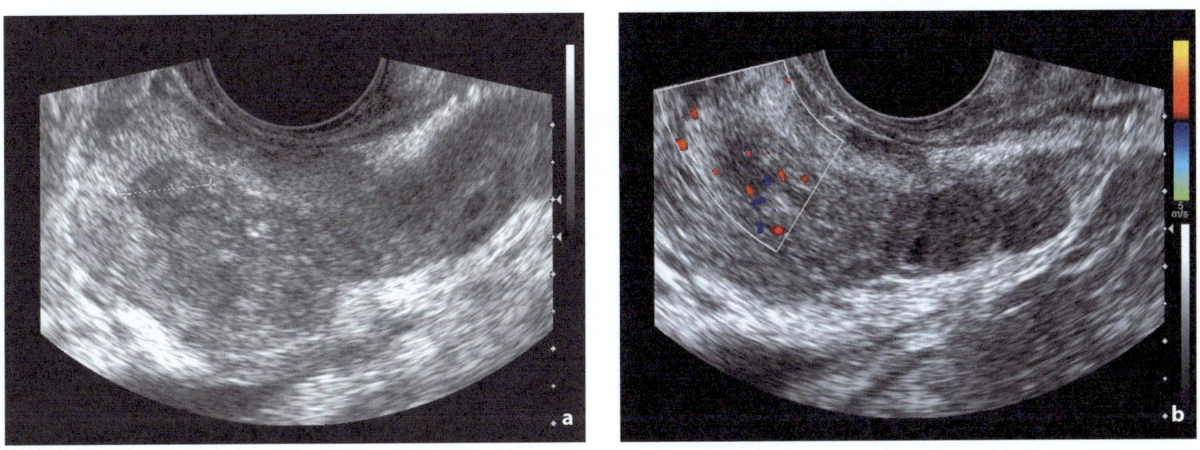

Fig. 6.109a,b Prostate cancer. Peripheral heterogeneous hypoechoic nodule (**a**, *between the calipers*) with some vascular signals at CD (**b**)

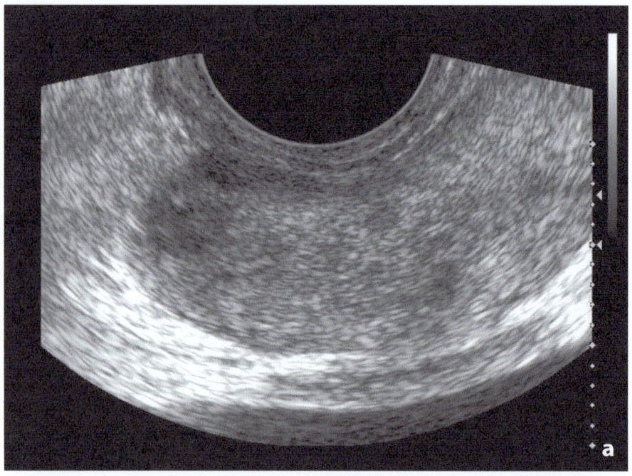

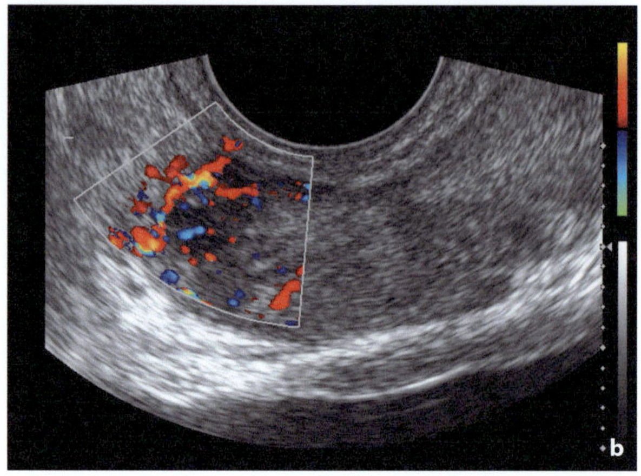

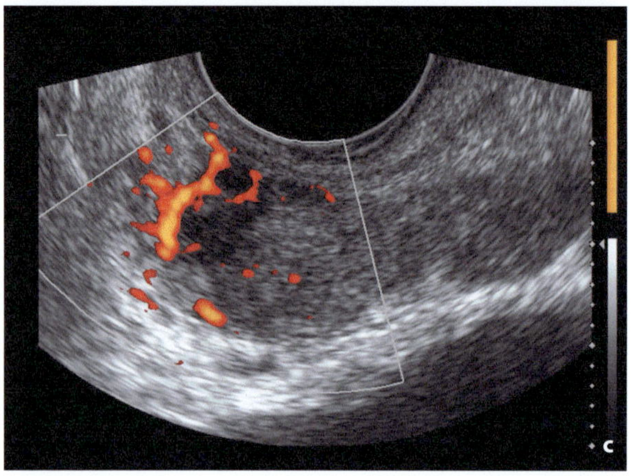

Fig. 6.110a-c Prostate cancer. Peripheral heterogeneous hypoechoic nodule (**a**) with moderate vascularity, especially peripheral and perilesional, at CD (**b**) and PD (**c**)

targeted (3–5 cores on the nodule identified at DRE and/or TRUS and/or CD) [111]. When US identifies a hypoechoic nodule, the biopsy is targeted at it. Otherwise, the cores are taken randomly, and although the results are less than brilliant, the technique is able to identify numerous tumors with negative TRUS [112]. When the biopsy finding is one of **prostatic intraepithelial neoplasm** (PIN), i.e. a dysplastic lesion which is a precursor of adenocarcinoma, the indication is to repeat the biopsy after several months (especially in the case of high-grade PIN). Cases indicated for surgery, or possibly hormone therapy, may require a staging MR examination.

TRUS can provide information for tumor **staging**, although this is not the principal aim and there are more reliable modalities such as MR (Fig. 6.111). As it grows the lesion induces broad changes to the echostructure of the prostate, possibly with the presence of a hypoechoic disruption including fibrotic or calcified echogenic areas. The lesion may also undergo extracapsular spread and invade the periglandular structures (the hyperechoic "capsule"). This may be suspected in the presence of focal deformation of the capsular profile, localized interruption of the capsule, extensive contact between the lesion and the capsule, interruption of the echoes of the periprostatic fat or obliteration of the rectoprostatic angle. In addition, anterior capsular invasion is often difficult to identify with TRUS, especially if the prostate is particularly enlarged [95,102,103]. Involvement of the seminal vesicles can be identified by their asymmetric size, shape and/or echogenicity, with the presence of a hypoechoic halo around the ejaculatory ducts or disappearance of the normal acute angle between the seminal vesicle and the prostate. The identification with TRUS of clear invasion is not easy, but US-guided biopsy may be performed if needed. In the event of invasion of other adjacent structures (bladder and rectum), which is for the most part possible for the larger tumors, continuity between the lesion and the wall involved may be seen. CD can be a help in identifying infiltration of the neurovascular bundle. The extracapsular extension is studied by TRUS particularly in the axial plane, whereas invasion of the seminal vesicles is evaluated in sagittal images [103]. Moreover, TRUS has shown a rather limited accuracy with regard to staging: 46% in localized forms and 66% in locally advanced forms (58–86% overall), with

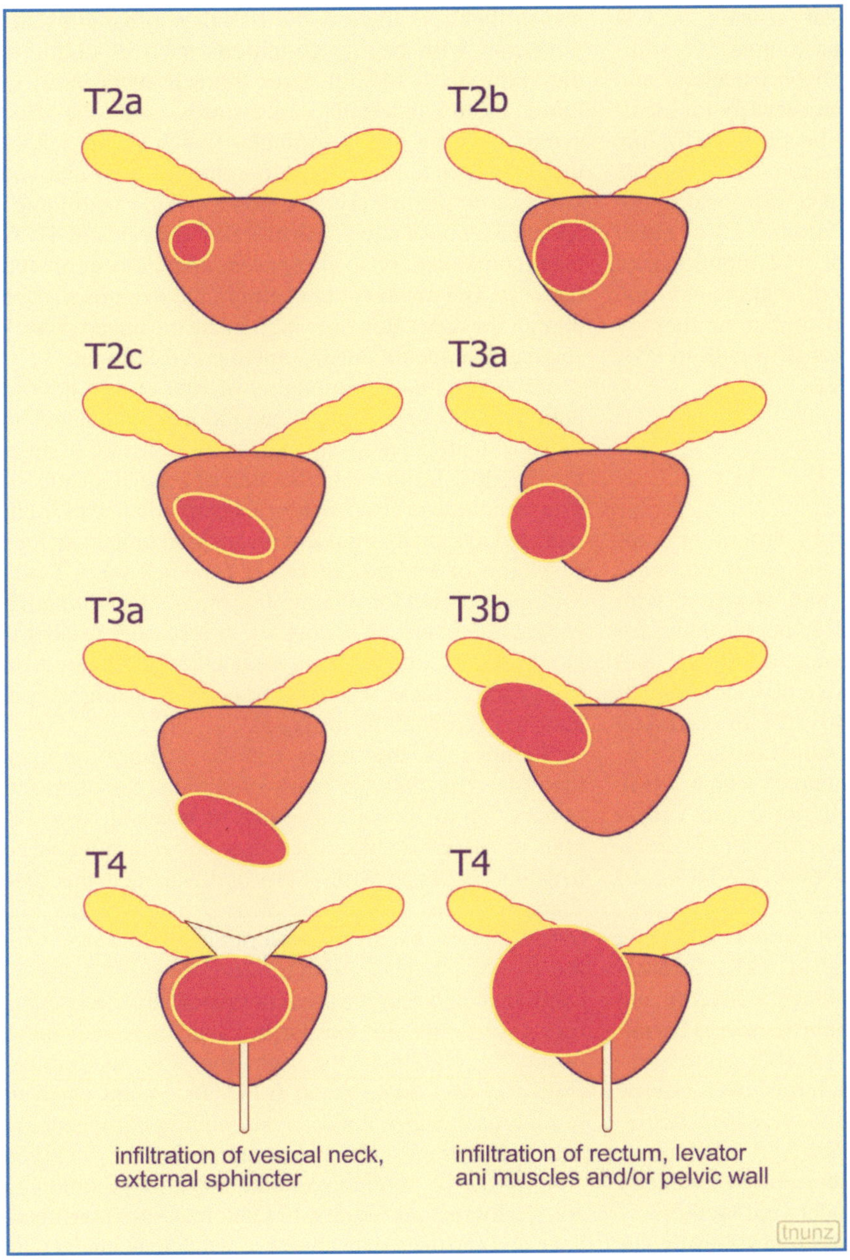

Fig. 6.111 Staging of prostate cancer. *T2a*, unilateral tumor extending to <50% of one lobe; *T2b*, unilateral tumor extending to >50% of one lobe; *T2c*, tumor involving both lobes; *T3a*, extracapsular extension, unilateral or bilateral; *T3b*, invasion of the seminal vesicles; *T4*, invasion of other pelvic structures other than the seminal vesicles (bladder neck, external sphincter, rectum, elevator ani muscles and/or pelvic wall). Modified from [31]

sensitivity of 27–86% and specificity of 58–94% for capsular invasion, sensitivity of 22–92% and specificity of 65–100% for invasion of the seminal vesicle and sensitivity of 66% and specificity of 78% for the identification of invasion of the neurovascular bundle [102,103]. The lymph nodes classified as regional are the nodes of the lesser pelvis, i.e. located below the plane passing through the bifurcation of the common iliac artery. Lymph node metastases (internal obturator lymph nodes, as well as hypogastric, presacral, common iliac and lumbar nodes) are present in >40% of patients with T4 but are only identified at US when sufficiently large.

The **follow-up** of treated and asymptomatic patients is generally not based on imaging but on the PSA assay, which does not distinguish between local and distant recurrence, and DRE, which is limited in accuracy. The prostate gland is mainly investigated when the PSA level has increased and bone scans are still negative [102]. TRUS can be useful in suspicious cases for identifying **recurrence** after radical prostatectomy and for guiding the biopsy. The appearance is of a hypoechoic area with vascular signals at CD surrounding the vesicourethral anastomosis. In addition, some 30% of recurrence can be isoechoic and difficult to identify. After **radiation therapy** for localized carcinomas, the prostate becomes atrophic, fibrotic and heterogeneously echogenic. TRUS is able to identify residual tumor/recurrence as a focal hypoechoic area with a sensitivity of around 50%. Focal lesions >5 mm and persistent for >12 months after radiation therapy are suspicious of malignancy and should be biopsied [95,113]. Postradiation therapy recurrence is defined as three consecutive rises in PSA level after postradiation nadir [102].

6.9 Testicular Tumors

Tumors of the testis account for around 1% of neoplasms in males (but it is the most common neoplasm between the ages of 15 and 44 years), with an increasing incidence. Germ cell tumors account for 95% of lesions, with a peak incidence between 25 and 35 years and a low incidence above 40 years. **Germ cell tumors** include seminoma (40–50% of germ cell tumors, bilateral in 2–5% of cases) and nonseminomatous tumors (60% of germ cell tumors) which are in general more aggressive than seminoma and with a slightly earlier onset: embryonic cell tumor (15–25%), choriocarcinoma (1–3%), teratomas (5–10%, of different grade of differentiation), yolk sac tumors, mixed tumors (20–40%, usually embryonic carcinoma + teratoma) [114,115]. **Non-germ cell**, stromal **tumors** are rarer (1–5% of testicular cancers) and include Leydig cell tumor, gonadoblastoma and Sertoli cell tumor. These tumors are of variable aggressiveness and can be functioning in terms of hormone production and bilateral. The risk factors of testicular malignancies include cryptorchidism (risk 2.5–8 times greater than in the subject with normally descended testicles, and even if the patient underwent orchiopexy but at an age >2 years), testicular dysgenesis, testicular atrophy of various origin, Klineferter syndrome, Down's syndrome, testicular microlithiasis (moderately), non-microlithiasic testicular calcifications (probably), maternal exposure to diethylstilbestrol and oral contraceptive during pregnancy [116,117]. The high curability of these tumors (>95%) requires particularly thorough diagnostic and therapeutic management. In most cases, however, the patient seeks medical advice at a rather late stage: almost 2/3 of subjects when the mass has been present for >3 months. The most common presentation is a mildly painful or painless testicular mass in a young male. However, around 10% of cases manifest with acute pain, probably secondary to intralesional hemorrhage, and in this case there is the risk of confusion by the physician with benign conditions such as orchiepididymitis. In 4–14% of cases thoracic metastases, or more often abdominal metastases, are the first symptom of an occult testicular tumor [115]. Tumor markers include AFP (nondifferentiated teratoma and yolk sac tumor, rarely seminoma), LDH (seminoma and nonseminomatous germ cell tumors) and HCG (seminoma and above all nonseminomatous germ cell tumors). The markers are useful in the diagnosis (even though they are often only high in the advanced phase), staging, therapeutic management and follow-up.

US is the imaging modality of first choice both in patients who present with an indolent mass and in those with atypical onset, and has a sensitivity of practically 100% for the identification of testicular cancers. The technique is also used for the surveillance of high-risk subjects such as those with cryptorchidism and for suspicion of burned-out tumor (see below). CT and PET can be used for staging. In general, discriminating between the various histotypes of testicular tumors is not possible, at least not with certainty. However, nearly all of these testicular tumors are malignant, at least the germ cell forms [116].

Tumors of the testis can be solitary or even multiple, especially in cases of seminomas or mixed tumors. Up to 10% of cases can be bilateral, synchronous or metachronous. They may be oval, rounded or irregular in shape with sharp or ill-defined margins. They appear as hypoechoic areas (iso- or hyperechoic forms are rare, occurring most often in teratomas) with more-or-less heterogeneous echotexture often due to hypo-anechoic necrotic areas or hemorrhagic echogenic foci (especially in the larger and more advanced forms, in particular the nonseminomatous tumors) (Figs. 6.112–6.118, Video 6.11). In typical cases of seminoma the appearance is particularly homogeneous and well circumscribed. Calcifications are found in around 1/3 of seminomas and are also common in nonseminomatous tumors. In teratomas, components of bone and cartilage may appear as echogenic nuclei with posterior acoustic shadowing. The surrounding testicular parenchyma as well as the contralateral testis is often the site of microlithiasis [115,118]. Teratomas with a cystic appearance need to be distinguished from dysplastic cysts [119]. Larger and more diffuse lesions may conserve only a shell of healthy surrounding testicular tissue or they may disrupt and totally invade the organ, which in massive cases may appear deformed or with an irregular contour due to involvement of the tunica albuginea. CD shows intralesional vascular signals in most testicular tumors and can demonstrate an increase in arterial and/or venous flows with respect to the surrounding parenchyma, with anarchic structures and irregular distribution.

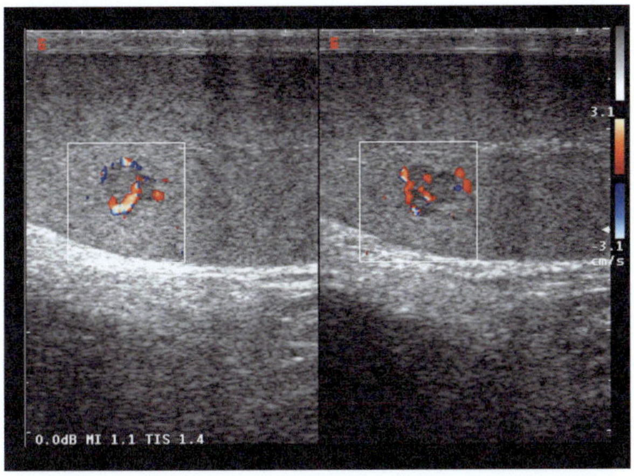

Fig. 6.112 Leydig cell tumor. Small hypoechoic testicular nodule appearing hypervascular at CD. Despite the small size and low aggressiveness of the histotype, the CD findings nonetheless require an "aggressive" diagnostic-therapeutic approach

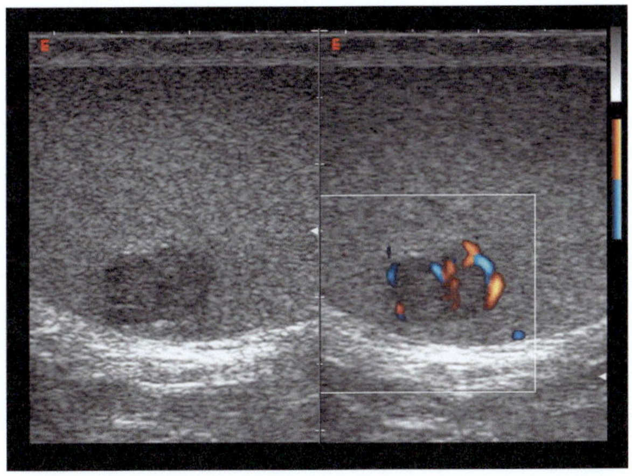

Fig. 6.113 Seminoma of the testis. Relatively well-defined and homogeneous hypoechoic nodule with moderate hypervascularity at directional PD

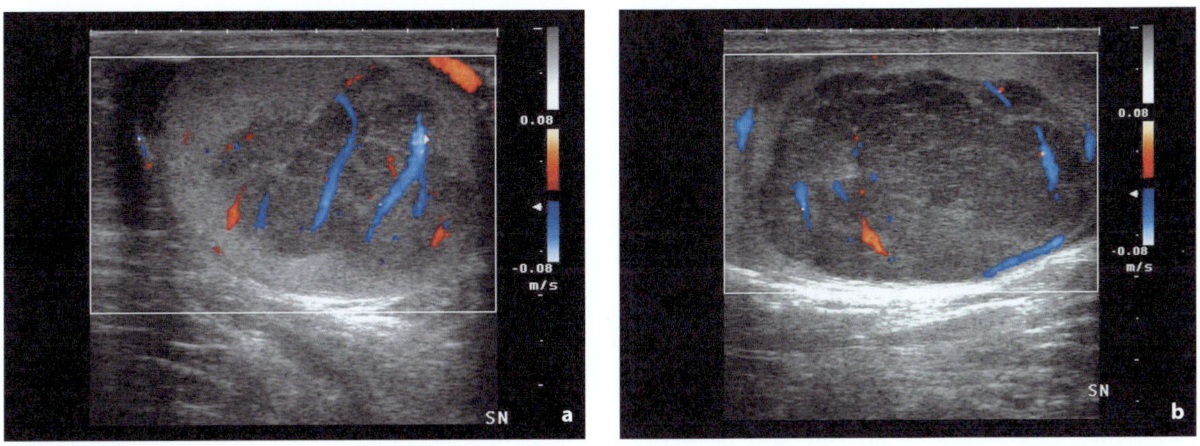

Fig. 6.114a,b Seminoma of the testis. Large heterogeneous hypoechoic nodule with moderate vascularity at CD

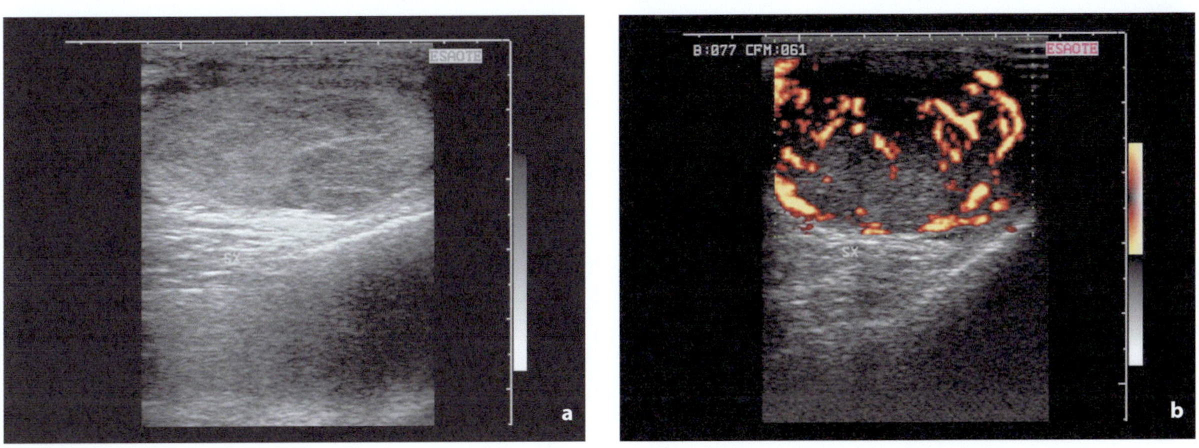

Fig. 6.115a,b Seminoma of the testis. Diffuse hypoechoic testicular infiltrate (**a**), with especially peripheral hypervascularity at PD (**b**)

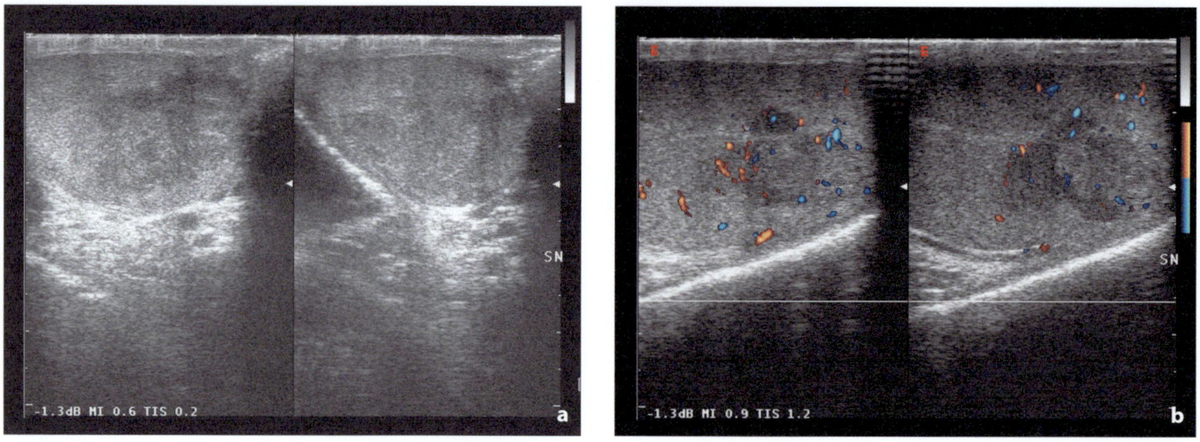

Fig. 6.116a,b Seminoma of the testis. Areas of mild and heterogeneous hypoechogenicity (**a**) with moderate vascularity at directional PD (**b**)

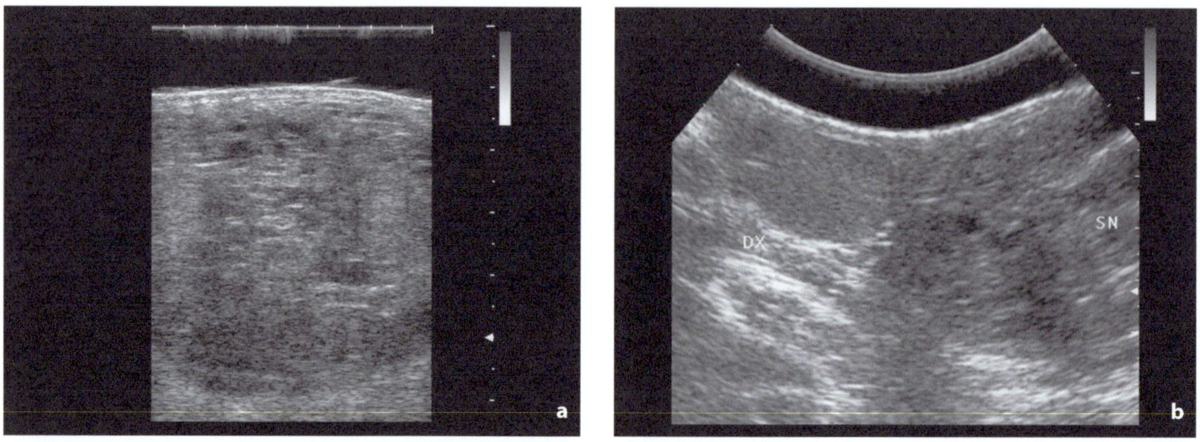

Fig. 6.117a,b Teratocarcinoma of the testis. Markedly widened and totally disrupted testicle due to the presence of heterogeneous hypoechoic tissue (**a**). The image with the abdominal transducer (**b**) shows the difference between the healthy right side

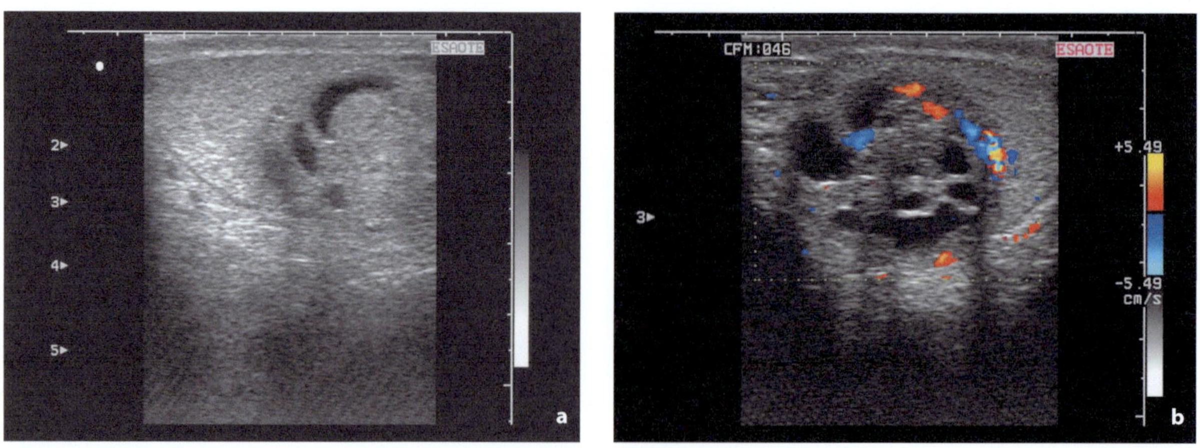

Fig. 6.118a,b Teratocarcinoma of the testis. Complex mass with multiple microcystic loculations (**a**) and solid vascular components at CD (**b**)

The mean RI is 0.7 and the peak velocity is around 10 cm/s [120] (Figs. 6.119, 6.120). In some cases the nodule, especially if small, appears iso-hypovascular to the rest of the testis, regardless of the histotype. Only Leydig cell tumors show a rather characteristic peripheral hypervascularity (in association with a small homogeneous hypoechoic nodule without calcifications), although this is not usually enough for a correct preoperative diagnosis (which if performed would make testicle-sparing surgery possible in this

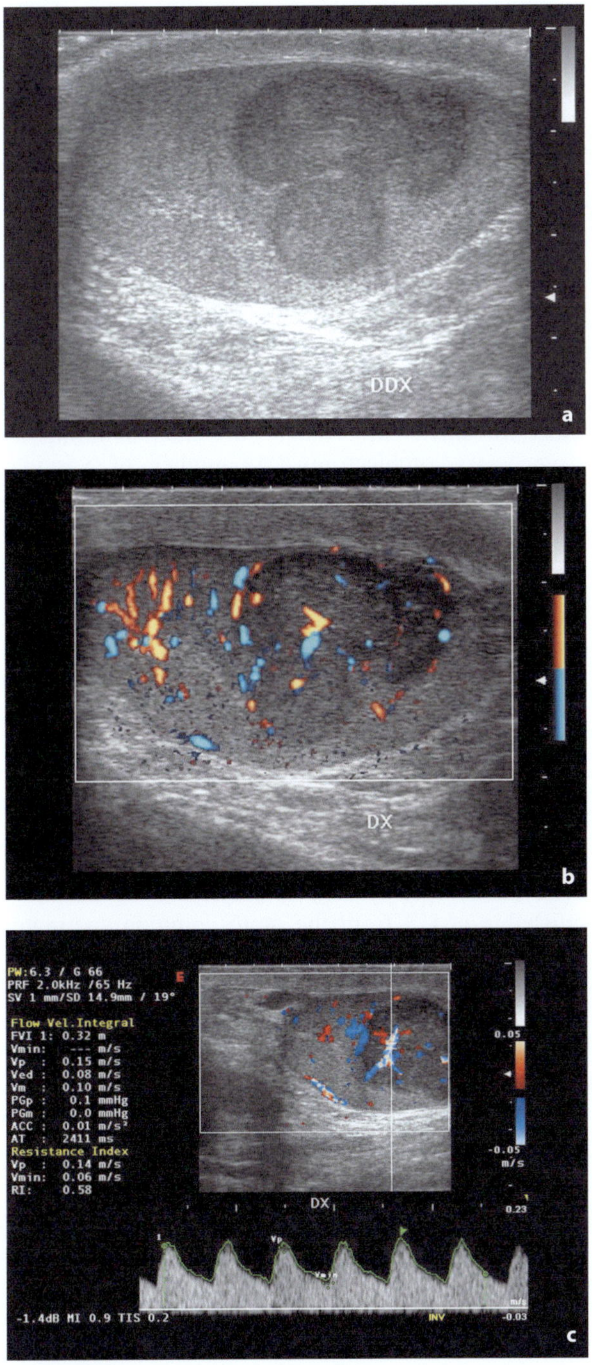

Fig. 6.119a-c Seminoma of the testis. Lobulated hypoechoic lesion of the testis (**a**), with moderate vascular signals at both the center and periphery of the lesion at directional PD (**b**), with V_{max} 15 cm/s and RI 0.58 at spectral Doppler (**c**)

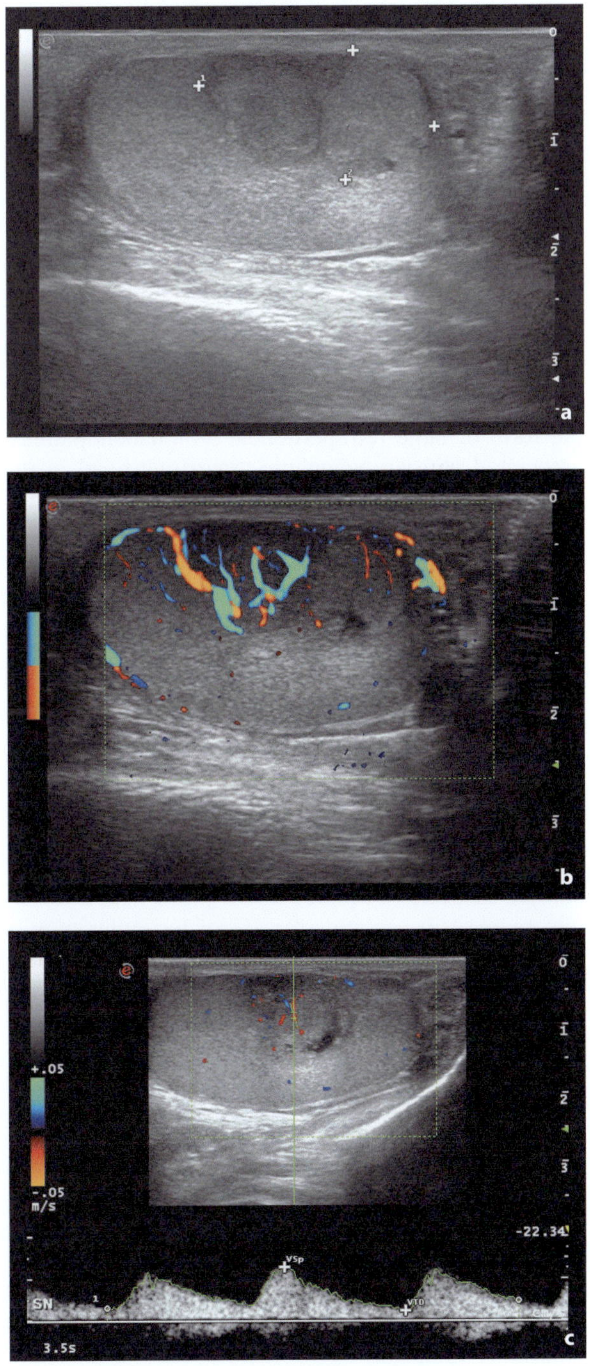

Fig. 6.120a-c Seminoma of the testis. Bilobulated hypoechoic nodule of the testis (**a**, *calipers*) with moderate vascularity at directional PD (**b**) and relatively high resistance at spectral Doppler (**c**)

fundamentally benign tumor) [114,120,121]. Although in general, CD provides no major additional information with respect to the morphologic findings, it can be useful in the identification of barely perceptible tumors and especially in differential diagnosis with infarction, fibrotic lesions or hematomas. CD can be misleading in focal orchitis, especially if the clinical presentation is atypical, because in this case the hypervascularity may be incorrectly interpreted by the sonographer. Nonetheless, in neoplastic nodules a pattern of vascular displacement can be identified which is not seen in inflammation [114,115,120].

The study of lumbar lymph node **metastases** is best performed with CT and MR (Fig. 6.121). Hematogenous metastases which can be detected with US are especially to the liver, as well as the kidneys, adrenal glands, spleen, prostate, peritoneum and muscles.

A particular characteristic is given by tumors which have undergone **spontaneous regression** (burned out). In this case metastatic lesions may be found, e.g. in the form of large retroperitoneal lymphadenopathies, associated with an echogenic "scarring" band in the testis, with posterior acoustic shadowing and possible hypoechoic halo. Although relatively infrequent, this is an important condition because the differential diagnosis includes the rare primary germ cell tumors of the abdomen and pelvis. Therefore, in the presence of a biopsy finding of an abdominal germ cell lesion a regressed primary testicular tumor should also be taken into consideration and searched for with US. The differential diagnosis includes the appearance of the normal mediastinum testis and fibrotic phenomena such as the outcome of segmental infarction [119,122,123] (Figs. 6.122, 6.123).

A lymphoma, generally non-Hodgkin's, should also be suspected in patients >50 years with a testicular mass, as it accounts for 4% of testicular tumors and is the second neoplastic cause of a testicular mass at this age. In **lymphomas** and **leukemias**, the appearance is one of an often bilateral testicular mass with hypoechoic areas, variable size, generally homogeneous echotexture, well-defined margins and numerous vascular signals at CD (regardless of size). Occasionally, alternating hypoechoic strips may be seen irradiating from the mediastinum testis, or diffuse involvement of the testis may be observed, either diffusely disrupted or homogeneously invaded with the risk of a false-negative diagnosis [114,115]. Differentiation from testicular inflammation can be challenging and should be based on the clinical and laboratory findings.

Testicular metastases are rare and can originate from cancers of the skin (melanomas), prostate, lung, kidney and gastrointestinal tract (including carcinoids). The US appearance is extremely variable and nonspecific, with single or multiple nodules or diffuse invasion [114,119].

The **differential diagnosis** of testicular tumors should also include a number of conditions which in general may have a different clinical presentation, or at any rate have the possibility of modifications at an examination performed after several days. These include testicular atrophy, partial necrotic outcomes from testicular torsion (without detorsion or with late detorsion), partial infarction, focal orchitis, granulomatous diseases (sarcoidosis, tuberculosis, idiopathic granulomatous orchitis, etc.), epidermoid cysts (formation of echogenic and often calcified wall with heterogeneous content), hematomas (personal history of trauma, even minor), outcomes of recent biopsy (hypoechoic) or old biopsy (echogenic), especially in patients studied for infertility (Figs. 6.124–6.128). In most of these cases, however, the patient history and clinical findings, together with the results of US, CD and a possible study performed after a short period of time are sufficiently diagnostic, thus avoiding an unnecessary orchiectomy. A number of vascular anomalies of the testis should also be taken into consideration. These include intratesticular varicocele, which nonetheless has a rather definite appearance, being associated with extratesticular varicocele and accentuation of the CD pattern during the Valsalva maneuver, and arteriovenous malformations, which mimic a hypervascular neoplastic lesion, having a hypoechoic appearance of a nodulation with intense internal color signals [116,124].

With regard to **extratesticular expansive disease** of the scrotum, the most important are fluid collections (hydrocele, pyocele, hematocele, etc.), hernias, spermatocele (cystic dilatation of the tubules in the head of the epididymis), epididymal cysts (indistinguishable at US from the more common spermatocele), cysts of the tunica albuginea, mesothelioma of the tunica vaginalis, fibrous pseudotumor, spermatic cord tumors, epididymal tumors and metastases of the scrotum wall [116,125] (Figs. 6.129–6.131). **Epididymal tumors** are in fact rare, with 75% being cases of benign adenomatoid tumor (generally arising from the tail, with hypoechoic or, more often, hyperechoic appearance with respect to the testis) and the remaining 25% being made up of papillary cystadenomas (von Hippel–Lindau syndrome), leiomyomas and other even rarer histotypes [115,119]. **Spermatic cord tumors** (lipomas, fibromas, liposarcomas, rhabdomyosarcomas, etc.) have onset in both children and adults and are generally identifiable as heterogeneous echogenic masses. **Metastases of the scrotum** are rare, generally originate from melanomas and carcinomas of the anal canal and have a heterogeneous hypoechoic appearance [116].

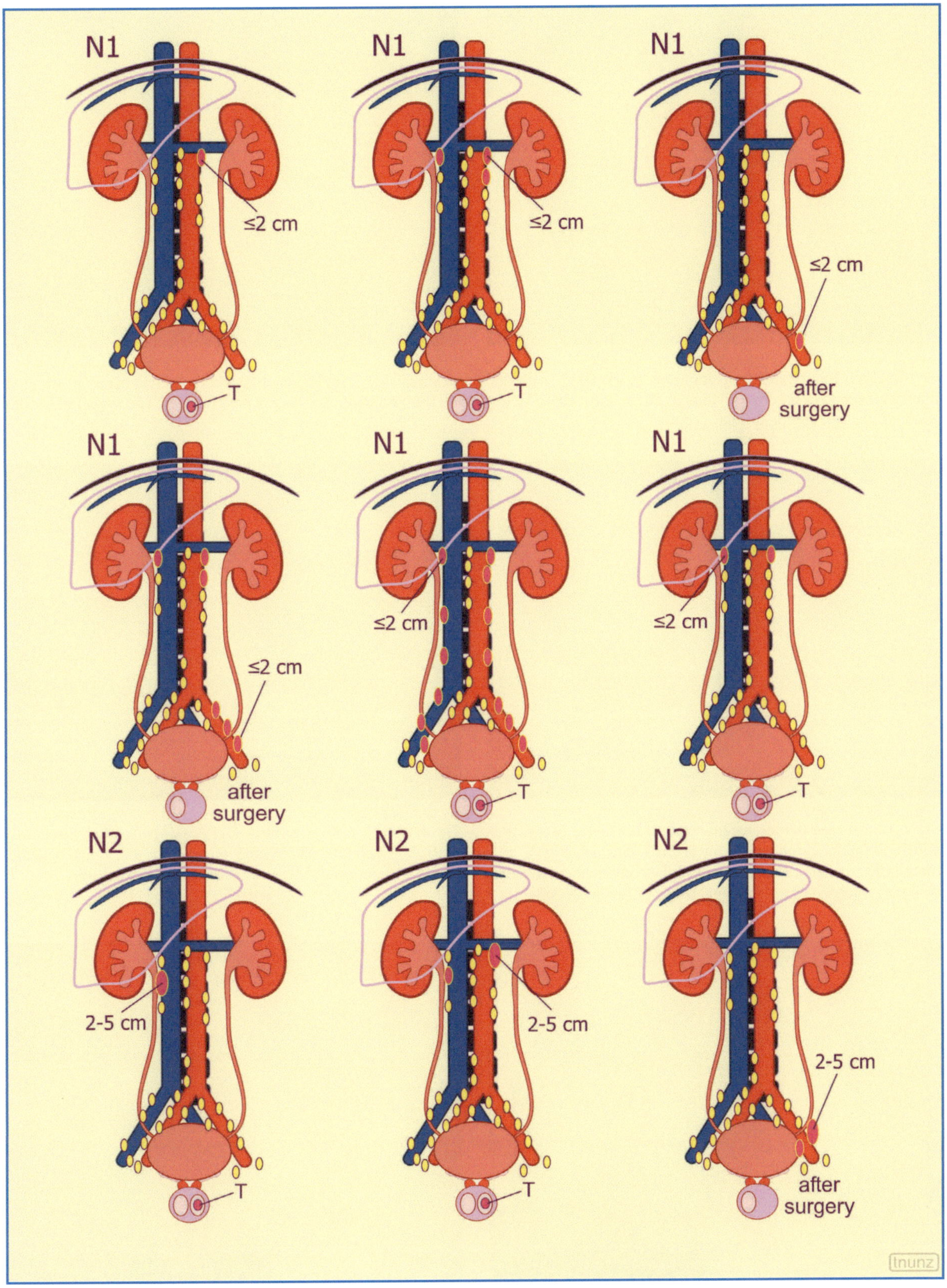

Fig. 6.121 N parameter for testicular cancer. Regional lymph nodes include para-aortic, pre-aortic, interaortocaval, precaval, paracaval, retrocaval, retro-aortic and lymph nodes located along the spermatic vein. *N1* refers to metastasis to one or more regional lymph nodes with all ≤2 cm, *N2* refers to metastasis to one or more regional lymph nodes with all ≤5 cm, *N3* (not shown) refers to metastasis in lymph node >5 cm. Modified from [31]

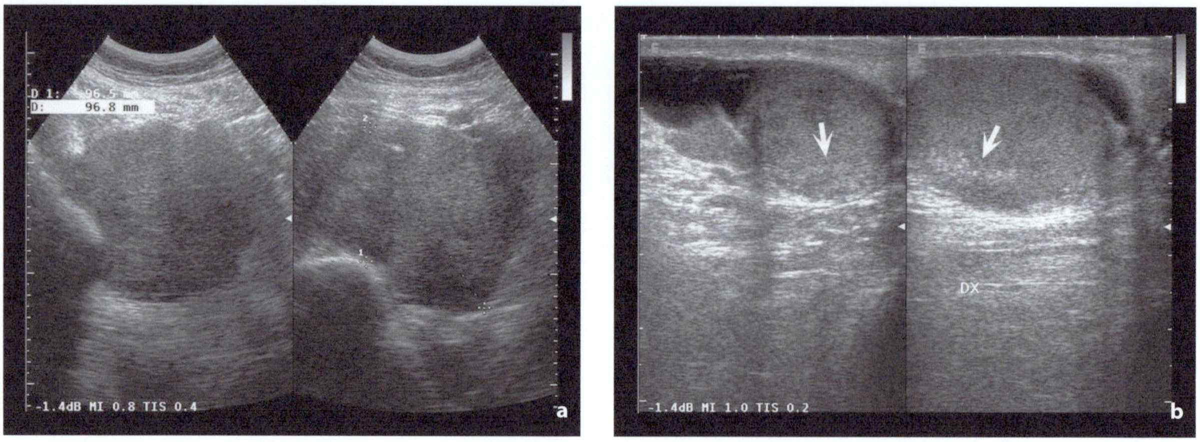

Fig. 6.122a,b Burned-out dysgerminoma of the testis, with pelvic metastasis. Heterogeneous hypoechoic pelvic mass (**a**) which at biopsy is seen to be a germ cell tumor. The subsequent testicular study shows a thin calcifying echogenic band (**b**, *arrow*) indicating residual of a primary neoplasm

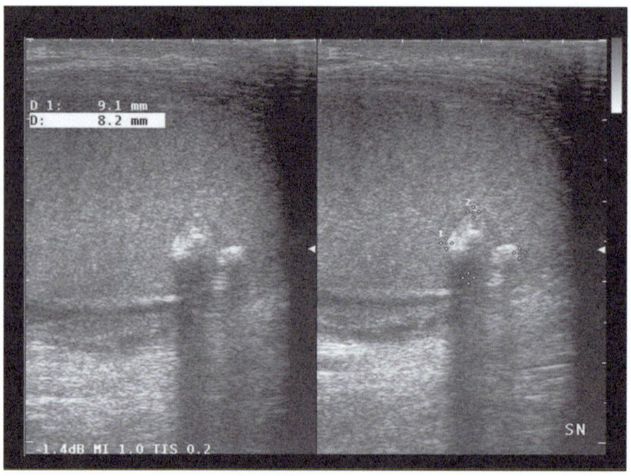

Fig. 6.123 Burned-out teratocarcinoma of the testis. In a patient with abdominal lymph node metastasis and secondary lung metastases, the testicular US study shows only a heterogeneous calcified patch indicating residual tissue of the neoplasm

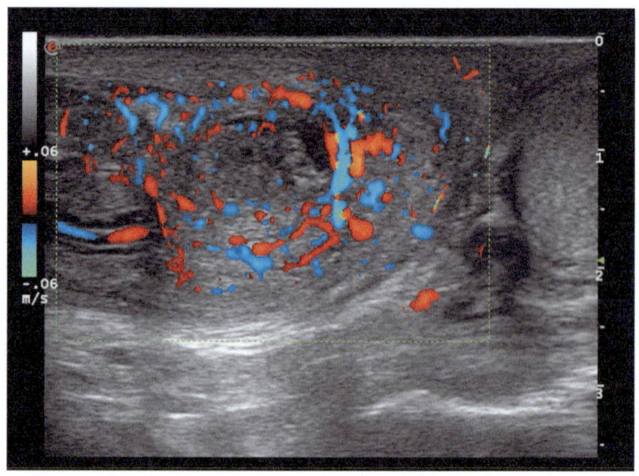

Fig. 6.124 Abscessed orchitis. CD shows peripheral vascularity of the hypoechoic area detected within the testis, which nonetheless is without central flow signals due to liquefaction

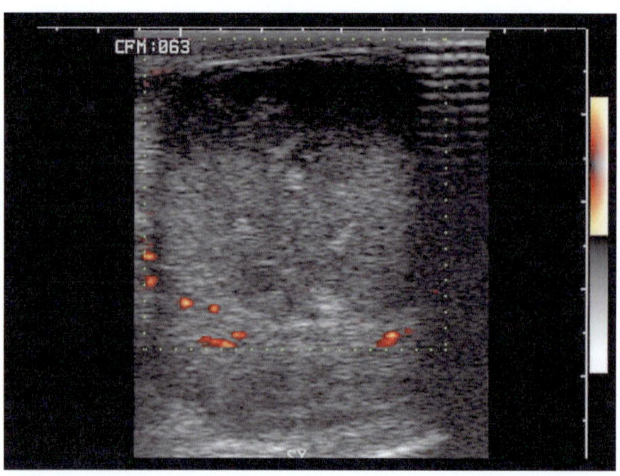

Fig. 6.125 Necrosis of the testis after testicular torsion. Heterogeneous hypoechoic remodeling of the testis, mimicking a neoplasm (apart from the clinical presentation) but avascular at PD

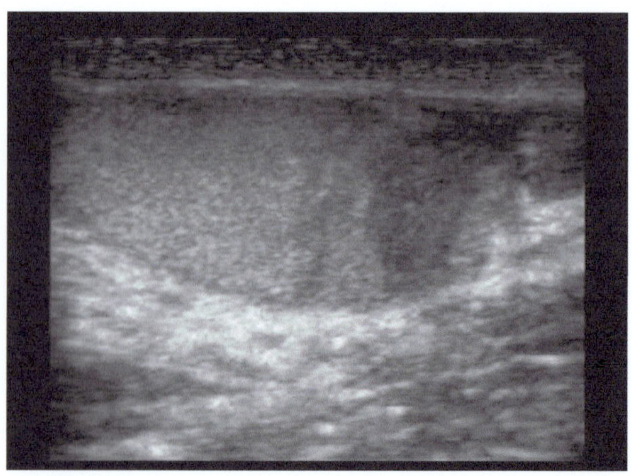

Fig. 6.126 Partial infarction of the testis. Heterogeneous hypoechoic band of the testis mimicking a neoplasm

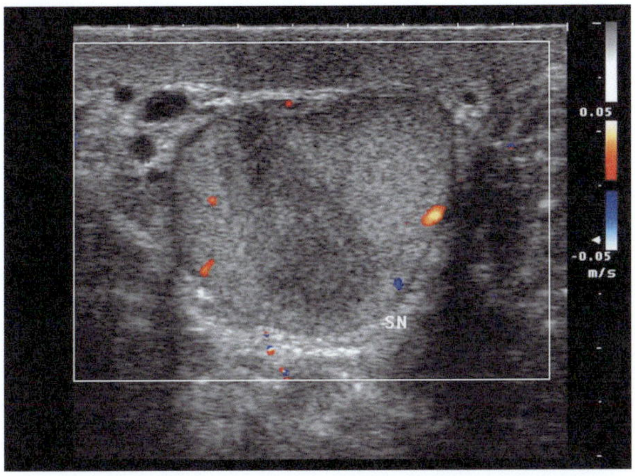

Fig. 6.127 Infarction on hypotrophic testicle. Dysmorphic testicle smaller than normal with internal heterogeneous hypoechoic band and no vascular signals mimicking a neoplasm

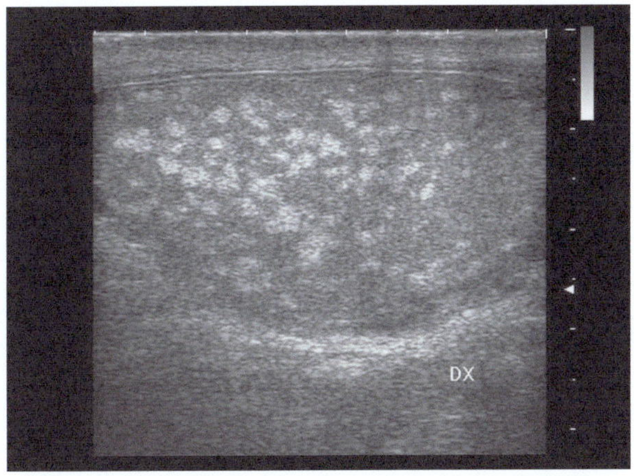

Fig. 6.128 Testicular angiomatosis. Unilateral, scattered, non-confluent echogenic patches

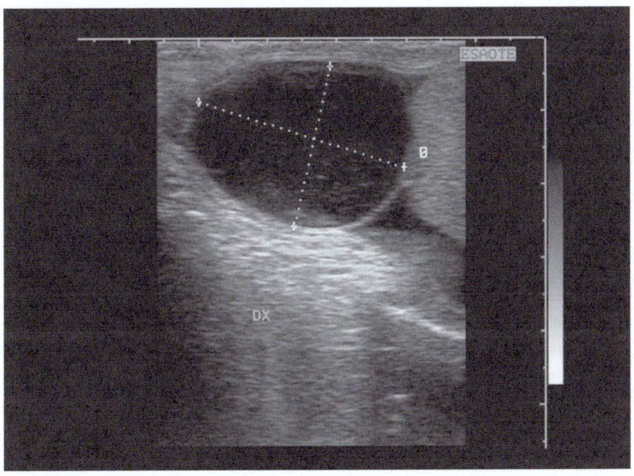

Fig. 6.129 Cyst of the epididymis. Homogeneous unilocular cystic mass at the level of the head of the epididymis

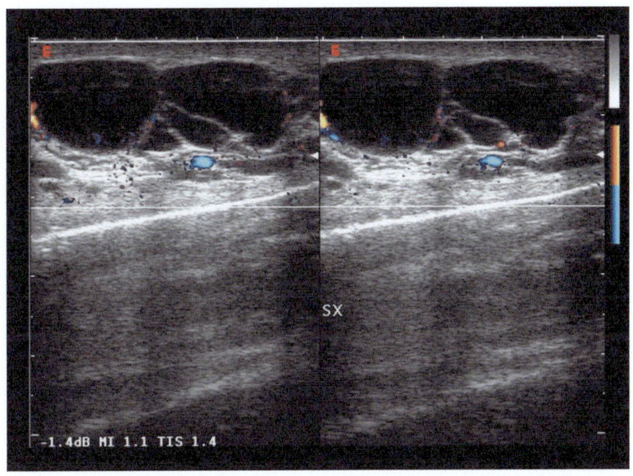

Fig. 6.130 Cysts of the epididymis. Multilocular cystic mass, with some slight septal vascular signals at directional PD

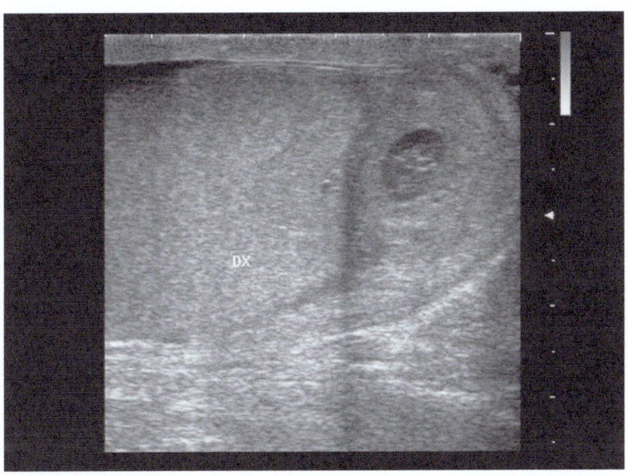

Fig. 6.131 Epididymitis. Echogenic thickening of the head of the epididymis with internal hypo-anechoic liquefactive area

References

1. Rüeger R (2005) Sonography of the adrenal glands. Praxis 94:343-348
2. Jeffrey RB et al (1995) Sonography of the abdomen. Raven Press, New York
3. Mitchell IC et al (2007) Adrenal masses in the cancer patient: surveillance or excision. Oncologist 12:168-174
4. Dunnick NR (1990) Adrenal imaging: current status. AJR Am J Roentgenol 154:927-936
5. de Bree E et al (1998) Cysts of the adrenal gland: diagnosis and management. Int Urol Nephrol 30:369-376
6. Trojan J et al (2000) Cystic adrenal lymphangioma: incidental diagnosis on abdominal sonography. AJR Am J Roentgenol 174:1164-1165
7. Reznek RH et al (2004) Primary adrenal malignancy. In: Husband JE et al (eds) Imaging in oncology, II Edition. Taylor & Francis, London, 307-323
8. Musante F et al (1988) Myelolipoma of the adrenal gland: sonographic and CT features. AJR Am J Roentgenol 151:961-964
9. Hugosson C et al (1999) Imaging of abdominal neuroblastoma in children. Acta Radiol 40:534-542
10. Siegel MJ (2004) Neuroblastoma. In: Husband JE et al (eds) Imaging in oncology, II Edition. Taylor & Francis, London, 953-972
11. Amundson GM et al (1987) Neuroblastoma: a specific sonographic tissue pattern. AJR Am J Roentgenol 148:943-946
12. Ghiatas AA et al (1996) Is sonography flow imaging useful in the differential diagnosis of adrenal masses? Br J Radiol 69:1005-1008
13. O'Kane P et al (2000) The adrenals. In: Shirkhoda A (ed) Variants and pitfalls in body imaging. Lippincott Williams & Wilkins, Philadelphia, 375-390
14. Dewbury KC (2001) The adrenals. In: Meire H et al (eds) Abdominal and general ultrasound, II Edition. Churchill Livingstone, London, 479-495
15. Amendola MA (2000) The kidneys. In: Shirkhoda A (ed) Variants and pitfalls in body imaging. Lippincott Williams & Wilkins, Philadelphia, 355-374
16. Hélénon O et al (2001) Ultrasound of renal tumors. Eur Radiol 11:1890-1901
17. Ascenti G et al (2001) Usefulness of power Doppler and contrast-enhanced sonography in the differentiation of hyperechoic renal masses. Abdom Imaging 26:654-660
18. Jamis-Dow CA et al (1996) Small (≤3-cm) renal masses: detection with CT versus US and pathologic correlation. Radiology 198:785-788
19. Setola SV et al (2007) Contrast-enhanced sonography of the kidney. Abdom Imaging 32:21-28
20. Bosniak MA et al (1995) Small renal parenchymal neoplasms: further observations on growth. Radiology 197:589-597
21. Curry NS (2002) Imaging the small solid renal mass. Abdom Imaging 27:629-636
22. Caskey CI (2000) Ultrasound techniques for evaluating renal masses, renal obstruction, and other upper tract pathology. Ultrasound Q 16:23-39
23. Webb JAW (2001) Renal masses and trauma. In: Meire H et al (eds) Abdominal and general ultrasound, II Edition. Churchill Livingstone, London, 549-568
24. Jinzaki M et al (1997) Small solid renal lesions: usefulness of power Doppler US. Radiology 209:549-550
25. Quaia E et al (2003) Characterization of renal tumours with pulse inversion harmonic imaging by intermittent high mechanical index technique: initial results. Eur Radiol 13:1402-1412
26. Lemaitre L et al (1995) Renal angiomyolipoma: growth followed up with CT and/or US. Radiology 197:598-602
27. Zhang J et al (2006) Imaging of kidney cancer. Radiol Clin North Am 45:119-147
28. Jewett MA et al (2008) Renal tumor natural history: the rationale and role for active surveillance. Urol Clin North Am 35:627-634
29. Siow WY et al (2000) Renal cell carcinoma: incidental detection and pathological staging. J R Coll Surg Edinb 45:291-295
30. Snyder ME et al (2006) Incindence of benign lesions for clinically renal masses smaller than 7 cm in radiological diameter: influence of sex. J Urol 176:2391-2396
31. Wittekind CH et al (2005) TNM atlas. Springer-Verlag Berlin
32. Robson CJ et al (1969) The results of radical nephrectomy for renal cell carcinoma. J Urol 101:297-301
33. Ascenti G et al (2004) Contrast-enhanced second-harmonic sonography in the detection of pseudocapsule in renal cell carcinoma. AJR Am J Roentgenol 182:1525-1530
34. Li G et al (2004) Characteristics of imaging-detected solid renal masses: implication for optimal treatment. Int J Urol 11:63-67
35. Raj GV et al (2007) Predicting the histology of renal masses using preoperative Doppler ultrasonography. J Urol 177:53-58
36. Tamai H et al (2005) Contrast-enhanced ultrasonography in the diagnosis of solid renal tumors. J Ultrasound Med 24:1635-1640
37. Hora M et al (2004) Rupture of papillary renal cell carcinoma. Scand J Urol Nephrol 38:481-484
38. Habboub HK et al (1997) Accuracy of color Doppler sonography in assessing venous thrombus extension in renal cell carcinoma. AJR Am J Roentgenol 168:267-271
39. Kallman DA et al (1992) Renal vein and inferior vena cava tumor thrombus in renal cell carcinoma: CT, US, MRI and venacavography. J Comput Assist Tomogr 16:240-247
40. Seong CK et al (2002) Hypoechoic normal renal sinus and renal pelvis tumors. Sonographic differentiation. J Ultrasound Med 21:993-999
41. Duncan AW et al (1996) Cysts within septa: an ultrasound feature distinguishing neoplastic from non-neoplastic renal lesions in children? Pediatr Radiol 26:315-317
42. Williams H et al (2004) Wilms' tumor and associated neoplasms of the kidney. In: Husband JE et al (eds) Imaging in oncology, II Edition. Taylor & Francis, London, 933-952
43. Reznek RH et al (2004) Lymphoma. In: Husband JE et al (eds) Imaging in oncology, II Edition. Taylor & Francis, London, 817-874
44. Duyndam DAC et al (2002) Bilateral perirenal lymphoma: imaging with ultrasound, CT and MRI. Clin Radiol Extra 57:1-2
45. Bosniak MA (1997) The use of the Bosniak classification system for renal cysts and cystic tumors. J Urol 157:1852-1853
46. Robbin ML et al (2003) Renal imaging with ultrasound contrast: current status. Radiol Clin North Am 41:963-978
47. Kim AY et al (1999) Contrast-enhanced power Doppler sonography for the differentiation of cystic renal lesions:

preliminary study. J Ultrasound Med 18:581-588
48. Ascenti G et al (2007) Complex cystic renal masses: characterization with contrast-enhanced US. Radiology 243:158-165
49. Quaia E et al (2008) Comparison of contrast-enhanced sonography with unenhanced sonography and contrast-enhanced CT in the diagnosis of malignancy in complex cystic renal masses. AJR Am J Roentgenol 191:1239-1249
50. Derchi LE et al (2002) Ultrasound in gynecology. Eur Radiol 11:2137-2155
51. Ascher SM et al (2002) Cancer of the adnexal organs. In: Bragg DG et al (eds) Oncologic imaging. WB Saunders Company, Philadelphia, 549-574
52. Jeong et al (2000) Imaging evaluation of ovarian masses. Radiographics 20:1445-1470
53. Kurtz AB et al (1999) Diagnosis and staging of ovarian cancer: comparative values of Doppler and conventional US, CT, and MR imaging correlated with surgery and histopathologic analysis – report of the Radiology Diagnostic Oncology Group. Radiology 212:19-27
54. Berlanda N et al (2002) Impact of a multiparameter, ultrasound-based triade on surgical management of adnexal masses. Ultrasound Obstet Gynecol 20:181-185
55. Sassone AM et al (1991) Transvaginal sonographic characterization of ovarian disease: evaluation of a new scoring system to predict ovarian malignancy. Obstet Gynecol 78:70-76
56. Brown DL et al (1998) Benign and malignant ovarian masses: selection of the most discriminating gray-scale and Doppler sonographic features. Radiology 208:103-110
57. Marret H et al (2002) Color Doppler energy prediction of malignancy in adnexal masses using logistic regression models. Ultrasound Obstet Gynecol 20:597-604
58. Guerriero S et al (2002) Complex pelvic mass as a target of evaluation of vessel distribution by color Doppler sonography for the diagnosis of adnexal malignancies. Results of a multicenter European study. J Ultrasound Med 21:1105-1111
59. Wilson WD et al (2006) Sonographic quantification of ovarian tumor vascularity. J Ultrasound Med 25:1577-1581
60. Hata K et al (1995) Intratumoral peak systolic velocity as a new possible predictor for detection of adnexal malignancy. Am J Obstet Gynecol 172:1496-1500
61. Kurjak A et al (1992) Transvaginal ultrasound, color flow, and Doppler waveform of the postmenopausal adnexal mass. Obstet Gynecol 80:917-921
62. Valentin L et al (2006) Which extrauterine pelvic masses are difficult to correctly classify as benign or malignant on the basis of ultrasound findings and is there a way of making a correct diagnosis? Ultrasound Obstet Gynecol 27:438-444
63. Fleischer AC et al (2008) Contrast-enhanced transvaginal sonography of benign versus malignant ovarian masses: preliminary findings. J Ultrasound Med 27:1011-1018
64. Testa AC et al (2005) The use of contrasted transvaginal sonography in the diagnosis of gynecologic diseases. A preliminary study. J Ultrasound Med 24:1267-1278
65. Arger PH (1996) Asymptomatic palpable adnexal masses. In: Bluth EI et al (eds) Syllabus: a special course in ultrasound. RSNA Publications, Oak Brook, 241-248
66. Jan KA et al (2002) Sonographic spectrum of hemorrhagic ovarian cysts. J Ultrasound Med 21:879-886
67. Patel MD et al (1999) Endometriomas: diagnostic performance of US. Radiology 210:739-745
68. Tongsong T et al (2006) Numerous intracystic floating balls as a sonographic feature of benign cystic teratoma. Report of 5 cases. J Ultrasound Med 25:1587-1591
69. Caspi B et al (2006) Variable echogenicity as a sonographic sign in the preoperative diagnosis of ovarian mucinous tumors. J Ultrasound Med 25:1583-1585
70. Lee MS et al (2001) Ovarian sclerosing stromal tumors. Gray scale and color-Doppler sonographic findings. J Ultrasound Med 20:413-417
71. Alcázar JL et al (2003) Transvaginal gray scale and color Doppler sonography in primary ovarian cancer and metastatic tumors to the ovary. J Ultrasound Med 22:243-247
72. Chen CY et al (2007) The power Doppler velocity index, pulsatility index, and resistive index can assist in making a differential diagnosis of primary ovarian carcinoma and Krukenberg tumors: a preliminary study. J Ultrasound Med 26:921-926
73. Akin O et al (2006) Imaging of uterine cancer. Radiol Clin North Am 45:167-182
74. Boles SM et al (2002) Carcinoma of the cervix and endometrium. In: Bragg DG et al (eds) Oncologic imaging. WB Saunders Company, Philadelphia, 523-548
75. Kitchener H (2006) Management of endometrial carcinoma. Eur J Surg Oncol 32:838-843
76. Valenzano M et al (2001) The role of transvaginal ultrasound and sonohysterography in the diagnosis and staging of endometrial adenocarcinoma. Radiol Med 101:365-370
77. Epstein E et al (2002) An algorithm including results of gray-scale and power Doppler ultrasound examination to predict endometrial malignancy in women with postmenopausal bleeding. Ultrasound Obstet Gynecol 20:370-376
78. Levine D et al (1995) Change in endometrial thickness in postmenopausal women undergoing hormone replacement therapy. Radiology 197:603-609
79. Coleman BG (1996) Imaging women receiving tamoxifene therapy. In: Bluth EI et al (eds) Syllabus: a special course in ultrasound. RSNA Publications, Oak Brook, 185-194
80. Bega G et al (2003) Three-dimensional ultrasonography in gynecology. Technical aspects and clinical applications. J Ultrasound Med 22:1249-1269
81. Takacs P et al (2005) Echogenic endometrial fluid collection in postmenopausal women is a significant risk factor for disease. J Ultrasound Med 24:1477-1481
82. Warming L et al (2002) Measurement precision and normal range of endometrial thickness in a postmenopausal population by transvaginal ultrasound. Ultrasound Obstet Gynecol 20:492-495
83. Peri N et al (2007) Sonographic evaluation of the endometrium in patients with a history or an appearance of polycystic ovarian syndrome. J Ultrasound Med 26:55-58
84. Fleischer AC (2003) Color Doppler sonography of uterine disorders. Ultrasound Q 19:179-189
85. Alcázar JL et al (2006) Reproducibility of endometrial vascular patterns in endometrial disease as assessed by transvaginal power Doppler sonography in women with postmenopausal bleeding. J Ultrasound Med 25:159-163
86. Alcázar JL et al (2005) Endometrial volume and vascularity measurements by transvaginal three-dimensional ultrasonography in stimulated and tumoral endometria: an interobserver reproducibility study. J Ultrasound Med 24:1091-1098

87. Mercé LT et al (2007) Clinical usefulness of 3-dimensional sonography and power Doppler angiography for diagnosis of endometrial carcinoma. J Ultrasound Med 26:1279-1287
88. Sarna A et al (2005) Computed tomographic and ultrasonographic findings of endometrial carcinoma appearing as a fungating inguinal mass. J Ultrasound Med 24:1579-1582
89. Gordon AN et al (1990) Depth of myometrial invasion in endometrial cancer: preoperative assessment by transvaginal ultrasonography. Gynecol Oncol 39:321-327
90. Takac I (2007) Transvaginal ultrasonography with and without saline infusion in assessment of myometrial invasion of endometrial cancer. J Ultrasound Med 26:949-955
91. Artner A et al (1994) The value of ultrasound in preoperative assessment of the myometrial and cervical invasion in endometrial carcinoma. Gynaecol Oncol 54:147-151
92. Del Maschio A et al (1993) Estimating the depth of myometrial involvement by endometrial carcinoma: efficacy of transvaginal sonography vs MR imaging. AJR Am J Roentgenol 161:595-538
93. Schmidt G (2006) Differential diagnosis in ultrasound imaging. Georg Thieme Verlag, Stuttgart
94. Zhang J et al (2006) Imaging of bladder cancer. Radiol Clin North Am 45:183-205
95. Rickards D et al (2001) The lower urinary tract. In: Meire H et al (eds) Abdominal and general ultrasound, II Edition. Churchill Livingstone, London, 585-612
96. Husband JE et al (2004) Primary adrenal malignancy. In: Husband JE et al (eds) Imaging in oncology, II Edition. Taylor & Francis, London, 343-374
97. Balci NC et al (2002) Cancer of the adnexal organs. In: Bragg DG et al (eds) Oncologic imaging. WB Saunders Company, Philadelphia, 629-645
98. Francica G et al (2008) Correlation of transabdominal sonographic and cystoscopic findings in the diagnosis of focal abnormalities of the urinary bladder wall: a prospective study. J Ultrasound Med 27:887-894
99. Kocakoc E et al (2008) Detection of bladder tumors with 3-dimensional sonography and virtual sonographic cystoscopy. J Ultrasound Med 27:45-53
100. Özden E et al (2007) A New parameter for staging bladder carcinoma: ultrasonographic contact length and height-to-length ratio. J Ultrasound Med 26:1137-1142
101. Karahan OI et al (2004) Color Doppler ultrasonography findings of bladder tumors: correlation with stage and histopatologic grade. Acta Radiol 45:481-486
102. Akin O et al (2006) Imaging of prostate cancer. Radiol Clin North Am 45:207-222
103. Yu et al (2002) Cancer of the prostate. In: Bragg DG et al (eds) Oncologic imaging. WB Saunders Company, Philadelphia, pp 575-602
104. Gleason DF (1977) The veterans administration cooperative urological research group. In: Tannenbaum M (ed) Urologic pathology: the prostate. Lea & Febiger, Philadelphia, 171-198
105. Turgut AT et al (2007) Power Doppler ultrasonography of the feeding arteries of the prostate gland: a novel approach to the diagnosis of prostate cancer? J Ultrasound Med 26:875-883
106. Halpern EJ et al (2001) Prostate cancer: use of contrast-enhanced US for detection. Radiology 219:219-225
107. Yi A et al (2006) Contrast-enhanced sonography for prostate cancer detection in patients with indeterminate clinical findings. AJR Am J Roentgenol 186:1431-1435
108. Pelzers A et al (2005) Prostate cancer detection in men with prostate specific antigen 4 to 10 ng/ml using a combined approach of contrast-enhanced color Doppler targeted and systematic biopsy. J Urol 173:1926-1929
109. Littrup PJ et al (1991) Determination of prostate volume by transrectal US for cancer screening. Part I. Comparison with prostate specific antigen assays. Radiology 178:537-542
110. Veneziano S et al (1990) Correlation between prostate specific antigen and prostate volume, evaluated by transrectal ultrasonography: usefulness in diagnosis of prostate cancer. Eur Urol 18:112-116
111. Clements R (2001) Ultrasound of prostate cancer. Eur Radiol 11:2119-2125
112. Lan S-K et al (2007) Diagnostic performance of a random versus lesion-directed biopsy of the prostate from transrectal ultrasound. Results of a 5-year consecutive clinical study in 1 institution in south Taiwan. J Ultrasound Med 26:11-17
113. Nudell DM et al (2000) Imaging for recurrent prostate cancer. Radiol Clin North Am 38:213-229
114. Akin EA et al (2004) Ultrasound of the scrotum. Ultrasound Q 20:181-200
115. Oyen RH (2002) Scrotal ultrasound. Eur Radiol 12:19-34
116. Dogra VS et al (2003) Sonography of the scrotum. Radiology 227:18-36
117. Miller FN et al (2007) Testicular calcification and microlithiasis: association with primary intra-testicular malignancy in 3,477 patients. Eur Radiol 17:363-369
118. Parenti GC et al (2007) Association between testicular microlithiasis and primary malignancy of the testis: our experience and review of the literature. Radiol Med 112:588-596
119. Fowler R (2001) The scrotum and penis. In: Meire H et al (eds) Abdominal and general ultrasound, II Edition. Churchill Livingstone, London, 627-658
120. Horstman WG et al (1992) Testicular tumors: findings with color Doppler US. Radiology 185:733-737
121. Maizlin ZV et al (2004) Leydig cell tumors of the testis. Gray scale and color Doppler sonographic appearance. J Ultrasound Med 23:959-964
122. Comiter CV et al (1996) Burned-out primary testicular cancer: sonographic and pathological characteristics. J Urol 156:85-88
123. Patel MD et al (2007) Sonographic and magnetic resonance imaging appearance of a burned-out testicular germ cell neoplasm. J Ultrasound Med 26:143-146
124. Kutlu R et al (2003) Intratesticular arteriovenous malformation. Color Doppler sonographic findings. J Ultrasound Med 22:295-298
125. Sudakoff GS et al (2002) Scrotal ultrasonography with emphasis on the extratesticular space: anatomy, embryology, and pathology. Ultrasound Q 18:255-273

US-Guided Intervention

7

7.1 US Guidance for Interventional Procedures

Thanks to the progress of modern imaging modalities a reliable noninvasive characterization of most focal lesions can today be obtained. In general, reaching a diagnosis with diagnostic techniques (radiologic as well as nuclear medicine, endoscopy, laboratory, etc.) rather than with cytologic or histologic biopsy is preferable, although the latter may avoid an excessive "spiral" between the different imaging techniques, with the associated costs in time and money. In most cases, however, a histologic or at least cytologic diagnosis of malignancy is still needed for appropriate patient management. In addition there are also medical-legal motives when undertaking treatment involving chemotherapy, radiation therapy and/or surgery. It should also be recalled that in many circumstances the collection of cytologic or histologic material does not serve diagnostic purposes but rather is done to obtain important information for beginning or continuing therapy, such as histologic type, grade of neoplasm, or its biochemical and functional characteristics.

For palpable superficial lesions the percutaneous procedures, at least FNAC, can be performed without diagnostic imaging guidance, whereas guidance is absolutely necessary in the presence of deep lesions. The **non-imaging-assisted** modality is in fact faster and more economic and is largely used especially for the thyroid. However, for palpable masses the use of imaging modalities, and in particular US, may be preferable or even indispensable.

US is useful first of all in the preliminary evaluation of a lesion, confirming its effective presence at the level of the "palpable mass" and easily identifying the lesions that are not to be aspirated (e.g. aneurysms). In addition, US guidance enables definition of the relations with the anatomic structures positioned around or deep to the lesion (vessels, lung, etc.), the aspiration of lesions which are mobile beneath the fingers, and multiple sampling in different points of the lesion (also avoiding necrotic or cystic areas). For example, in one study on FNAC of the cervical lymph nodes, use of the US-guided procedure involved 1% of false positives and 1% of false negatives compared with 5% and 8% respectively for the procedure without US guidance [1].

With the exclusion of areas that are poorly accessible or inaccessible to ultrasound, such as the skull, bone and chest, all other body regions are preferentially reached with US guidance. With respect to CT and MR, US is ubiquitously available, faster, more flexible in its range of applications, more economical and above all has the considerable advantage of being performed in real time, with the possibility of continuous monitoring of the needle, the lesion and the adjacent structures, and being able to do so in multiple scan planes. Moving targets are therefore less of a problem than in the setting of CT or MR guidance. With particular respect to CT, US does not use ionizing radiation or iodinated contrast media. It is also worth noting that US is the only transportable guidance technique, and can therefore be used for diagnostic or therapeutic procedures both at the patient's bedside and in the operating room. The possibility of rotating the transducer and changing the angle of insonation at will provides an optimal visualization of small and deep lesions and therefore makes it possible to follow the needle tip during the entire procedure. In the liver, and in general in the abdominal structures accessible with ultrasound, US guidance is preferable to CT or MR whenever the lesion can be adequately visualized with US. US has proven to be particularly useful in biopsies of small and very small hepatic lesions [2,3]. In particular, biopsy of subphrenic hepatic lesions, which in CT would require an inclined approach, is preferably done with US

O. Catalano, A. Nunziata, A. Siani, *Fundamentals in Oncologic Ultrasound*.

guidance. In general, with some variations for the individual preferences of the operator, CT guidance is reserved for the adrenal glands, deep lymph nodes and possibly the pancreas, as well as for lesions that are not identifiable with US. When the lesion, especially if a hepatic lesion, is barely visible or not visible at all with US, it may be made out with CEUS, which increases the lesion–parenchyma contrast [4–6]. Alternatively, several navigation systems have been proposed in which the volume acquired with CT or MR, whose images have been uploaded onto the support hardware of the US system, is exploited to guide the "virtual" US targeting, for both sampling and percutaneous ablation. This means that significant advantages of US guidance do not need to be sacrificed even when the lesion is barely identifiable if at all [7,8]. It should, however, be noted that in up to 45% of patients referred for RF ablation, the treatment is not feasible, mainly because of tumor inconspicuousness [9].

With regard to procedures of core biopsy or vacuum biopsy in the breast, US is in competition with mammography. Stereotactic mammographic biopsy, however, involves the use of ionizing radiation, requires dedicated and immediately available systems, causes greater discomfort for the patients, is not able to reach all the areas (e.g. the axillary tail), is unable to visualize both the lesion and the needle in real time, takes longer and is more expensive. It should also be noted that stereotactic guidance is fundamentally unidirectional, whereas with US the insonation angle can be varied as desired and multiple biopsies according to different trajectories can be performed [10]. The fundamental advantage of stereotactic guidance is the possibility of its use in the event of microcalcifications, a highly important indication which in itself is often not accessible to US guidance. However, if appropriately guided by mammography, US can in some cases identify clusters of microcalcifications not associated with nodules, and therefore enable US-guided biopsy [11]. In other cases, mammographic biopsy should be reserved especially for lesions that cannot be accessed with US.

The use of US guidance may be difficult or impossible in the case of thoracic masses which do not reach the base of the neck or the thoracic wall or which at any rate are separated from the transducer by a layer of air (lung).

At the level of the extremities, US is by far the most utilized guide for biopsies of soft tissue solid lesions and drainage of collections (inguinal region, thigh, axilla, gluteus, etc.) [12]. Even superficial bone lesions or thin bone segments (e.g. ribs) can be reached with US guidance, as can areas of bone tumor spread into the soft tissues.

The various diagnostic and therapeutic procedures can be performed freehand, or by constantly exploiting the guidance of the US transducer but with no attachment between needle and transducer (US-assisted technique) or attaching the needle to the transducer (US guidance proper), which can be the normal method used in diagnostic procedures. In general, none of these options is better than the others and often the choice depends on the preference of the individual operator. In the end it will be the result in terms of "pathologic judgment" which dictates the correctness of the procedure used on each occasion. In the **freehand** technique used for large and superficial targets, the role of US is limited to localizing the area to be targeted, measuring its depth and marking the corresponding point on the skin. Then without the use of US the puncture is performed, such that the needle is not attached to the transducer. The **US-assisted** procedure uses the transducer normally utilized for diagnostic imaging to constantly monitor the progression of the needle (Fig. 7.1, Video 7.1). Particularly for FNAC of superficial structures, in fact, the transducer can only be used to assist the procedure without a needle guide. With the transducer held in one hand and the needle in the other, the needle is pushed immediately lateral to the transducer itself (coaxial approach), with an inclination which varies depending on the depth to be reached and the presence of sensitive structures located lateral to the target. The more superficial the lesion, the greater the inclination of the needle with respect to the transducer (therefore the penetration of the needle is deep, ending up being located right beneath the transducer). When the lesion is located deeply, the needle is inclined less and even placed lateral to the center of the ultrasound beam. An alternative is the tangential approach, whereby the needle is inserted in a direction perpendicular to the insonation angle and therefore to the position of the transducer on the skin. In this case the visualization of the needle and its tip can be more difficult, particularly in the first tract of penetration. Nonetheless, this approach can allow deep structures that are at risk to be avoided (e.g. pleural surface in the case of breast lesions) and may even make it possible to use shorter needles for structures that would need long needles if approached perpendicularly – long needles are subject to greater deformation and deviation when penetrating tissues, especially deep tissues. Experimentally it has been shown that the optimal conditions for an effective and safe US-assisted puncture include a distance between transducer and needle of 2–3 cm, in combination with an angle between the two of 55–60°: this enables an early and a reasonable visualization of the needle tip together with a short track of the needle itself [13]. The **US-guided** technique uses small needle-guide attachments (biopsy kit) inserted laterally

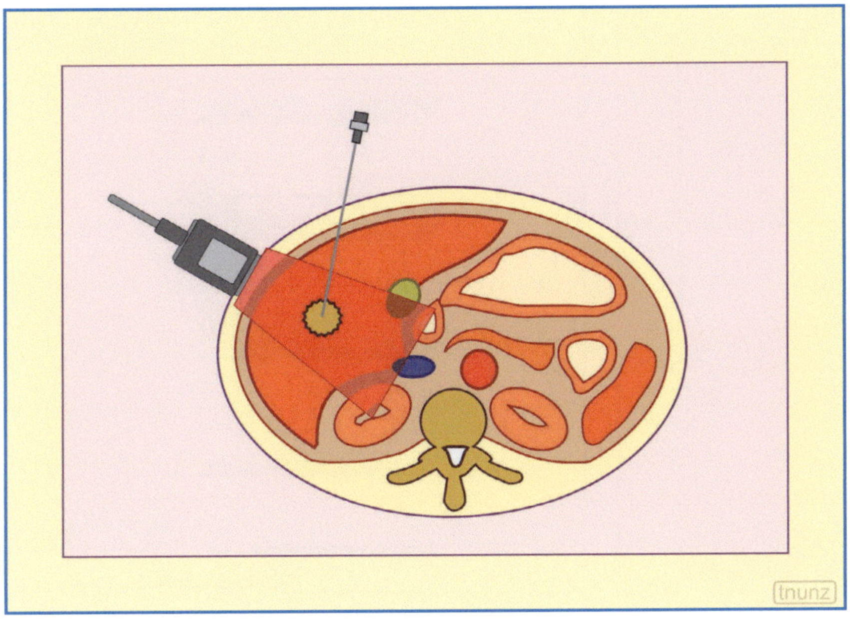

Fig. 7.1 US-assisted percutaneous procedure. The needle is not attached to the transducer, which only serves to verify the needle trajectory and the position of the needle in the target are correct

onto the transducer, which are different according to the angle to be obtained, or with the possibility of varying the angle itself. The diameter of the canal of the device depends on the diameter of the needle to be used. The needle is therefore attached to the transducer, thus requiring a correspondence between the predisposed electronic trace on the monitor and the needle track, which is inevitably oblique to be able to enter into the field of view. The US system in fact makes it possible to select a trajectory angle corresponding to the chosen adaptor, and one or more dotted lines appear on the monitor indicating the exact path the needle will follow. These dedicated devices are especially used for deep structures as they increase the precision of the biopsy and reduce the problem of deviation of the needle along its track, even though at the same time they reduce the possibility of correcting the trajectory of the needle itself (although the needle can be removed and repositioned at a different angle). In addition they do not allow the needle to be followed in the first few centimeters of its progression or to puncture particularly superficial structures (Fig. 7.2). Given the greater obliqueness with respect to the tangential approach, this system also requires longer needles. An alternative US-guided technique is to use special transducers which are dedicated to the interventional procedure being performed and have a central hole and an eccentric canal for the passage of the needle. The transducer-needle system, which is rather cumbersome and poorly adapted to the curved regions of the skin surface, is therefore coaxial and very precise with respect to even small and deep targets and with little likelihood that the system suffers deviations. However, at least some of the models of transducers do not allow inclination of the needle with respect to the ultrasound beam to be adjusted, which can be a hindrance when certain anatomic structures need to be avoided [14]. Experimentally, a slight distortion of the image has been encountered with the dedicated abdominal transducers, which the operator should bear in mind during procedures of diagnostic or therapeutic targeting of lesions. A positioning error linked to the geometry of the transducer from –10.9 to 3.8 mm was encountered with the dedicated transducers and a shift from –11.3 to 3.8 mm with the systems with lateral attachment. As a result, when dedicated transducers are used for liver puncture in general, the use of a transducer with a larger radius through the center hole is recommended with the puncture angle as obtuse as possible, whereas for lesions of the hepatic dome the use of more tightly curved transducers with a more acute angle is advisable [15].

The **needles** are used for diagnostic sampling, therapeutic aspiration of fluids and injection of therapeutic substances. The needles may be generically classified according to size (fine and large), tip configuration (aspiration and cutting/core biopsy), and sampling mechanism (manual, semiautomated and automated). With regard to the diameter (external diameter), the needles are distinguished in fine if <1 mm (20 G or above) and large if >1 mm (21 G and below). In general, fine aspiration needles are used for cytologic sampling and larger-gauge aspiration needles are used for drainage of fluid collections and cutting for biopsy. There is a clear correlation between needle diameter and diagnostic accuracy, but also

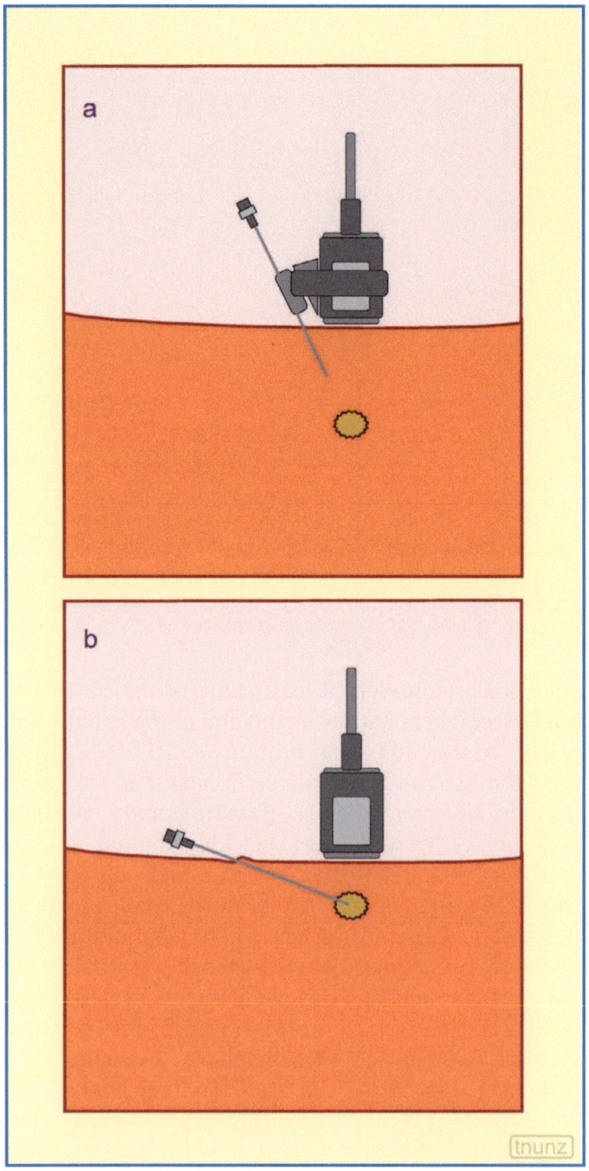

Fig. 7.2a,b US-guided percutaneous procedure. The needle is attached to the transducer with a dedicated device (a). The puncture of a particularly superficial target (b) can, however, be better performed by detaching the needle

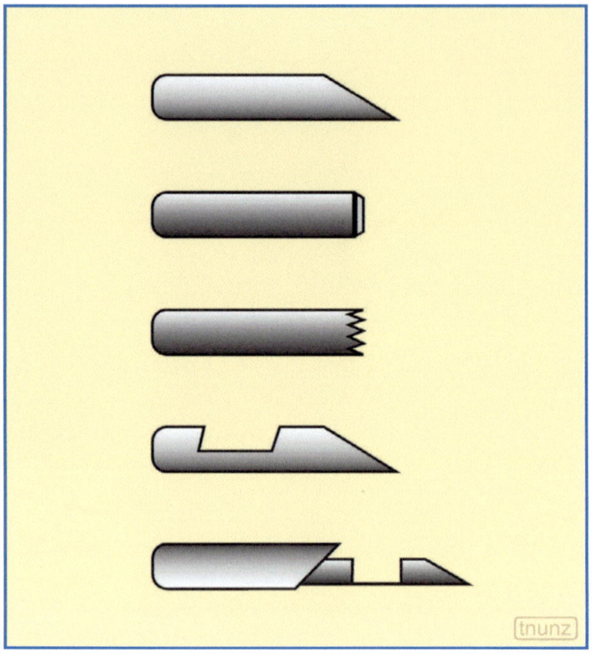

Fig. 7.3 Cutting needles. Different conformations of cutting needle tips, with apical or lateral cutting surfaces

between needle diameter and complications. The choice depends on many factors, such as the indication for sampling or puncture, the type of material expected, the experience and confidence of the operator, the preference of the pathologist, the degree of patient compliance and the presence of risk factors (e.g. bleeding diathesis). **Aspiration needles** have a tip that is beveled at different angles in different models but generally from 25 to 30°, which operates not so much by cutting the tissue but rather by shearing it. Examples include Chiba and spinal needles. **Cutting needles** operate with a cutting mechanism and are equipped with a stylet, which may or may not be removable, a conical, trocar or bevel tip with an angle varying from 45° to 90° which allows it to penetrate into the tissues, possibly with a screw-tip mechanism (Fig. 7.3). Smaller-gauge cutting needles (18–22 G) have a removable stylet and a syringe for aspiration of the material. Examples include Greene, Franseen, Otto, Madayag, Surecut and modified Menghini. The stylet may also reach the plunger of the syringe, as in the modified Menghini needle, so that the core remains in the syringe and does not fragment (Fig. 7.4). Large-gauge cutting needles such as TruCut, Lee, Wescott and Menghini (14–19 G) have the same conformation as the smaller-gauge needles or have a guillotine-like mechanism with which an outer cannula cuts the tissue trapped in the notch on the stylet (Fig. 7.5). There are also cutting needles connected to automated devices like the biopsy pistol, which is equipped with a spring-firing mechanism enabling the needle to fire and rapidly penetrate the tissue. The **pistol systems** make possible the simple and rapid performance of sampling and obtain a significant quantity of tissue, also less degraded by fragmentation than with conventional needles. In this case, the tip of the cannula is advanced to the superficial margin of the target and then the needle is made to "fire" within (Fig. 7.6). The choice of the diameter of trocar needles depends on the disease being evaluated and

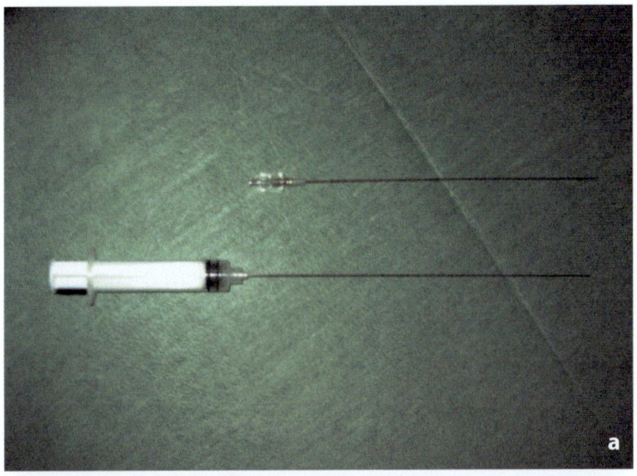

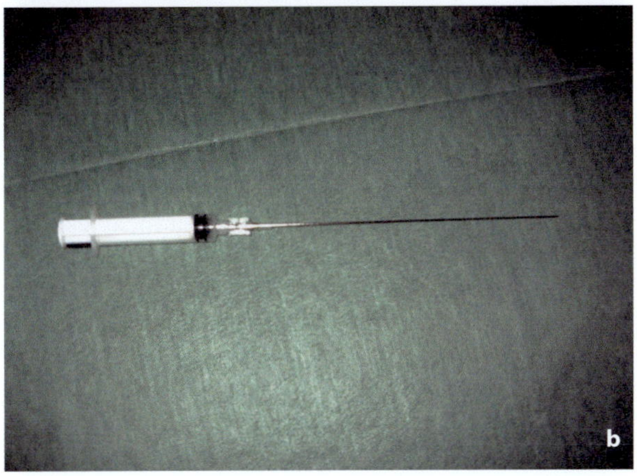

Fig. 7.4a,b Biopsy needle. System with premounted syringe and 20-cm-long 17 G needle. Image with needle separate from the stylet (**a**) and with needle mounted (**b**)

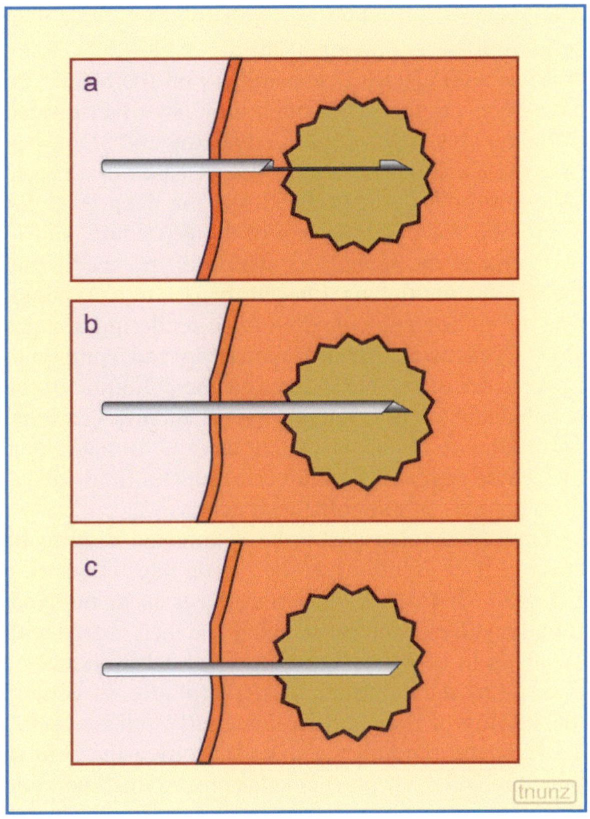

Fig. 7.5a-c Cutting needle, sampling mechanism. With a guillotine-like system the tip of the needle is placed on the surface of the target (**a**) and then plunged into the lesion, removing a tissue core and then aspirating it (**b**,**c**)

therefore on the quantity of material required by the pathologist [14].

The presence of the needle within the area to be sampled should be constantly verified by exploiting the real-time characteristic of the technique. In general, if the transducer-needle alignment is correct, the US visualization of the needle is good even though not comparable to CT or radioscopy. The possible obliqueness of the needle-ultrasound beam incidence can be verified by observing the orientation of the part of the needle that is still external to the patient, with respect to the transducer. If the needle tip cannot be seen, even after varying the position of the transducer, a number of expedients may be resorted to: multiple passes can be done in order to visualize it, or backwards and forwards movements with the stylet while leaving the needle in place, or alternatively small quantities of air or saline solution can be introduced in order to generate echoes [14]. In addition, the dedicated needles usually have polymer coatings or dimples on the distal surface which increase the

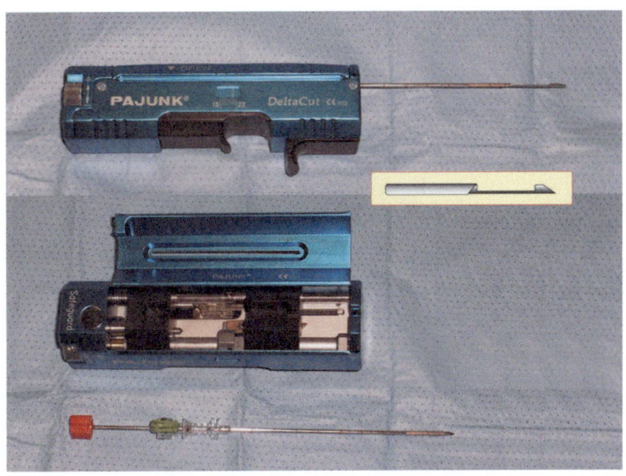

Fig. 7.6 Automated pistol. Multiuse pistol system with dedicated 14 G cutting needle. The device is illustrated assembled with and without the needle, and the internal mechanism is visible. The inset shows the conformation of the cutting tip

echogenicity and which prove particularly useful in conditions of a suboptimal needle angle (20°). Even systems with electrical transmitters on the needle tip have been proposed, although they have had limited diffusion [16]. The use of 3D modality and 3D in real time (4D) can be useful (in 34% of cases in a recent series) at both the superficial and the deep level for improving the US definition of the procedure, and in particular of the spatial orientation of the needle and the lesion – multiplanar images are used or a combination of tomographic and volume-rendering images [17]. Even tissue harmonic imaging and compound imaging are often able to improve the definition of the needle, and in general are useful in interventional procedures to the superficial structures. In particular, the needle positioned within effusion and fluid collections appears as a double linear echo.

Transducers that cannot be disinfected need to be covered by a sheath or sterile plastic bags containing US gel. Alternatively the transducer is disinfected, usually with mechanical cleaning and then treated with aldehyde in solution. The transducer cable should be covered by a long sheath of sterile plastic. In general the sterility of field and the materials used is crucial. To facilitate running the transducer over the skin in puncture and other percutaneous procedures, the same liquid disinfectant can be used or a specific sterile gel, which although more expensive improves visualization. All of the diagnostic and therapeutic techniques described below require informed consent, as well as an adequate patient history to evaluate the specific risks of the procedure and possible allergies to the materials used.

7.2 Needle Aspiration – Superficial Structures

Fine needle aspiration cytology (**FNAC**) involves the sampling of material with a fine needle (maximum 20 G, i.e. with external diameter <1 mm) for the purposes of cytologic evaluation (therefore, the term fine needle aspiration biopsy and correlated abbreviation FNAB, although widely used in practice, should be avoided), as well as cytochemical and immunocytochemical evaluation. Malignant tumors, especially those with a limited stromal component, are particularly rich in cellular material and therefore the analysis of these cells is generally sufficient for reaching a diagnosis of their nature. In general, FNAC is also enough for a diagnosis of tumor recurrence or metastasis from a known primary tumor [18].

Local anesthesia is generally not used, and only disinfection of the skin is performed (possibly with chlorhexidine and ethanol) [18]. By applying compression with the transducer the distance between the skin and the target can be reduced and therefore the distance the needle needs to travel.

Sampling can be performed using the needle alone – a simple syringe needle for sampling with a diameter varying from 21 to 27 G (generally 21–23 G). In general, the greater the diameter, the greater the amount of cellular material sampled, but the greater the amount of blood in the sample may be. The sampling technique can exploit the passive diffusion of the material within the needle lumen (capillarity), possibly accompanied by multiple and rapid to-and-fro movements at various angles (multidirectional technique) together with simultaneous rotational movements. The aim is to sample all the areas of the lesion, which can have a variable distribution of tumor cells or tumor cells with varying grades of dedifferentiation. The accuracy of the sample is notably influenced by the number and breadth of the needle passes. Moreover, it seems perfectly clear that US guidance also allows the most suspicious part of a focal lesion, a pathologic area or a lymph node, to be targeted. Alternatively, active aspiration can be done with a syringe connected to the needle, with the needle motionless or undergoing small jiggling movements, and then delicately interrupting the suction and withdrawing the needle. The needle is not withdrawn in aspiration, to avoid the sampling of contaminating material along the needle track and to avoid damaging the quality of the material sampled with excessive suction (Fig. 7.7). Some operators only rely on active aspiration when with capillarity no material is seen entering the transparent portion of the syringe. Systems of remote aspiration may also be used, with dedicated syringes or pumps. In general, however, the systems of forced aspiration can increase the quantity of material sampled but may also damage the quality of the cells and increase the blood component [14].

Maintaining the needle overly long in the tissue is not recommended, especially in highly vascular lesions or organs, since this significantly increases the blood component in the sample with the risk of the blood, over time, coagulating. In larger, both superficial and deep masses, taking the samples from a peripheral location is advisable, because the presence of central necrosis can reduce the cellularity of the material sampled. CD can be useful in these cases, by not only offering a vascular map of the tissues to be transited and therefore enabling improved detection of the important vessels adjacent to the lesion, but also enabling the sampling procedure to be directed towards the more vascular regions and therefore, presumably, those that are richer with material useful for diagnostic purposes. The same also holds for biopsies.

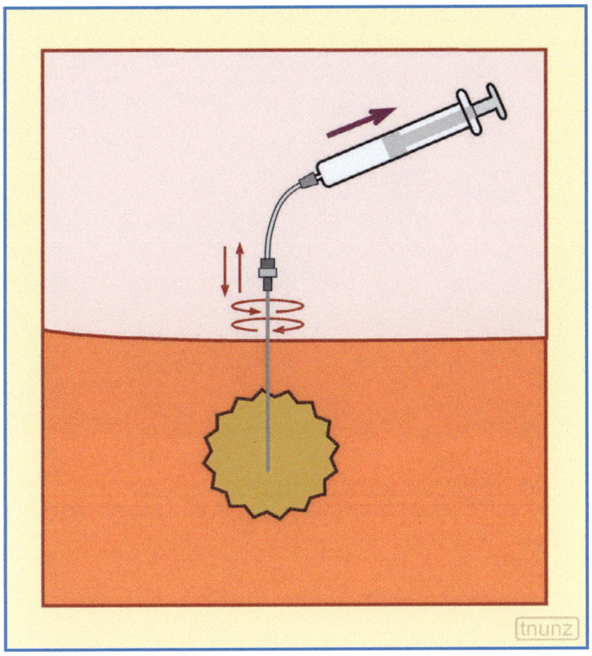

Fig. 7.7 Needle aspiration. Suction with the plunger of the syringe associated with rotation and multiple passes of the needle

A correct **preparation** of slides is vital. The pathologist should have available all the information regarding the clinical history of the patient in order to be able to use special stains or cytochemical analyses if required. The preparation of the needle aspiration involves immediately depositing the material onto clean glass slides possibly treated with cleaning solution, through the aspiration of a small quantity of air with a syringe which is then attached to the needle and used to expel the material from the needle, which is almost placed in contact with the slide. The needle holder can be tapped against a slide to obtain all the residual material, or the stylet can be inserted into the needle lumen or another smaller gauge needle, or some heparinized saline solution can be used. The material is then immediately smeared in a delicate but precise and uniform manner with the use of another slide held at an angle of around 10° with respect to the former upon which the material was placed. In general, the slide is left to air dry (or is fixed with methanol) for May–Grünwald–Giemsa staining (partly substituted by Diff–Quick) or, especially when immunohistochemical evaluations are required, it can be fixed immediately with immersion in 95% ethanol (10–15 min in appropriate closed containers) or with spray for Papanicolaou staining or special staining. Sprays can cause a nonuniform fixation with the creation of possible artifacts and therefore are not recommended by pathologists [18]. When the sampled material is particularly abundant, prior to smearing on the slide the most consistent part can be embedded in paraffin (cell block) and then cut with the microtome. This system is able to obtain information relating to the tissue on the basis of the agglomeration of the cells with poor stromal content obtained. In the case of prevalently liquid material, this is placed in the form of drops on the slide and then smeared, while the residual fluid in placed in a test-tube containing a prefixative (50% methanol), and immediately sent to the laboratory where it is centrifuged and the resulting sediment analyzed. In the case of a microhistologic sample obtained with a cutting needle, the tissue core is fixed with 10% formalin for a maximum time of 4 h and then dehydrated and embedded in paraffin.

During slide preparation a number of problems may arise. An excessive blood component can dilute the cellularity, rendering the cytologic material insufficient for diagnostic purposes. In addition, the material should not be contaminated by US gel or skin disinfectant liquid as this can cause deterioration of the cells [18]. There are also a number of artifacts related to an incorrect smear procedure. The adequacy of the sample, i.e. the presence in the material of cells to be analyzed, should be confirmed immediately with a rapid stain. Should the cytopathologist declare the sample inadequate, a repeat aspiration should be performed. The presence of the cytologist is therefore very important, reducing the number of inadequate samples and increasing the specificity and accuracy of the technique. In the absence of a pathologist it may be preferable to perform multiple FNAC or utilize core biopsy to guarantee the sampling of a sufficient quantity of material.

The **diagnostic classes** are standardized particularly for the breast: C1, inadequate or unsatisfactory smear; C2, benign cells present; C3, mild atypia within some cells but probably benign; C4, suspicious of malignancy, with indication for work-up; C5, malignant cells present (cells unequivocally malignant, possibly identifiable at low-power microscopy).

FNAC is encumbered by a moderate rate of inadequate findings, in which the material is unsatisfactory for reaching a diagnostic result. It should also be recalled that FNAC is encumbered by a certain percentage of false positives and especially false negatives, such that a positive result is highly convincing in affirming the malignancy of a lesion, whereas the same cannot be said for a negative result. **Complications** of the procedure are very limited. Hematomas may occur, especially in subjects with clotting disorders, or infections. Cases of needle-track seeding are rare.

FNAC of the **breast** has a sensitivity of 83–98%, with a specificity of 93–97%. The percentage of inadequate results varies from 5% to 40% in different centers, but it is less than 10% in the presence of cancer. False negatives, in subcentimeter lesions, vary from 2% to 36%. The predictivity of class C5 for carcinoma is >99%, but false positives can reach 6% and are essentially due to atypical proliferative lesions. A benign appearance of a solid breast nodule at combined US, mammography and FNAC evaluation virtually excludes malignancy [19]. The diagnosis of benign lesions is more difficult and in particular the identification of phyllodes tumor is often incorrect. FNAC has proven to be useful in verifying the state of the axillary lymph nodes both during staging of breast cancer when the axillary US finding is indeterminate and during neoadjuvant treatment for LABC [20]. A positive FNAC of an axillary lymph node identified as suspicious at US can avoid the need for the sentinel lymph node procedure. The complications include pain, hematomas, infection, pneumothorax (deep lesions or lesions in operated patients). Seeding is rare, exceptional with thin needles.

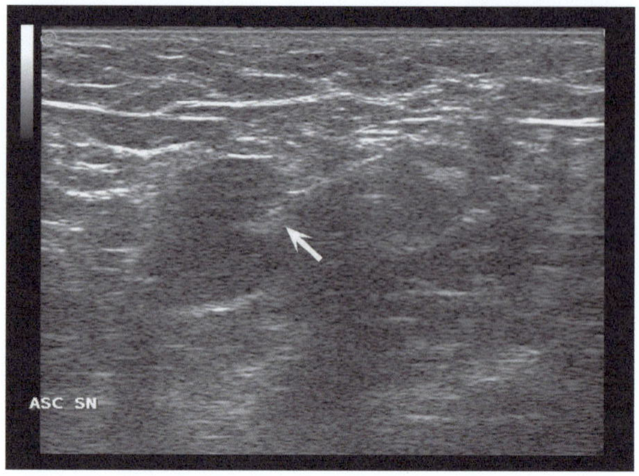

Fig. 7.8 Needle aspiration, axillary lymph node metastasis from melanoma. The needle tip can be seen in the lymph node cortex (*arrow*)

FNAC is practically an integral part of the US approach to the **thyroid** nodule. The procedure is economical, widespread, easy to perform and substantially without complications (pain and small hematomas). Cases of tumor seeding after FNAC are rare. Although it is possible to puncture even very small lesions, thyroid FNAC is used particularly for hypoechoic nodules >10 mm, or nodules which for one reason or another cannot definitely be considered benign (and which are not "hot" at scintigraphy). Nodules <10 mm are aspirated, especially if cervical lymphadenopathies of unknown origin are present, in the case of multiple lesions for planning the extent of surgical resection, and in the event the analysis of a surgical specimen from a partial thyroid resection has shown a tumor. Palpable nodules can even be punctured with the freehand technique, but US guidance is recommended for poorly palpable or non-palpable nodules, small nodules or nodules which have already been punctured without US guidance with unsatisfying results [21]. The procedure uses 22–25 G fine aspiration needles. Sensitivity ranges from 65% to 98% and specificity from 72% to 100% [22]. The rate of inadequate sampling is significant, reaching as high as 34% [18]. The preoperative predictive accuracy is above 90%, although this clearly depends on the experience of the physician who gathers the sample and the cytologist who examines it [23]. In general, FNAC is unable to differentiate adenoma from follicular carcinoma. False positives are reported in 0–7% of cases. False negatives are more frequent (0.5–12% of cases) and can be reduced with a careful needle-aspiration technique, meticulous follow-up and series FNAC. If the sonographer observes a nodule with suspicious characteristics in a patient with a prior negative FNAC, a request to repeat the sample seems appropriate [21,23].

The **parathyroid glands** are aspirated with 21 or 22 G needles, especially in cases where there is doubt between an exophytic thyroid nodule and a parathyroid nodule or in the case of primary or secondary hyperparathyroidism. Limited hematomas may occur. In patients undergoing hemodialysis, the puncture is best not performed on the same day as the dialysis session since this would require anticoagulant therapy.

FNAC of the **superficial lymph nodes** is accurate in the diagnosis of metastases, whereas it is not sufficient for lymphomas (Fig. 7.8). US and CD guidance can orient the procedure towards the most suspicious lymph nodes or towards the most suspicious portion of atypical lymph nodes. The main limitations are small lymph nodes and lymph nodes immediately adjacent to large vessels. A sensitivity of 89–98% and specificity of 95–98% have been reported for cervical lymph nodes [24].

In the suspicion of a malignant tumor of the **soft tissues** a core biopsy is required (e.g. 20 G needle), whereas for the diagnosis of postoperative recurrence FNAC is generally sufficient (18–25 G needles) [25]. In sarcomas the cellularity is lower than in carcinomas and therefore correct preparation of the material becomes even more important [18].

FNAC of **bone** lesions with suspicion for metastasis is usually performed with US guidance, especially at the level of the thoracic cage and pelvis. The technique has proven to be effective when the accessibility of the lesions is adequate, with a sensitivity of 93% [26].

7.3 Needle Aspiration – Internal Structures

FNAC of thoracic or abdominal organs is usually performed as an outpatient procedure. The site of access is first established, then it is sterilized and local anesthesia is performed in cases where the approach is intercostal or the subject is particularly anxious and in children. The need for long needles to reach deep lesions means that simple syringe needles cannot be used. In these cases dedicated needles are required which cannot be excessively fine, otherwise they would deviate along their track. Generally 20–23 G Chiba stylet needles are used.

Safety parameters for the procedure generally include a platelet count >40,000/mm^3 (>50,000 in the case of HCC or chronic liver disease), a PT >40–50%, a PTT <45 s, a PT ratio <1.7 (<1.6 in the case of HCC on chronic liver disease) and a time to bleeding <10 min [27,28]. However, in patients in good general conditions these laboratory evaluations are not always required, since the probability of bleeding is quite low. A case of a particularly low platelet count or a state of clotting deficiency can be corrected before the procedure with platelet transfusion or fresh frozen plasma. Antiplatelet therapy is often interrupted 2–5 days prior to the procedure, although in subjects without other risk factors it may even not be interrupted [29]. Antibiotic therapy is only used in immunodepressed subjects or when there is a high probability of transiting a septic field, e.g. in transcolonic procedures. In the presence of marked ascites pre-biopsy paracentesis may be appropriate [27]. The puncture of a functioning adrenal lesion requires specific premedication [14]. The risk of anaphylaxis in the case of a hydatid cyst usually contraindicates the procedure, unless it is performed for therapeutic purposes. It is always correct to have a peripheral venous access available, especially for biopsies but also for FNAC. In anxious patients sedation can be administered, although in especially agitated patients, or the absence of a sufficiently safe access, the procedure should not be performed. Fasting prior to the procedure is not necessary. For lesions adjacent to the gallbladder, inducing contraction of the organ with a fatty meal may be advisable.

The tip of the needle is directed under US guidance. Subsequently the stylet is removed and the sample is taken, which may be done with the capillarity technique or with aspiration, the latter being performed manually or with dedicated pistol systems. In general, however, excessive active aspiration tends to be avoided in favor of multiple intralesional passes of the needle to obtain abundant material with a low blood component.

Strictly speaking, performing a control 30–60 min after the procedure is advisable to rule out a hemoperitoneum. For patients with a clotting disorder an overnight stay in hospital may be preferable, with discharge the morning after [29].

Major **complications** of deep FNAC are rare but possible events. In large patient populations with abdominal procedures, severe complications have been registered in 0.04–0.05% of cases and death in 0.004–0.008%. The risk of hemorrhage increases in the presence of a clotting disorder, highly vascular tumor (HCC, hemangioma, angiosarcoma), highly vascular organ (spleen), superficial lesion, particular extension of the disease, very tangential course of the needle with respect to the organ capsule, use of large-gauge needles (see core biopsy) and repeated passes. Tumor seeding is very rare: for HCC it ranges between 0.6% and 5.1% [27].

Imaging-guided FNAC has proven effective and minimally invasive in the diagnosis of thoraco-abdominal masses, being diagnostic in 93% of cases, with an accuracy of 100% in the benign-malignant distinction, 54% in the characterization of benign lesions and 64% in the characterization of malignant lesions [30]. The pre-FNAC clinical-radiologic diagnosis has been shown to be correct in 80% of malignant lesions. The major limitations include small lesions, sites that are particularly difficult to access and lymphomatous lesions (which require biopsy).

When anatomically possible, the approach to **hepatic** lesions is best when the needle passes through a certain amount of healthy parenchyma, especially in the case of hemangiomas, HCC or hypervascular metastases, with the aim of avoiding possible post-procedural bleeding directly into the peritoneal cavity. In the presence of multifocal lesions, the most appropriate choice for FNAC is a deep lesion, and not necessarily the largest lesion, rather than a subcapsular lesion (Video 7.2). A diagnostic algorithm for FNAC has recently been developed. FNAC is performed first, and the on-site pathologist makes a preliminary diagnosis. When a malignant lesion is diagnosed, immediate subtyping is attempted and core biopsy is mainly obtained when FNAC subtyping is still undefined or when FNAC is negative but the clinical suspicion for malignancy remains [31].

Lesions of the **pancreas** are generally reached with a direct anterior approach, since passing through the liver, stomach or colon does not generally create problems. Nonetheless, CT guidance is often preferred, especially due to the difficulty with US in avoiding the peripancreatic vascular structures. The sensitivity of FNAC for the diagnosis of pancreatic cancer is 67–90% and false negatives are often due to an occasionally intense desmoplastic and inflammatory reaction in these tumors [14]. The rate of inadequate procedures is considerable, and notably higher than in other abdominal organs [18]. Complications are not frequent (<3%) and include acute pancreatitis, septicemia and, in rare cases, seeding. Due to the latter event, FNAC tends to be avoided in patients who are potential candidates for surgical resection.

Puncture of the **spleen** was in the past considered ill-advised due to the hypervascularity of the organ and the thinness of its capsule. However, puncture can be safely practiced with the use of a fine needle (usually 22–25 G). US guidance is preferable with lateral access and the patient in the right lateral or supine position. The main indication is a dubious lesion in the subject with an extrasplenic tumor, and the main complication is hemoperitoneum.

The abdominal **lymph nodes** are aspirated especially in the suspicion of metastasis, even postoperative, in patients with gastrointestinal, urologic or gynecologic tumors. The diagnosis of lymphoma in subjects without available superficial metastases nonetheless requires core biopsy, since FNAC is insufficient.

The **adrenal glands** are generally punctured under CT guidance, especially in the case of small lesions. A direct posterior approach may be adopted through the paraspinal muscles and the perirenal fat, although with an inclined trajectory, especially on the left to avoid the posterior costophrenic sinus. Alternatively, a lateral approach may be used on either the right or the left, or even a transhepatic approach for the right adrenal gland. The main indication is in cases of dubious differential diagnosis between benign and metastatic lesions in subjects with an extra-adrenal lesion or in the case of an incidental finding of an adrenal lesion with a dubious appearance. The positive and negative predictive value for the diagnosis of malignancy is 100% and 92%, respectively. It should, however, be borne in mind that the diagnosis of adenoma or hyperplasia is challenging with FNAC alone. The complications of the procedure can reach 13% of cases and include hemorrhage, pneumothorax and hypertensive crisis [32].

Renal lesions are generally not biopsied since they can usually be adequately characterized with imaging and lesions that are not clearly benign require surgical excision in any case. Nonetheless a sample may be indicated in special circumstances – in the case of differential diagnostic doubt (e.g. focal inflammation and angiomyolipoma), for the confirmation of an RCC in a high surgery risk patient, in the subject with metastatic RCC to confirm the primary nature of the lesion or in the suspicion of metastasis (e.g. differential diagnosis between metastasis and second tumor in a subject with extrarenal neoplasm), and in the suspicion of a lymphoma (although in this case histologic biopsy is preferable) [33]. The procedure is done with the patient in the prone or opposite lateral position, also on the basis of the position of the lesion to be reached. Hypervascular lesions should be punctured with caution. Complications range from 0% to 12% of cases and include hematuria (3–12%), intrarenal, subcapsular or perirenal hematoma, arteriovenous fistula and seeding (Video 7.3).

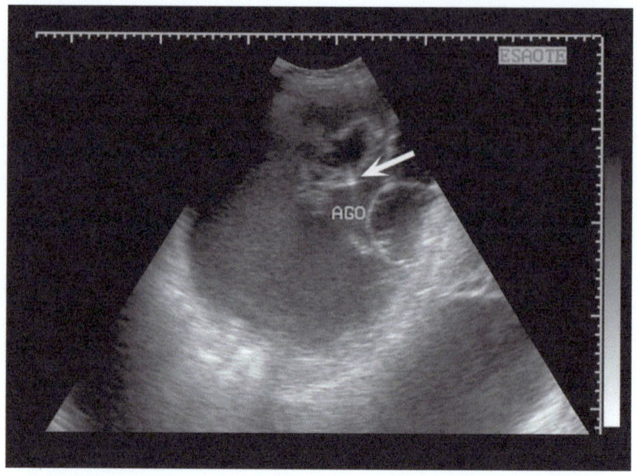

Fig. 7.9 Biopsy of adnexal mass. Visualization of the needle tip (*arrow*) within the complex, prevalently fluid mass

In primary and secondary **bowel** lesions, FNAC is generally performed with 22 G Chiba needles with a length of 11–15 cm. Multiple passes are performed with the needle directed according to a plane tangential to the intestinal wall so as to obtain an abundant sample but at the same time without violating the integrity of the mucosa, with the consequent risks of complications and tumor seeding [34]. If the FNAC sample is insufficient, 1–2 core biopsies are performed with 18 G needles.

The **uterus** and **adnexa** can be punctured with a suprapubic approach (possibly also transvesical), transvaginal or transrectal, with 20–22 G needles. The indication is pelvic masses of uncertain nature or origin, suspicion of an ovarian origin of a peritoneal carcinosis, suspicion of ovarian metastasis (e.g. from stomach cancer) or suspicion of postoperative recurrence of a gynecologic tumor (Fig. 7.9).

Pelvic and **retroperitoneal** lesions can be reached, according to the cases, with both an anterior and posterior approach. Pelvic lesions can be reached through the ischial foramen and in particular its inferomedial portion, immediately lateral to the wing of sacrum. Deep pelvic lesions can benefit from a US-guided low lateral approach through the psoas muscle, or transrectal or transvaginal. Thoracic masses can generally be reached with an intercostal approach, with the choice of the most appropriate patient position (Video 7.4).

7.4 Core Biopsy – Superficial Structures

True **biopsy** involves the acquisition of a greater quantity of tissue with respect to fine needle aspiration and therefore enables a microhistologic rather than cytologic analysis of the material itself, with the possibility of obtaining information on the invasiveness and grade of the tumor as well as defining certain biologic, histochemical and immunohistochemical parameters (Fig. 7.10). Whereas FNAC has the fundamental aim of distinguishing between benignity and malignancy, biopsy can be used in various conditions. These include characterizing a lesion which has not been sufficiently defined with imaging, evaluating the grade, the histologic type or the biologic characteristics of a frankly neoplastic lesion for the purposes of treatment planning, evaluating a particularly suspicious lesion in a cancer patient (e.g. differential diagnosis between metastasis and second tumor) and evaluating the tumor component after treatment (neoplastic residual, recurrence, etc.).

With respect to FNAC, the use of larger-gauge needles reduces the risk of an inadequate sample (5% of cases in a large multiorgan series vs. 29% of FNAC), provided that an adequate number of samples is taken, but does involve increased invasiveness and complications [18]. While it is true that biopsy tends to be more expensive than US-guided FNAC, it is also true that this trend can be reversed if the number of inadequate FNACs is high and therefore a significant number of patients needs to subsequently undergo US-guided core biopsy (which instead is only rarely inadequate, e.g. 1% of breast biopsies). Another advantage of biopsy over FNAC is the possibility of producing material that is useful for more advanced evaluation than the simple but fundamental benign-malignant distinction. The experience of the operator is extremely important, even more so than for FNAC: the rate of inadequate samples among nonexpert operators is twice that of the operator with consolidated experience [18].

With regard to the more-or-less large gauge of the needle, local anesthesia may be required prior to the procedure, together with a skin incision to facilitate the penetration of the cutting needle (especially if large gauge). After the sample has been taken, manual compression or dry ice should be applied to the skin. Some authors prefer to use intravenous sedation [33].

Fine 21 G needles may be used for the procedure, or larger-bore 18 G or even up to 14 G cutting needles [35]. The tip of the needle is positioned on the anterior margin of the lesions. Then, in the manual system the stylet is partially withdrawn and the needle is pushed forward and backward twice into the lesion and then withdrawn after a rotational movement (to avoid deep anchorage of the core). With special regard to the breast, cutting needles (14–20 G) with automatic or semiautomatic systems are used [10]. The number of samples taken varies from center to center, but is generally at least 3 (usually 4–5, on the basis of the size of the lesion, which if small requires a greater number of samples to avoid inadequacy). This number is considered necessary to maximize the diagnostic accuracy of the procedure. There are even systems with **coaxial needles** – used less – whereby an external larger-gauge cannula needle is positioned and left in place while multiple samples are taken with the internal smaller needle. This can theoretically reduce the risks associated with multiple biopsies, with repeated needle passes, with regard to both the mechanical complications and the risk of tumor seeding [33]. Alternatively the tandem technique can be used, whereby an initial needle is inserted and left in place during subsequent repeated biopsies, thus acting as a guide for introduction of the necessary needles.

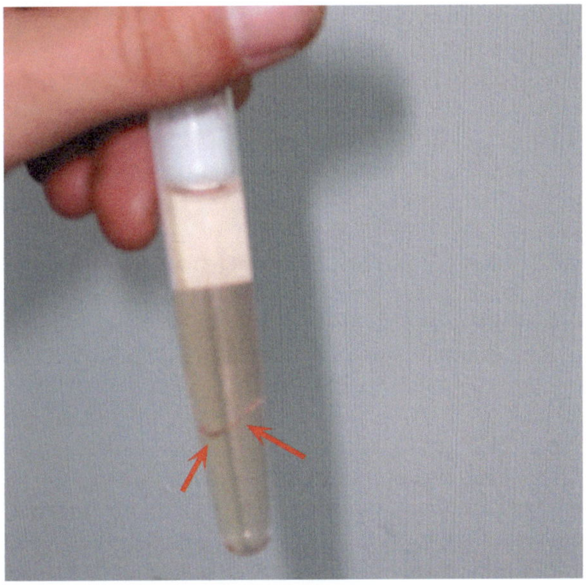

Fig. 7.10 Tissue core for microhistology. The material sampled with the cutting needle (*arrows*) can be seen within the test-tube

The material is generally fixed in 10% formalin, which is compatible with most routine and special stains, even though it is not always optimal for immunohistochemical analysis [18]. Other fixatives used by the pathologist include Carnoy's solution (acetic acid and chloroform), B5 (formalin and mercuric chloride) and Bouin's fixative (acetic acid and picric acid). If the material is particularly abundant, a part of it can be wrapped in aluminum paper and frozen by rapid immersion in liquid nitrogen and kept for possible further evaluations, e.g. histochemical or molecular biology analyses.

Core biopsy has demonstrated elevated accuracy similar to that of surgical biopsy, although less invasive and less expensive. In one series, 14 G core needle biopsy results were concordant with surgical excision findings in 96% of 975 nonpalpable lesions and all false negatives were prospectively identified because of the discordance between imaging results and histologic findings [36]. Repetition of the sampling or performance of surgical biopsy is in fact recommended in cases of disagreement between imaging and histologic findings. In addition, follow-up of negative cases at core biopsy is required in order to identify possible false negatives (3.7% of cases in the breast) [10]. With respect to FNAC, core biopsy is especially useful for the precise pathologic definition of benign lesions, for diagnosing certain histotypes and for attempting to distinguish between precancerous and atypical lesions and carcinoma. The main indications are the inadequacy of a prior FNAC, a discrepancy between clinical, radiologic or cytologic findings, and the need for more detailed histologic and biologic information for the correct therapeutic management of the patient. It should nonetheless be noted that with respect to the definitive histologic findings, biopsy can underestimate the degree of malignancy and invasiveness of the tumor.

Several **diagnostic classes** can be identified: B1, normal tissue (possibly due to incorrect sampling); B2, benign lesion, B3, lesion with uncertain malignant potential; B4, suspicious lesion; B5, malignant lesion. A biopsy procedure can in fact be nondiagnostic for a variety of reasons. These include acellularity, unsatisfactory material, an atypical but not definitive finding or a finding suspicious for a certain lesion but not conclusive.

Biopsy in the **breast** is used especially when FNAC of a nodule is inadequate or discordant with the clinical or mammographic and US findings, as well as in the precise characterization of fibroadenomas and possibly high-risk atypical proliferative lesions (atypical lobular hyperplasia, lobular carcinoma in situ and papillary lesions). It should nonetheless be noted that biopsy may be of little help in some differential diagnoses, such as between fibroadenoma and benign phyllodes tumor [37]. The correspondence between core biopsy and the histopathologic evaluation of the entire surgical specimen is 95% in invasive carcinomas and 71% of those in situ, with overall sensitivity of 96% and specificity of 93%. This renders extemporaneous biopsy useless in positive cases, unless there is disagreement between the core biopsy finding and the imaging data. However, surgical biopsy is still indicated in the event of radiologic suspicion but core biopsy negative for malignancy [38]. In patients with carcinoma, a false-negative result may depend on failure to recognize the lesion at US, technical or sampling errors (dense and fibrotic breast, deep or poorly defined nodule, needle or lesions poorly identified, etc.), US-histology disagreement (the histologic finding appears relatively incompatible with the US finding and should therefore induce the repetition of the sampling), absent imaging-histologic correlation or absent follow-up after a negative histologic finding [35,39]. In the case of particularly deep lesions or lesions adjacent to the thoracic wall, pistol systems with large-gauge needles (e.g. 14 G) can be used to reach the surface of the lesion with the tip of the cannula, to slightly raise it by inclining the portion of the cannula external to the patient, and lastly to fire the needle into the target. This makes a vertical approach possible even for very deep lesions, which in some cases would require an approach parallel to the thoracic wall but with a particularly long needle track. Radiography of the sampled material may be advisable to document the presence of microcalcifications. Another possible indication as an alternative to FNAC is the sampling of suspicious axillary lymph nodes with the aim of avoiding the intraoperative sentinel lymph node procedure. More invasive alternatives to breast core biopsy are vacuum-assisted biopsy and large-core biopsy. The latter technique uses a pistol-like device with an internal circular blade to perform excision biopsy of the nonpalpable breast lesion in a single pass under stereotactic mammographic guidance. Small breast lesions can in this way be entirely removed intact, and possibly with the addition of a surrounding disease-free margin.

Biopsy can be useful for **lymph node** metastases of various origins especially when guided by US and CD towards the most suspicious nodes or towards the most suspicious portion of the nodes, while bearing in mind the difficulties in the case of small or necrotic lymph nodes. A core biopsy with a 16–18 G needle can sample sufficient material for an evaluation of the lymphomatous disease and thus avoid excision biopsy [24].

Core biopsy is very rare in the **thyroid**, with repeat FNAC being preferable, although sometimes core biopsy is needed to characterize primary lymphomas [40]. Biopsy may, however, be advantageously used for superficial lymph nodes, both in patients with carcinoma in the afferent lymph node group and in patients with lymphoma. The procedure generally uses 14–16 G cutting needles [41].

Lesions of the **salivary glands** are generally punctured with 18–20 G needles, possibly with pistol systems, using on average two passes per patient [42]. In the benign-malignant distinction, core biopsy has demonstrated an accuracy of 97–100%, with advantages over FNAC in terms of the diagnosis and grading

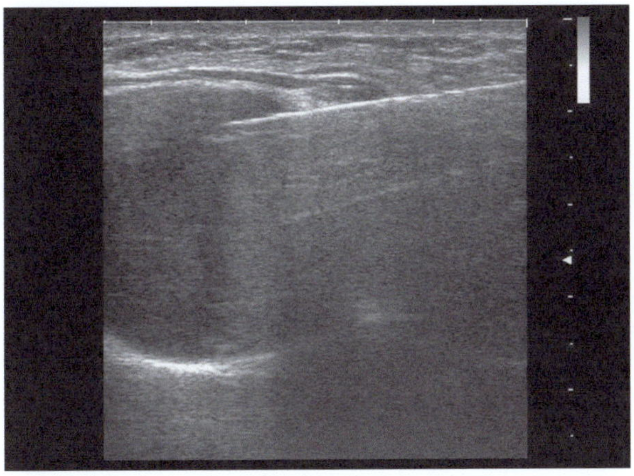

Fig. 7.11 Biopsy of liposarcoma of the thoracic wall. The cutting needle can be seen inside the hypoechoic mass

of lymphomas and carcinomas and in terms of the differentiation between lymph node hyperplasia and lymphoma itself. Complications are rare.

With regard to **soft tissue** tumors, large-gauge needles are generally preferred (14–18 G) for use especially with pistol systems, because the characterization of sarcomas may require large quantities of tissue (Fig. 7.11). The diagnosis of recurrence of soft-tissue tumors, however, can be done with FNAC [43]. The risk of seeding and postoperative recurrence can be minimized by performing the biopsy in the point where the surgeon will make the surgical incision for excision, or at least the procedure should involve only one pathologic muscular compartment, without passing through others. CT- or US-guided biopsy has also proven useful in the distinction between subtypes of liposarcoma, and in particular in the identification of nondifferentiated foci in the context of the mass, a characteristic which can influence prognosis and treatment management [44].

7.5 Core Biopsy – Internal Structures

Microhistologic **biopsy** is usually performed at the abdominal level with cutting needles ranging from 14 G to 22 G. There are many more-or-less well-founded reasons for the use of large-gauge needles, including the possibility of obtaining a greater quantity of tissue (especially in relation to certain diseases such as lymphomas), the greater possibility of US to visualize these needles and the lower risk of deviation. Lower, gauge needles are preferable in subjects where the procedure appears at greater risk of complications, such as in cirrhotic patients or in the case of hypervascular/superficial lesions. In reality the findings of the literature are controversial and a large single center study on abdominal-pelvic biopsies showed that both fine and large needles provided similar diagnostic results and a similar percentage of incorrect diagnosis and nondiagnostic findings. Given that finer needles often involve a smaller number of passes and lower risks, they should not be rejected *a priori* in favor of larger-gauge needles. This is another area which underlines the importance of interaction between the sonographer and the pathologist [45].

In general, subcutaneous anesthesia is performed (taking care not to puncture vessels) along the trajectory that the needle will take. In the case of liver biopsy, an attempt should be made to induce anesthesia also in the hepatic capsular region involved, since this is particularly sensitive. With larger-gauge needles it may be necessary to perform a small incision in the skin with the tip of a scalpel.

If the trajectory of the needle inserted with the freehand technique appears incorrect, withdrawing it slightly and rotating it is advisable, so that cutting side is facing towards the target. Subsequently the needle is advanced with a different inclination of the external part, possibly applying pressure on the adjacent skin. Unlike a trocar needle, which has a symmetrical tip and tends to follow a straight path, Chiba-type biopsy needles have an asymmetrical tip which is beveled on one side such that the smooth side does not modify the tissues during advancement, whereas the cutting side tends to displace them. This tendency of the needle to deviate in the direction of the cutting edge should be borne in mind when advancing the needle and can be exploited to correct the trajectory (Fig. 7.12). There is also the possibility of using coaxial systems or the tandem technique, perhaps by leaving a fine needle in place and using it as a guide for the advancement of a larger-gauge needle over it. Alternatively, a large-bore but short cannula needle can be used to direct the internal, finer and much longer biopsy needle correctly without deviations.

With regard to the risk of hemorrhage, the limitations indicated for deep FNAC are even more valid here. Especially in conditions of particular risk it may also be appropriate to inject a bioabsorbable coagulant into the needle track, such as Gelfoam or fibrin, or a nonabsorbable one, such as Gianturco spirals. In patients with biliary obstruction there is an increased risk of causing the formation of bilomas or biliary peritonitis, so prior to liver biopsy biliary decompression may be appropriate.

The incidence of **complications** is low, but greater than with fine needles for FNAC. The reported incidence of mortality with cutting needles was 0.027% and with 19 G needles or finer 0.031% [46]. The complications of abdominal biopsy generally manifest

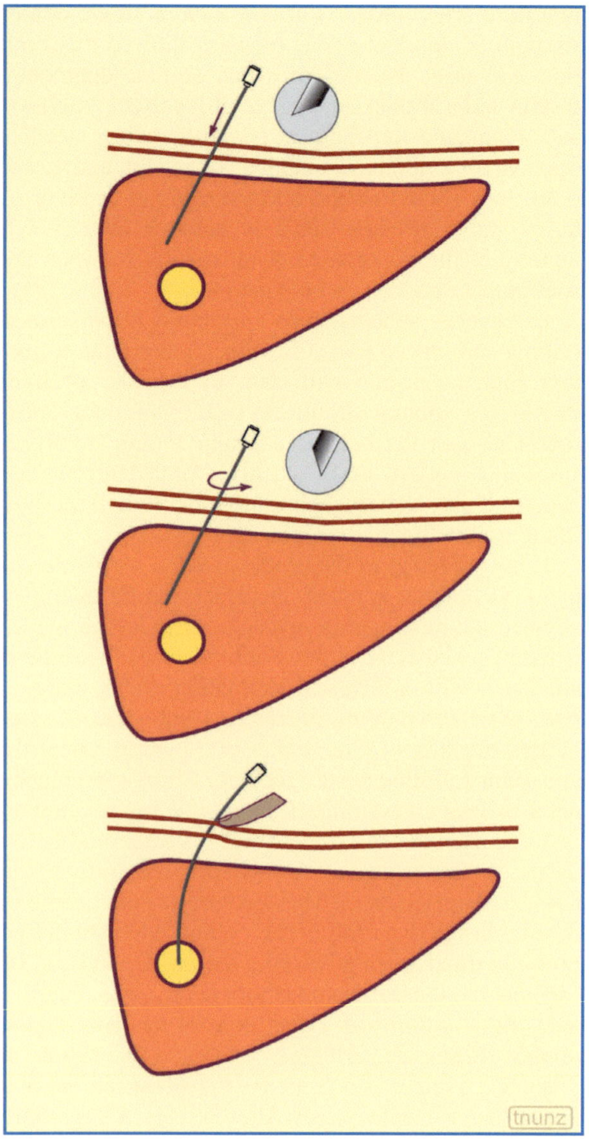

Fig. 7.12 Correction of the trajectory. An inadequate trajectory can be corrected by exploiting the orientation of the beveled side of the tip, which once rotated can be redirected towards the target, also with inclination of the needle itself outside of the patient's body

in the first three hours after the procedure. In general, the procedure should be performed with inpatient admission and discharge the day after [29]. Major complications and death are rare events, but certainly more common than with FNAC. An increased risk exists in subjects with coagulation disorders and hepatic cirrhosis, especially in the case of puncture of hypervascular lesions such as HCC or hemangioma. The risks associated with biopsy of a hepatic hemangioma have certainly been overestimated in the past, and biopsy in doubtful cases at noninvasive imaging can be performed with efficacy and low incidence of complications [47]. The incidence of seeding after biopsy for HCC has been reported at 0.8–3.4% with cutting needles. The use of a coaxial cutting needle technique has made it possible to eliminate this risk, because the external needle remains in place and therefore protects the parenchyma from the implant of tumor cells during the multiple passes of the internal cutting needle [27]. Abdominal biopsies are always followed by a US study 10–30 min after the procedure, with exploration of the main peritoneal recesses in search of a possible fluid layer [29].

Peripheral lesions of the **lung** and parietal **pleura** can be adequately reached and biopsied with US guidance, usually with the use of 18 G modified Menghini or semiautomated Trucut needles. US has proven effective, and comparable with standard radiography, in identifying, but not in quantifying, postbiopsy pneumothorax. This manifests with the disappearance of lung sliding and loss of comet-tail artifacts, findings which enable identification of the aerated lung, and with the development of reverberation artifacts produced by free air in the pleural cavity. Clearly, the inability to visualize the biopsied lesion is also a suspicious finding [48].

Liver biopsy is performed principally in the suspicion of malignancy, even though in recent years the development of imaging modalities able to identify enhancement of HCC in the arterial phase (CEUS, dynamic MRI, CT) has in many cases made possible a simple "radiologic" diagnosis followed directly by treatment [49]. Liver biopsy is also performed to verify the diagnosis of benign lesions, such as hemangiomas, adenomas and FNH, as well as for metastases (Video 7.5–7.7).

Deep **lymph nodes**, which are more often reached with CT- rather than US-guidance, are sampled with FNAC (20–22 G) in the case of suspicious lesions in patients with a primary neoplasm, but require core biopsy in patients with lymphoma. This is because the low-grade non-Hodgkin's forms in particular are poorly defined by FNAC (Video 7.8).

FNAC may be sufficient in the **spleen** for confirming a diagnosis of metastases, but for lymphomas, in the absence of a superficial lymph node to excise, a core biopsy with a cutting needle (e.g. 21 G) is required. This is an important use in that it can avoid the need for a diagnostic splenectomy. Unlike the liver, the percentage of parenchyma to be transited by the needle should be reduced to a minimum to minimize the risk of hemorrhage, and therefore the most direct approach to the lesion should be sought (Video 7.9).

Biopsy of the **pancreas** may be necessary to confirm the diagnosis of carcinoma, especially in the forms that are considered nonoperable, and to distinguish adenocarcinoma from a neuroendocrine tumor, since the latter group is characterized by a different prognosis and different treatment plan. In the presence of liver metastases, the biopsy of these lesions rather than the pancreatic mass may be preferable, especially given the risks of the procedure.

The biopsy of the **kidney** is performed principally in the suspicion of a lymphoma. The other limited indications for diagnostic renal puncture can generally be met with FNAC. In the suspicion of oncocytoma, the biopsy is usually avoided due to the risk of not recognizing possible areas of malignant degeneration. Recently, however, a large series reported the diagnostic efficacy of renal core biopsy performed with a coaxial technique (18 G needle with pistol and 17 G introducer) and the safety of the procedure (1.3% of postprocedural hematomas and 0.7% of late pseudoaneurysms) in characterizing renal lesions. The sensitivity and specificity of the US- or CT-guided procedure for the diagnosis of malignancy were 98% and 100%, respectively, with the procedure significantly affecting the clinical management of the patient in 60.5% of cases [33] (Video 7.10, 7.11).

Biopsy of the **adrenal gland** has a sensitivity for the diagnosis of malignancy >90%, although it does have some difficulty in distinguishing between adenomatous and carcinomatous tissue (sensitivity of 54–86%) and in differentiating between primary carcinoma and metastasis from RCC [32].

The **prostate** can be punctured with palpation guidance or US guidance, with either a transperineal or occasionally transrectal approach. Core biopsy is generally performed, and only rarely FNAC. Linear transrectal transducers are able to visualize the entire needle track. Usually 15–18 G cutting needles are used, especially with automatically triggered devices. Focal lesions are targeted and then the remainder of the gland is sampled systematically (sextant, octant or more) [50]. The principal indications for US-guided biopsy are the presence of hypoechoic areas >10 mm and the presence of a hypoechoic area 5–10 mm but with pathologic values of serum PSA or PSAD. In some centers all patients with a serum PSA between 4 and 10 ng/mL undergo biopsy, whereas in others only those with a suspicious PSAD do. If the pathologic values are not associated with structural alterations at US, a random biopsy is performed, although in this case US guidance is generally not required.

7.6 Vacuum-Assisted Biopsy

The systems of **vacuum-assisted** biopsy (VB) such as Mammotome are based on the aspiration of tissue cores with the use of needles and dedicated systems under mammographic (stereotactic) or US guidance. The system involves the introduction of a needle and is able to take several histologic samples of a lesion assisted by the vacuum.

The system consists of an operating arm which supports a **single-use** 8, 11 or 14 G needle, and a control module on a cart which contains the software for performing the procedure, as well as a pump for the aspiration and a small screen to follow the maneuvers. The procedure is performed in the outpatient clinic under local anesthesia. The tip of the needle is positioned near the area to be sampled, but not within the lesion, because if the lesion is small the needle may conceal it, whereas if the lesion is hard or calcified the needle may dislodge it (Fig. 7.13). The tangential position of the needle with respect to the lesion enables EUS visualization of the effective capture of the tissue to be sampled within the transducer. The tissue material is drawn by the vacuum system into a lateral channel (histologic window) of the distal end of the needle, then sectioned by a high-speed rotating blade and lastly brought out of the sampling chamber (while the introducer system remains in place) [51]. The procedure can be done either automatically or semiautomatically using the commands present on the operating arm (advancement of the blade, retraction of the blade and aspiration of the material). By rotating the arm, different tissue portions can be sampled at different angles, thus obtaining each time 15–20 mm cores which are fixed in 10% formalin for 4–6 h and then embedded in paraffin and hematoxylin-eosin stained for histologic examination. At the end of the procedure, which has an overall duration of 10–15 min, a metal clip or an echogenic marker can be placed in the path as an anatomic landmark (since the lesion has been partly or totally removed), possibly together with a bioabsorbable coagulant to guarantee hemostasis.

US-guided VB has proven to be more accurate than mammography, US and FNAC in predicting the benignity of a breast nodule, thus suggesting it should be the option of choice in indeterminate or doubtful cases. In this way surgical biopsy can be avoided in cases with doubtful results or discrepancies between previous examinations and the persisting suspicion of malignancy. Clearly in many cases VB should be preceded by FNAC, since if the latter proves to be positive the former will no longer be necessary.

With respect to core biopsy, VB does in fact have the advantage of not requiring multiple passes of the needle (which is left in place as the various vacuum-assisted samples are taken), although it should be recalled that at least in theory the use of coaxial needles for core biopsy avoids repeated passes for sampling different portions of a nodule. In addition,

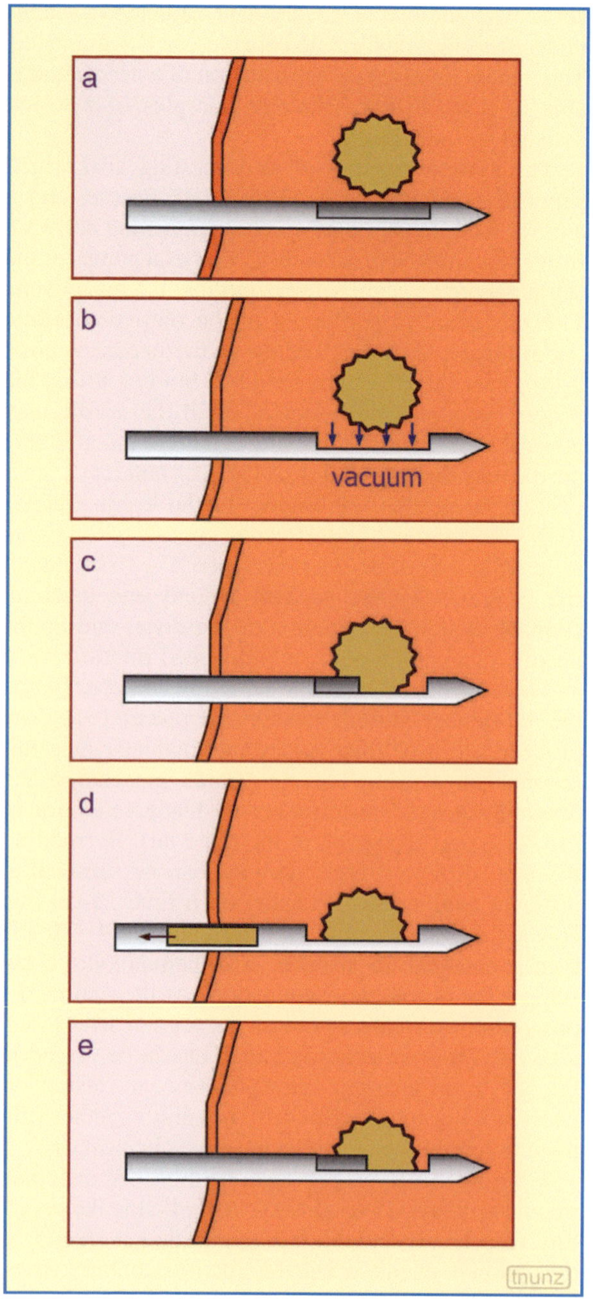

Fig. 7.13a-e Vacuum-assisted biopsy. The tip of the dedicated needle is brought immediately tangental to the target (**a**), which is then attracted by suction into the histologic window (**b**). A portion of the target is then cut (**c**), inserted into the lateral channel and brought to the outside (**d**). Lastly, the system is ready to sample additional tissue (**e**)

with respect to core biopsy, the VB cores are more consistent and can be more easily analyzed with anatomopathologic, immunohistochemical and biologic techniques (hormone receptors, proliferative indices, etc.), which is also important for therapeutic management of the patient, especially in cases of LABC [19]. VB has a diagnostic accuracy of >99% and a high correlation with surgical biopsy. This biopsy technique is more accurate than the classic percutaneous biopsy performed with automatic needles (14 G), especially for small (<15 mm) nodular lesions (visible therefore also or only with US). The greater accuracy derives from the possibility of obtaining numerous and larger cores of tissue from the lesion even to the point of its disappearance at imaging, with a significant reduction in false negatives (3–11% of cases) which are present when US guidance is used [52]. VB does have elevated costs, linked to the need for a dedicated device with dedicated needles, and it is also more invasive with a higher risk of complications than core biopsy [10]. Even though the lesions may on occasions be entirely removed, the procedure in itself is not a therapeutic modality. Because the nodule is fragmented by the procedure, the measurement of its size can no longer be made on the resection material and therefore the T parameter with its importance for prognosis can only be based on the pre-VB imaging findings.

Compared with vacuum-assisted biopsy performed under mammographic (**stereotactic**) guidance, the US-guided procedure has advantages and disadvantages. It is indicated in all lesions that are adequately visible at US, because it enables real-time monitoring, it is faster and more economic and does not use ionizing radiation. It should also be recalled that not all lesions which are well visualized at mammography can be technically biopsied with mammographic guidance. However, conditions such as isolated microcalcifications and structural distortions, which are currently among the leading indications for VB, usually require stereotactic guidance.

Complications of the procedure are mild and include bleeding, which can generally be limited with appropriate compression, and vasovagal reactions.

7.7 Placement of Presurgical Markers

US can be used for the preoperative or even intraoperative localization of small, superficial, nonpalpable lesions, as well as the immediate postexcision evaluation of the surgical site or of the surgical specimen, in order to define the effective completeness of the resection. With regard to preoperative localization, this is important because in many cases it enables the skin incision to be minimized and the lesion to be reached with greater safety and less trauma for the anatomic parts in question. Occasionally the site of the lesion may be simply marked with a dermographic pencil ("cutaneous" landmark). On other occasions intralesional **marker wire** is used, especially for breast cancers, lymph nodes and soft tissue tumors [53]. In the breast this procedure may also be used to surgically reach clusters of microcalcifications or to guide excision biopsy, although in recent years the nonsurgical procedures (core biopsy and VB) have largely substituted these applications [10]. In soft tissues the use may be associated with small lesions, lesions situated in anatomic areas disrupted by prior surgery, lesions adjacent to vulnerable structures or at any rate situated in a site which is otherwise difficult to access [53].

The US-guided placement of metallic guidewire can be used, as stated above, in the phase preliminary to the excision of a small and/or deep nodule (Video 7.12). The procedure is generally done without general or local anesthesia, given the extremely small bore (e.g. 21 G) [53]. Needles of different lengths are used, taking into account the site and depth of the lesion, as well as the need for the needle to reach the center of the lesion before opening the hook. **Repositionable needles** such as Homer or Hawkins may be used, with the possibility of modifying the position of the wire if it does not appear to be optimal. In the case of **non-repositionable needles** such as Kopans, the anchorage system does not allow for modifications in position [54] (Fig. 7.14). In both cases, once the wire has been anchored with the hook system, the part outside of the patient's body is wrapped in gauze to minimize discomfort and to reduce the risk of them becoming dislodged (a non-rare event, especially with repositionable systems) (Fig. 7.15). Under ideal circumstances, the procedure is performed with the patient on the transfer trolley in the hours immediately prior to surgery. A mammography can be done to confirm the correct position of the landmark, but this is generally not required. Instead, mammographic evaluation of the resected surgical specimen with the wire still in place is important.

An alternative to tumor resection guided by a marker wire, which is more complex but probably more precise, is **radioguided occult lesion localization** (ROLL) [55,56]. In this procedure a radiotracer is used (particles of human serum albumin labeled with Tc^{99m}) to mark the nodule, the position of which can then be identified in the operating room with the use of a manual gamma camera, thus making the resection of the lesion possible. Clearly, since the lesions are nonpalpable, the radiotracer needs to be injected with stereotactic or, better still, US guidance [55]. It is also possible to combine this procedure with the search for the axillary sentinel lymph node and therefore perform radioguided resection in both the breast and the axilla [57].

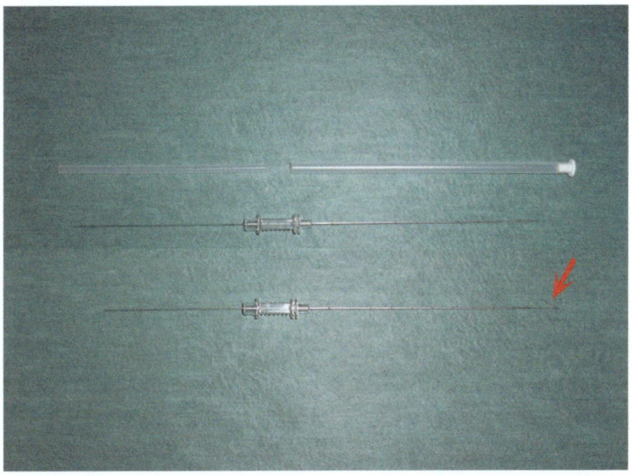

Fig. 7.14 Surgical wire marker. The 21 G guidewire is shown both closed and with the small hook open (*arrow*)

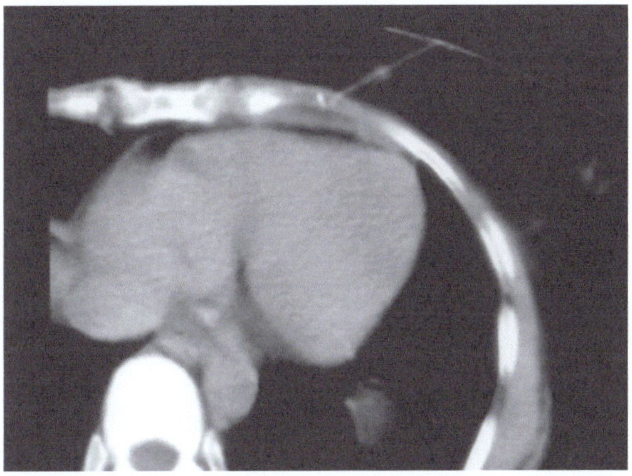

Fig. 7.15 Incorrect placement of the wire marker. CT scan shows how the guidewire, targeted at a small breast nodule, has been placed and opened (a small hook is visible) in the depth of the thoracic wall at the level of the costal plane, immediately adjacent to the pericardial surface (which shows a limited fluid reaction of blood thickening)

7.8 Drainages

The evacuation of fluids, whether free or collections, can be done according to the case with simple needle aspiration or as a first-or second-choice option with the placement of a drainage catheter [28]. **Percutaneous aspiration** is easier and is able to obtain material for cell culture and a possible antibiogram in the case of an abscess. The drained material can be pus, bile, blood, chyle or intestinal juice and according to the situation is used for microscopic evaluation (hemoglobin content, leukocyte fraction), biochemical evaluation (bilirubin, urea, triglycerides, glucose, LDH, amylase, etc.), microbiologic evaluation (cell culture, etc.) or cytologic evaluation. However, aspiration does not completely drain the abscess, especially if it is particularly large and/or multichambered and/or with densely corpuscular contents. **Percutaneous drainage** with one or more catheters has largely replaced surgical drainage due to its lower morbidity. It should always be preceded by an explorative puncture, which on the one hand allows the diagnosis to be confirmed and on the other enables the consistency of the fluid to be tested so as to choose the most appropriate catheter. The materials required include needles, guidewires, introducers, dilators, catheters, drainage systems and securing systems, all of which are generally included in dedicated kits (Fig. 7.16). Local anesthesia is performed once peripheral venous access has been guaranteed and with efforts to avoid structures such as vessels, spleen and bowel loops. The catheters come in a variety of materials (silicon, polyethylene, polyurethane, latex, Teflon, etc.) and are measured in French (F), where 3 F correspond to 1 mm. They are classified into fine (5–8 F for small collections of serous, biliary, lymphatic, etc. material), medium (9–11 F for denser, corpuscular or necrotic material or larger collections) and large (12–14 F for particularly dense material or particularly large collections). The catheters consist of a tip, either open or closed and with a varying configuration, a body and a connective system, either screw on (luer lock) or conical. This last portion allows the catheter to be connected to the drainage containers such as syringes or bags or securement devices of needles or stylets (Fig. 7.17). The tip may be J-shaped, pigtail, basket or balloon. Multiple lateral holes guarantee adequate drainage of even corpuscular fluids. The holes may be located for a variable length along the distal tract of the catheter with a unilateral, spiral or facing alignment, although the latter tends to render the distal portion of the catheter more fragile. Some large-bore catheters have a double lumen for simultaneously performing drainage and irrigation of the cavity with saline, antibiotic or fluidifying solution (Fig. 7.18).

There are various **techniques** for the **deployment** of catheters, all of which require local anesthesia and possibly the administration of sedatives or analgesics. The Seldinger technique was adapted from angiography and consists of the placement of a needle in the collection, possibly of medium gauge (18 G), then a guidewire (0.035–0.038 inches), possibly followed by dilators of increasing diameter and lastly the catheter itself over the guidewire. Once the guidewire has been withdrawn, the catheter is connected to the drainage system and fixed to the skin with some simple sutures or special silicon discs. This widely used system is precise and causes little trauma (Fig. 7.19). The modified Seldinger technique uses a reinforced catheter over a cylindrical metal guide. The simple but potentially more traumatic one-stop technique does not use a guidewire: instead a reinforced catheter is placed directly with a trocar cannula inserted through a small surgical incision in the skin (Fig. 7.20). Particularly flexible or balloon-tipped catheters can be placed using the introducer technique: the introducer is positioned with one of the previous modalities and consists of an external sheath mounted on a dilator.

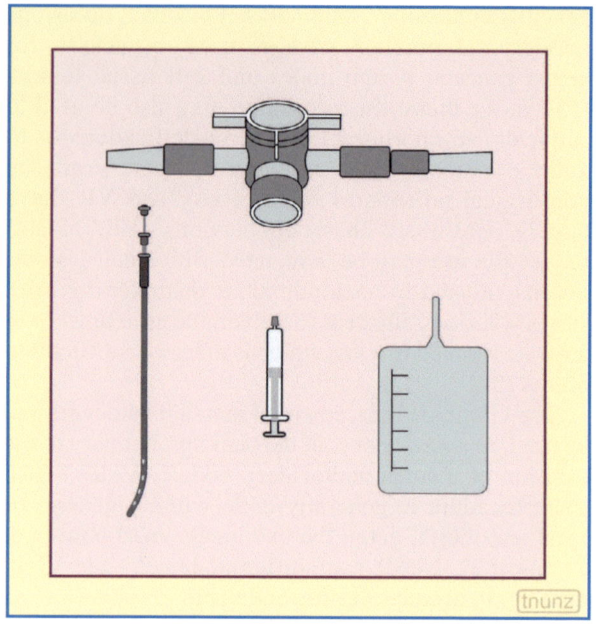

Fig. 7.16 Drainage kit. Catheter, syringe, collection bag, three-way stopcock

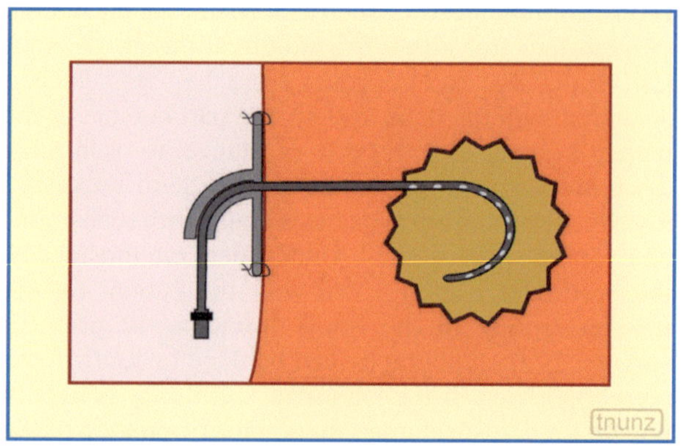

Fig. 7.17 System of skin securement of a catheter. The drainage catheter placed with the tip within a collection is secured to the skin with a special disc and sutures

The **needles** used for the deployment of these

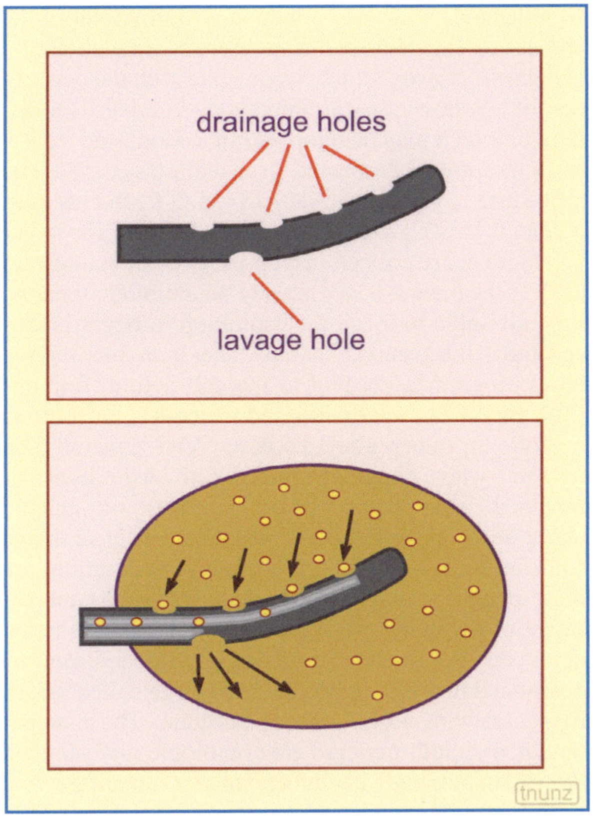

Fig. 7.18 Catheter with double lumen. The two internal canals enable simultaneous irrigation and drainage of the collection

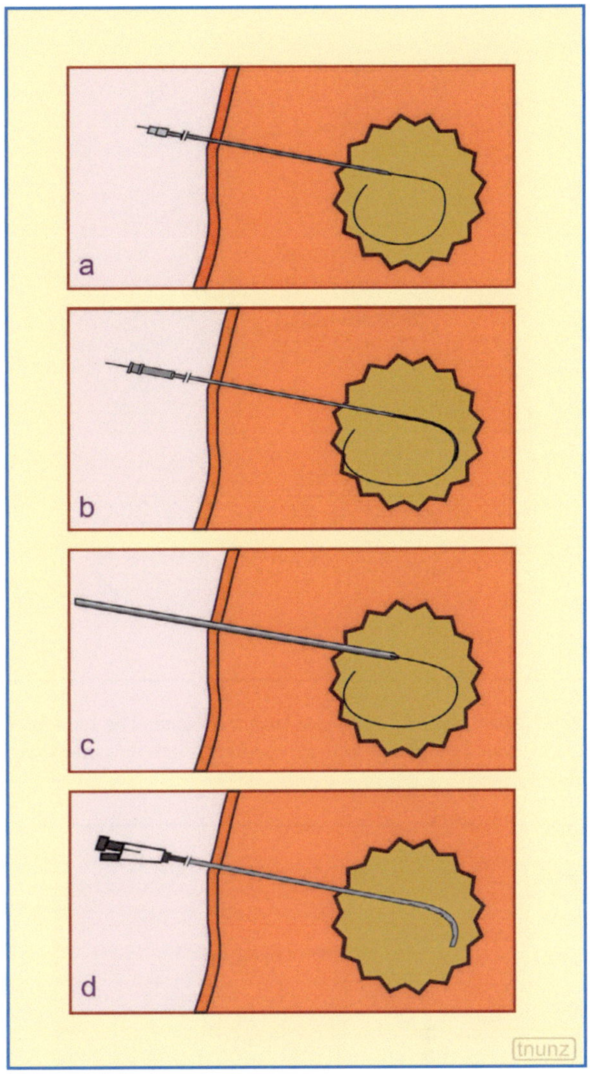

Fig. 7.19a-d Drainage with Seldinger technique. After puncture of the collection and placement of the guidewire, the catheter is advanced over the guidewire, which is then removed

catheters are generally Chiba or spinal needles, with a diameter that varies according to the guidewire that will need to be introduced inside it. The **guidewires** can be metallic, Teflon-coated steel, plastic or hydrophilic, depending on to the case, with a diameter from 0.016 to 0.038 inches and variable length. They may be stiff or flexible with a straight, J-shaped or even retractable tip.

An internal system with traction wire, which reaches right up to the proximal end outside the patient's body, allows the catheter to be adjusted according to the characteristic distal shape after it has been positioned. The content of the collection can be drained by passive flow or by active aspiration. It is advisable to maintain the system in slight aspiration to avoid collapse of the walls of the cavity, which could hinder the complete drainage of the collection or obstruct the catheter itself. The position of the multiple holes in the distal end of the catheter should also be considered, so that they are not positioned outside the collection and thus hampering effective suction and above all spreading its contents to inappropriate areas (Fig. 7.21). The cone of the catheter is particularly delicate, since it is susceptible to traction and inclination both during the procedure and in the following days, especially due to improper movements by the patient. Correct maintenance of the catheter is crucial for the complete success of the treatment. In addition, monitoring of symptoms, laboratory findings and US appearance is a fundamental part of the evaluation of the involution of the collection. The catheter should be kept connected until the flow falls below 10–15 mL a day after which, possibly after 1–2 days with the closed system, it can be removed.

In the cancer patient the formation of intra-

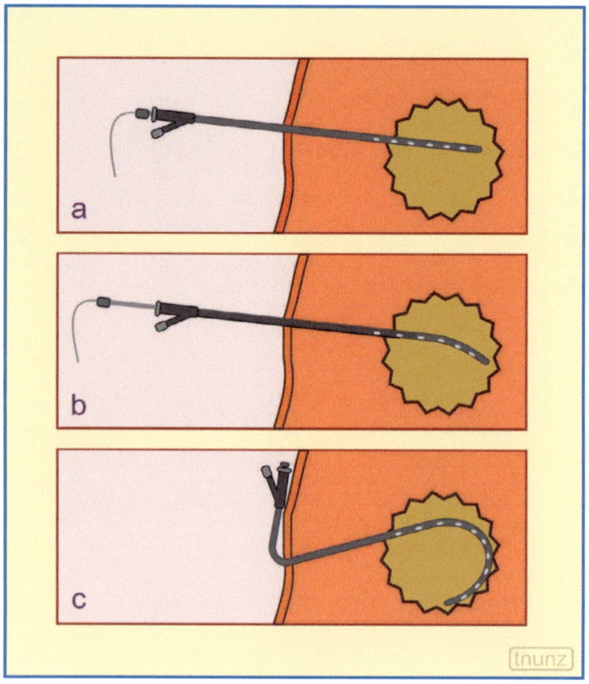

Fig. 7.20a-c Drainage with one-stop technique. The reinforced trocar-tipped catheter is introduced directly into the collection

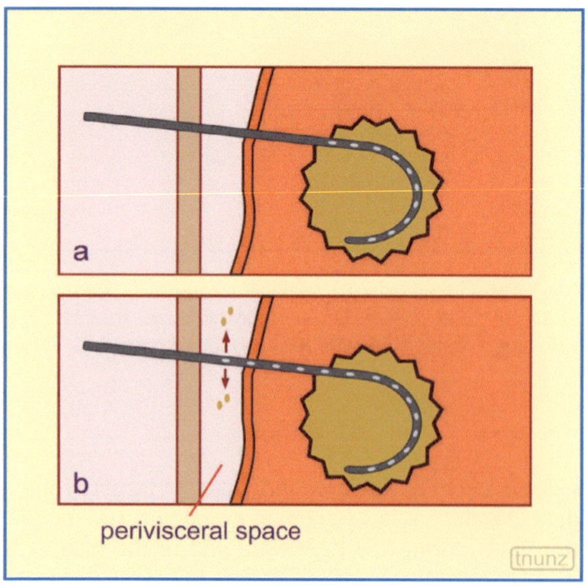

Fig. 7.21a,b Incorrect placement of the catheter. The catheter in (**a**) can be seen with all the holes within the collection to be drained, whereas in (**b**) holes can be seen external to the collection, which is responsible for the leakage of material

peritoneal and intraparenchymal **abdominal abscesses** is principally associated with radical surgery or therapeutic procedures of another kind, including interventional radiologic procedures, which can become complicated with an infection. Alternatively, the abscess or empyema can be a direct complication of a neoplastic growth, which may evolve with the perforation of a hollow organ or internal or external fistulization, or which may develop within a neoplastic cavity, as in the case of abscessed liver metastases [58]. The procedure is performed with 18–22 G Chiba needles, although larger-gauge needles may be used for larger and more dense collections (corpuscular or echogenic) [29]. If the patient is not already on antibiotic therapy, it is advisable to await the aspiration to begin broad-spectrum intravenous therapy and then modify the basic program according to the cell culture findings [29]. Small and medium-sized abscesses, as well as mycotic or tubercular abscesses, can generally be treated with diagnostic/therapeutic aspiration or repeated aspiration. Large, bacterial or amebic abscesses often require the placement of a drainage catheter, usually 8–10 F [58]. When the collections are multilocular, it may be possible to break the thinner septations with the tip of the catheter when it is being deployed. Alternatively, multiple catheters can be positioned in different portions of a large collection, or irrigation with urokinase can be done. The material obtained should undergo microbiologic analysis and often also cytologic and biochemical evaluation.

Pelvic collections or **abscesses** situated deep within the rectouterine pouch may be accessed with a transvaginal approach, especially in the absence of adequate alternatives (US- or CT-guided suprapubic access and transgluteal access, fundamentally with CT guidance) [59]. There are in fact dedicated intravaginal transducers with an attachable guide for the placement of needles or drainage catheters (Fig. 7.22). Preliminary TVUS is able to accurately define the relations between the collection, the vaginal dome and the adjacent pelvic structures. The procedure, and especially the placement of the needle or guidewire in the collection, is monitored in real time with the transducer in place. Subsequently this is removed and the guidewire is exploited for the deployment of the catheter. A further alternative is given by US-guided transperineal access, which may be indicated in male subjects having undergone abdominoperineal resection, where this approach can be the only nonsurgical method of draining deep pelvic collections [60].

The causes of failure of percutaneous treatment procedures include an inappropriate access site, insufficient number of drains, an insufficient gauge of the needle, early suspension of the aspiration, or premature removal of the catheter [58]. **Complications** of the drainage of abdominopelvic abscesses are limited, with an incidence of 4–5%, but since cancer patients may be more-or-less immunodepressed they are clearly at a higher risk. Minor complications include

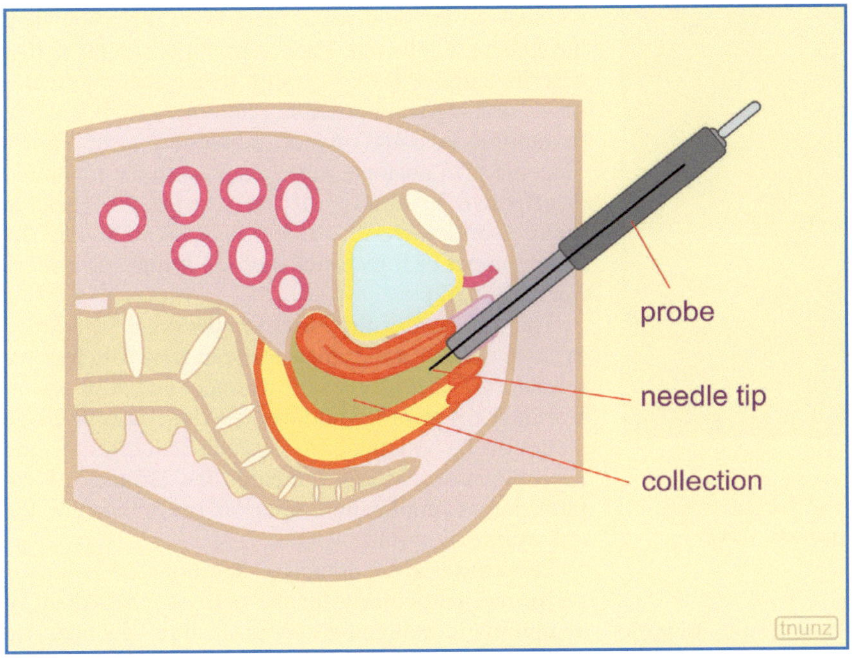

Fig. 7.22 Transvaginal drainage. Dedicated intraluminal transducer enables the transvaginal puncture of a collection in the rectouterine pouch

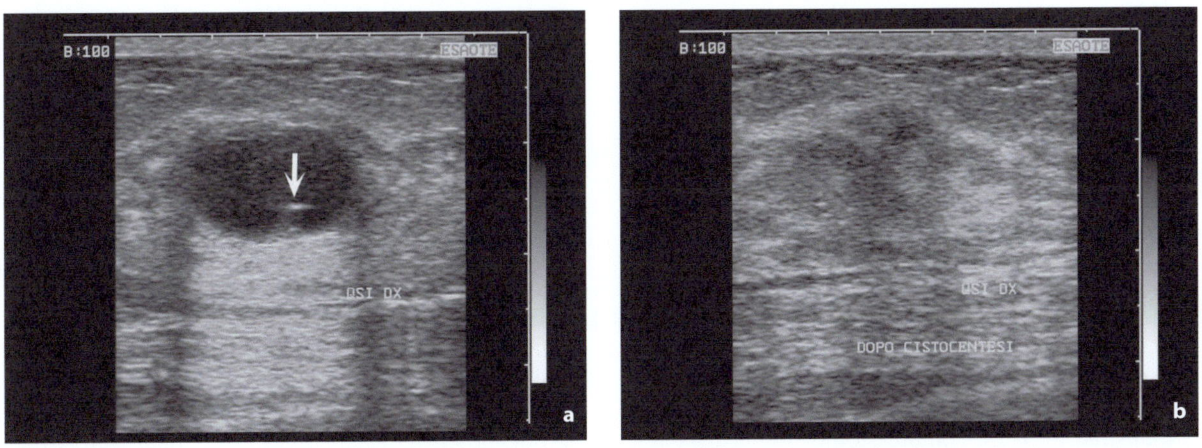

Fig. 7.23a,b Breast cyst drainage. The scan during the procedure (**a**) shows the homogeneous unilocular cystic mass with the needle tip inside (*arrow*). The scan after drainage (**b**) demonstrates the complete collapse of the mass

fever (transitory bacteremia), pain, cutaneous infection at the access site of the catheter and mild bleeding. Major complications include generalized sepsis and septic shock, disseminated intravascular coagulation, hemoperitoneum (vascular lesion), pneumothorax (lung puncture), pyothorax (contamination of the pleural cavity), choleperitoneum (lesion of the bile ducts), peritonitis and fistulas (digestive organ lesion).

The treatment of **cysts** with drainage or possible sclerotherapy is performed in benign or at least presumed benign masses in the thyroid, breast, liver, pancreas (pseudocysts), spleen and kidney. The therapeutic indication, as an alternative to surgery (laparoscopy or open air) should be based on the presence of significant symptoms, but clearly there can under certain circumstances be other motivations, including the need to confirm the nature of a benign lesion [61]. With regard to **breast cysts**, the procedure is indicated in large and/or symptomatic forms (Figs. 7.23, 7.24). Cytologic evaluation should be performed for all cysts that are not completely drained and for those in which the drained fluid has the

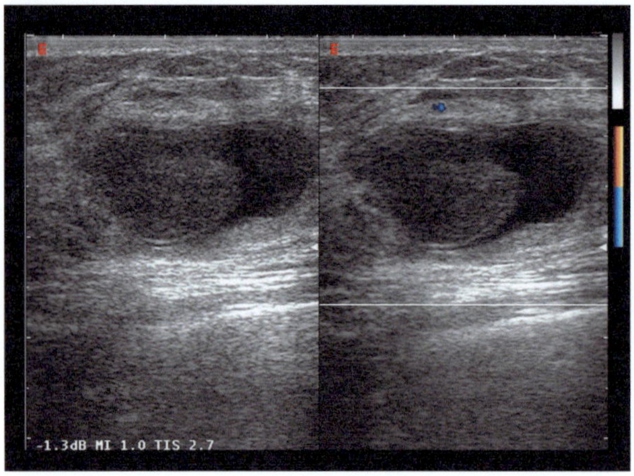

Fig. 7.24 Intracystic hemorrhage after breast cyst drainage. The CD study shows a large clot within a cyst drained without US guidance three days earlier. No flow signals are visible

appearance of blood [62]. If large, simple **hepatic cysts** can be treated when symptomatic (5–17% of cases) and causing pain, hepatomegaly, jaundice or digestive problems or when they produce acute complications such as internal hemorrhage or infection. Simple aspiration may be done, although this is often a source of recurrence, or aspiration and subsequent sclerosis with ethanol or even tetracycline, phenol, glucose, fibrin glue or still other agents. Sclerotherapy with ethanol can be performed in a single session, with US-guided deployment of the catheter and intracystic retention of the alcohol for 60 min or, in a recent series, just 10 min (with a variable quantity of ethanol from 10% to 96% of the cystic volume but never greater than 100 mL) [61,63]. The percutaneous treatment of simple **renal cysts** can be done when these are particularly large or when they are deemed responsible for pain, compression of the urinary tract (or an obstacle to the expulsion of calculi within the tract) or nephrovascular hypertension. Simple aspiration may be performed with drainage of the cyst, but to avoid recurrence, sclerosis with ethanol (with a quantity of 30% of the cystic volume), tetracycline, atossisclerol or fibrin glue is preferable. The Seldinger technique is used for puncture, as well as needle-trocar catheter systems, with the drainage catheter left in place for a week. In addition, there are also multisession protocols. Complications are rare and include hemorrhage, infections, pneumothorax, arteriovenous fistulas and intestinal perforation [64,65].

The drainage of sterile postoperative collections, such as **lymphocele**, **urinoma** or **biloma**, is especially done when these are large, when they compress the adjacent structures (e.g. hydronephrosis) or when they raise doubts regarding differential diagnosis from residual tumor or disease recurrence, or when they have become infected. The treatment is similar to that described above for cysts, with transcatheter percutaneous drainage and possible sclerotherapy in a single or multiple sessions (ethanol, antibiotics, talcum, fibrin glue, etc.). In postoperative lymphocele the treatment is effective in almost all cases, with the possible requirement, however, of new sessions following the development of a recurrence of the lymphatic collection [61,66,67].

The drainage of **liquefactive tumors** is performed in cases of large and symptomatic masses which prove refractory to other types of treatment and with palliative intent. The procedure may be limited to drainage alone or be extended to include sclerosis of the necrotic cavity, which increases the efficacy of the procedure. Complications are principally linked to the risk of infection [68].

Paracentesis, i.e. drainage of peritoneal effusion, is performed particularly for the palliative treatment of symptomatic malignant ascites, in turn secondary to peritoneal carcinosis. Malignant ascites, which is associated with very poor prognosis (<6 months life expectancy), involves symptoms such as abdominal distension, nausea, anorexia, early satiety, and in extreme cases respiratory problems. Abundant peritoneal effusion markedly reduces the quality of life of these patients and may therefore require an adjunct to pharmacologic therapy. Paracentesis is an outpatient procedure which can generally be performed blind: It is predominantly done in the left lower quadrant of the abdomen with the patient slightly turned towards that side. However, it is not unusual for US guidance to be required because the quantity of effused material is not abundant or is irregularly distributed due to blocked diffusion between the various peritoneal compartments. In addition, there are often phenomena of adhesion of the bowel loops to the abdominal wall, which increase the risk of a non-guided procedure [69]. US guidance can at the same time avoid complications such as the puncture of a bowel loop and increase the efficacy of the procedure by identifying the most appropriate site for performing the puncture. The aim is to drain as much fluid as possible and therefore reduce the number of periodic paracentesis sessions required (Fig. 7.25). An accurate preliminary US study is therefore vital for identifying the most appropriate needle track. The approach can be anterior, anterolateral or lateral, with measurement using the calipers of the distance between the skin and the center fluid area to be drained. The drainage catheter with multiple side holes is placed with the tip inclined, and the patient is asked to slightly change position during aspiration to facilitate drainage. At least 0.5 L should be drained to obtain some improvement in symptoms. It

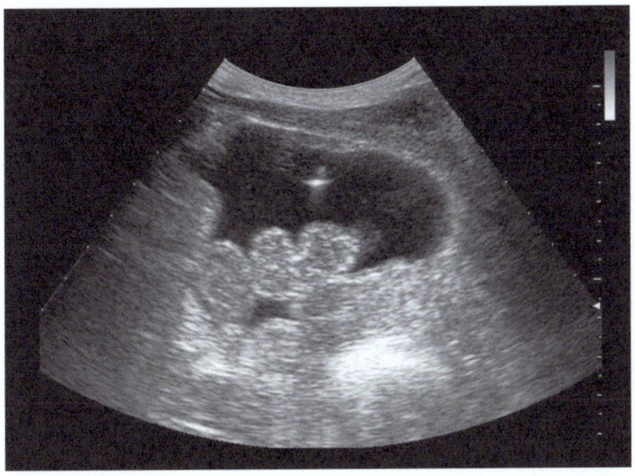

Fig. 7.25 Paracentesis. The needle tip is recognizable within the fluid

should nonetheless be borne in mind that the drainage of large volumes of fluid in very short periods of time can create a condition of imbalance in the patient, e.g. in the form of a loss of pressure. Some authors have suggested monitoring pressure during and immediately after the procedure, as well as drainage of the fluid without excessive velocity [69]. At the end of the procedure the needle is removed, or occasionally the catheter is left indwelling for 24 h or several days, although with the possible risk of bacterial infection of the abdominal cavity. In special cases long-term catheters may be deployed (e.g. subcutaneous tunneled catheters) which are able to function for months with the daily drainage of small quantities of fluid. This eliminates the need for the frequent inpatient admissions for repeated procedures of paracentesis. In this case US guidance can be useful for possible periodic repositioning of the catheter itself [70,71].

7.9 Percutaneous Ethanol Injection

Percutaneous ethanol injection (PEI) is the most widespread ablation procedure for the treatment of hepatic lesions and in particular HCC, and can also be used in the treatment of autonomous thyroid nodules, hyperparathyroidism (primary, secondary or tertiary), hyperfunctioning adrenal adenomas, cysts of the liver, kidney or other sites and Morton neuromas [72–74]. The ablation effect is linked to both diffusion of ethanol in the cells, with dehydration and coagulative necrosis, and penetration into the small intralesional vessels, with damage to the endothelial cells and consequent luminal thrombosis and ischemia. HCC has characteristics which render it particularly susceptible to this treatment. These include relatively slow growth, well-circumscribed or frankly capsulated appearance, with relatively poor consistency, high vascularity and location in compact parenchyma which limits the extranodular diffusion of the ethanol such as in the patient with chronic liver disease. In addition, the appearance of extrahepatic metastases occurs only in a minority of typically advanced cases. PEI is especially used to treat small lesions, particularly in patients who are not candidates for surgical resection or with postoperative recurrence [49,75]. In nodules <3 cm, the technique is able to obtain complete necrosis in around 70% of cases. The direct ablation of malignant thrombi is also possible, especially if segmental or subsegmental, in order to avoid progression towards the major portal branches. In liver metastases the results have instead been poor and treatment of these lesions with PEI has been abandoned.

PEI is generally performed as an outpatient procedure on an empty stomach, without sedation and without local anesthesia. The only absolute contraindication is severe hemorrhagic diathesis, whereas ascites is not a contraindication in itself, unless it is marked and located along the chosen needle track. Anxious subjects may be given pharmacologic treatment for both sedation and pain. Having peripheral venous access in all patients is advisable. The treatment is performed once or, more commonly, twice a week for 4–6 weeks. Dedicated 21–22 G Chiba needles are used (PEIT, with a closed conical tip and three distal side holes) with 95% ethanol. With the patient in the supine or lateral position and with a subcostal or intercostal approach, ethanol is slowly injected into the lesion, possibly into more than one place in the lesion. For example, a deep area and a superficial area of the lesion can be identified, with the deep portion being initially treated and then the superficial portion afterwards, withdrawing the needle somewhat. Alternatively, multiple needles may be simultaneously inserted, with the injection of the ethanol beginning from the deepest needle. If the nodule is particularly small, placing the needle at its center is generally sufficient to obtain evenly distributed necrosis. Some authors advocate CD guidance, with the injection of ethanol in relation to the intralesional arteries. CEUS may be utilized in the case of lesions not visualized at conventional US. The ethanol is readily identifiable because it appears as a clear "cloud" of hyperechogenicity, with possible posterior acoustic shadowing, which fills the lesion for 2–3 cm around the needle tip and which diffuses in the vessels surrounding the nodule in the form of some small intraluminal echogenic nuclei. If the intravascular diffusion of the alcohol appears excessive, the injection should be interrupted. Respiration should be stopped during the insertion and withdrawal of the needle, whereas it should be calm and shallow during the injection of ethanol. When the injection is finished, the needle is generally left in place for an additional 30–60 s to avoid the reflux of ethanol, after which it is slowly withdrawn with care to avoid the diffusion of ethanol along the needle track, which can be particularly painful for the patient. Should this occur the withdrawal is halted for half a minute or so and the needle is then definitively removed. Some authors advocate the injection of an analgesic during withdrawal of the needle [29,73,76].

Overall, the procedure lasts 10–20 min and the patient remains in the waiting room for the subsequent 1–2 h. The quantity of ethanol used is generally a few milliliters (1–8/session), although as much as 14 mL may be used per session, possibly in fractions with several minutes' interval. The quantity depends not only on the size of the lesion but also on the tolerance shown by the patient and the greater or lesser ease with which the ethanol diffuses in the lesion. The quantity in mL of ethanol to be injected for a complete treatment cycle can be calculated with the formula for a sphere, $4/3\ \Pi\ (r + 0.5)^3$, where r is the radius of the nodule in cm (e.g. at least 14 mL for a 2 cm lesion and at least 32 mL for a 3 cm lesion). The number of sessions and the quantity of ethanol to be injected nonetheless depend on the initial volume of the nodule and the compliance of the individual patient. In general, 2–3 sessions are required for nodules <2 cm, 4–6 for nodules 2–3 cm and 6–8 sessions for nodules 3–4 cm (the number of sessions is approximately twice the diameter of the nodule). The part of the nodule which needs to be treated in the sessions subsequent to the first can be chosen by targeting a more vascular area at CD, or with greater contrast enhancement at CEUS. In the event of residual tumor even after various sessions more destructive percutaneous procedures such as RFTA can be used [73,76].

There are a limited number of side-effects to the procedure, including pain possibly radiating to the epigastrium or right shoulder and possible mild fever in the days subsequent to PEI. The leakage of ethanol into the peritoneal cavity is particularly painful, and reflux into the bile ducts can cause significant stenosis. Penetration into the portal branches usually causes chemical thrombosis, which nonetheless regresses in 1–3 months. Major **complications** include hemoperitoneum, hemobilia, chemical cholangitis, cholecystitis, abscess formation, hepatic infarction, caval thrombosis, intestinal injury, hydrothorax and pneumothorax [77] (Fig. 7.26). Mortality is 0.09% in multisession PEI. Intra- and extrahepatic tumor seeding is relatively rare – 1.1% in a targeted study [78], 0.01% in a large patient population with PEI treatments and one-shot PEI [29] (Fig. 7.27). There is nonetheless the

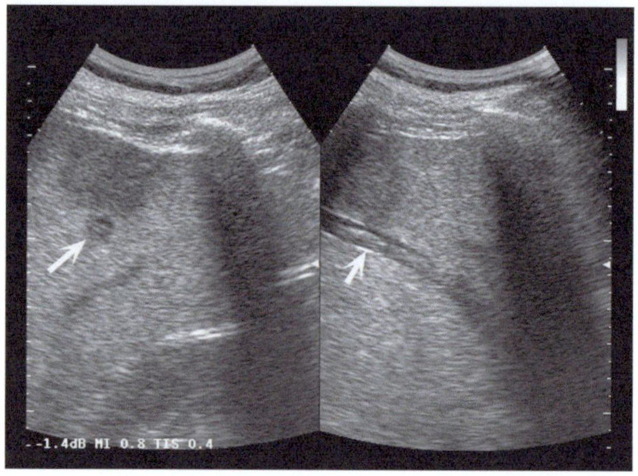

Fig. 7.26 Portal thrombosis after PEI. The treated hypoechoic lesion can be seen together with a luminal defect within a segmental portal branch, sectioned in both longitudinal and transverse views (*arrows*)

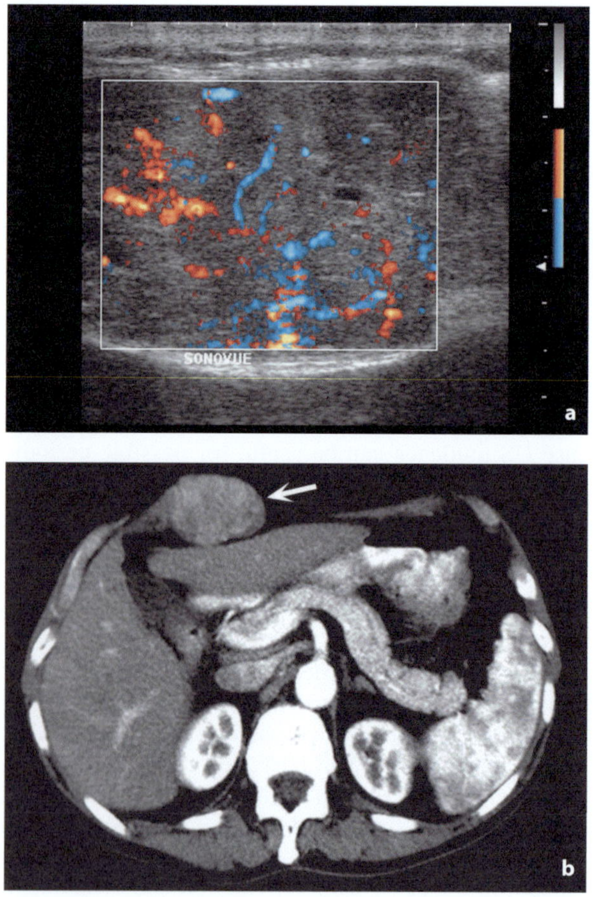

Fig. 7.27a,b Mural seeding of HCC after PEI. The scan with directional PD after intravenous contrast medium injection (**a**) shows a large hypervascular mural nodulation at the level of the thoracic wall. CT scan in the arterial phase confirms the diagnosis (**b**, *arrow*)

problem, encountered relatively frequently in various series, of residual tumor and local recurrence, as well as the limitations in the treatment of multiple and/or large lesions. Local **recurrences** are in fact found in 33% of HCC <3 cm and as many as 43% of those >3 cm [79]. The ethanol diffuses heterogeneously in the lesions, particularly in relation to the internal septations, and in extracapsular tumor diffusion: residual tumors and recurrences are typically at the periphery of the treated lesion.

An alternative is offered by **PEI** performed in a **single session** (one-shot) with the injection of an increased quantity of ethanol [73]. Under general anesthesia, multiple passes are performed with introduction into the lesion (>5 cm) of a quantity of ethanol corresponding to the size of the lesion itself [29,80]. Given the complications recorded in the past, including cardiovascular problems associated with acute ethylism (especially if significant quantities of alcohol inadvertently diffuse into the vessels), the proponents of the procedure have recently divided it into two or more sessions, with an interval of two weeks [29].

7.10 Radiofrequency Ablation and other Ablation Therapies

Subsequent to the introduction of PEI numerous other **percutaneous ablation therapies** (PATs) have been developed which all have the characteristic of inducing local destruction of a lesion in a minimally invasive and nonsurgical manner and which limit the damage to the healthy hepatic parenchyma and therefore only marginally influence the functional reserve of the organ. PATs are based on the effect of chemical substances (PEI, injection of acetic acid), heat (radiofrequency thermoablation, coagulation with microwaves, laser therapy, injection of boiling saline solution), cold (cryotherapy) or radioactivity (injection of microspheres labeled with yttrium-90). **Radiofrequency thermal ablation** (RFTA) in particular exploits the effect of coagulative necrosis induced in the tumor by resistive heating produced by electromagnetic waves (radiofrequencies – RF), thus producing a spheroidal necrotic area around the electrode tip. The RF originate from the electrode tip, which is connected to a generator which converts electric current into electromagnetic energy. Heat is produced directly in the tissue surrounding the non-isolated portion (exposed tip) of the active electrode and is dependent on the difference between the heat produced by the electrode and the heat dissipated by the tissue due to the cooling effect of blood circulation. It should also be noted that in the cirrhotic liver the perinodular parenchyma tends to act as thermal insulation, forming a sort of protection from the dissipation of the heat outside of the nodule ("oven effect") [75,81].

RFTA was originally used mainly for HCC and liver metastases, although its applications have significantly broadened. Currently it is indicated for benign hepatic lesions (benign tumors, hydatidosis) and lesions of the thyroid (e.g. hot nodules and recurrences of carcinoma), parathyroid (hyperfunctioning adenomas), lung (some non-small-cell carcinomas and some metastases), bone (painful metastases and osteoid osteoma), adrenal gland (metastases), kidney (primary lesions), uterus (myomas) and even the breast, pancreas, prostate and spinal-paraspinal lesions [81,82]. Like other ablation procedures, RFTA can be used in the setting of laparoscopic or laparotomic procedures and not only with a percutaneous approach [61,81]. In some cases the intent is radical treatment, at least locally, while in others it is palliative. In both events, however, it seems clear that for the same results PATs are preferable to surgery given their lower morbidity, mortality and costs.

There are currently numerous **possibilities for the treatment of HCC**, which can be integrated in a synchronous or sequential manner (multimodal treatment), although to date it has not been possible to make definitive choices. Surgical resection is curative, but cannot be applied in all patients and does not eliminate the problem of an "organ" disease. Organ transplant is the only treatment which really solves the hepatic problem, but it can only be done in select patients. Transcatheter intra-arterial procedures (chemotherapy, embolization, radioembolization, chemoembolization) are generally reserved for larger lesions with a palliative intent. PATs are minimally invasive and repeatable, but they have only a local effect and are characterized by high rates of recurrence, especially PEI. Last of all, systemic treatments (chemotherapy with agents such as sorafenib, doxorubicin, immunotherapy with interferon, hormone therapy with tamoxifen, gene therapy, etc.) are little effective or still undergoing experimentation [73,75,83,84]. The choice depends on the general conditions of the patient, the stage of the disease and the residual liver function, as well as the individual choice of the patient and the specific experience and preference of the individual center [84]. Conceptually, the use of PAT should be considered merely as a bridging procedure to transplant, but clearly the number of patients able to benefit from liver transplantation is far below the number of subjects with hepatic lesions [61]. In theory, surgical resection is still considered the treatment of choice, even though there are no significant randomized controlled trials comparing resection and percutaneous ablation. The option of surgery should be offered to all patients with a single lesion, a non-cirrhotic liver or cirrhotic but with good residual function, normal bilirubin and a pressure gradient in the hepatic vein <10 mmHg. However, only 9–27% of patients are eligible for surgery due to limited hepatic functional reserve, multifocal lesions and lesions in both hepatic lobes, and the presence of extrahepatic metastases and/or portal invasion. In addition, resection is encumbered by a rate of recurrence (including new nodules in other segments) >70% within five years [49,85]. This explains the current diffusion of percutaneous ablation procedures, which are less invasive and are repeatable and therefore ideal in patients with early-stage HCC who are not candidates for surgery (although in most centers this option is offered as first choice). RFTA, which is at least as effective as PEI for lesions >2 cm but with a lower number of sessions, is without doubt superior for larger lesions and able to obtain good control of the lesions, thus proving to be "locally curative" [75]. One long-term study reported a survival of 78% at three years and 54% at five years for patients with effectively ablated HCC [86].

With regard to **liver metastases**, those treated with RFTA or other percutaneous procedures (except PEI, which is ineffective) have predominantly been suggering from colorectal cancer. Without surgical resection these patients have a median survival <12 months, which is little modified by chemotherapy or radiation therapy, whereas surgical series with adequately selected patients have reported a five-year survival rate of 20–45% [87]. What is expected from PATs, which are undeniably less invasive and therefore more repeatable than surgical resection, is to obtain similar results, thus prolonging disease-free survival with a reasonable quality of life [61,81,88].

There are various **systems for RFTA** which vary with regard to the type of needle-electrode, the number of electrodes at the tip and the power of the generator. The RITA system (RITA Medical Systems, USA) uses a current generator connected to an external 12–15 G insulated needle with a variable number of terminal hooks, each 1–2 cm in length and equipped with an active electrode at the tip. When the needle is in place, the hooks are deployed and form a sort of an inverted umbrella with a diameter of around 5 cm. The Elektrotom HiTT 106 (Berchtold, Germany) "perfusion system" uses a 275 kHz generator and a 12–14 G monopolar needle-electrode with a 15 mm active tip able to reach temperatures of up to 100 degrees. The hollow electrode needle is perfused with an outward flow of isotonic saline solution. The "cool tip" system (Radionics, USA) typically uses a 480 kHz generator and a 14–18 G monopolar "cluster" needle. Three parallel electrodes are spaced 5 mm from each other with 10–30 mm of active tip (to be chosen in relation to the breadth of necrosis desired). The internal refrigeration of the electrode is achieved with a saline solution at 2–5° C introduced by a peristaltic pump. The RF 3000 system (Radiotherapeutics, USA) characteristically uses a 480 kHz generator and an expandable LeVeen monopolar needle which contains 12 retractable curved tips, which, when open, form a 4-cm-wide "umbrella" [29,89–93]. Experimentally it has been shown that the perfusion cool-tip electrodes induce larger volumes of necrosis than those provoked by other systems, although the cool-tip and 12-hook needle systems induce more regular and repeatable volumes than the perfusion and 9-hook needle systems [89,94].

The **diameter of the lesion** produced depends largely on the diameter of the electrode and the duration of the RF application, even though it tends to be greater in vitro than in vivo, because in the latter case the cooling produced by blood perfusion in the treated region has an antagonistic effect. The heating of the tissues is greatest at the level of the area of greatest density of the current, i.e. around the tip of the electrode. The main factor limiting necrosis is the phenomenon of carbonization, which is created around the electrode at high temperatures and limits further diffusion of the heat into the surrounding tissues. The area of necrosis can be increased with additional electrodes used either simultaneously or alternately, or with the injection of cooling saline solution before and/or during the procedure (thus enabling the energy generated to be increased without inducing excessive phenomena of boiling or cavitation around the tip). Systems with bipolar electrodes have also been proposed (single bipolar electrode or double electrode) [81].

To obtain complete necrosis and avoid recurrence at the periphery of the treated lesion, necrosis of not only the lesion but also a layer of tissue surrounding it is required for HCC and especially for metastases. The "ablation zone" is defined as the radiologically identifiable region in which the ablation effect was directly induced, whereas the "ablation margin" is defined as a tissue area of 5–10 mm around the lesion [95] (Fig. 7.28). The failure to extend necrosis to the entire ablation margin increases the risk of recurrence, evidently caused by microscopic extension of the tumor cells beyond the radiologically identifiable ablation zone or due to the intrinsic limitations of the imaging technique in defining the real extension of the lesion [80].

In general, RFTA uses needles with a much larger gauge than those used in other ablation techniques, such as laser photocoagulation. The latter may there-

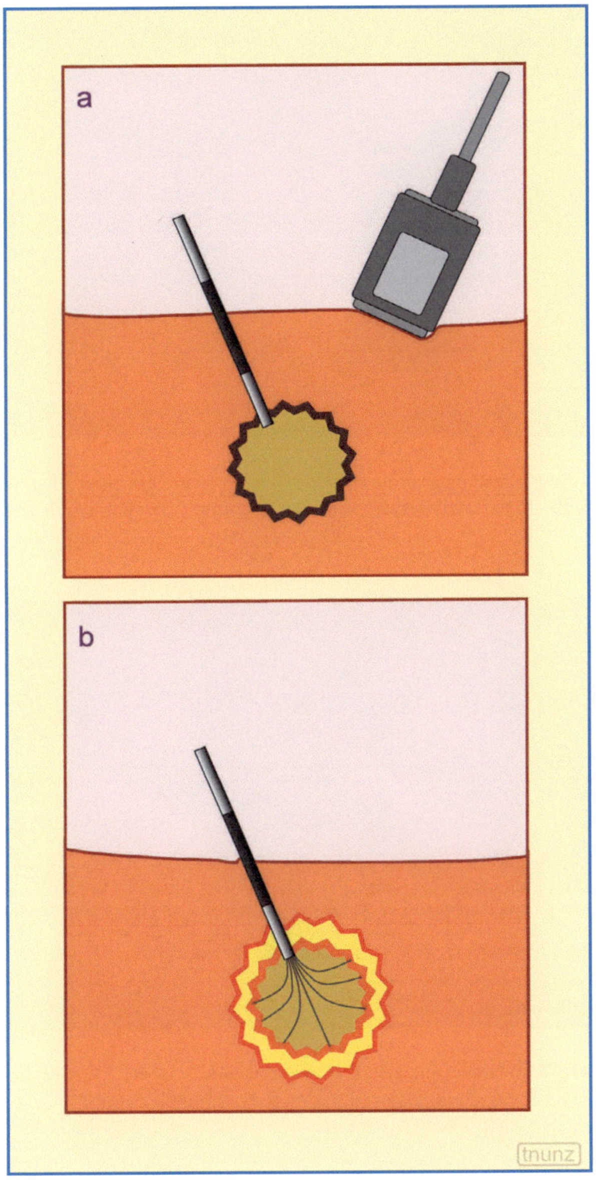

Fig. 7.28a,b Concept of safety margin. Percutaneous ablation should aim to obtain not only nodular necrosis (**a**), but also a 5–10 mm halo of perinodular tissue necrosis (**b**)

fore be preferable for deep lesions which are poorly defined at US and/or which require multiple passes [29]. Some lesion sites increase the risk of complications at RFTA, such as peripheral locations, especially if adjacent to the diaphragm (risk of perforation), or exophytic (risk of tumor rupture), or adjacent to the gallbladder, the major vessels (risk of hemorrhage) and especially the parahilar bile ducts (risks of biliary stenosis) [29]. Even myelin is sensitive to thermal insults and therefore RFTA should be used with care in the treatment of lesions that are particularly close to nerves. In patients with a pacemaker, care should be taken to avoid the pacemaker being found along the course between the electrode and the grounding pad. In patients with hip prostheses too, the grounding pad should not be placed adjacent to the prosthesis.

Typical **inclusion criteria** for HCC are a single nodule <5 cm diameter or 3 nodules <3 cm diameter, and for liver metastases <6 lesions with <5 cm diameter or <10 lesions with <4 cm diameter [96]. Kidney lesions are generally treated in patients with a single kidney (anatomically or functionally) or in patients with multiple tumors (e.g. patients with von Hippel–Lindau syndrome).

In most centers RFTA, like the other percutaneous ablation procedures with the exception of multisession PEI, is performed as an inpatient procedure in a single session, unless the subsequent control reveals residual tumor. Generally the treatment is performed in the operating room under general anesthesia. Occasionally the procedure is performed with simple sedation when the patient is particularly compliant and the number of insertions is one or at most two [29,81]. Tracheal intubation enables, among other things, the modification of the "height" of the diaphragm, and therefore facilitates the treatment of subdiaphragmatic lesions. With the monopolar techniques a grounding pad is applied below the thigh of the patient, whereas with bipolar systems a second, passive electrode is used which is positioned 5 cm from the active electrode [81]. The RF are applied for a variable length of time – several minutes – in relation to the RFTA technique used, the power of the generator available and the need for multiple insertions (Video 7.13). Once the procedure has been completed, the still hot (70–80°) electrode needle is slowly withdrawn so as to decontaminate the needle track of possible tumor cell seeding and at the same time guarantee a form of hemostasis. Clearly this maneuver should be done in this way even when the needle needs to simply be repositioned, e.g. because it was placed in a suboptimal site. In general, US guidance is sufficient for the ablation of primary and secondary hepatic lesions which have not yet undergone percutaneous treatment, whereas in the recurrence of HCC the superiority of CEUS in targeting treatment on the area of tumor recurrence has been demonstrated [97].

The evaluation of hematocrit and liver enzymes 6 h after the treatment is advisable, as well as a repetition of laboratory tests the morning after, prior to discharge, which in some centers occurs on the third day. A reduction in hemoglobin by as much as 1–2 g and of platelets by 10–15% is possible, especially in the case of large lesions with multiple insertions of the

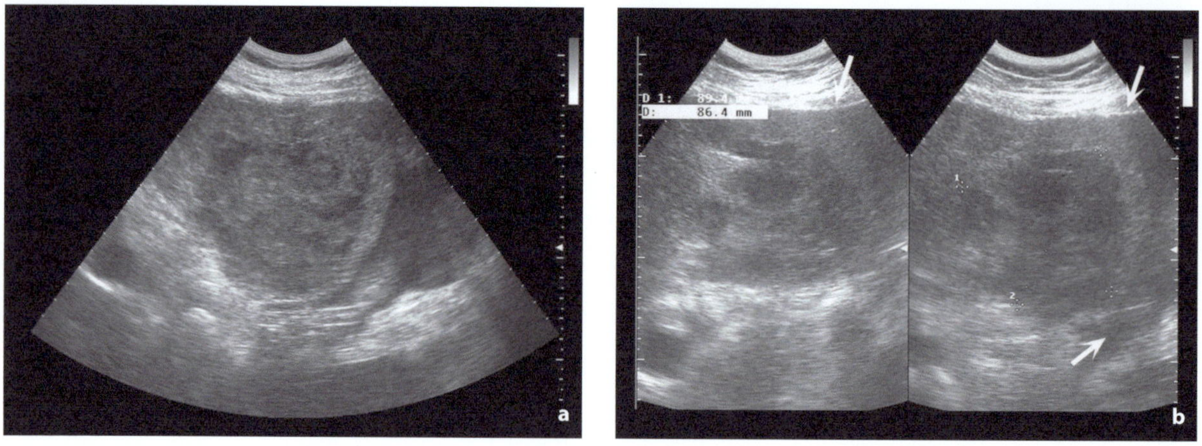

Fig. 7.29a,b Hemoperitoneum after treatment of HCC with RFTA. The follow-up examination performed five days after ablation shows a heterogeneous hypoechoic lesion in the left hepatic lobe with adjacent moderate peritoneal effusion (*arrows*) which was absent prior to treatment. Onset of anemia in the previous days

needle: the condition stabilizes after 2–3 days. An increase by as much as ten times the pretreatment level of serum transaminase is also possible, which then gradually falls over the following days. Bilirubin may also be increased, returning to initial levels after 4–5 days [96]. In the following days the necrosis induced is almost constantly associated with symptoms of malaise, muscle soreness and mild fever (around 38°), which cannot be considered complications but rather an expected event. Occasionally the intraperitoneal opening of the cavity with the ablated material, which has come into contact with the hepatic capsule, can cause acute abdominal pain several days after the treatment. Real **complications** can be distinguished as local and systemic and are fundamentally linked either to the insertion of the needle-electrode or to thermal damage produced by the RF (Figs. 7.29, 7.30). The incidence of major complications after hepatic RFTA is greater than that of multisession PEI and reported at 2–4% with a mortality of 0–1.4%. A large single-center study on cases of HCC and metastases treated with the expandable RITA system [90] identified early major complications in 5% of cases, late major complications in 2% of cases and minor complications in 32.5%. It should, however, be recalled that hepatic resection still has a morbidity >26% and mortality of 3%, with these figures being derived from centers where patients are carefully selected for surgery [86,96]. Hemorrhage (hemoperitoneum) after RFTA is not a rare event but usually limited (<2 units) with onset within several hours of the procedure. Transfusions may be required, but only in rare cases is embolization or surgery necessary. In cirrhotic livers, however, with the additional problem of clotting disorder and low platelet count, not

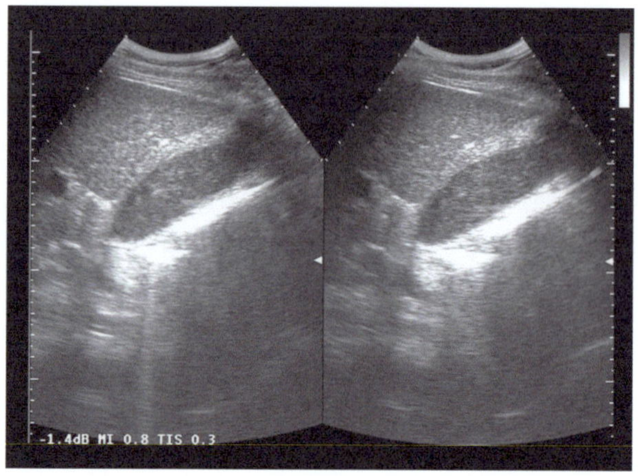

Fig. 7.30 Hemohilia after treatment of HCC with RFTA. Corpuscular hypoechoic material within the gallbladder lumen

inducing excessively large volumes of necrosis is advisable to limit the risk of hemorrhage [96]. Infection of the treated zone usually occurs late, when pathogens penetrating from an even distant portal of entry reach the lesion by a hematogenous or ascending route. Antibiotic therapy is advisable for three months after RFTA in patients with biliary stent or biliary-intestinal anastomosis [96]. In addition to clinical suspicion, abscess formation may be suspected due to the visibility at US of a treated lesion which increases in size or shows internal reverberation artifacts due to gas. Diagnostic aspiration confirms the diagnosis and can indicate antibiotic treatment or drainage. Lesions due to the penetration of the needle in adjacent anatomic structures can lead to pneumothorax, intestinal perforation (especially of the colon), formation of fistulas and/or abscesses, diaphragmatic laceration, occlusion of the hepatic artery and ureteral lesion (for renal RFTA). To avoid these events, some authors have adopted the technique of transcatheter instillation of 0.3–1 L of 5% dextrose between the area to be treated and the adjacent vulnerable structure, i.e. the right pleural cavity or the perihepatic spaces [96,99]. Lesion of the bile duct can produce inflammation, bilomas and stricture and can be prevented by cannulation and cooling of the common bile duct. In general, however, it is advisable to avoid the ablation of lesions located too close to the common bile duct or the gallbladder. Thrombosis of the portal vein or of its lobar or segmental branches can on the one hand increase the ablation effect on the lesion but on the other can cause irreversible failure in the cirrhotic liver [96]. Ablation treatment can in fact lead to temporary or permanent failure of liver function. In particular, in patients with Child C there is the real risk of bleeding from esophageal varices, which generally occurs 15–20 days after treatment. Renal RFTA, in contrast, does not cause a deterioration of kidney function. The ablation of metastases from functional neuroendocrine tumors can induce a marked increase in the blood serum levels of the hormones produced. In carcinoid a possibly fatal hypertensive crisis may be induced and therefore periprocedural treatment with octreotide and thorough postablation monitoring is advisable. Adrenal ablation can lead to hypertensive crises due to the release of catecholamine by the functioning healthy glandular tissue, and therefore arterial pressure should be constantly monitored during the procedure [96].

The incidence of tumor seeding along the needle track is estimated at 0–5% [96]. A multicenter study on 2542 patients treated with RFTA (cool-tip technique) for HCC reported an incidence of 0.9% [74]. In an isolated series, however, a much higher incidence was reported: 12.5% in patients with HCC <5 cm treated with RFTA [100]. As surgery has already shown, the risk is higher with liver metastases than with HCC. The heating of the needle-electrode prior to its withdrawal from the liver can, as stated above, avoid the seeding of tumor cells in the needle track.

One of the main limits of PATs is the volume of necrosis, which does not allow the treatment of large tumors, due to the risk of considerable residual tumor. The percentage recurrence of HCC after RF ablation has been reported at 63% (local in 26% and distant in 53%) [85]. The risk factors for local recurrence are tumor >3 cm, contact of the tumor with a vessel and insufficient safety margin, whereas for recurrence in other hepatic segments the only risk factor reported is elevated AFP levels prior to treatment. This suggests that larger HCCs with elevated serum AFP levels should be treated more aggressively and monitored more closely [85].

Determining the number of ablations required in larger lesions can be difficult, as can establishing the exact location of the needles or the electrodes so as to induce homogeneous distribution of the necrotizing agent, whether it is ethanol or heat, unless multiple overlapping ablations are performed or different ablation therapies are combined. Relying on multiple ablation sessions or using multiple ablation needles tends to complicate the procedure, such that to overcome these limitations **combined treatments** have been used over the years. These modalities see the simultaneous or sequential use of the combined antitumor effects of two different types of locoregional treatment: PEI + chemoembolization (TACE), RFTA + TACE, microwave thermocoagulation + TACE, laser photocoagulation + TACE, ablation with high-intensity focalized ultrasound + TACE, external beam radiation therapy + TACE, PEI + RFTA, percutaneous procedure + obstruction of the arterial or venous flow [98,101–104]. The combination with TACE is able to reduce the negative effects of the latter on liver function, with it being done in a segmental or subsegmental rather than global manner. In addition, the clotting necrosis induced by TACE makes the increased diffusion of ethanol possible in the event of a subsequent PEI [103]. In a recent series of patients with early-stage HCC, RF combined with TACE produced a 5-year survival rate comparable with that from hepatectomy [105].

Combined treatment with PEI and RFTA is able to produce a larger necrosis volume than the simple arithmetic addition of the destructive effect of the two techniques, due to mutual strengthening. In fact the ethanol induces coagulative necrosis which facilitates the diffusion of the heat, in part due to the thrombosing effect on the small intralesional vessels (the effect of the RF is in fact reduced in areas with persistent perfusion). In addition, it is thought that the ethanol is heated by the subsequent application of the RF, with an increase in its necrotizing effect and diffusion in the tumor areas without RFTA [106]. In some centers the ethanol is injected centrally and the thermoablation is performed peripherally, whereas in others the opposite is done, but always with PEI preceding RFTA (although the RFTA electrodes are placed first since the hyperechogenicity induced by the ethanol would make it difficult to do at a later time) (Fig. 7.31, Video 7.14). The combined procedure PEI + RFTA is able to reduce the number and duration of the applications of RF per session and is even able to make

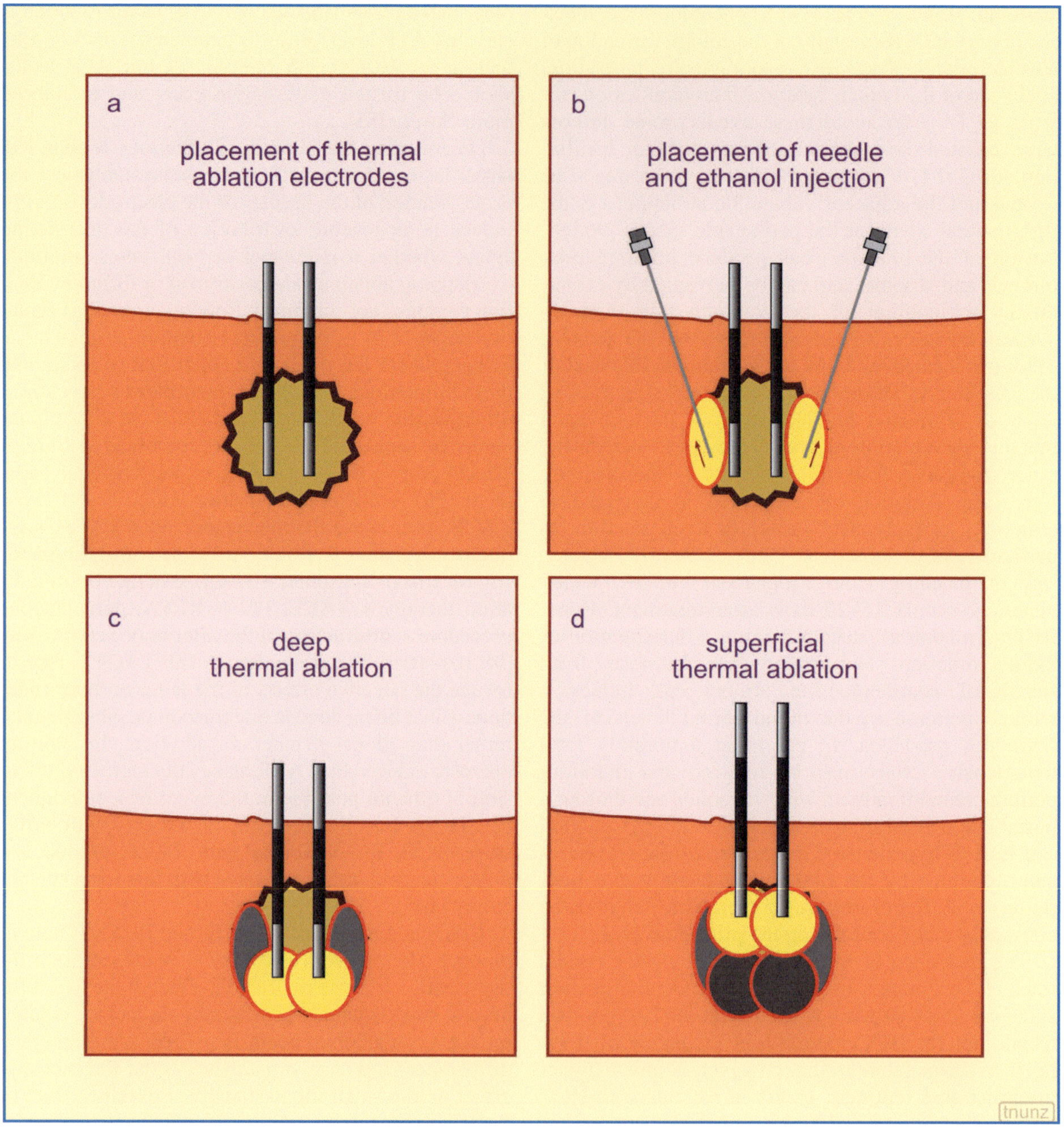

Fig. 7.31a-d Combined treatment with RFTA and PEI for HCC >4 cm. The RF electrodes are first positioned (**a**). Then the needles are inserted and ethanol injected (**b**). Lastly the thermoablation is performed on the deep portion (**c**) and superficial portion (**d**) of the lesion. Modified from [98]

lesions in "difficult" locations accessible to treatment, such as subcapsular, paracholecystic and paradiaphragmatic lesions (although a recent study failed to reveal differences in the complications after RF between subcapsular and deep lesions [107]). In these cases ethanol is used on the side of the lesion adjacent to the zone at risk and RF on the other [98,108].

7.11 Assessment of Liver Lesions Treated with Ablation Therapies

Diagnostic imaging performs numerous tasks in the evaluation of lesions treated with PATs. These include determining the effective destruction of all the neoplastic tissue (completeness of necrosis), identifying possible complications and the early identification of disease recurrence, both in the site of treatment (true recurrence) and in other portions of the organ in question (appearance of new nodules). Follow-up is clearly fundamental both in the patient with HCC and in the patient with metastasis from an extrahepatic tumor, because the natural tendency is towards the development of new lesions. The early identification of **residual**, **recurrence** or **new lesions** is important, at least in the patient treated with radical intent, because it improves the possibility of early treatment and therefore disease control.

Tumor markers, in particular AFP for HCC and CEA for metastases from colon cancer, are a parameter indicating the general state of the disease, but they have limited value in describing the state of viability of the individual treated nodule [81].

US has difficulty demonstrating necrosis. The hyperechogenicity produced by the diffusion of ethanol in PEI, or by heat in RFTA or other similar therapies, only very approximately indicates the extension of the necrotic area and cannot be used as an effective estimate of possible residual tumor during the course of ablation therapy [81] (Fig. 7.32). In addition, the echogenicity produced by the treatment of the superficial part of the lesion conceals the visualization of the deep portions, unless the deep portion is systematically treated first and then the superficial portion of the lesion. In reality, the ablation is often continued until the broadest possible area of necrosis is achieved, within the limits of patient safety and compliance.

US is unable to distinguish between necrotic tissue and healthy tissue within the lesion treated, the post-treatment appearance of which is in fact variable and nonspecific. Hypoechoic lesions tend to become iso-hyperechoic and hyperechoic lesions tend to become heterogeneous, but this clearly is not sufficient for establishing whether there is a component of residual active tumor tissue or not (Figs. 7.33, 7.44). The focal necrotic outcome repeats the shape and size of the original lesion, occasionally appearing more ellipsoid, i.e. elongated towards the direction of the source of ablation. Especially after RF and laser photocoagulation, the study may reveal bands of greater echogenicity within the necrotic lesions, at least in the larger lesions. These bands are sign of the carbonization produced by the electrode or the needle [81].

CD and **PD** have been proposed in the past for evaluation of the effectiveness of PATs, but their role has been limited since the introduction of CEUS. PD is without doubt more sensitive than CD, and both techniques increase their sensitivity with the injection of US contrast medium. However, the value of the Doppler techniques is on balance positive, as they can indicate residual tumor when they identify

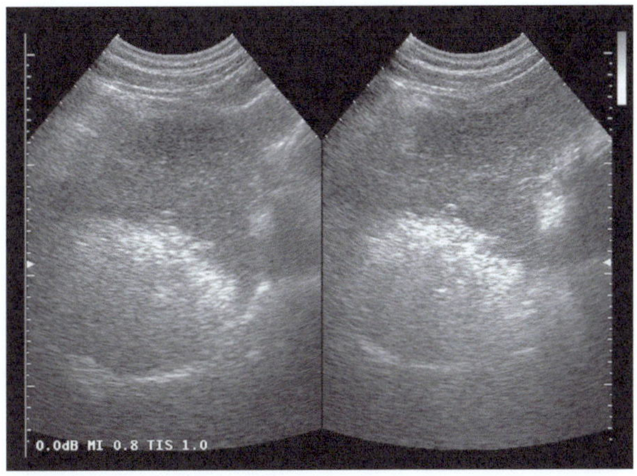

Fig. 7.32 HCC after treatment with PEI in single session. US scan performed two days after the one-shot session shows diffuse gaseous and artifactual hyperechogenicity

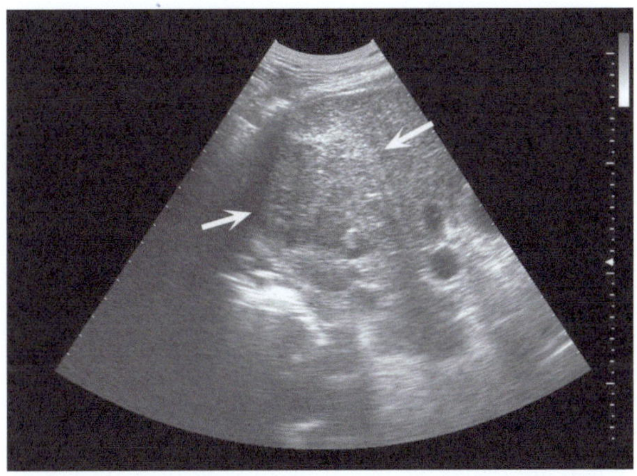

Fig. 7.33 HCC after RFTA. Nonspecific heterogeneous echogenic appearance of the large nodular hepatic lesion (*arrows*)

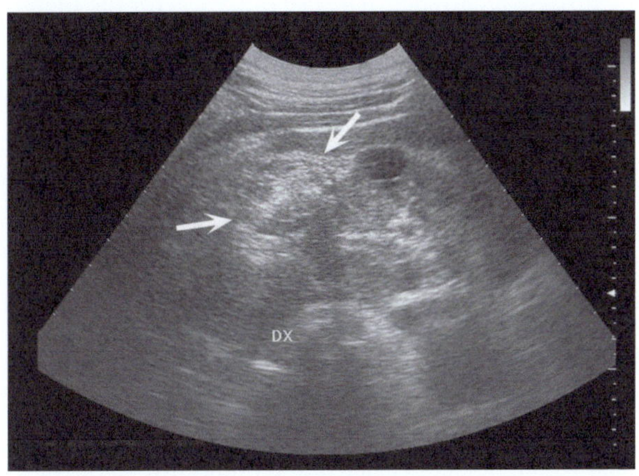

Fig. 7.34 Necrotic renal cell carcinoma after RFTA in patient with single kidney. The scan at six months from ablation treatment shows an exophytic heterogeneous echogenic lesion of the right kidney (*arrows*)

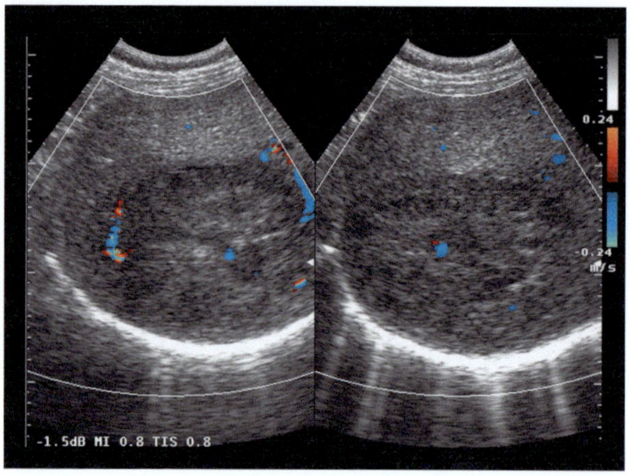

Fig. 7.35 Active residue of HCC after combined treatment with transcatheter chemoembolization and PEI. CD study of the large hepatic lesion shows some residual arterial signals

intra-lesional vascular signals after treatment. In this case CD can be useful in the guidance of percutaneous retreatment targeted at the areas of residual vascularity [109–111] (Fig. 7.35). Instead in the case of absent flows, concluding that there has been complete necrosis is indubitably arbitrary, although each case should be evaluated on its own merits. At any rate, several series have demonstrated that CT is superior to the Doppler techniques in defining the results of treatment [112].

CEUS is useful for guiding the treatment of lesions which are barely visible if at all at gray-scale US, or for guiding the ablation of already treated lesion with local recurrence. In this case US may encounter difficulties in recognizing the necrotic component caused by disease recurrence. The use of CEUS for the identification of residual tumor immediately after ablation and during the same treatment session is conceptually very interesting, particularly in the treatment of larger lesions which require the insertion of multiple electrodes and in which the hyperechogenicity developed from the treatment may conceal certain areas of residual tumor.

In both PEI and other PATs, an extemporaneous ablation targeted at the residual active tissue identified by CEUS can be done. In practice, however, other factors need to be considered, such as the consequential increase in the total time of the ablation session and the hyperechogenicity induced by the ethanol or heat which hinders visualization of the still viable parts of the tumor, which also appear hyperechoic [6]. Postprocedural CEUS, performed in the first 24 h after the treatment, is useful in that it can define the need for retreatment and plan it early, without needing to wait for the CT or MR study at 2–3 weeks. However, CEUS performed within an hour of the ablation procedure has proven to be less accurate than follow-up at two weeks with CT or MR (sensitivity 40%, specificity 94%), with a concordant result in 76% of cases [113]. CEUS is especially useful in multisession PEI. CEUS study can in fact define the number of sessions and the quantity of ethanol still required, thus avoiding undertreatment in the case of residual tumor and overtreatment when the lesion appears completely necrotic and therefore the therapeutic protocol can be interrupted and the patient scheduled for follow-up. Even in the kidney CEUS has demonstrated its utility in postablation evaluation, at least for lesions which are accessible for the depth of exploration [82].

Residual tumor is located peripherally, where the ethanol has more difficulty diffusing due to the presence of intralesional septations and where the heat or the cold used by the other PATs is obstructed by the cooling or warming action, respectively, of the perilesional vessels. The residual tumor, both HCC and metastases, is also often eccentric, being more commonly located on the deep side of the lesion treated, with a crescent shape or, more rarely, a nodular appearance (Fig. 7.36). In HCC it is markedly hyperechoic in the arterial phase, whereas in metastases it is more difficult to identify, appearing as a more-or-less mild vascularity in both the arterial phase and the portal-sinusoidal phase (Figs. 7.37–7.40). Often the viable tumor tissue can be identified adjacent to a larger paranodular vessel which is visible as it protrudes marginally towards the area of necrosis ("perivascular cuff"). The agreement between CEUS follow-up and CT or MR follow-up is 91% [113]. CEUS has difficulty in differential diagnosis between residual tumor and large residual vessels adjacent to the lesion, as well as with the postablation granulation tissue, which nonetheless tends to be thin and circumferential and furthermore to disappear at the subsequent controls.

Early CT is today used only in the suspicion of complications. Multiphase CT is the most used imaging modality for the evaluation of lesions treated with percutaneous procedures, since it is panoramic, standardized and reliable [114,115]. The study, with **CT** or **dynamic MR** (possibly with liver-specific contrast media) is performed within six weeks of treatment [95]. Prior to this time earlier information could be obtained regarding the persistence of viable tissue and therefore regarding the need for retreatment. However, an examination performed in the first 15 days from the ablation session often creates interpretation difficulties, since reactive phenomena are present which can mimic the persistence of neoplastic tissue. It should also be borne in mind that CEUS is

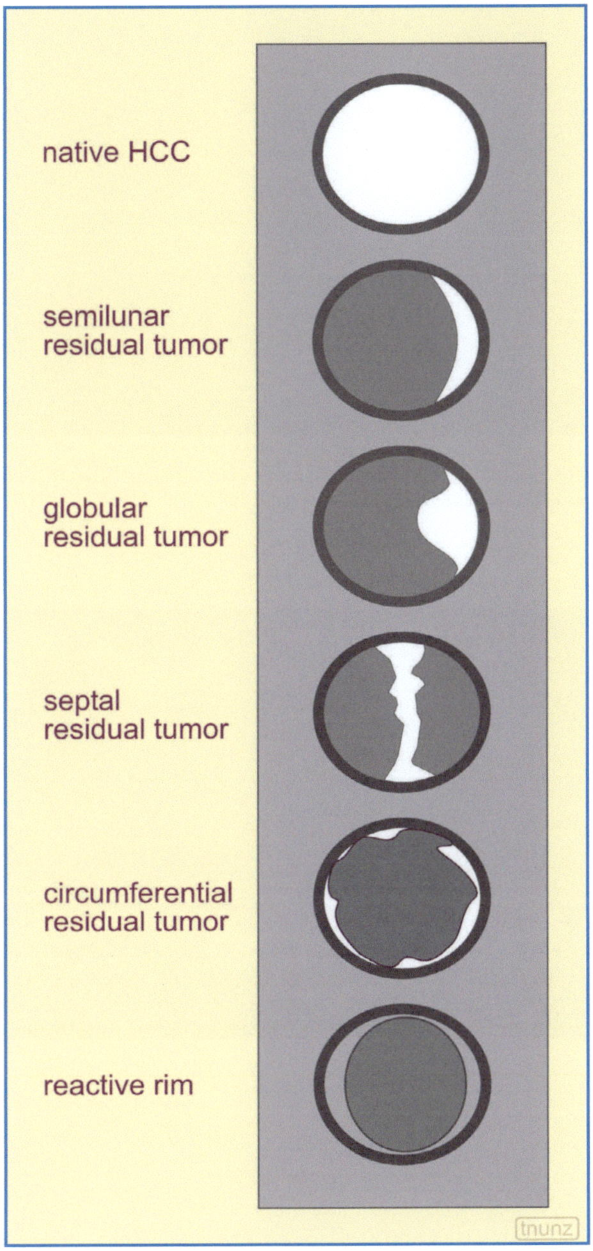

Fig. 7.36 Main CEUS patterns of residual tumor after percutaneous ablation. The hypervascular (hyperechoic) residue of HCC can be crescent shaped, nodular, hourglass shaped along internal septations, or circumferential. Particularly in the latter case reactive tissue should be distinguished from perilesional granulation tissue

increasingly being used in early post-treatment evaluation, with indication for retreatment in the case of identification of residual disease. In the case of complete necrosis, the patient is sent to CT or MR follow-up, which is performed increasingly late (even 3–6 months at some centers with significant

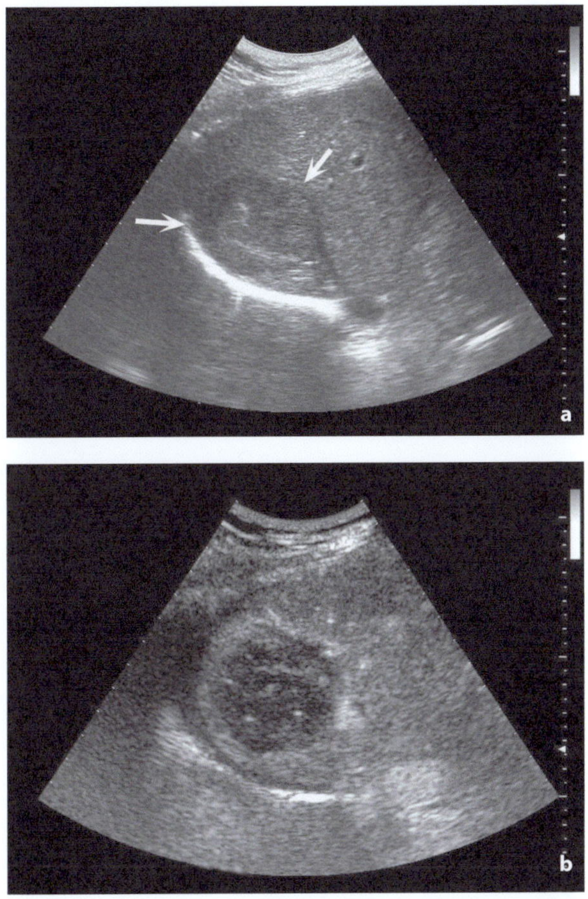

Fig. 7.37a,b HCC treated with RFTA. The pretreatment scan shows a large, nodular, hypoechoic lesion (**a**, *arrows*). CEUS scan after ablation (**b**) shows substantial avascularity of the lesion, with mild perilesional reactive phenomena

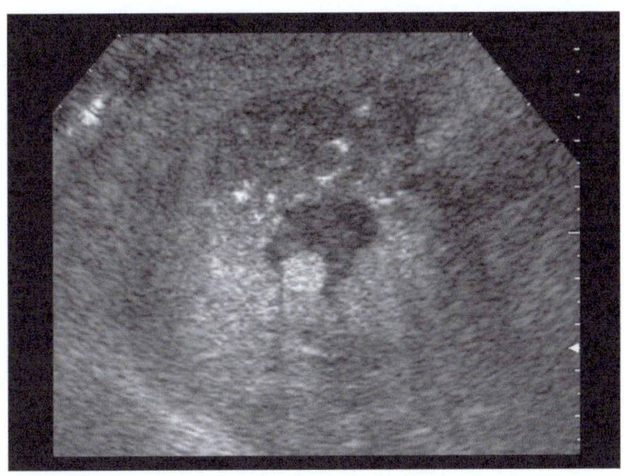

Fig. 7.38 HCC, residual tumor after treatment with PEI. CEUS scan with intermittent system in the arterial phase shows a necrotic hypoechoic lesion with an eccentric nodularity of persistent enhancement

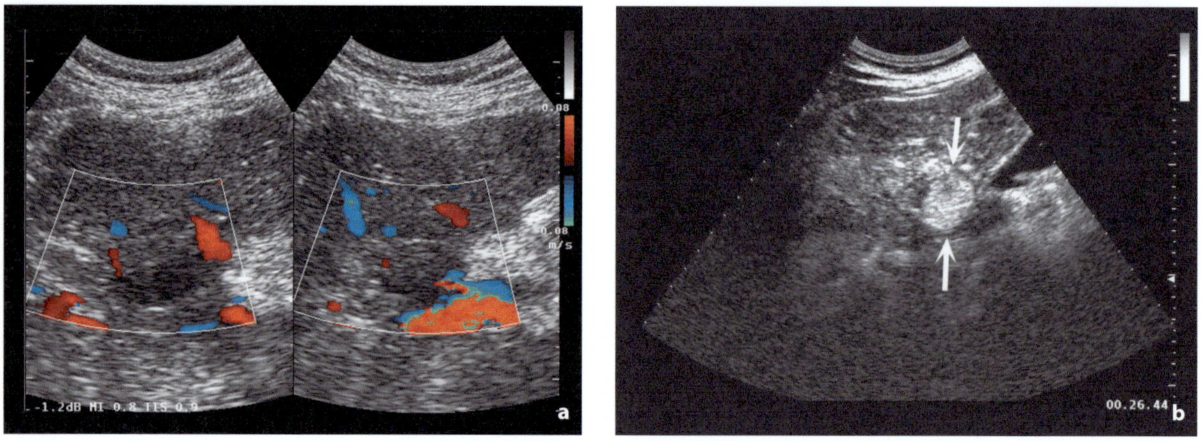

Fig. 7.39a,b Residue of HCC after treatment with PEI. CD study after treatment shows some residual vascular signals (**a**). CEUS evaluation in the arterial phase identifies large hypervascular nodular residue (**b**, *arrows*)

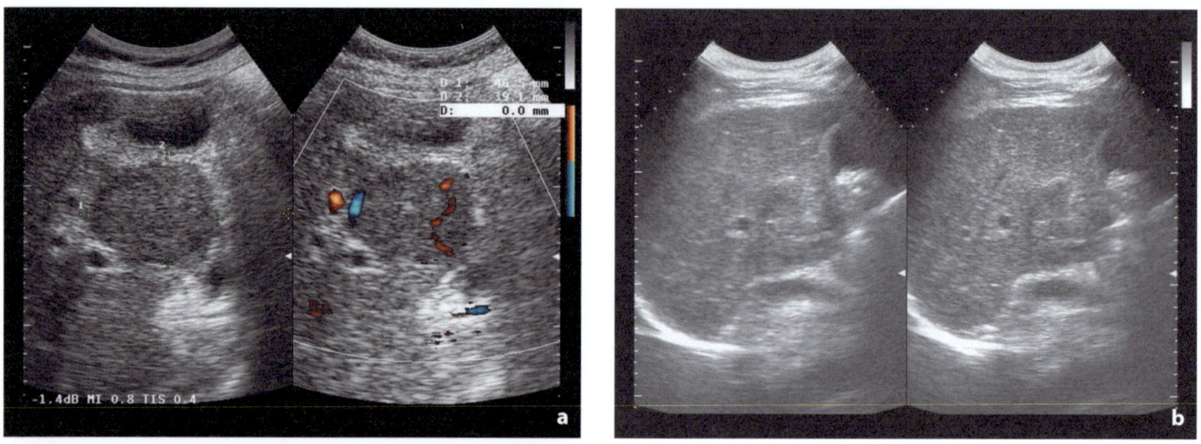

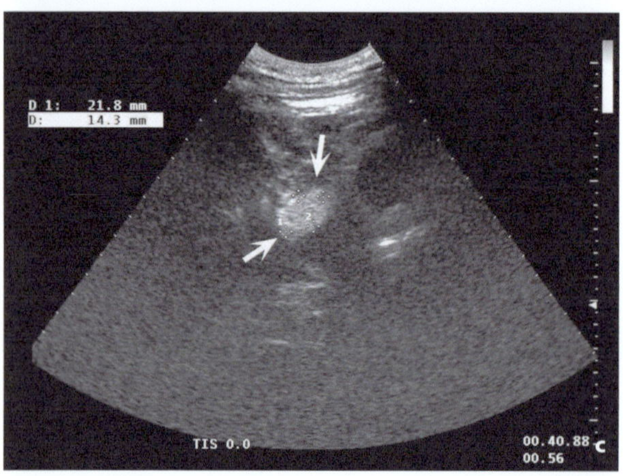

Fig. 7.40a-c Residue of HCC after combined treatment with PEI and RFTA. Hepatic nodule adjacent to gallbladder with internal arterial signals at directional PD (**a**). The portion adjacent to the gallbladder is treated with PEI and the rest with RFTA. Nonspecific heterogeneous hypoechoic appearance after treatment (**b**). Nodularity of residual viable tissue (*arrows*) in the CEUS study in the arterial phase (**c**)

experience with CEUS). The interval of long-term follow-up is 3–6 months which becomes one year in subjects treated a long time ago. The follow-up is based on tumor markers and US, with the use of CEUS or the heavy machines in select cases and especially in the presence of changes of the known picture. Recurrence can be within the treated areas (clearly due to the persistence of microscopic tumor foci), on the margins

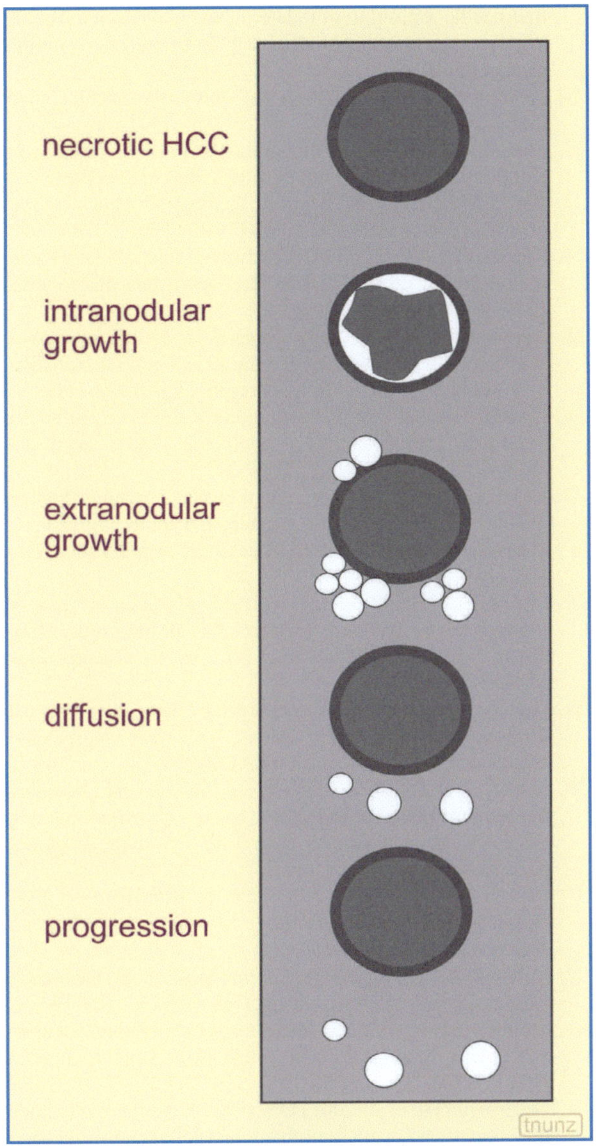

Fig. 7.41 Main CEUS patterns of tumor recurrence after percutaneous ablation. Patterns include growth within the treated nodule, growth marginally external to the treated nodule, diffusion within the same segment as the treated nodule and progression with new nodules in segments other than the treated segment. Modified from [116]

of the necrotic lesion, in the same segment but not in contact with the original necrotic region (also possibly due to the growth of a microscopic satellite nodule) or in another segment (more as a consequence than a recurrence of the same organ nature of HCC) [116] (Figs. 7.41–7.43).

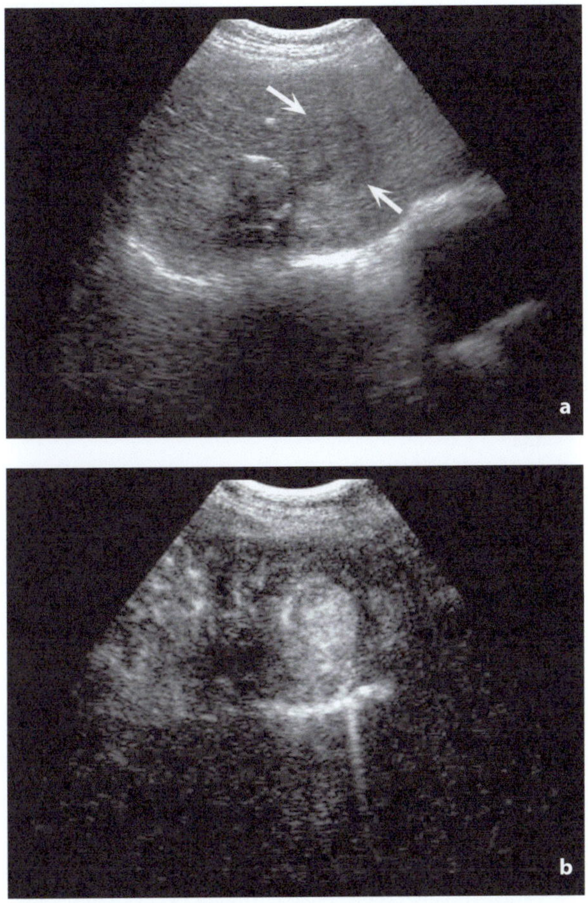

Fig. 7.42a,b Recurrence of HCC after PEI. US (**a**) shows a heterogeneous hypoechoic nodularity (*arrows*) adjacent to a treated lesion with marginal calcifications. CEUS in the arterial phase (**b**) demonstrates the hypervascularity of the paranodular recurrence and the persistent avascularity of the treated nodule

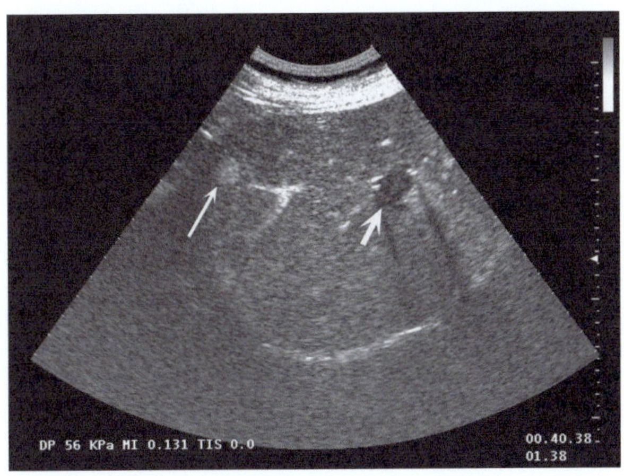

Fig. 7.43 New nodule of HCC in patient with necrotic nodule after PEI. CEUS study in the arterial phase shows an anechoic necrotic nodule (*short arrow*) and a new nodule with hypervascular appearance in another segment (*long arrow*)

References

1. Baatenburg de Jong RJ et al (1991) Ultrasound-guided fine-needle aspiration biopsy of neck nodes. Arch Otolaryngol Head Neck Surg 117:402-404
2. Middleton WD et al (1997) Small (1.5 cm or less) liver metastases: US-guided biopsy. Radiology 205:729-732
3. Yu SCH et al (2001) US-guided percutaneous biopsy of small (1-cm) hepatic lesions. Radiology 218:195-199
4. Numata K et al (2008) Ablation therapy guided by contrast-enhanced sonography with sonazoid for hepatocellular carcinoma lesions not detected by conventional sonography. J Ultrasound Med 27:395-406
5. Skjoldbye B et al (2002) Improved detection and biopsy of solid liver lesions using pulse-inversion ultrasound scanning and contrast agent infusion. Ultrasound Med Biol 28:439-444
6. Solbiati L et al (2004) Guidance and monitoring of radiofrequency liver tumor ablation with contrast-enhanced ultrasound. Eur J Radiol 51(suppl)S19-S23
7. Hirooka M et al (2006) Virtual sonographic radiofrequency ablation of hepatocellular carcinoma visualized on CT but not on conventional sonography. AJR Am J Roentgenol 186:S255-S260
8. Minami Y et al (2004) Treatment of hepatocellular carcinoma with radiofrequency ablation: usefulness of contrast harmonic sonography for lesions poorly defined with B-mode sonography. AJR Am J Roentgenol 183:153-156
9. Rhim H et al (2008) Planning sonography to assess the feasibility of percutaneous radiofrequency ablation of hepatocellular carcinomas. AJR Am J Roentgenol 190:1324-1330
10. Crystal P et al (2005) Accuracy of sonographically guided 14-gauge core-needle biopsy: results of 715 consecutive breast biopsies with at least two-year follow-up of benign lesions. J Clin Ultrasound 33:47-52
11. Soo MS et al (2003) Sonographic detection and sonographically guided biopsy of breast microcalcifications. AJR Am J Roentgenol 180:941-948
12. Wu HP et al (1998) Percutaneous drainage of fluid collections in the extremities. Radiology 208:159-165
13. Bradley MJ (2001) An in-vitro study to understand successful free-hand ultrasound guided intervention. Clin Radiol 53:495-498
14. Wojtowycz M (1995) Handbook of interventional radiology and angiography. II edition. Mosby, St. Louis
15. Konno K et al (2003) Image distortion in US-guided liver tumor puncture with curved linear array. Eur Radiol 13:1291-1296
16. Hopkins RE et al (2001) In-vitro visualization of biopsy needles with ultrasound: a comparative study of standard and echogenic needles using an ultrasound phantom. Clin Radiol 56:499-502
17. Albrecht H et al (2006) Real-time 3D (4D) Ultrasound-guided percutaneous biopsy of solid tumours. Ultraschall in Med 27:324-328
18. Orsi F et al (2004) Factors affecting the results of ultrasound-guided percutaneous biopsy in oncology. Radiol Med 107:252-260
19. Bonifacino A et al (2005) Accuracy rates of US-guided vacuum-assisted breast biopsy. Anticancer Res 25:2465-2470
20. Krishnamurthy S et al (2002) Role of ultrasound-guided fine-needle aspiration of indeterminate and suspicious axillary lymph nodes in the initial staging of breast carcinoma. Cancer 95:982-988
21. Wong KT et al (2005) Ultrasound of thyroid cancer. Cancer Imaging 5:157-166
22. Solbiati L et al (2001) Ultrasound of thyroid, parathyroid glands and neck lymph nodes. Eur Radiol 11:2411-2424
23. Walsh RM et al (1999) The management of solitary thyroid nodule: a review. Clin Otolaryngol Allied Sci 24:388-397
24. Rubaltelli L et al (2004) Ultrasonography of superficial lymph nodes: results acquired and new trials. Radiol Med 107:388-400
25. Alexander AA et al (1997) Superficial soft-tissue masses suggestive of recurrent malignancy: sonographic localization and biopsy. AJR Am J Roentgenol 169:1449-1451
26. Civardi G et al (1994) Lytic bone lesions suspected for metastasis: ultrasonically guided fine-needle aspiration biopsy. J Clin Ultrasound 22:307-311
27. Maturen KE et al (2006) Lack of tumor seeding of hepatocellular carcinoma after percutaneous needle biopsy using coaxial cutting needle technique. AJR Am J Roentgenol 187:1184-1187
28. McGahan JP (2008) Invasive ultrasound principles (biopsy, aspiration, and drainage. In: McGahan JP et al (eds) Diagnostic ultrasound, II edition. Informa Healthcare, New York, 81-104
29. Giorgio A et al (2003) Complications after interventional sonography of focal liver lesions. A 22-year single-center experience. J Ultrasound Med 22:193-205
30. Sheikh M et al (2000) Deep-seated thoracic and abdominal masses: usefulness of ultrasound and computed tomography guidance in fine needle aspiration cytology diagnosis. Australas Radiol 44:155-160
31. Pupulim LF et al (2008) Algorithm for immediate cytologic diagnosis of hepatic tumors. AJR Am J Roentgenol 190:W208 - W212
32. Mitchell IC et al (2007) Adrenal masses in the cancer patient: surveillance or excision. Oncologist 12:168-174
33. Maturen KE et al (2007) Renal mass core biopsy: accuracy and impact on clinical management. AJR Am J Roentgenol 188:563-570
34. Ledermann HP et al (2001) Diagnosis of symptomatic intestinal metastases using transabdominal sonography and sonographically guided puncture. AJR Am J Roentgenol 176:155-158
35. Youk JH et al (2008) Sonographically guided 14-gauge core needle biopsy of breast masses: a review of 2,420 cases with long-term follow-up. AJR Am J Roentgenol 190:202-207
36. Schueller G et al (2008) US-guided 14-gauge core-needle breast biopsy: results of a validation study in 1352 cases. Radiology 248:406-413
37. Zuiani C et al (2005) Proliferative high-risk lesions of the breast: contribution and limits of US-guided core biopsy. Radiol Med 110:589-602
38. Cipolla C et al (2006) Validity of needle core biopsy in the histological characterisation of mammary lesions. The Breast 15:76-80
39. Youk JK et al (2007) Missed breast cancers at US-guided core needle biopsy: how to reduce them. Radiographics 27:79-94
40. Kwak JY et al (2007) Primary thyroid lymphoma: role of ultrasound-guided needle biopsy. J Ultrasound Med 26:1761-1765

41. Nori J et al (2005) Role of axillary lymph node ultrasound and large core biopsy in the preoperative assessment of patients selected for sentinel node biopsy. Radiol Med 109:330-344
42. Howlett DC et al (2007) Sonographically guided core biopsy of a parotid mass. AJR Am J Roentgenol 188:223-227
43. Fornage BD (2000) Soft-tissue masses: the case for increased utilization of sonography. Appl Radiol 10:8-22
44. Nikolaidis P et al (2005) Liposarcoma subtypes: identification with computed tomography and ultrasound-guided percutaneous needle biopsy. Eur Radiol 15:383-389
45. Stockberger SM et al (1999) Abdominal and pelvic needle aspiration biopsies: can we perform them well when using small needles? Abdom Imaging 24:321-328
46. Smith EH (1991) Complications of percutaneous abdominal fine-needle biopsy. Radiology 178:253-258
47. Heilo A et al (1997) Liver hemangioma: US-guided 18-gauge core-needle biopsy. Radiology 204:719-722
48. Sartori S et al (2007) Accuracy of transthoracic sonography in detection of pneumothorax after sonographically guided lung biopsy: prospective comparison with chest radiography. AJR Am J Roentgenol 188:37-41
49. Bruix J et al (2001) Clinical management of hepatocellular carcinoma. Conclusions of the Barcelona-2000 EASL conference. European Association for the Study of the Liver. J Hepatol 35:4214-30
50. Akin O et al (2006) Imaging of prostate cancer. Radiol Clin North Am 45:207-222
51. Parker SH et al (1996) Ultrasound guided mammotomy. A new breast biopsy technique. J Diagn Med Sonogr 12:113-118
52. March DE et al (2003) Breast masses: removal of all US evidence during biopsy by using a handheld vacuum-assisted device: initial experience. Radiology 227:549–555
53. Tregnaghi A et al (2005) Usefulness and limits of ultrasound-guided hook-wire positioning for localisation of soft tissue lesions prior to surgery. Radiol Med 110:646-654
54. Kopans DB et al (1989) Preoperative imaging-guided needle placement and localization of clinically occult breast lesions. AJR Am J Roentgenol 152:1-9
55. De Cicco C et al (2002) Radioguided occult lesion localisation (ROLL) and surgical biopsy in breast cancer. Technical aspects. Q J Nucl Med 46:145-151
56. Nadeem R et al (2005) Occult breast lesions: a comparison between radioguided occult lesion localisation (ROLL) vs. wire-guided lumpectomy (WGL). Breast 14:283-289
57. Strnad P et al (2006) Radioguided occult lesion localisation in combination with detection of the sentinel lymph node in non-palpable breast cancer tumours. Eur J Gynaecol Oncol 27:236-238
58. Caremani M et al (2004) US guided percutaneous treatment of hepatic infectious lesions. Giorn It Ecogr 7:223-232
59. Abbitt PL et al (1990) Endovaginal sonography for guidance in draining pelvic fluid collections. AJR Am J Roentgenol 154:849-850
60. Sperling DC et al (1998) Deep pelvic abscess: transperineal US-guided drainage. Radiology 208:111-115
61. Lucey BC et al (2006) Radiologic management of cysts in the abdomen and pelvis. AJR Am J Roentgenol 186:562-573
62. Mehta TS (2003) Current uses of ultrasound in the evaluation of the breast. Radiol Clin North Am 41:841-856
63. Larssen TB et al (2003) Single-session alcohol sclerotherapy in symptomatic benign hepatic cysts performed with a time of exposure to alcohol of 10 min: initial results. Eur Radiol 13:2627-2632
64. Agostini S et al (2004) Percutaneous treatment of simple renal cysts with sclerotherapy and extended drainage. Radiol Med 108:522-529
65. Chung BH et al (2000) Comparison of single and multiple sessions of percutaneous sclerotherapy for simple renal cyst. Br J Urol 85:626-627
66. Caliendo MV et al (2001) Sclerotherapy with use of doxycycline after percutaneous drainage of postoperative lymphoceles. J Vasc Interv Radiol 12:73-77
67. Karcaaltincaba M et al (2005) Radiologic imaging and percutaneous treatment of pelvic lymphocele. Eur J Radiol 55:340-354
68. Gorich J et al (1995) Percutaneous drainage of refractory necrotizing tumors: experience in 9 patients. Rofo 163:527-531
69. Ross GJ et al (1989) Sonographically-guided paracentesis for palliation of symptomatic malignant ascites. AJR Am J Roentgenol 153:1309-1311
70. Brooks RA et al (2006) Long-term semi-permanent catheter use for the palliation of malignant ascites. Gynecol Oncol 101:360-362
71. Rosenberg S et al (2004) Comparison of percutaneous management techniques for recurrent ascites. J Vasc Interv Radiol 15:1129-1131
72. Bartolozzi C et al (1996) Ethanol injection for the treatment of hepatic tumours. Eur Radiol 6:682-696
73. Livraghi T (2003) Radiofrequency ablation, PEIT, and TACE for hepatocellular carcinoma. J Hepatobiliary Pancreat Surg 10:67-76
74. Livraghi T et al (2005) Risk of tumour seeding after percutaneous radiofrequency ablation for HCC. Br J Surg 92:856-858
75. Livraghi T et al (1999) Small hepatocellular carcinoma: treatment with radio-frequency ablation versus ethanol injection. Radiology 210:655-661
76. Livraghi T (2001) Treatment of hepatocellular carcinoma by interventional methods. Eur Radiol 11:2207-2219
77. Di Stasi M et al (1997) Percutaneous ethanol injection in the treatment of HCC. A multicenter survey of evaluation practices and complication rates. Scand J Gastroenterol 32:1168-1173
78. Ishii H et al (1998) Needle tract implantation of HCC after percutaneous ethanol injection. Cancer 82:1638-1642
79. Lencioni R et al (2005) A critical appraisal of the literature on local ablative therapies for hepatocellular carcinoma. Clin Liver Dis 9:301-314
80. Giorgio A et al (1996) One-shot percutaneous ethanol injection of liver tumors under general anesthesia: preliminary data on efficacy and complications. Cardiovasc Intervent Radiol 19:27-31
81. Scott Gazelle G et al (2000) Tumor ablation with radiofrequency energy. Radiology 217:633-646
82. Meloni MF et al (2008) Follow-up after percutaneous radiofrequency ablation of renal cell carcinoma: contrast-enhanced sonography versus contrast-enhanced CT or MRI. AJR Am J Roentgenol 191:1233-1238
83. Giorgio A et al (2000) Interstitial laser photocoagulation under ultrasound guidance of liver tumors. Eur J Ultrasound 11:181-188

84. Lau WY (2002) Management of hepatocellular carcinoma. J R Coll Surg Edinb 47:389-399
85. Kim Y-S (2006) Intrahepatic recurrence after percutaneous radiofrequency ablation of hepatocellular carcinoma: analysis of the pattern and risk factors. Eur J Radiol 59:432-441
86. Tateishi R et al (2005) Percutaneous radiofrequency ablation for HCC. An analysis of 1000 cases. Cancer 103:1201-1209
87. Choi J (2006) Imaging of hepatic metastases. Cancer Contr 13:6-12
88. Solbiati L et al (1997) Hepatic metastases: percutaneous radiofrequency ablation with cooled-tip electrodes. Radiology 205:367-373
89. Brieger J et al (2003) In vivo efficiency of four commercial monopolar radiofrequency ablation systems: a comparative experimental study in pig liver. Invest Radiol 38:609-616
90. Buscarini L et al (2004) Radiofrequency thermal ablation with expandable needle of focal liver malignancies: complication report. Eur Radiol 14:31-37
91. Curley SA et al (1999) Radiofrequency ablation of unresectable primary and metastatic hepatic malignancies: results in 123 patients. Ann Surg 230:1-8
92. Francica F et al (1999) Ultrasound-guided percutaneous treatment of hepatocellular carcinoma by radiofrequency hyperthermia by "cooled-tip needle": a preliminary clinical experience. Eur J Ultrasound 9:145-153
93. Lee JM et al (2004) Saline-enhanced hepatic radiofrequency ablation using a perfused-cooled electrode: comparison of dual probe bipolar mode with monopolar and single probe bipolar modes. Korean J Radiol 5:121-127
94. De Baere T et al (2001) Radio-frequency liver ablation: experimental comparative study of water-cooled vs. expandable systems. AJR Am J Roentgenol 176:187-192
95. Goldberg BB (2005) Contrast-enhanced sonographic imaging of lymphatic channels and sentinel lymph nodes. J Ultrasound Med 24:953-965
96. Gillams AR (2005) Complications of percutaneous therapy. Cancer Imaging 5:110-113
97. Minami Y et al (2007) Contrast harmonic sonography-guided radiofrequency ablation therapy versus B-mode sonography in hepatocellular carcinoma: prospective randomized controlled trial. AJR Am J Roentgenol 188:489-494
98. Vallone P et al (2006) Combined ethanol injection therapy and radiofrequency ablation therapy in percutaneous treatment of hepatocellular carcinoma larger than 4 cm. Cardiovasc Intervent Radiol 29:544-551
99. Rhim H et al (2008) Planning sonography to assess the feasibility of percutaneous radiofrequency ablation of hepatocellular carcinomas. AJR Am J Roentgenol 190:1324-1330
100. Llovet JM et al (2001) Increased risk of tumour seeding after percutaneous radiofrequency ablation of a single hepatocellular carcinoma. Hepatology 33:1336-1337
101. Buscarini L et al (1999) Percutaneous radiofrequency thermal ablation combined with transcatheter arterial embolization in the treatment of large hepatocellular carcinoma. Ultraschall Med 20:47-53
102. Gasparini D et al (2002) Combined treatment, TACE and RF ablation, in HCC: preliminary results. Radiol Med 104:412-420
103. Lencioni R et al (1998) Combined transcatheter arterial chemoembolization and percutaneous ethanol injection for the treatment of large hepatocellular carcinoma: local therapeutic effect and long-term survival rate. Eur Radiol 8:439-444
104. Qian J et al (2003) Combined interventional therapies of hepatocellular carcinoma. World J Gastroenterol 9:1885-1891
105. Yamakado K et al (2008) Early-stage hepatocellular carcinoma: radiofrequency ablation combined with chemoembolization versus hepatectomy. Radiology 247:260-266
106. Goldberg SN et al (2000) Percutaneous tumor ablation: increased coagulation by combining radio-frequency ablation and ethanol instillation in a rat breast tumor model. Radiology 210:655-661
107. Sartori S et al (2008) Subcapsular liver tumors treated with percutaneous radiofrequency ablation: a prospective comparison with nonsubcapsular liver tumors for safety and effectiveness. Radiology 248:670-679
108. Kurokohchi K et al (2002) Combination therapy of percutaneous ethanol injection and radiofrequency ablation against hepatocellular carcinomas difficult to treat. Int J Oncol 21:611-615
109. Bartolozzi C et al (1998) Hepatocellular carcinoma treatment with percutaneous ethanol injection: evaluation with contrast-enhanced color Doppler US. Radiology 209:387-393
110. Choi D et al (2000) Hepatocellular carcinoma treated with percutaneous radio-frequency ablation: usefulness of power Doppler US with a microbubble contrast agent in evaluating therapeutic response – preliminary results. Radiology 217:558-563
111. Lencioni R et al (2005) A critical appraisal of the literature on local ablative therapies for hepatocellular carcinoma. Clin Liver Dis 9:301-314
112. Vallone P et al (2003) Local ablation procedures in primary liver tumors: Levovist US versus spiral CT to evaluate therapeutic results. Anticancer Res 23:5075-5079
113. Dill-Macky MJ et al (2006) Radiofrequency ablation of hepatocellular carcinoma: predicting success using contrast-enhanced sonography. AJR Am J Roentgenol 186:S287-295
114. Catalano O et al (2000) Helical CT findings in patients with hepatocellular carcinoma treated with percutaneous ablation procedures. J Comput Assist Tomogr 24:748-754
115. Catalano O et al (2000) Multiphase helical CT findings after percutaneous ablation procedures for hepatocellular carcinoma. Abdom Imaging 25:607-614
116. Catalano O et al (2001) Hepatocellular carcinoma recurrence after percutaneous ablation therapy: helical CT patterns. Abdom Imaging 26:375-383

Subject Index

A

B

C

D

E

M

N

O

P

Q

R

S

T

U

V

W

MIX
Papier aus verantwortungsvollen Quellen
Paper from responsible sources
FSC® C105338

If you have any concerns about our products,
you can contact us on
ProductSafety@springernature.com

In case Publisher is established outside the EU,
the EU authorized representative is:
Springer Nature Customer Service Center GmbH
Europaplatz 3, 69115 Heidelberg, Germany

Printed by Libri Plureos GmbH
in Hamburg, Germany